Neurointervention

Published and forthcoming Oxford Specialist Handbooks

General Oxford Specialist Handbooks
Cardiopulmonary Transplantation and Mechanical Circulatory Support
Infection in the Immunocompromised Host
Pharmaceutical Medicine
Postoperative Complications, 2e
Prison Medicine and Health
Retrieval Medicine

Oxford Specialist Handbooks in Anaesthesia
Anaesthesia for Emergency Care
Global Anaesthesia
Obstetric Anaesthesia Paediatric Anaesthesia
Regional Anaesthesia, Stimulation, and Ultrasound Techniques
Thoracic Anaesthesia
Vascular Anaesthesia

Oxford Specialist Handbooks in Cardiology
Adult Congenital Heart Disease
Cardiac Catheterization and Coronary Intervention
Cardiovascular Computed Tomography
Cardiovascular Imaging
Cardiovascular Magnetic Resonance
Echocardiography, 3e
Fetal Cardiology, 2e
Heart Disease in Pregnancy
Inherited Cardiac Disease, 2e
Nuclear Cardiology, 2e
Pacemakers and ICDs, 2e
Paediatric Cardiology
Pulmonary Hypertension
Valvular Heart Disease

Oxford Specialist Handbooks in End of Life Care
End of Life Care in Dementia
End of Life Care in Heart Failure
End of Life Care in Kidney Disease
End of Life Care in Respiratory Disease

Oxford Specialist Handbooks in Neurology
Parkinson's Disease and Other Movement Disorders, 2e
Stroke Medicine, 3e

Oxford Specialist Handbooks in Obstetrics and Gynaecology
Fetal Medicine
Obstetric Medicine
Urogynaecology

Oxford Specialist Handbooks in Oncology
Myeloproliferative Neoplasms
Practical Management of Complex Cancer Pain, 2e
Radiotherapy Planning

Oxford Specialist Handbooks in Paediatrics
Management of Childhood Infections: The Blue Book, 4e
Neurodisability and Community Child Health
Paediatric Dermatology, 2e
Paediatric Endocrinology and Diabetes, 2e
Paediatric Gastroenterology, Hepatology, and Nutrition, 2e
Paediatric Haematology and Oncology, 2e
Paediatric Intensive Care
Paediatric Nephrology, 3e
Paediatric Palliative Medicine, 2e
Paediatric Respiratory Medicine, 2e
Paediatric Rheumatology, 2e

Oxford Specialist Handbooks in Psychiatry
Eating Disorders
Forensic Psychiatry
Medical Psychotherapy

Oxford Specialist Handbooks in Radiology
Head and Neck Imaging
Interventional Radiology
Musculoskeletal Imaging
Thoracic Imaging

Oxford Specialist Handbooks in Surgery
Burns
Cardiothoracic Surgery, 2e
Colorectal Surgery, 2e
Current Surgical Guidelines, 2e
Gastric and Oesophageal Surgery
Hand Surgery
Oral and Maxillofacial Surgery, 3e
Otolaryngology and Head and Neck Surgery
Paediatric Surgery, 2e
Plastic and Reconstructive Surgery, 2e
Urological Surgery, 2e
Vascular Surgery, 2e

Neurointervention

EDITED BY

Jeremy Lynch

Consultant Interventional and Diagnostic Neuroradiologist
Department of Neuroradiology
King's College Hospital, London
Queen's Hospital, Romford
London, United Kingdom

Shelley Renowden

Consultant Neuroradiologist
Department of Neuroradiology
Southmead Hospital
North Bristol NHS Trust
Bristol, United Kingdom

Philip White

Professor of Interventional and Diagnostic Neuroradiology
Translational and Clinical Research Institute
Newcastle University, Henry Wellcome Building,
Framlingham Place
Newcastle upon Tyne, United Kingdom

OXFORD
UNIVERSITY PRESS

OXFORD
UNIVERSITY PRESS

Great Clarendon Street, Oxford, OX2 6DP,
United Kingdom

Oxford University Press is a department of the University of Oxford. It furthers the University's objective of excellence in research, scholarship, and education by publishing worldwide. Oxford is a registered trade mark of Oxford University Press in the UK and in certain other countries.

Published in the United States of America by Oxford University Press
198 Madison Avenue, New York, NY 10016, United States of America.

British Library Cataloguing in Publication Data

Data available

Library of Congress Control Number: 2026930335

ISBN 978–0–19–888971–7

DOI: 10.1093/med/9780198889717.001.0001

Printed in India by
Replika Press Pvt. Ltd.

Preface

Neurovascular disorders are a major global health burden, with stroke alone causing over 6 million deaths annually and affecting one in four people aged 25 or older during their lifetime. Neurointervention has emerged as a transformative discipline, with mechanical thrombectomy alone being one of the most effective medical treatments in any branch of medicine available today.

The complexity of our field demands a collaborative approach both locally, through multidisciplinary teamwork, and globally, through international cooperation. Practitioners from diverse clinical backgrounds, including radiologists, neurosurgeons, and neurologists, converge within this specialty, each bringing unique skills and perspectives. This diversity is reflected in the range of names used for the field: interventional neuroradiology, neurointervention, endovascular neurosurgery, and surgical neuroangiography. Being part of this relatively small but growing community is a privilege and source of inspiration.

Neurointerventional radiology continues to be a rapidly evolving specialty and although its origins date back to the 1960s and 1970s, it really took off in the 1990s following the introduction of the GDC coil, which revolutionised the treatment of intracranial aneurysms. Since then, the field has experienced major advancement in imaging technology, devices, and techniques, accounting for its massive expansion in scope and capability, particularly currently in the treatment of ischaemic stroke, but also by novel treatments such as middle meningeal artery embolisation for chronic subdural haematomas and cerebrospinal fluid–venous fistula embolisation, and emerging technologies like the Stentrode neural interface and the eShunt device.

Neurointerventional techniques range significantly in both complexity and risk. Some procedures, such as lumbar punctures, can be mastered within weeks, whereas others, particularly embolisation of spinal or brain vascular malformations, require many years of meticulous study and practice. The intricate anatomy, need for technical precision, and inherent risk of serious complications make the more complex procedures particularly challenging to master.

To ensure the optimal practice of neurointervention and its continued future development and evolution, a broad and detailed knowledge is mandatory—not only of neurovascular anatomy (microvascular and angiographic), functional neuroanatomy, techniques (including complications, and their management and avoidance), and devices but also of neuropathophysiology, neurovascular physiology, neurointensive care, and aspects of pharmacology and haematology. This handbook therefore aims to provide this comprehensive education and is a concise, evidence-based, and accessible resource suitable for daily practice, structured to address the most common clinical situations encountered in neurointervention. With introductory chapters, clear terminology, and practical guidance, our goal is for it to become a trusted, well-used companion, supporting clinicians in delivering safe, effective care to patients with complex neurovascular conditions.

Contents

Contributors *ix*

Abbreviations *xiii*

1. Introduction 1
2. Neurovascular anatomy 7
3. Drugs and analgesia 93
4. Equipment and devices 115
5. Non-vascular procedures 145
6. Vascular access 175
7. Diagnostic angiography 193
8. Cerebral aneurysms 227
9. Ischaemic stroke 317
10. Atherosclerotic disease 399
11. Cranial dural arteriovenous fistulas 415
12. Brain arteriovenous malformations 447
13. Venous procedures 475
14. Spinal vascular lesions 493
15. Tumour embolisation 513
16. Epistaxis and middle meningeal artery embolisation 535

Index *545*

Contributors

Ronit Agid
Professor, University of Toronto, Section Head Interventional Neuroradiology, Toronto Western Hospital, JDMI, UHN, Toronto, Ontario, Canada
Chapter 5: Non-vascular procedures

Tommy Andersson
Professor of Neurointervention, Department of Medical Imaging, AZ Groeninge Hospital, Kortrijk, Belgium; Department of Neuroradiology, Karolinska University Hospital, and Department of Clinical Neuroscience, Karolinska Institutet, Stockholm, Sweden
Chapter 9: Ischaemic stroke

Consoli Arturo
Head of Department, Department of Diagnostic and Therapeutic Neuroradiology, Hôpital Foch, Suresnes, France
Chapter 2: Neurovascular anatomy

Momodou G. Bah
Michigan State University College of Human Medicine, Lansing, Michigan, USA
Chapter 15: Tumour embolisation

Dodi Boccardi
Director of the Department of Neuroradiology, ASST Grande Ospedale Metropolitano Niguarda, Milan, Italy
Chapter 12: Brain arteriovenous malformations

Karl Boyle
Department of Geriatric and Stroke Medicine, ESO Certified Comprehensive Stroke Centre, The National Neurosciences Centre, Beaumont Hospital, Dublin, Ireland; Royal College of Surgeons of Ireland, Ireland
Chapter 9: Ischaemic stroke

William Brown
Post-CCT Diagnostic Neuroradiology Fellow, Bristol, UK
Chapter 5: Non-vascular procedures

Neeraj Chaudhary
Professor of Neurointervention and Neuroimaging, Chief, Neurointerventional Radiology (Adult and Pediatric), Director, Neurointerventional Radiology Fellowship Program, Lead, Neurointervention and Stroke, Comprehensive Stroke Center, Departments of Radiology, Neurosurgery, Neurology, and Otorhinolaryngology, Michigan Medicine, University of Michigan, Ann Arbor, Michigan, USA
Chapter 15: Tumour embolisation

Andrew Clifton
Consultant Interventional Neuroradiologist, St George's Hospital, London, UK
Chapter 10: Atherosclerotic disease

Matthew Common
Specialist Registrar in Radiology, Beaumont Hospital, Dublin, Ireland
Chapter 9: Ischaemic stroke

Mazen Elwishi
Consultant Anaesthetist, St George's University Hospitals NHS Foundation Trust, London, UK
Chapter 3: Drugs and analgesia

Richard Farb

Associate Professor, Division of Neuroradiology, Department of Medical Imaging, University of Toronto, Toronto, Ontario, Canada
Chapter 5: Non-vascular procedures

Joseph Gemmete

Professor of Radiology, Neurosurgery, Neurology, and Otolaryngology, Department of Radiology, University of Michigan Hospitals, Ann Arbor, Michigan, USA
Chapter 9: Ischaemic stroke; Chapter 15: Tumour embolisation

Tony Goddard

Leeds Teaching Hospitals NHS Trust, Leeds, UK
Chapter 8: Cerebral aneurysms

Shawn Halpin

Chief Medical Officer and Medical Director, DMC Imaging Ltd, UK; Former Consultant Interventional Neuroradiologist, University Hospital of Wales, Cardiff, UK
Chapter 1: Introduction

Eef Hendriks

Division of Neuroradiology, Joint Department of Medical Imaging, University Health Network, Toronto Western Hospital, Toronto, Ontario, Canada; Department of Medical Imaging, Temerty Faculty of Medicine, University of Toronto, Toronto, Ontario, Canada
Chapter 11: Cranial dural arteriovenous fistulas

Shah Islam

Consultant Interventional and Diagnostic Neuroradiologist, National Hospital for Neurology and Neurosurgery, London, UK
Chapter 6: Vascular access; Chapter 7: Diagnostic angiography; Chapter 8: Cerebral aneurysms; Chapter 12: Brain arteriovenous malformations; Chapter 13 Venous procedures

Anne Marie Liddy

Consultant Geriatrician and Stroke Physician, Beaumont Hospital, Dublin, Ireland
Chapter 9: Ischaemic stroke

Leanne Lin

Diagnostic and Interventional Neuroradiologist, Riverside Radiology and Interventional Associates, Adjunct Faculty Department of Radiology, University of Michigan, Ann Arbor, Michigan, USA
Chapter 15: Tumour embolisation; Chapter 16: Epistaxis and middle meningeal artery embolisation

Jeremy Lynch

Consultant Interventional and Diagnostic Neuroradiologist, Department of Neuroradiology, King's College Hospital, London, UK; Queen's Hospital, Romford, UK
Chapter 1: Introduction; Chapter 2: Neurovascular anatomy; Chapter 3: Drugs and analgesia; Chapter 4: Equipment and devices; Chapter 6: Vascular access; Chapter 7: Diagnostic angiography; Chapter 8: Cerebral aneurysms; Chapter 9: Ischaemic stroke; Chapter 11: Cranial dural arteriovenous fistulas; Chapter 13 Venous procedures; Chapter 14: Spinal vascular lesions; Chapter 15: Tumour embolisation

Juan Miguel Macho Fernández

Department of Angioradiology, Hospital Clínic de Barcelona, Barcelona, Spain
Chapter 11: Cranial dural arteriovenous fistulas

Steve Morgan

Consultant Diagnostic and Interventional Spinal Radiologist, Southmead Hospital, Bristol, UK
Chapter 5: Non-vascular procedures

Alex Mortimer
Consultant Interventional Neuroradiologist, North Bristol NHS Trust, Southmead Hospital, Bristol, UK
Chapter 9: Ischaemic stroke

Prakash Muthusami
Interventional Neuroradiologist, Department of Diagnostic Imaging, The Hospital for Sick Children, Toronto, Ontario, Canada
Chapter 6: Vascular access; Chapter 7: Diagnostic angiography; Chapter 8: Cerebral aneurysms; Chapter 12: Brain arteriovenous malformations

Patrick Nicholson
Consultant Neurointerventional Radiologist, Beaumont Hospital, Dublin, Ireland
Chapter 9: Ischaemic stroke; Chapter 13 Venous procedures

Sreehari Panicker
Radiology Resident, Henry Ford Health System, Detroit, Michigan, USA
Chapter 16: Epistaxis and middle meningeal artery embolisation

Tufail Patankar
Consultant Interventional Neuroradiologist, Queen's Hospital, Romford, London, UK; Visiting Professor, KEM Hospital, Mumbai, India; Honorary Senior Lecturer, University of Leeds, Leeds, UK; Reader in Radiology and Director of Radiology, University of Bolton, Bolton, UK
Chapter 4: Equipment and devices

Mariangela Piano
Neuroradiologist, Department of Neuroradiology, ASST Grande Spedale Metropolitano Niguarda, Milan, Italy
Chapter 12: Brain arteriovenous malformations

Benjamin Pinsky
Department of Radiology, University of Michigan, Ann Arbor, Michigan, USA
Chapter 15: Tumour embolisation

Sarah Power
Consultant Diagnostic and Interventional Neuroradiologist, Department of Radiology, Beaumont Hospital, Dublin, Ireland
Chapter 9: Ischaemic stroke

Ayman Qureshi
Consultant Neuroradiologist, National Hospital for Neurology and Neurosurgery, London, UK
Chapter 7: Diagnostic angiography; Chapter 13 Venous procedures

Mads Rasmussen
Consultant in Neuroanaesthesia, Department of Anaesthesiology, Aarhus University Hospital, Aarhus, Denmark
Chapter 9: Ischaemic stroke

Adam Rennie
Consultant Diagnostic and Interventional Neuroradiologist, Department of Radiology, Great Ormond Street Hospital, London, UK
Chapter 2: Neurovascular anatomy

Shelley Renowden
Consultant Neuroradiologist, Department of Neuroradiology, Southmead Hospital, North Bristol NHS Trust, Bristol, UK
Chapter 3: Drugs and analgesia; Chapter 7: Diagnostic angiography; Chapter 8: Cerebral aneurysms; Chapter 12: Brain arteriovenous malformations; Chapter 14: Spinal vascular lesions

Marc Ribó
Assistant Professor, Stroke Unit, Department of Neurology, Hospital Vall d'Hebron, Barcelona, Spain
Chapter 9: Ischaemic stroke

Fergus Robertson
Consultant Interventional and Diagnostic Neuroradiologist, Great Ormond Street Hospital for Children, London, UK
Chapter 6: Vascular access; Chapter 7: Diagnostic angiography; Chapter 8: Cerebral aneurysms; Chapter 12: Brain arteriovenous malformations

Georges Rodesch
Department of Diagnostic and Therapeutic Neuroradiology, Hôpital Foch, Suresnes, France
Chapter 2: Neurovascular anatomy

Sara Sciacca
Consultant Interventional Neuroradiologist, Ruskin Wing Department of Neuroradiology, King's College Hospital, London, UK
Chapter 7: Diagnostic angiography

Brian Sifrig
Department of Radiology, University of Michigan, Ann Arbor, Michigan, USA
Chapter 15: Tumour embolisation

Oliver Spooner
North East London Stroke Operational Lead, Mechanical Thrombectomy and Research Lead for Stroke Medicine, Consultant Stroke Physician, The Royal London Hospital Hyperacute Stroke Unit, Barts Health, London, UK
Chapter 9: Ischaemic stroke

George Tse
Consultant Interventional Neuroradiologist, Sheffield Teaching Hospitals NHS Foundation Trust, Sheffield, UK
Chapter 12: Brain arteriovenous malformations

Philip White
Professor of Interventional and Diagnostic Neuroradiology, Translational and Clinical Research Institute, Newcastle University, Newcastle upon Tyne, UK
Chapter 8: Cerebral aneurysms

Zachary M. Wilseck
Department of Radiology, University of Michigan, Ann Arbor, Michigan, USA
Chapter 16: Epistaxis and middle meningeal artery embolisation

Leonard Yeo
National University of Singapore, Yong Loo Lin School of Medicine, Singapore
Chapter 9: Ischaemic stroke

Abbreviations

3D	three-dimensional
4D	four-dimensional
a.	artery
ACA	anterior cerebral artery
ACOM	anterior communicating artery
ACT	activated clotting time
ACTH	adrenocorticotropic hormone
ADP	adenosine diphosphate
AI	artificial intelligence
AICA	anterior inferior cerebellar artery
AMA	accessory meningeal artery
AP	anteroposterior
APA	ascending pharyngeal artery
APTT	activated partial thromboplastin time
ARU	Aspirin Reaction Unit
ASA	anterior spinal artery
aSAH	aneurysmal subarachnoid haemorrhage
ASC	acute stroke centre
ASPECTS	Alberta Stroke Program Early CT Score
AT	antithrombin
AVF	arteriovenous fistula
AVM	arteriovenous malformation
BAO	basilar artery occlusion
bAVM	brain arteriovenous malformation
BBB	blood–brain barrier
BD	twice daily
BGC	balloon guide catheter
BP	blood pressure
BTO	balloon test occlusion
BVR	basal vein of Rosenthal
CAS	carotid artery stenting
CBF	cerebral blood flow
CCA	common carotid artery
CEA	carotid endarterectomy
CFV	common femoral vein
CN	cranial nerve
CO_2	carbon dioxide
COX	cyclo-oxygenase
CRH	corticotrophin-releasing hormone
CSC	comprehensive stroke centre
cSDH	chronic subdural haematoma
CSF	cerebrospinal fluid
CT	computed tomography
CTA	computed tomography angiography/angiogram
CTP	computed tomography perfusion
CVR	cortical venous reflux
CVST	cerebral venous sinus thrombosis
DAPT	dual antiplatelet therapy
DAVF	dural arteriovenous fistula
DCI	delayed cerebral ischaemia
DIDO	door-in to door-out
DiVO	distal vessel occlusion
DMSO	dimethyl sulfoxide
DOAC	direct-acting oral anticoagulant
DSA	digital subtraction angiography
DSM	digital subtraction myelography
DWI	diffusion-weighted imaging
ECA	external carotid artery
ECG	electrocardiogram
EJV	external jugular vein
EVD	external ventricular drain(age)
EVOH	ethylene vinyl alcohol
EVT	endovascular treatment
FCA	focal cerebral arteriopathy
FDS	flow-diverting stent
FLAIR	fluid-attenuated inversion recovery
GA	general anaesthesia/anaesthetic
GABA	gamma-aminobutyric acid
GCS	Glasgow Coma Scale
GP	glycoprotein
GTN	glyceryl trinitrate
h	hour(s)
HDU	high dependency unit
HEMA	hydroxyethyl methacrylate
HU	Hounsfield unit(s)

ICA	internal carotid artery
ICAD	intracranial atherosclerotic disease
ICH	intracranial haemorrhage
ICP	intracranial pressure
ICU	intensive care unit
IIH	idiopathic intracranial hypertension
IJV	internal jugular vein
ILT	inferolateral trunk
IM	intramuscular(ly)
IMA	internal maxillary artery
INR	international normalised ratio
IPS	inferior petrosal sinus
IPSS	inferior petrosal sinus sampling
ISAT	International Subarachnoid Aneurysm Trial
ITU	intensive therapy unit
IU	international unit(s)
IV	intravenous(ly)
IVT	intravenous thrombolysis
JNA	juvenile nasopharyngeal angiofibroma
LA	local anaesthesia/anaesthetic
LE	liquid embolic
LMWH	low-molecular-weight heparin
LP	lumbar puncture
LVO	large vessel occlusion
MCA	middle cerebral artery
mcg	microgram(s)
MDT	multidisciplinary team
MeVO	medium vessel occlusion
MHT	meningohypophyseal trunk
min	minute(s)
MIP	maximal intensity projection
MMA	middle meningeal artery
MMAE	middle meningeal artery embolisation
MPV	median prosencephalic vein
MR	magnetic resonance
MRA	magnetic resonance angiography
MRI	magnetic resonance imaging
mRS	modified Rankin Scale
MT	mechanical thrombectomy
n-BCA	*n*-butyl-2-cyanoacrylate
NCCT	non-contrast computed tomography
NICE	National Institute for Health and Care Excellence
NIHSS	National Institutes of Health Stroke Scale
NMDA	*N*-methyl-D-aspartate
NSAID	non-steroidal anti-inflammatory drug
OD	once daily
PCA	posterior cerebral artery
PCOM	posterior communicating artery
PICA	posterior inferior cerebellar artery
PRU	P2Y12 Reaction Unit
PSC	primary stroke centre
PT	prothrombin time
PTA	percutaneous transluminal angioplasty
PVA	polyvinyl alcohol
PVO	parent vessel occlusion
PVS	parent vessel sacrifice
RA	rotational angiography
RCT	randomised controlled trial
RHV	rotating haemostatic valve
rtPA	recombinant tissue plasminogen activator
s	second(s)
RPH	retroperitoneal haematoma
SAH	subarachnoid haemorrhage
SCA	superior cerebellar artery
SIADH	syndrome of inappropriate antidiuretic hormone secretion
sICH	symptomatic intracranial haemorrhage
SLEC	spinal longitudinal extradural collection
SMV	superficial middle cerebral vein
SNIS	Society of NeuroInterventional Surgery
SNRI	serotonin and noradrenaline reuptake inhibitor
SPECT	single-photon emission computed tomography
SSRI	selective serotonin reuptake inhibitor
STA	superficial temporal artery
STIR	short tau inversion recovery
STRS	stereotactic radiosurgery
SWI	susceptibility weighted imaging
TCD	transcranial Doppler ultrasound

TIA	transient ischaemic attack.
TICI	Thrombolysis in Cerebral Infarction
T_{max}	time to maximum
tPA	tissue plasminogen activator
UFH	unfractionated heparin
UIA	unruptured intracranial aneurysm
UN	United Nations
v.	vein
VOGM	vein of Galen malformation
vWF	von Willebrand factor
WEB	Woven Endobridge
WFNS	World Federation of Neurosurgical Societies
WHO	World Health Organization

Chapter 1

Introduction

History of neurointervention *2*
Ethics *3*
Consent *4*

History of neurointervention

1918	Walter Dandy develops pneumoencephalography
1919	Walter Dandy develops ventriculography
1927	António Egas Moniz and Pedro Almeida Lima perform the first cerebral angiogram
1938	First endosaccular coiling of an aneurysm using 30 feet (9 metres) of silver wire via a transorbital approach
1941	Farinas describes femoral catheterisation for angiography
1953	Seldinger introduces the percutaneous catheterisation technique
1960	Luessenhop and Spence report the first endovascular embolisation of a brain arteriovenous malformation (AVM) by insertion of methyl methacrylate spherical emboli directly into the carotid artery
1964	Luessenhop and Velasquez perform the first catheter-based embolisation of an intracranial aneurysm
1970	Serbinenko performs the first endovascular therapeutic occlusion using a detachable latex balloon catheter to treat a carotid-cavernous fistula
1980	Mathias performs the first carotid angioplasty for atherosclerotic stenoses
1990	Théron implants the first carotid stent
1990	Guglielmi detachable coils first used in human patients
1991	First usage of an ethylene vinyl alcohol copolymer for treatment of an AVM by Terada et al.
1997	Moret introduces the balloon remodelling technique (balloon-assisted coiling) for wide-necked cerebral aneurysms
1997	Higashida reports the first usage of stent-assisted coiling for an intracranial aneurysm
2002	The International Subarachnoid Aneurysm Trial (ISAT) demonstrates endovascular coiling delivers superior clinical results to surgical clipping for ruptured aneurysms
2002	Higgins first implants a venous sinus stent for idiopathic intracranial hypertension
2007	First clinical use of flow diverters for intracranial aneurysms
2011	The Woven Endobridge (WEB) intrasaccular device enters clinical use
2015	Major randomised controlled trials (RCTs) confirm mechanical thrombectomy's benefit for acute ischaemic stroke
2019	First human implantation of the Stentrode brain–computer interface
2021	First-in-human endovascular implantation of the eShunt device for communicating hydrocephalus
2024	RCTs demonstrate that middle meningeal artery (MMA) embolisation significantly reduces recurrence of chronic subdural haematoma

Ethics

Endovascular therapy risks serious injury. Moral, ethical, and legal principles must be taken into account when balancing risk and benefit and in deciding whether to proceed with any procedure.

- Beauchamp and Childress, in their seminal work *Principles of Biomedical Ethics* (1979), established three key principles:
  1. Respect for autonomy: this principle emphasises respecting the decision-making capacity of autonomous persons. In healthcare, this means respecting the choices and actions of patients, provided they are informed and voluntary.
  2. Beneficence: this involves the obligation to act for the benefit of others, promoting their welfare, and taking positive steps to prevent and remove harms.
  3. Non-maleficence: often summarised by the phrase 'do no harm', this principle requires healthcare providers to refrain from causing harm to patients.
- In this framework, the morality of an action is more important than the outcome. Paternalism is rejected, because of the primary importance of the autonomy of each individual. Doctors must respect the decisions of their patients, even if they believe the decisions are unwise.
- The autonomy of the individual is the dominant consideration in many international laws and treaties.
- The Universal Declaration on Bioethics and Human Rights (UNESCO, 2005) mandates that United Nations member states uphold human dignity, rights, and fundamental freedoms. It reinforces individual autonomy and responsibility, providing safeguards for those unable to exercise autonomy. The declaration asserts that medical interventions should only occur with the prior, free, and informed consent of the individual, contingent upon sufficient information.
- The principle of individual freedom and autonomy is strongly upheld in the international agreements of the United Nations Universal Declaration of Human Rights (1948), the Nuremberg Code (1949), and the International Covenant on Civil and Political Rights (1967).
- The European Convention on Human Rights (1950), bolstered by the Charter of Fundamental Rights of the European Union (2000), advocates for the inviolability of human dignity, demanding its respect and protection. In the medical field, this translates to the requirement for free and informed consent. Individuals are entitled to privacy and physical integrity, as well as the right to autonomy.

Consent

- The Council of Europe (1997), through the Oviedo Convention, specifies that a health intervention is permissible only following free and informed consent. It is essential that the person involved is previously informed about the intervention's purpose, nature, consequences, and risks.
- The Oviedo Convention also clarifies the crucial distinction between consent and informed consent. Informed consent must be granted based on objective information from the responsible healthcare professional, including details about the intervention's purpose, nature, consequences, alternatives, and associated risks, and must be free from any external pressure.
- This information should also encompass risks specific to the patient's individual characteristics, such as age or the presence of other medical conditions. Any additional information requested by patients must be sufficiently addressed.
- For many years, accusations of negligence against a doctor could be defended by showing that the doctor acted in accordance with a body of opinion provided by a group of reasonable, responsible, and respectable colleagues, termed the 'Bolam test', deriving from the landmark case *Bolam vs Friern Hospital Management Committee* (1957) in the UK. This test has been a foundational element in medical negligence law, particularly in the UK.

Requirements for informed consent

- More recently, UK case law has shifted towards a more patient-centred approach. Instead of questioning, 'What would a prudent doctor say in this situation?', the focus has moved to 'What would a prudent patient want to know?'
- In the case of *Montgomery vs Lanarkshire Health Board* (2015) and *Birch vs University College London Hospital NHS Foundation Trust* (2008), the courts defined what a 'proper' consent process must entail:
    - The doctor is required to clearly explain the nature, purpose, and alternative options of the procedure.
    - Patients must be given sufficient time and space to contemplate their decision. This suggests that, except in emergencies, consent should be a two-stage process. Initially, the doctor explains and responds to questions, but formal consent is not obtained until a subsequent meeting, allowing the patient time to consider and ask additional questions.
    - The amount of information provided to the patient should reflect their individual needs, which can vary from person to person. While written information can be useful, it may be overwhelming for some and insufficient for others.
    - Doctors should disclose all risks that a prudent patient might wish to be informed about, regardless of their rarity.
    - Ethically and legally, there is leeway to withhold certain information if the doctor firmly believes that full disclosure would severely harm the patient's health. However, this does not permit withholding information that might dissuade a patient from undergoing a procedure deemed necessary by the doctor.

- It is essential for the doctor to verify that the patient has the capacity to comprehend the information.
- All discussions should be thoroughly documented in the patient's notes. Merely obtaining a signature on a consent form does not safeguard against potential litigation.

Further reading

Miller F, Wertheimer A, eds. The Ethics of Consent: Theory and Practice. Oxford University Press; 2009.
Varkey B. Principles of clinical ethics and their application to practice. Med Princ Pract. 2021;30(1):17–28.

Chapter 2

Neurovascular anatomy

Thoracic aorta *8*

External carotid artery (ECA) I: superior thyroid, lingual, facial, posterior auricular, and superficial temporal branches *12*

ECA II: occipital and ascending pharyngeal branches *17*

ECA III: internal maxillary artery *21*

Internal carotid artery *30*

Circle of Willis *38*

Anterior cerebral artery *40*

Middle cerebral artery *44*

Vertebral artery *47*

Basilar artery *51*

Posterior cerebral artery *54*

'Dangerous' cranial anastomoses *58*

Cranial nerve supply *61*

Extracranial veins *62*

Dural venous sinuses *64*

Supratentorial and medullary veins *69*

Infratentorial veins *74*

Summary of spinal vascular anatomy *77*

Embryology of the spinal vascular system *82*

Spinal arterial anatomy *84*

Spinal venous anatomy *89*

Thoracic aorta

Aortic arch

(See Figure 2.1.)

- The ascending aorta arises from the aortic vestibule of the left ventricle, then ascends superiorly and slightly to the right for about 5 cm, giving rise to the right and left coronary arteries.
- It becomes the aortic arch at the transthoracic plane of Ludwig, a horizontal line joining the manubriosternal joint to the inferior endplate of T4, before curving backwards and over the left main bronchus.
- There are normally three main branches: the brachiocephalic trunk, the left common carotid artery (CCA), and the left subclavian artery.
- The aortic arch ends as it again intersects the transthoracic plane to become the descending aorta. It runs inferiorly and initially to the left but then veers towards the midline, ending at the aortic hiatus of the diaphragm. This segment has paired posterior intercostal, subcostal, and superior phrenic branches, and unpaired bronchial, mediastinal, pericardial, and oesophageal branches.

Brachiocephalic artery

- The first and largest branch of the arch ascends posteriorly and to the right before bifurcating into the right subclavian artery and the right CCA.

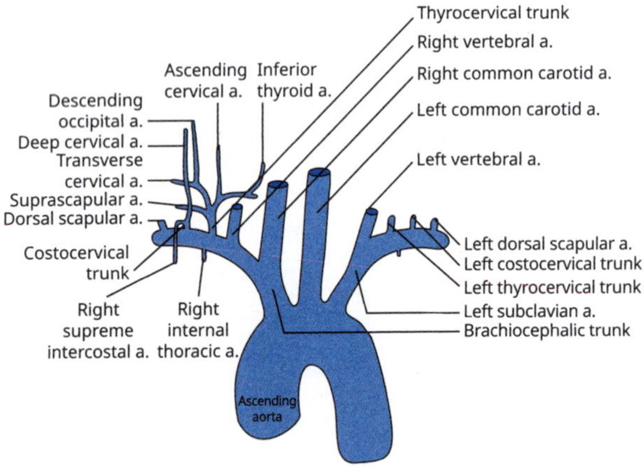

Figure 2.1 Branches of the aortic arch.

Right subclavian artery

- Arises from the brachiocephalic artery behind the right sternoclavicular joint.
- It can be divided into three parts: medial, behind, and lateral to scalenus anterior. It becomes the axillary artery at the lateral border of the first rib.

Branches from medial to lateral

- Vertebral artery: this arises from the posterosuperior aspect of the first part and ascends superiorly, usually entering the foramen of the transverse process of C6.
- Internal thoracic (or mammary) artery: this originates from the anterior aspect of the first part and is directed inferiorly behind the upper six costal cartilages. It terminates by dividing into the superior epigastric and musculophrenic branches.
- Thyrocervical trunk: this arises superiorly and anteriorly, opposite the internal thoracic artery from the first subclavian part. It divides into inferior thyroid, suprascapular, and transverse cervical branches. The ascending cervical artery usually arises from the inferior thyroid branch and has anastomoses with vertebral (C3, C4), ascending pharyngeal, occipital, and deep cervical arteries, in addition to multiple spinal branches.
- Costocervical trunk: the costocervical trunk arises posteriorly and superiorly from the second part of the subclavian artery distal to the thyrocervical trunk. It divides into the supreme intercostal and deep cervical arteries.
    - The supreme intercostal artery, the first branch, gives off the upper two posterior intercostal arteries. These, in turn, have radicular (and sometimes radiculomedullary/radiculopial) spinal branches. Alternatively, this artery may arise from the thyrocervical trunk, the internal thoracic artery, or directly from the aortic arch. There are also anastomoses with the vertebral artery.
    - The deep cervical artery runs close to the spinous processes and supplies the posterior deep cervical muscles. Similar to the ascending cervical, it has multiple important anastomoses including with the vertebral arteries (at C2, C3, and C4) and may reconstitute the vessel if absent or occluded. It often also gives off spinal branches, importantly the artery of the cervical enlargement at around C5/6.
- Dorsal scapular artery: supplying levator scapulae and the rhomboid muscles.

Right common carotid artery

- The right CCA arises from the brachiocephalic trunk behind the sternoclavicular joint. It ascends in the carotid space adjacent to the internal jugular vein (IJV) and vagus nerve and bifurcates into its internal and external branches usually at the upper border of the thyroid cartilage at C4.
- At the bifurcation, the vessel dilates into the carotid sinus (or bulb), which is a baroreceptor, sensitive to pressure changes in arterial blood pressure (BP). Stimulation (particularly during balloon angioplasty) may result in pronounced bradycardia and peripheral vasodilatation.

- On the posterior edge of the bifurcation is the carotid body, a chemoreceptor which is mainly responsive to changes in the arterial respiratory gases O_2, CO_2, and pH.
- Usually, no branches arise from the CCA itself; however, occasionally the superior thyroid, ascending pharyngeal, or occipital arteries may do so.

Left common carotid artery

- The left CCA arises just distal to the brachiocephalic artery from the aortic arch. It ascends posteriorly and laterally before bifurcating into its internal and external branches.

Left subclavian artery

- The left subclavian artery arises just posterior and slightly to the left of the left CCA. It ascends superiorly and then curves laterally to become the axillary artery at the lateral border of the first rib.
- Its branches are identical to those of the right subclavian artery.

Aortic arch variants

(See Figure 2.2.)

- The normal branch pattern is found in about 80% of individuals, but there are many variations:
  - Common origin of the brachiocephalic artery and left CCA, or left CCA branching from the brachiocephalic artery (about 13%): this is sometimes (incorrectly) referred to as a 'bovine' arch. Normally a Simmons tip or similar is required to catheterise the left CCA in this configuration.
  - Left vertebral artery origin from the aortic arch (about 3%): the vessel is found between the left CCA and the left subclavian artery and enters the foramen transversarium at C4. It is usually fairly straightforward to select the vessel with a Berenstein or Ver tip catheter.
  - Vertebral arteries from the internal or external carotid arteries: very rare.
- Some other anomalies are illustrated in Figure 2.2.

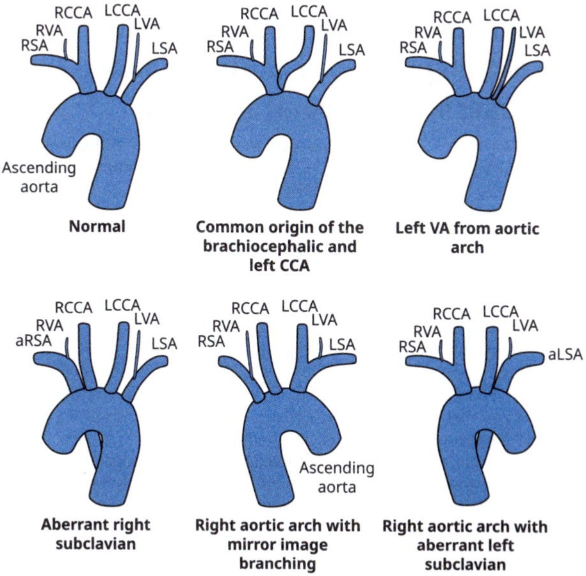

Figure 2.2 Aortic arch variants. aLSA, aberrant left subclavian artery; aRSA, aberrant right subclavian artery; LCCA, left common carotid artery; LSA, left subclavian artery; LVA, left vertebral artery; RCCA, right common carotid artery; RSA, right subclavian artery; RVA, right vertebral artery.

Further reading

Hanneman K, Newman B, Chan F. Congenital variants and anomalies of the aortic arch. Radiographics. 2017;37(1):32–51.

Moore KL, Dalley AF, Agur AMR. Clinically Oriented Anatomy. 8th ed. Lippincott Williams & Wilkins; 2018.

External carotid artery (ECA) I: superior thyroid, lingual, facial, posterior auricular, and superficial temporal branches

- The ECA (Figures 2.3 & 2.4) arises from the CCA, typically at the level of the C4 vertebra (varying from C2 to T2). In 75%, the internal carotid artery (ICA) lies posterolateral to the ECA.
- It supplies structures of the head, neck, and face, including muscles, skin, and bones, as well as the pharynx, oral cavity, larynx, thyroid gland, cranial nerves (CNs), and dura mater.
- To safely embolise branches of the ECA, it is essential to have a comprehensive understanding of its numerous anastomoses with cerebral arteries (internal carotid, ophthalmic, and vertebral arteries) and supply to CNs.
- Course:
  - Near its origin, the inferiorly directed superior thyroid artery arises.
  - The ECA then runs superiorly towards the parotid gland, giving off the lingual and facial arteries anteriorly, and the occipital, ascending pharyngeal, and posterior auricular arteries posterosuperiorly.
  - It bifurcates into the superficial temporal artery (STA) and internal maxillary artery (IMA) after piercing the parotid gland, behind the neck of the mandible.

Superior thyroid artery

- **Supply:** upper thyroid gland, infrahyoid, sternocleidomastoid, and cricothyroid muscles, superior larynx, and the parathyroids. It has rich anastomoses with the inferior thyroid branch of the thyrocervical trunk.
- **Origin:** anteriorly at the origin of the ECA. Occasionally it originates from the CCA and rarely from a common origin with the lingual artery.
- **Course:** it is directed acutely downward and continues lateral to the larynx before reaching the thyroid gland.

Lingual artery

- **Supply:** ipsilateral tongue and buccal and oral mucosa. It can also supply the submandibular and sublingual salivary glands. Conservative embolisation is necessary because the tongue often does not receive additional arterial supply and iatrogenic tongue injury can be very debilitating.
- **Origin:** the lingual artery originates anteriorly from the ECA just below the facial artery, although it occasionally shares a common origin. Rarely, it can share a common origin with the superior thyroid.
- **Course:** initially, anterosuperior to the greater horn of the hyoid, it then turns inferiorly and then anteriorly, crossed by the hypoglossal nerve. It then runs horizontally along the hyoid before diving under the hyoglossus.

Facial artery

- **Supply:** the submandibular gland, musculocutaneous tissue of the face, and the mandible.

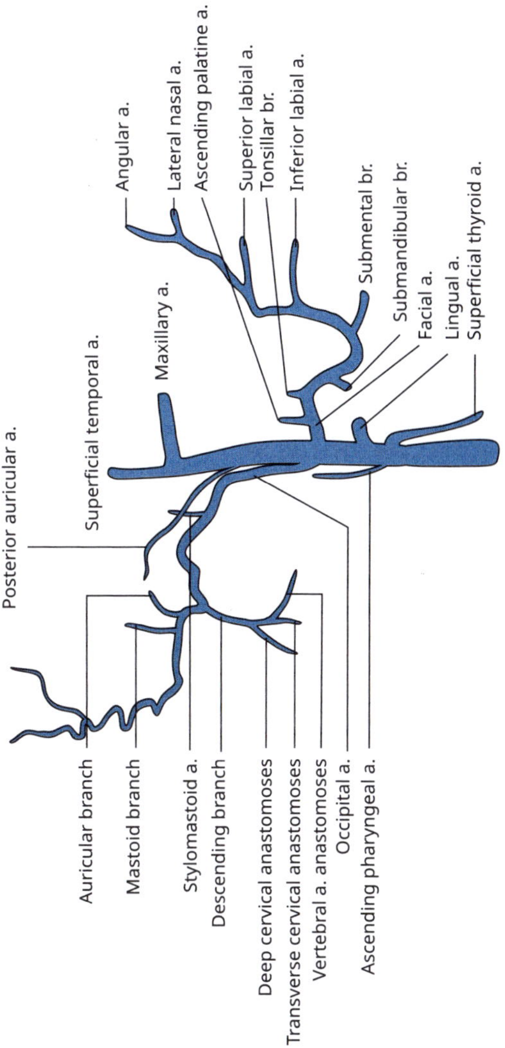

Figure 2.3 Proximal branches of the ECA.

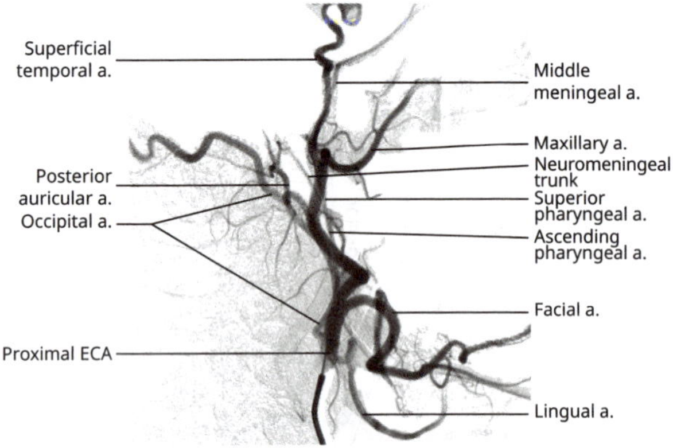

Figure 2.4 Lateral ECA angiogram.

- **Origin:** the facial artery usually arises just above the lingual artery, although sometimes it shares a common origin.
- **Course:** initially anterosuperiorly directed it turns inferiorly and descends in the parapharyngeal space to reach the submandibular gland. It runs anterolaterally, crossing the deep aspect of the gland and giving off the submental artery before crossing the mandible in front of the masseter. The artery terminates at the level of the ala of the nose in about 50% and gives rise to the superior labial artery and alar branches. Alternatively, it becomes the angular artery, running in the nasolabial fold to reach the angle of the eye.

Branches

- Ascending palatine artery: this originates most frequently from the apex of the proximal segment of the facial artery or from the ascending pharyngeal or lingual arteries. It ascends superiorly between the styloglossus and stylopharyngeus, giving off tonsillar branches. The artery reaches and supplies the soft palate and the Eustachian tube superiorly. It anastomoses with the pharyngeal branches of the ascending pharyngeal, descending palatine, and accessory meningeal arteries. Damage to this vessel is often implicated in post-tonsillectomy haemorrhage.
- Tonsillar branch: this arises from the proximal descending part and ascends between the internal pterygoid muscle and styloglossus. It courses anteromedially to supply the palatine tonsil and tongue. It can also be injured during tonsillectomy.
- Submandibular gland branches: these originate inferiorly from the submandibular and submental segments of the artery.
- Submental artery: this originates at the submandibular segment of the artery and courses anteriorly on mylohyoid, delivering branches to the submandibular gland and regional musculocutaneous tissue and the mandible.

- Masseteric muscular and buccal mucosal branches: these originate superiorly from the facial artery.
- Inferior and superior labial arteries: the inferior labial artery runs along the lower lip whereas the superior labial artery follows the upper. They supply the labial glands, mucous membranes, and regional musculature. The superior labial artery also delivers branches to the nasal septum and ala and can anastomose with the sphenopalatine artery (the terminal branch of the IMA).
- Lateral nasal artery: this originates distal to the superior labial branch (or from the superior labial artery) and runs superiorly along the side of the nose. Occasionally, it is the terminal branch of the facial artery.
- Angular artery: if present, this is the terminal branch of the facial artery. It may also originate from the ophthalmic or infraorbital arteries. The vessel courses in the nasojugal fold giving off the medial palpebral artery supplying the eyelids, and anastomoses with the lateral palpebral artery (lacrimal artery) to form the palpebral arcade. There are anastomoses with the ophthalmic, lateral nasal, and infraorbital arteries in addition to its counterpart across the midline.

Posterior auricular artery

- **Supply:** musculocutaneous tissue of the face, scalp, pinna, and parotid gland. It is in haemodynamic balance with the occipital artery and STA. There are anastomoses with the anterior auricular artery (a branch of the STA) above the ear.
- **Origin:** the vessel arises from the distal ECA posteriorly at the level of the inferior parotid gland. Alternatively, it may share a common trunk with the occipital artery.
- **Course:** the artery is directed posterosuperiorly beneath the parotid gland and runs on the superior surface of the posterior belly of the digastric muscle. It turns superficially at the mastoid process and courses posterosuperiorly in the posterior auricular sulcus, between the mastoid process and the pinna.

Branches

- Stylomastoid branch: this artery arises from the posterior auricular artery slightly less frequently than the occipital artery. It is an important component of the facial arcade, supplying the facial nerve in the temporal bone and an anastomosis in the tympanic cavity involving the inferior, anterior, superior, and caroticotympanic arteries.
- Parotid branches.
- Muscular branches.

Superficial temporal

- **Supply:** the lateral aspect of the scalp and face.
- **Origin:** this is one of the two terminal divisions of the ECA (the other being the IMA).
- **Course:** the artery originates behind the neck of the mandible in the parotid gland. It ascends laterally along the superficial surface of the temporalis muscle, over the posterior aspect of the condylar process, and passes superficially over the zygomatic process of the temporal bone. After a few centimetres it divides into its frontal and parietal terminal branches.

Branches

- Transverse facial artery: this arises within the parotid gland near the origin of the STA and divides into superior and inferior branches. The superior division passes through and supplies the parotid gland before running anteriorly and supplying the face, parotid duct, regional musculature, and the facial nerve. It anastomoses with the infraorbital, zygomaticomalar, inferior palpebral, buccal, and facial arteries. The inferior trunk also supplies the parotid gland and runs superficially over the masseter, which it supplies. It anastomoses with branches of the IMA.
- Anterior tympanic artery: this small artery arises from the proximal STA or IMA. It supplies the mandibular joint and the tympanic cavity, where it anastomoses with the inferior tympanic, superior tympanic, and caroticotympanic arteries.
- Anterior auricular branches: superior, middle, and inferior branches supply the external ear.
- Zygomatico-orbital artery: this arises just proximal to the bifurcation and is directed anteriorly along the upper border of the zygomatic arch towards the lateral angle of the orbit. The artery supplies the anterior temporal and malar region and orbicularis orbis.
- Posterior deep temporal artery: this arises at the level of the zygoma and is directed posteroinferiorly. Rarely it originates from the IMA or from a common trunk with the zygomatico-orbital arteries. It supplies the temporalis muscle and anastomoses with the middle and anterior temporal arteries.
- Frontal and parietal terminal divisions: these two large terminal branches arise a couple of centimetres above the superior margin of the zygomatic arch, supplying muscle, skin, and bone. The frontal division curves anterosuperiorly towards the superior orbital rim. It anastomoses with the supraorbital and frontal branches of the ophthalmic artery. The parietal division runs posterosuperiorly and anastomoses with the occipital, deep middle temporal, and posterior auricular arteries.

Further reading

Kiyosue H, ed. External Carotid Artery: Imaging Anatomy Atlas for Endovascular Treatment. Springer Nature; 2020.

Lasjaunias P, Berenstein A. Surgical Neuroangiography: 1 Functional Anatomy of Craniofacial Arteries. Springer Science & Business Media; 2012.

Upile T, Jerjes W, Nouraei SA, et al. The stylomastoid artery as an anatomical landmark to the facial nerve during parotid surgery: a clinico-anatomic study. World J Surg Oncol. 2009;7:71.

ECA II: occipital and ascending pharyngeal branches

Occipital artery

(See Figure 2.3)

- **Supply:** musculocutaneous tissue and bone, dura mater of the posterior cranial fossa, and CNs.
- **Origin:** posterosuperiorly from the proximal ECA usually just above or below the ascending pharyngeal artery (occasionally they share a common trunk). In some cases, it arises from the internal carotid, vertebral, deep cervical, or posterior auricular arteries.
- **Course:**
    - First segment: runs posterosuperiorly to reach the occipital groove of the temporal bone.
    - Second segment: horizontal to the superior nuchal line (a bony ridge sweeping laterally from the external occipital protuberance).
    - Third segment: ascends the distal occiput.

Branches

- Proximal sternocleidomastoid branches.
- Stylomastoid artery: this arises from the first segment of the occipital artery or the posterior auricular artery. It enters the stylomastoid foramen with the facial nerve, which it supplies, contributing to the facial arcade in the temporal bone with the petrosal branch of the middle meningeal artery (MMA). It enters the tympanic cavity and anastomoses with the superior tympanic artery from the petrosal branch of the MMA, anterior tympanic branch of the IMA, the inferior tympanic branch of the ascending pharyngeal, the caroticotympanic branch of the ICA, and the arcuate branch of the anterior inferior cerebellar artery (AICA). It also supplies the tympanic antrum, mastoid bone, and semicircular canal.
- Jugular branch: this variant origin of the jugular artery (which usually originates from the neuromeningeal trunk) may arise from the first segment and runs through the jugular foramen into the posterior condylar canal. The artery supplies meninges of the posterior fossa and vasa nervorum of CNs 9, 10, and 11. The hypoglossal artery, neuromeningeal trunk, or pharyngeal trunk may also arise from the occipital artery.
- Descending muscular branches: there are superficial and deep muscular branches arising from the second segment that run inferiorly to supply the back muscles, such as the splenius and trapezius. Importantly, the deep branch anastomoses with the vertebral artery and branches of the costocervical trunk at the C1–C2 level and the cervical arteries at C3–C4.
- Mastoid branches: these arise from the second segment and supply the mastoid bone and skin. A large mastoid branch often continues superiorly and then enters the cranium through the mastoid foramen to supply the posterior fossa dura mater—the posterior meningeal artery. It divides into descending, ascending, and posteromedial branches. The descending branch courses along the sigmoid sinus and anastomoses with the sigmoid sinus branch of the ascending pharyngeal. The ascending branch runs posterosuperiorly along the sigmoid sinus

before anastomosing with the petrosquamous branch of the MMA and sometimes the subarcuate branch of the AICA. The posteromedial branch courses inferomedially and anastomoses with the hypoglossal, jugular, and musculospinal branches of the ascending pharyngeal, or the jugular branch of the posterior meningeal artery from the vertebral artery.

- Muscular, cutaneous, and transosseous branches: these contribute to a rich regional anastomosis. Some of the osseous branches penetrate the skull to enter the cranial cavity.

Ascending pharyngeal artery

(See Figure 2.5.)

- **Supply:** nasopharynx, Eustachian tube, middle ear, oropharynx, soft palate, abducens, glossopharyngeal, vagus, accessory, and hypoglossal nerves.
- **Origin:** this long needle-thin artery arises posteromedially from the proximal ECA, close to the occipital artery origin, sometimes sharing an origin. It can also arise from a common trunk with the lingual and facial arteries, the carotid bifurcation, internal carotid, or ascending cervical artery. There are numerous potential anastomoses with the vertebrobasilar artery and ICA.
- **Course:** it runs straight up medial to the ICA, giving off small muscular branches before dividing into anterior pharyngeal and posterior neuromeningeal trunks.

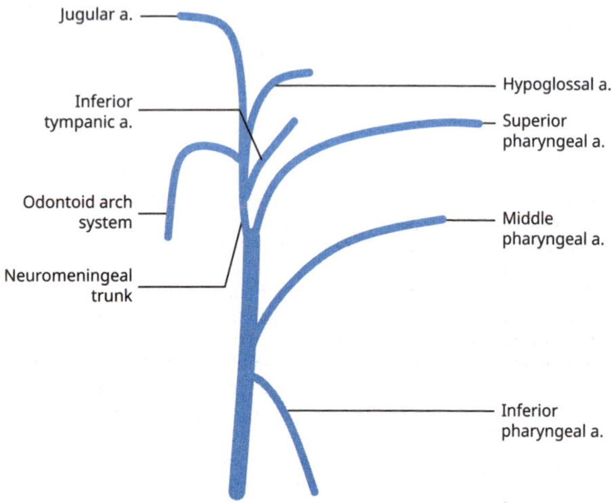

Figure 2.5 Ascending pharyngeal artery.

Branches

- Superior, middle, and inferior pharyngeal branches: these branches supply the pharyngeal submucosal spaces and contribute to a rich anastomotic network with the contralateral ascending pharyngeal artery and IMA.
    - The superior branch is directed upwards and supplies the nasopharynx and soft palate. It anastomoses with the artery of the pterygoid canal and middle meningeal and accessory meningeal arteries (from the IMA), and the vidian and mandibular arteries (ICA cavernous segment). The superior branch gives off Eustachian tube and carotid branches. The former supplies the Eustachian tube and submucosa of the fossa of Rosenmüller while the latter traverses the foramen lacerum to anastomose with the recurrent artery of the foramen lacerum (inferolateral trunk (ILT) of the ICA, both ipsilateral and contralateral).
    - The middle branch is directed anteromedially and supplies the nasopharynx and soft palate. It is an important source of bleeding in refractory epistaxis and post-tonsillectomy haemorrhage. It may anastomose with the pterygovaginal, accessory meningeal, and descending and greater palatine arteries.
    - The inferior branch, also of importance in post-tonsillectomy haemorrhage, courses anteroinferiorly and supplies the oropharynx. It may anastomose with the ascending palatine artery.
- Inferior tympanic artery: this may arise from the pharyngeal or neuromeningeal trunks, or at the bifurcation. It is directed superiorly through the canal of Jacobson (inferior tympanic canaliculus) to enter the tympanic cavity. Here the artery supplies the facial and accessory nerves and anastomoses with the anterior tympanic artery (from the IMA), petrosal branch of the MMA, and the stylomastoid, and caroticotympanic arteries. The latter is normally a tiny branch of the petrous ICA but may enlarge and form the anatomical variant of the 'aberrant ICA' in the absence of normal cervical ICA development.
- Musculospinal branch: this passes posteroinferiorly at the C3 level. It supplies the spinal accessory nerve and the superior sympathetic ganglion. Important anastomoses connect with the ascending and deep cervical arteries and vertebral artery.
- Neuromeningeal trunk: this branch is important because of its supply of CNs. It enters the posterior fossa via the foramen magnum. It may also arise from the occipital or posterior auricular arteries. The trunk bifurcates into jugular and hypoglossal and branches:
    - The jugular is the more superior and lateral and enters the cranium through the jugular foramen. It supplies the glossopharyngeal, vagus, and accessory nerves in addition to meninges. It has an ascending medial branch that accompanies the inferior petrosal sinus and anastomoses with the lateral clival artery (meningohypophyseal trunk (MHT)). Clival branches also anastomose with branches of the ILT and other clival branches of the meningohypophyseal artery and can supply the abducens nerve in Dorello's canal. A sigmoid branch accompanies the sigmoid and transverse sinuses and anastomoses with the middle meningeal and occipital arteries. An additional

ascending branch supplies dura mater of the internal auditory canal and may anastomose with the AICA. The posterior meningeal artery may originate from the jugular branch.

- The hypoglossal branch is more posterior, inferior, and medial and enters the cranium through the hypoglossal canal to supply the hypoglossal nerve and meninges. A medial branch runs over the medial clivus and anastomoses with the medial clival artery (MHT of the ICA). A descending branch anastomoses with its contralateral counterpart and forms the odontoid arch arcade, together with bilateral C3 radicular branches of the vertebral arteries. Posterior branches course inferomedially along the floor of the posterior fossa, medially as the artery of the falx cerebelli and laterally as the posterior meningeal artery. Both of these may also arise from the vertebral or posterior inferior cerebellar arteries. Rarely, the posterior inferior cerebellar artery (PICA) may arise from the hypoglossal artery.

- Muscular branches: multiple tiny muscular branches originate from any of the above branches.

Further reading

Hacein-Bey L, Daniels DL, Ulmer JL, et al. The ascending pharyngeal artery: branches, anastomoses and clinical significance. AJNR Am J Neuroradiol. 2002;23(7):1246–1256.

Kiyosue H, ed. External Carotid Artery: Imaging Anatomy Atlas for Endovascular Treatment. Springer Nature; 2020.

Lasjaunias P, Berenstein A. Surgical Neuroangiography: 1 Functional Anatomy of Craniofacial Arteries. Springer Science & Business Media; 2012.

ECA III: internal maxillary artery

- The internal maxillary artery (IMA) and STA are the terminal divisions of the ECA. The IMA can be referred to as simply the *maxillary* artery.
- IMA branches supply the organs and muscles of the head and neck, mouth, paranasal sinuses, dura, and CNs (Figures 2.6 & 2.7).
- **Origin:** the IMA originates within the parotid gland behind the neck of the mandible.
- **Course:**
  - The first (mandibular) segment runs deep to the neck of the mandible and runs anterior just lateral to the inferior alveolar nerve towards the border of the lateral pterygoid muscle. It gives off the deep auricular, anterior tympanic, middle meningeal, accessory meningeal, and inferior alveolar (dental) arteries.
  - The second (zygomatic or pterygoid) segment curves anteromedially, either superficial or deep to the pterygoid muscles, to reach the pterygopalatine fossa. It gives off middle deep temporal, pterygoid, masseteric, buccal, and anterior deep temporal branches.
  - The third (pterygopalatine) segment runs medially in the pterygopalatine fossa giving off the posterior superior dental, infraorbital, descending palatine, and pharyngeal arteries and the arteries of the foramen rotundum, pterygoid canal (vidian artery), and superior orbital fissure. It terminates as the sphenopalatine artery at the medial border of the fossa, in the sphenopalatine foramen.

Deep auricular artery

- **Origin:** this tiny artery is the first maxillary branch. It may share a common origin with the anterior tympanic artery.
- **Course:** it ascends within the parotid behind the temporomandibular joint. It passes through the wall of the external acoustic meatus to supply the skin of the canal and the outer surface of the tympanic membrane.

Anterior tympanic artery

- **Origin:** another small vessel, sometimes shares a common origin with the deep auricular artery. It also occasionally arises from the STA, the distal ECA, or other proximal maxillary arteries such as the inferior dental or middle meningeal.
- **Course:** the artery ascends behind the temporomandibular joint and bifurcates into anterior and posterior branches. The anterior branch supplies the temporomandibular joint, and the posterior branch enters the tympanic cavity through the petrotympanic fissure to supply the mucosa of the tympanic cavity and the tympanic membrane.
- **Anastomoses:** stylomastoid artery, the artery of the pterygoid canal (vidian artery), and anastomoses within the tympanic cavity including the caroticotympanic branch of the ICA.

Middle meningeal artery

- The MMA is an extremely important vessel because it is often a route for embolisation of dural arteriovenous fistulas, tumours, and subdural haematomas. The artery supplies more than two-thirds of the cranial dura. Confusingly, the nomenclature of its parts and branches varies between texts. We use that described by Kiyosue et al.

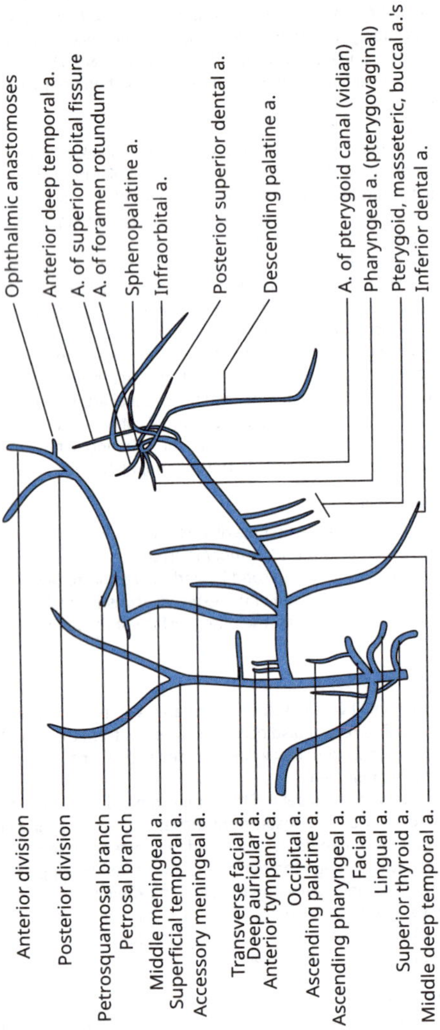

Figure 2.6 External carotid and internal maxillary branches.

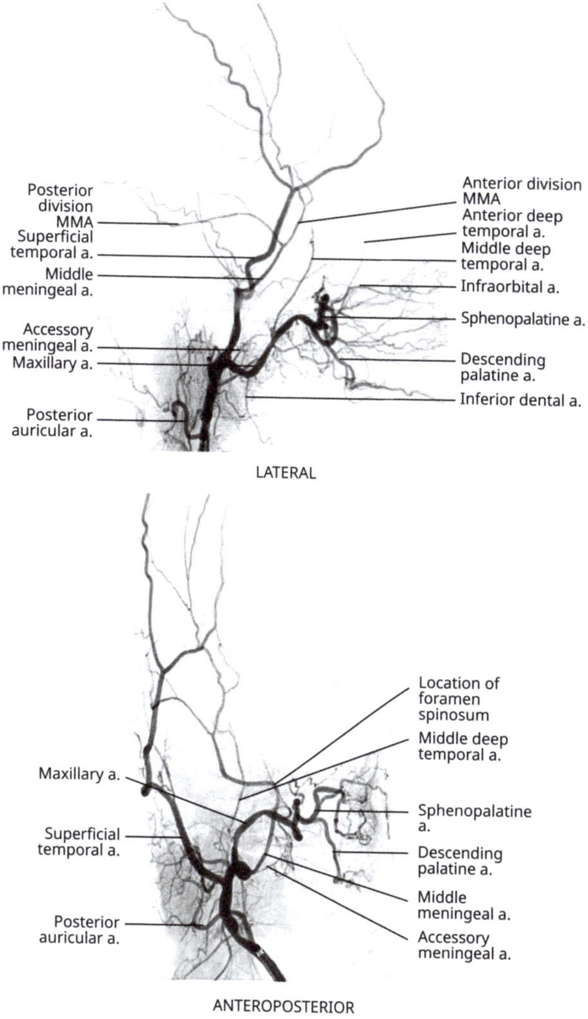

Figure 2.7 Distal ECA angiogram.

- **Origin:** the MMA arises from the superomedial surface of the first segment of the IMA. Often it shares a common trunk with the accessory meningeal artery. The MMA may also rarely originate from the ophthalmic artery (the 'recurrent meningeal artery'), the cavernous ICA via the ILT, the petrosal ICA via the persistent stapedial or vidian arteries, the cervical ICA, the basilar artery (usually distal third), or the occipital artery.
- **Course:**
  - Extracranial segment: the artery passes superiorly and medially and enters the cranial cavity via the foramen spinosum.
  - Horizontal segment: it then turns abruptly laterally and runs horizontally giving off wispy petrosal and cavernous sinus branches. The vessel continues to reach the petrosquamous suture, delivering a petrosquamosal branch.
  - Temporal segment: it then courses anteriorly on the greater wing of the sphenoid to reach the pterion (the convergence of the frontal, parietal, temporal, and sphenoid bones).
  - Pterional segment: this segment curves around the pterion.
  - Coronal segment: this segment runs superomedially along the coronal suture towards the midline, becoming the paramedian artery supplying the superior sagittal sinus.

Branches

- Cavernous sinus branches: anterior and posterior branches originate from the horizontal segment to supply the lateral wall of the cavernous sinus. The anterior branch runs anteromedially to supply the anterior cavernous sinus and anastomoses with the artery of the foramen rotundum. The posterior branch is directed posteromedially to supply the posterior cavernous sinus and anastomoses with the medial clival artery and the carotid branch of the superior pharyngeal branch of the ascending pharyngeal artery.
- Petrosal branches: these arise posteriorly at the level of the foramen spinosum from the proximal horizontal segment. The branches should be protected during embolisation particularly because the superficial petrosal branch passes through the facial nerve canal contributing to the facial arcade to supply the facial nerve. They run medially to supply regional dura mater. The proximal petrosal branch, immediately distal to the foramen spinosum, supplies the cavernous sinus, trigeminal nerve, and Gasserian ganglion and anastomoses with the ILT. This artery also supplies the superior tympanic cavity and anastomoses in the tympanic cavity with the caroticotympanic, superior tympanic (another petrosal branch supplying the tensor tympani muscle and superior part of the tympanic cavity), inferior tympanic, subarcuate (anterior inferior cerebellar branch) arteries, and the tubal branch of the accessory meningeal artery. There are also numerous important anastomoses including with the accessory meningeal artery, tentorial arteries from the inferolateral or MHTs of the ICA, dural branches from the AICA and ascending pharyngeal artery.
- Petrosquamosal branch: this arises from the horizontal segment slightly more distally than the petrosal branches. On the lateral view it can be difficult to distinguish from the petrosal branches, but this is easy on anteroposterior (AP) views as the petrosquamosal is directed laterally

(and is usually more prominent) whereas the petrosal branches course medially and are wispy. The distinction is important during embolisation because this branch is generally safe to occlude, unlike the petrosal.

- Posterior convexity branches: a variable number of posterior branches arise from the temporal and coronal segments, and the petrosquamosal branches, supplying a large region of convexity dura mater. Note that all peripheral branches of the MMA have potential anastomoses with more superficial arteries such as the STA and occipital artery via transosseous branches, which become evident under pathological conditions, in particular, dural arteriovenous fistulas. There are also potential anastomoses with dural branches of cortical arteries.
- Anterior convexity branches: these originate from the temporal, pterional, and coronal segments and course medially along the lesser wing of the sphenoid bone. There are important anastomoses with the ophthalmic artery. The MMA may be the sole supply of the orbit (the 'meningo-ophthalmic artery') or supply the lacrimal gland and lateral orbit via a recurrent branch traversing the foramen of Hyrtl (found in the spheno-orbital foramen, in the orbital roof). This latter branch usually also has ophthalmic artery anastomoses. Anterior branches from the coronal segment anastomose with the anterior ethmoidal branch of the ophthalmic artery.
- Paramedian arteries: these are the terminal branches of the MMA. They are directed anteriorly or posteriorly along the superior sagittal sinus and anastomose with the anterior (from the anterior ethmoidal artery) or posterior (from the ascending pharyngeal) falcine arteries. They deliver small branches to the superior sagittal sinus and falx cerebri. They also anastomose with dural branches of the posterior cerebral artery (PCA; Davidoff and Schechter) and the superior cerebellar artery (SCA; artery of Wollschlaeger and Wollschlaeger).

Accessory meningeal artery

- **Origin:** this artery has an oblique anterior and medial slant, arising anterosuperiorly from the first segment of the IMA or from the extracranial MMA. It supplies the CNs, the pharynx, the Eustachian tube, meninges and has several important anastomoses.

Branches

- Anterior branch: courses along the Eustachian tube reaching the torus tubaris, supplying regional mucosa, bone, and the tensor veli palatini muscle. There are anastomoses with the vidian artery, mandibular artery, the artery of the pterygoid and pharyngeal canals, and the pharyngeal branch of the ascending pharyngeal.
- Posterior branch: ascends superiorly and enters the skull through the foramen ovale or foramen vesalius. The vessel supplies the mandibular division of the trigeminal nerve, trigeminal ganglion and dura mater of Meckel's cave and the middle cranial fossa. There are anastomoses with inferolateral and MHTs of the ICA, recurrent meningeal branch of the ophthalmic artery, cavernous branches of the MMA, the artery of the foramen rotundum, and the subarcuate artery of the AICA.
- Superior branch of the ILT: the accessory meningeal artery is occasionally the origin for this important artery that supplies the

oculomotor, trochlear, trigeminal and abducens nerves, dura of the superior wall of the cavernous sinus and tentorium.

Inferior dental (or alveolar) artery

- **Origin:** inferiorly from the first segment of the IMA. Occasionally arises from a common trunk with the middle deep temporal artery.
- The vessel supplies the roots of the lower teeth and can be the source of bleeding after extraction of molar teeth, requiring embolisation.
- **Course:** it runs inferiorly accompanying the inferior alveolar nerve and vein. It enters the mandibular canal through an opening on the medial surface of the mandibular ramus and then courses anteroinferiorly and medially towards the mental foramen on the anterior surface of the mandible, anastomosing with mental branches of the facial artery.

Branches

- Extramandibular branches: multiple small branches supply the pterygoid and mylohyoid muscles and the lingual nerve.
- Terminal branches: it divides into the incisor (supplying the pulp of the teeth) and mental (supplying the lower lip and chin) terminal branches opposite the first premolar tooth.

Middle deep temporal artery

- **Origin:** this is from the proximal aspect of the second maxillary segment. It may share a common origin with the inferior dental artery.
- **Course:** superiorly on the temporal bone giving off small branches to bone and the temporalis muscle.
- **Anastomoses:** anterior deep temporal and superficial temporal arteries. There are transosseous anastomoses with the MMA and distal lacrimal branch of the ophthalmic artery.

Pterygoid artery

- **Origin:** inferiorly from the second maxillary segment.
- The artery supplies the medial and lateral pterygoid muscles.

Masseteric artery

- **Origin:** proximal part of the segment maxillary segment.
- **Course:** inferiorly through the mandibular notch, between the coronoid and condyloid processes, to supply the masseter muscle.
- **Anastomoses:** masseteric branches of the facial artery and transverse facial artery.

Buccal artery

- **Origin:** distal part of the second maxillary segment.
- **Course:** inferiorly to supply buccal mucosa, buccinator, the parotid duct, and skin.
- **Anastomoses:** ascending branch of the facial artery and the superior masseteric branch of the transverse facial artery. It is an important route for facial artery reconstitution after proximal facial artery ligation.

Anterior deep temporal artery

- **Origin:** the anterior deep temporal artery takes its origin from the distal aspect of the second segment. It may share a common origin with the buccal artery.

- **Course:** anterosuperiorly along the temporalis muscle which it supplies. It contributes an important branch to the lateral orbit which it reaches either via the zygomatic temporal fissure or inferior orbital fissure.
- **Anastomoses:** middle deep and superficial temporal arteries and also distal lacrimal branches of the ophthalmic artery.

Posterior superior dental artery

- **Origin:** this artery takes its origin from the proximal part of the third maxillary segment, just inside the pterygopalatine fossa. It often shares a common trunk with the infraorbital artery.
- **Course:** anteroinferiorly on the lateral surface of the maxilla, giving off osseous branches, supplying the mucosa of the maxillary sinus and buccal cavity, and buccinator. The vessel then enters the superior alveolar canal in the maxilla running towards the incisor foramen.
- **Anastomoses:** infraorbital, transverse facial, and descending palatine arteries.
- **Clinical relevance:** this vessel can also be a source of bleeding after molar teeth extraction.

Infraorbital artery

- **Origin:** this terminal branch of the IMA arises anteroinferiorly from the proximal part of the third maxillary segment. It may share a common origin with the posterior superior dental artery. It supplies the inferior rectus and inferior oblique muscles and lacrimal sac.
- **Course:** laterally, it looks like an upturned boat hull. It ascends on the posterior wall of the maxillary sinus and then traverses the inferior orbital fissure to enter the orbit. The vessel runs forward on the orbital floor in the infraorbital groove (together with the infraorbital nerve and vein), giving off osseous and muscular branches and anastomosing with the inferior muscular branches of the ophthalmic artery. It then exits through the infraorbital foramen (again with the infraorbital nerve and vein) to supply the lateral aspect of the nose, upper lip, and the lower eyelid.
- **Anastomoses:** the terminal branches anastomose with the superficial temporal, ophthalmic, facial, and transverse facial arteries.

Artery of the foramen rotundum

- **Origin:** posterosuperiorly from the third maxillary segment. It courses posteriorly accompanied by the maxillary nerve, which it supplies, and enters the cranium through the foramen rotundum to supply dura mater. It has a characteristic corkscrew appearance.
- **Anastomoses:** there is an important anastomosis with the anterolateral branch of the ILT (from the cavernous ICA). Care must be taken during embolisation to prevent embolisation through this anastomosis, to prevent CN damage and ischaemic stroke.

Artery of the superior orbital fissure

- **Origin:** superomedially from the third maxillary segment. It may share a common trunk with the artery of the foramen rotundum.
- **Course:** superiorly through the sphenopalatine foramen towards the superior orbital fissure.
- **Anastomoses:** anteromedial branch of the ILT and recurrent meningeal branch of the lacrimal branch of the ophthalmic artery.

Artery of the pterygoid canal (vidian artery)

- **Origin:** posterosuperiorly from the third maxillary segment. It may share a common origin with the artery of the foramen rotundum or the pharyngeal artery.
- It supplies the mucosa of the pterygopalatine fossa and nasopharyngeal cavity.
- **Course:** the vessel has a horizontal course, running posterolaterally through the vidian canal accompanied by the vidian nerve to reach the foramen lacerum where it anastomoses with the other vidian artery arising from the petrous ICA. Along its course it gives off mucosal branches to the nasal and oropharyngeal cavities and osseous branches within the pterygoid canal and Eustachian tube.
- **Anastomoses:** vidian artery of the ICA, pterygovaginal artery, mandibular artery, ascending pharyngeal (superior pharyngeal branch), accessory meningeal, and ascending palatine arteries (the pharyngeal/ Eustachian tube anastomosis).

Pharyngeal (pterygovaginal) artery

- **Origin:** third maxillary segment proximal to the sphenopalatine foramen. It sometimes shares a common trunk with the artery of the pterygoid/vidian canal or the sphenopalatine artery.
- **Course:** posteromedially and inferiorly through the pharyngeal (pterygovaginal) canal to supply the roof of pharynx and pharyngeal end of the Eustachian tube.
- **Anastomoses:** branches of the ascending pharyngeal artery, vidian artery, and accessory meningeal artery (pharyngeal/Eustachian tube anastomosis).

Descending palatine artery

- **Origin:** inferiorly from the third maxillary segment. It may share a common origin with the posterior lateral nasal branch of the sphenopalatine artery.
- **Course:** it descends and enters the greater palatine (pterygopalatine) canal accompanied by the great palatine nerve. Within the canal it gives off the lesser palatine artery which supplies the soft palate. The artery becomes the greater palatine artery as it exits the canal through the greater palatine foramen. It courses anteriorly beneath the hard palate to supply the hard plate, gingiva, and nasal septum.
- **Anastomoses:** posterior septal arteries (from the sphenopalatine) and the ascending palatine artery.
- **Clinical relevance:** the artery may become injured and bleed profusely after maxillary bone fracture.

Sphenopalatine artery

- **Origin:** the sphenopalatine is a terminal branch of the maxillary artery.
- **Course:** medially through the sphenopalatine foramen to enter the nasal cavity, which it supplies in addition to the paranasal sinuses. It is best seen on the anteroposterior projection angiographically due to its medial course.
- **Clinical relevance:** the artery is targeted in recurrent intractable epistaxis and during juvenile nasal angiofibroma embolisation.

Branches

- Posterior lateral nasal artery (or lateral sphenopalatine artery): this vessel sometimes originates from the descending palatine artery. It supplies the middle and inferior turbinates and maxillary and ethmoidal sinuses. It may anastomose with branches of the descending palatine artery, nasal branches of the facial artery, and ethmoidal branches of the ophthalmic artery.
- Posterior septal (or medial sphenopalatine) artery: this vessel is medially directed towards the superior turbinate and gives off a branch to the sphenoid ostium. It divides into superior and inferior branches. The superior branch supplies the superior turbinate before coursing medially to the nasal septum where it curves anteriorly. It anastomoses with branches of the anterior ethmoidal artery and descending palatine and contributes to Kiesselbach's plexus. This plexus is located on the anterior inferior quadrant of the nasal septum ('Little's area') and is a common site for epistaxis. It is supplied by five vessels: the sphenopalatine, superior labial, greater palatine, anterior ethmoidal, and posterior ethmoidal arteries.

Further reading

Bonasia S, Smajda S, Ciccio G, Robert T. Middle meningeal artery: anatomy and variations. AJNR Am J Neuroradiol. 2020;41(10):1777–1785.

Kiyosue H. External Carotid Artery: Imaging Anatomy Atlas for Endovascular Treatment. Springer Nature; 2020.

Lasjaunias P, Berenstein A. Surgical Neuroangiography: 1 Functional Anatomy of Craniofacial Arteries. Springer Science & Business Media; 2012.

Internal carotid artery

The ICA (Figure 2.8) originates at the bifurcation of the CCA. This is usually at C4 but may be as low as T2.

Segmental classification

Cincinnati segmental classification

The disadvantage of this classification (Bouthillier et al., 1996) is that not all the levels can be distinguished angiographically and the 'C' may be confused with cervical vertebral levels.

- C1: cervical, from the origin.
- C2: petrosal, starting at the carotid canal.
- C3: laceral, starting at the posterolateral margin of the foramen lacerum.
- C4: cavernous, starting at the superior margin of the petrolingual ligament.
- C5: clinoid, starting at the proximal dural ring.
- C6: ophthalmic, starting at the distal dural ring (where the ICA becomes intradural).
- C7: communicating, starting just proximal to the origin of the posterior communicating artery (PCOM) and ending at the bifurcation of the ICA.

New York University segmental classification

Optimised for angiography (Shapiro et al., 2014), hence used preferentially for this chapter:

- Cervical: from the origin.
- Petrosal: starting at the proximal margin of the carotid canal.
- Cavernous: starting at the superior margin of the petrolingual ligament (the anterior aspect of the petrous ridge is used as a landmark).
- Paraophthalmic: starting at the estimated location of the proximal dural ring, just proximal to the ophthalmic artery.
- Communicating: starting at the PCOM.
- Choroidal: starting at the anterior choroidal artery.
- Terminus: starting slightly distal to the anterior choroidal artery and ending at the carotid bifurcation.

Cervical segment

- This begins at the bifurcation of the CCA and ends as the artery enters the carotid canal.
- **Course:** the ICA is contained within the carotid sheath, anteromedial to the IJV. The ECA is also usually anteromedial initially, before it veers laterally. The vagus nerve and the cranial root of the accessory nerve are located posteriorly.

Branches

Usually, this segment does not have any branches.

Variants

- In the 'aberrant ICA' variant, the first ICA segment does not develop and the inferior tympanic branch of the ascending pharyngeal artery and its anastomosis with the caroticotympanic artery reconstitute the horizontal petrosal segment of the ICA. The appearance is of a lateralised, posterior, petrosal segment of the ICA and absence or hypoplasia of the vertical carotid canal. There is deficiency of the bony plate along the tympanic part of the ICA and this may be associated with pulsatile tinnitus and conductive hearing loss.

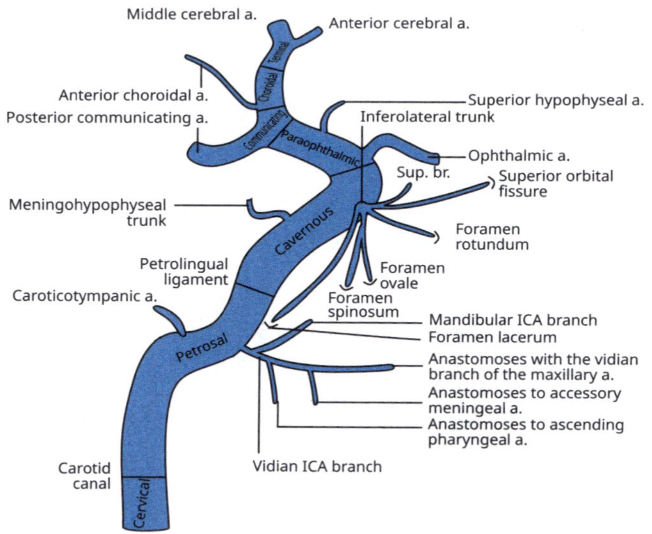

Figure 2.8 Internal carotid artery segments (New York University classification) and branches.

- Persistent hypoglossal artery: this variant, the second most common persistent vertebrobasilar anastomosis, arises from the distal cervical ICA and passes through an enlarged hypoglossal canal to join the vertebral or basilar arteries. If large, there may be hypoplasia of the ipsilateral vertebral and PCOM.
- Proatlantal arteries: these are remnants of the two most cranial intersegmental cervical segmental arteries. Type 1 corresponds to the first intersegmental artery. It arises from the posterior wall of the ICA between the C2 and C4 levels and travels dorsally to the first cervical space and through the occipitocervical space, joining the V3 segment of the vertebral artery in the suboccipital area. Type 2 corresponds to the second intersegmental artery. It originates from the ECA, follows a superoposterior path, and ascends to pierce the dura at the C1 level. It passes through the transverse foramen of the atlas and anastomoses with the contralateral vertebral V3 segment to form the basilar artery.

Petrosal segment

- From the carotid canal to the petrolingual ligament (approximately the anterior aspect of the petrous ridge).
- **Course:** the segment starts vertically in the carotid canal before turning anteromedially and running over the cartilage covering the foramen lacerum. It is accompanied by sympathetic fibres from the stellate ganglion and a venous plexus.

Branches

- Mandibulovidian artery: this artery has vidian and mandibular branches, both of which may arise separately from the ICA.
  - The vidian branch, horizontally orientated, passes anteriorly through the vidian canal and then into the pterygopalatine fossa to meet its counterpart vidian branch of the IMA. The branch is not always visible angiographically but may enlarge in certain situations, e.g., when supplying a juvenile nasopharyngeal angiofibroma.
  - The mandibular branch runs anteroinferiorly exiting the temporal bone to supply regional soft tissues and contributes to pharyngeal vascular anastomoses.
- Caroticotympanic: this small branch (the vestigial remnant of the hyoid artery) enters the middle ear cavity and anastomoses with the inferior tympanic branch of the ascending pharyngeal, the anterior tympanic and superior tympanic arteries, and a branch of the stylomastoid artery. As described above, it forms the cranial part of the 'aberrant ICA'.

Variants

- Persistent stapedial artery: this rare remnant of the hyoid artery is found in about 0.5%. Usually the stapedial artery regresses at the level of the caroticotympanic branch. The persistent artery arises from the distal cervical or proximal petrosal ICA segment and ascends vertically posterolateral to the ICA to enter the middle ear cavity. It passes through the crura of the stapes and then enters the middle cranial fossa to become the MMA. The foramen spinosum is usually hypoplastic or absent (although it is also possible to have an absent spinosal foramen without a persistent stapedial variant). It may cause pulsatile tinnitus. The persistent stapedial artery may also give rise to other ECA branches and/or have significant connections to the ophthalmic circulation.

- Otic artery: the existence of the otic artery is debated. If it exists, it is thought to originate from the lateral part of the petrosal segment of the ICA near the medial turn of the petrous carotid canal. Its course would then take it through the internal acoustic meatus, accompanying the facial and vestibulocochlear nerves, to connect with the basilar artery caudally.

Cavernous segment

- From the petrolingual ligament to the proximal dural ring.
- **Course:** the vessel runs superiorly along the posterior clinoid process to the anterior clinoid process before passing through the dural ring. Within the cavernous sinus it lies superomedially to the abducens nerve, and medial to CN III, CN IV, and the ophthalmic and maxillary divisions of CN V and the trigeminal (Gasserian) ganglion.

Carotid cave

- Although the cavernous segment of the ICA is extradural, aneurysms in this area can extend into the subarachnoid space if they are large or if they occur in the anatomically complex 'carotid cave' region, even when small.
- As the ICA makes its 180° posterior turn at the anterior genu of the siphon, it leaves the cavernous sinus and is transiently extradural. It then becomes subarachnoid and gives off the ophthalmic artery. The anterior clinoid process is superolateral to the genu of the ICA. Dural coverage extends medially to the tuberculum sellae from the anterior clinoid process. The dural ring is denser and more tightly adherent superolaterally and slopes inferomedially across the ICA so the medial and posterior aspects of the ICA genu can lie in the subarachnoid space. This is the carotid cave. Due to this anatomical variability, aneurysms pointing medially at this site may be intradural even if proximal to the distal dural ring. On angiography, it is advisable to consider all aneurysms distal to the anterior genu of the cavernous artery as potentially intradural, especially if pointing medially.

Branches

- The meningohypophyseal trunk (MHT): this projects posteriorly and laterally from the proximal cavernous ICA to supply the posterior pituitary, clivus, CNs III–VI, the trigeminal ganglion, the tentorium cerebelli, and other adjacent dura mater. It may exist as a single trunk or as multiple branches directly from the ICA (or, indeed, the ILT). There are four major branches:
  - The marginal tentorial artery of Bernasconi and Cassinari is a dural vessel that traverses the medial, free, edge of the tentorial leaf towards the torcular.
  - The basal (or lateral) tentorial artery, also a dural vessel, courses more laterally and inferiorly along the lateral edge of the tentorium cerebelli and sigmoid sinus and anastomoses with branches of the ascending pharyngeal, occipital, and middle meningeal arteries.
  - The lateral clival artery supplies the dura of the clivus. It has lateral and inferolateral branches which follow, respectively, the superior and inferior petrosal sinuses. There are anastomoses with its contralateral counterpart, the jugular branch of the ascending pharyngeal, and the MMA.

- The posterior inferior hypophyseal artery: anastomoses with its contralateral counterpart and supplies the posterior (and sometimes part of the anterior) lobe of the pituitary. It gives off an inferior clival artery that anastomoses with clival branches of the hypoglossal artery. The posterior inferior hypophyseal and medial clival arteries are remnants of the primitive IMA which can persist and enlarge in agenesis of the cervical ICA, so reconstituting the intracranial carotid circulation.
- Inferolateral trunk (ILT): originates on the lateral part of the mid-horizontal cavernous ICA and is directed inferiorly. It is an important vascular network connecting the middle meningeal, accessory meningeal, internal carotid, ophthalmic, and ascending pharyngeal arteries. The branches are:
  - The superior branch, which veers medially to supply CNs III, IV, and V1 (the ophthalmic division of the trigeminal nerve) in the cavernous sinus.
  - The anterior branch, which is divided into medial and lateral rami. The anteromedial ramus is directed towards the superior orbital fissure, supplying CNs III, IV, V1, and the abducens nerve (CN VI), and forming an anastomosis with the ophthalmic artery as the deep recurrent ophthalmic artery. The anterolateral ramus, directed laterally over the trochlear nerve and under the ophthalmic division of the trigeminal nerve, enters the foramen rotundum to anastomose with the IMA via the artery of the foramen rotundum.
  - The posterior branch, which is also split into medial and lateral rami. The posteromedial ramus is directed towards the foramen ovale and anastomoses with the accessory meningeal artery to supply the abducens nerve, the trigeminal ganglion, and the motor root of CN V. The posterolateral branch supplies the trigeminal ganglion and anastomoses with the MMA at the foramen spinosum.
  - The recurrent artery of the foramen lacerum, which forms an anastomosis in the foramen lacerum with the superior pharyngeal branch of the ascending pharyngeal artery.
  - Capsular arteries of McConnell—these small vessels provide a systemic supply to the anterior pituitary lobe and sella dura.
  - The MHT may arise partly or entirely from the ILT.

Variants

- Persistent trigeminal artery (seen in < 1%):
  - This variant, usually presellar although it can also run intrasellar, is the most common persistent vertebrobasilar anastomosis and usually arises from the posterior wall of the cavernous ICA (but may also arise from its lateral or anterior walls, the distal ICA petrosal segment, or the carotid siphon). There are three types: (i) Saltzman 1: the vessel joins the basilar distal to the AICA, there is an absent ipsilateral PCOM, and the vessel supplies the distal vertebrobasilar arteries. (ii) Saltzman 2: the vessel joins distal to the AICA, but there is an ipsilateral fetal PCOM which supplies the posterior cerebral arteries. (iii) Saltzman 3: does not join the basilar artery and instead terminates as the SCA (type a), AICA (type b), or PICA (type c).
  - The basilar artery caudal to the anastomosis is hypoplastic.
- The ophthalmic artery originates from the cavernous ICA in 8% ('dorsal ophthalmic artery').

Paraophthalmic segment

- From the estimated distal border of the cavernous segment, just proximal to the ophthalmic artery ostium, to the ostium of the PCOM.
- This segment incorporates the proximal and distal dural rings (the clinoid ICA segment); however, the dural anatomy in the anterior clinoid region is complex, variable, and impossible to reliably define on imaging, making it difficult to differentiate intradural and extradural aneurysms in this region.

Branches

- Ophthalmic artery: originates anteriorly from the ICA and traverses the orbital canal initially inferolateral and then arching superomedially over the optic nerve, adopting an American Civil War bayonet shape at the origin of the central artery of the retina and posterior choroidal arteries. Its branches are:
  - The central retinal artery: this, the most important branch, arises within the optic canal and travels alongside the optic nerve to supply the retina. It is a terminal branch without anastomoses and occlusion may result in permanent and severe visual loss. Note that if the choroid blush is visible on angiography, your catheter is in an artery which connects with the central retinal artery and it is therefore unsafe position to embolise. Absence of the choroidal blush on ICA injection implies that the ophthalmic artery arises from an external carotid branch (usually the MMA).
  - Ciliary arteries: supply the rectus muscles, conjunctiva, and sclera, and are responsible for the choroidal blush. These arise proximal to the central retinal artery.
  - Lacrimal artery: laterally placed, supplies the lacrimal gland, eyelids, and conjunctiva. The recurrent meningeal branch courses through the superior orbital fissure to connect with the MMA. Other anastomoses include branches of the infraorbital and deep temporal arteries.
  - Anterior and posterior ethmoidal arteries: the former distributes to the superior nasal septum and into the anterior meningeal branches (the artery of the falx cerebri), the latter to the posterosuperior nasal septum. These anastomose with the sphenopalatine artery.
  - Supratrochlear artery: supplies the skin of the forehead/scalp, and underlying pericranium and frontalis.
  - Dorsal nasal artery: supplies the lacrimal sac, face, and nose.
  - Superior hypophyseal arteries: these small vessels typically arise medially along the paraophthalmic ICA segment and supply the pituitary gland, optic chiasm, and optic nerve and some may supply the hypothalamus. There are anastomoses with their contralateral counterparts and ipsilateral PCOM.

Variants of orbital blood supply

- Dorsal ophthalmic: ophthalmic origin from the horizontal cavernous segment (a hypertrophied anteromedial branch of the ILT which normally regresses embryonically) that enters the orbit via the superior orbital fissure.
- Ventral ophthalmic: supraclinoid ICA/anterior communicating artery (ACOM)/A1 origin of the ophthalmic, entering the orbit via the optic canal.

- Meningo-ophthalmic: supply of the orbit is entirely from the MMA via the superior orbital fissure.
- Meningolacrimal artery: partial supply only of the lacrimal gland from the MMA via the foramen of Hyrtl.
- Recurrent meningeal: MMA origin from the ophthalmic artery.

Posterior communicating segment

- From the PCOM ostium to the anterior choroidal artery ostium.
- The PCOM insertion defines the PCA P1–P2 segments. Embryonically, the PCOM represents the caudal division of the ICA (contrasting with the adult description of the ICA division into the middle cerebral artery (MCA) and anterior cerebral artery (ACA)).
- A 'fetal type' PCOM, seen in approximately 25%, means the vessel is larger than the P1, or that it supplies most of the flow to the PCA territory. Complete absence of the PCOM is very rare; however, a very hypoplastic vessel may not be appreciated angiographically.
- Branches: the PCOM gives off numerous small perforators to the ventral thalamus. These may be present even if the vessel is hypoplastic. Therefore, even if there is a large P1 and small PCOM it cannot be assumed that the PCOM origin can be sacrificed as this may result in a ventral thalamic infarct which can be disabling.

Anterior choroidal segment

- From the anterior choroidal artery ostium and immediately adjacent.
- The anterior choroidal artery supplies highly eloquent tissue.[1] It is rarely absent. It usually arises posterolaterally from the ICA, 2–4 mm distal to the origin of the PCOM. It may uncommonly arise from the MCA, a joint origin with the PCOM, or the PCOM itself. It may also be larger than the PCOM, and thus occasionally mistaken for this vessel.
- The anterior choroidal artery runs posteriorly beneath the optic tract and then around the cerebral peduncle in the carotid, crural, and ambient cisterns before again crossing the optic tract from medial to lateral at the level of the lateral geniculate body. It then enters the choroidal fissure and terminates in the choroid plexus of the lateral ventricle. Occasionally, it may sweep around the pulvinar to reach the foramen of Monro. It anastomoses with the posterior choroidal artery via its intraventricular terminal branches and also with the middle and posterior cerebral arteries.
- The crucial branches are cisternal. They supply the optic tract, cerebral peduncle (corticospinal tracts, red nucleus, subthalamus), the posterior limb of the internal capsule, the optic radiation, the lateral geniculate body, proximal optic radiations, the hippocampus, the amygdala, the uncus, dentate gyrus, piriform cortex, globus pallidus, and the ventral thalamic nuclei. Although a small artery, its occlusion may cause significant neurological deficit, including contralateral hemiplegia, contralateral hemisensory loss, contralateral homonymous hemianopia, hemineglect, and aphasia.

1 An early treatment for Parkinson's disease involved clipping the anterior choroidal artery, but this method was eventually abandoned due to unacceptable complications.

- No vessels supplying brain parenchyma are found distal to the point at which it enters the lateral ventricle (the 'plexal point'). The artery often exhibits a sharp curve followed by a posterior turn at this location. It is generally safe to embolise distal to here, although it might be difficult to confidently identify the segment on angiography (cone beam computed tomography (CT) may be helpful).
- By definition, there is always just one anterior choroidal artery, i.e. the artery that supplies the choroid plexus. Multiple branches arising from the choroidal segment of the ICA represent perforating branches that would otherwise originate from the main stem of the anterior choroidal artery.
- Variants: the artery may persist as the main supply to the temporal, parietal, and occipital lobes. Embryonically, this represents failure of regression of territory normally annexed by the PCA.

Terminal segment

- From just distal to the anterior choroidal artery to the ICA bifurcation.
- This segment contains a variable number of perforating arteries to the anterior perforating substance, which contribute to the collateral reconstitution in Moyamoya disease. Anastomoses are found with the posterior choroidal arteries and ACA.

Further reading

Bouthillier A, van Loveren HR, Keller JT. Segments of the internal carotid artery: a new classification. Neurosurgery. 1996;38(3):425–432.

Byrne JV. Tutorials in Endovascular Neurosurgery and Interventional Neuroradiology. Springer; 2012.

Krings T, Geibprasert S, Cruz JP, ter Brugge KG. Neurovascular Anatomy in Interventional Neuroradiology: A Case-Based Approach. Springer; 2015.

Shapiro M, Becske T, Riina HA, et al. Toward an endovascular internal carotid artery classification system. AJNR Am J Neuroradiol. 2014;35(2):230–236.

Circle of Willis

- Variation is common in the circle of Willis (Figure 2.9) due to the numerous embryological steps involved in its formation. A symmetrical fully formed circle is found in only about 20% of the population.
- Variation is in accordance with haemodynamic principles. For example, there is usually a compensatory inverse relationship between the size of the P1 PCA segment and the PCOM to adequately supply the PCA territory.
- Complete absence of any one component is rare. More commonly, segments are so small that they cannot be visualised on conventional angiography. In addition to aplasia or hypoplasia there may be unusual geometric configurations, non-fusions, duplications, and fenestrations.[2]
- There is an association between these variations and the development of aneurysms due to increased haemodynamic stress contributing to their formation. The direction in which the aneurysm points is usually also related to the vessel direction. For example, an ACOM aneurysm will usually develop with the neck facing a dominant A1 segment.

2 **Non-fusion**: normally, many paired structures fuse during vascular development. This process can fail, leaving two channels joined at both the proximal and distal ends. **Duplication**: results from the failure of regression of embryologically distinct vessels that course next to each other and are joined proximally and distally. **Fenestration**: a single artery with two luminal channels. This occurs when a nerve or another structure present at the site of development forces the vessel to split around this structure.

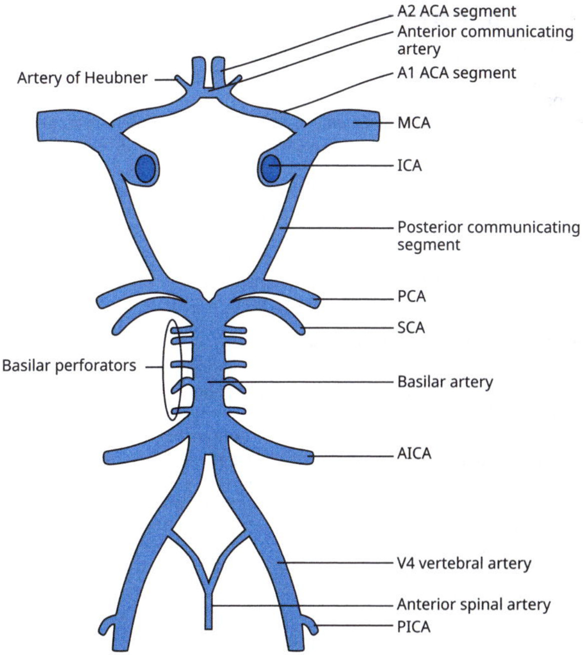

Figure 2.9 The circle of Willis.

Anterior cerebral artery

- The ACA (Figures 2.10 & 2.11) is the medial terminal division of the ICA, originating lateral to the optic chiasm and beneath the anterior perforating substance.
- ACA territory includes the medial frontal and parietal lobes, extending variably over the convexity, in equilibrium with distal MCA branches. Occlusion results in infarction of the medial cerebral hemispheres up to the parietal lobe, causing contralateral leg weakness and sensory impairment, executive dysfunction, urinary incontinence, behavioural changes, and gait apraxia.
- Cortical branches, from anterior to posterior include orbitofrontal, frontopolar, internal frontal (anterior, middle, posterior), paracentral, superior parietal, and inferior parietal branches.

A1 (pre-communicating) segment

- The A1 segment is directed forwards and medially above the optic nerve and chiasm towards the anterior interhemispheric fissure.
- Branches:
  - Medial lenticulostriate arteries: superior branches supply the anterior basal ganglia, anterior commissure, and anterior limb of the internal capsule. Medial branches supply the anterior aspect of the lateral wall of the third ventricle, hypothalamus, and septum pellucidum. Inferior branches infiltrate the optic nerves and chiasm. They vary in size and number.
  - The recurrent artery of Heubner: the largest laterally projecting perforating branch arising from the A1 or proximal A2 segment, travelling above the A1 and M1 segments, supplies the anterior hypothalamus, anteroinferior caudate head, anterior lentiform nucleus, and the anterior limb of the internal capsule. It is optimally

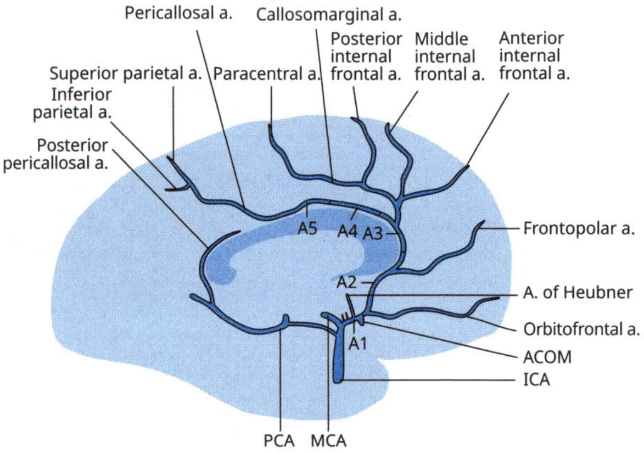

Figure 2.10 The anterior cerebral artery.

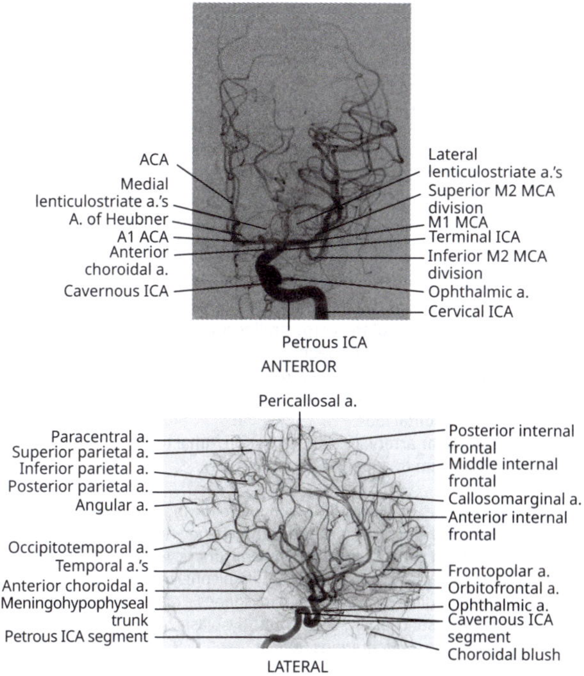

Figure 2.11 Angiogram of the anterior circulation.

demonstrated angiographically by a contralateral carotid injection. It is in haemodynamic balance with the medial lenticulostriates.

- Variations:
  - Variations in relative size are common and 10% are hypoplastic.
  - The interoptic or infraoptic A1, which may be due to a persistent ventral ophthalmic artery. This arises from the ICA at the level of the ophthalmic artery and runs below the optic nerve to supply normal ACA territory via an anastomotic segment. The anomaly may be either secondary to a persistent anastomosis between the primitive maxillary artery and the ACA or a persistent enlarged anastomotic channel between the primitive dorsal and ventral ophthalmic arteries.

Anterior communicating artery

- The ACOM varies in size and multiplicity and joins the A1 segments across the midline in the chiasmatic cistern above the optic chiasm. Usually, multiple small perforating branches arise from it supplying the septum pellucidum, corpus callosum, lamina terminalis, optic chiasm, and hypothalamus. The subcallosal artery, which supplies the rostrum and genu of the corpus callosum, is usually the largest single such branch.

- Variations:
  - Fenestrations are present in <4%. In cases of fenestration or duplication, both limbs may have perforators arising from them.
  - The primitive olfactory artery is a rare variant due to failure of regression of the terminal rostral division of the primitive ICA (olfactory artery). There are two variants. Type 1 originates from the ICA and courses anteriorly along the olfactory groove, making a characteristic hairpin turn to give rise to the distal ACA. Type 2 arises from the ACA and supplies the nasal cavity via the ethmoidal artery.

A2 (post-communicating) segment

- The A2 segment arises distal to the ACOM and extends to the junction of the rostrum and genu of the corpus callosum.
- The main branches of the A2 segment are:
  - The orbitofrontal artery: arising proximally and coursing anteriorly in the interhemispheric fissure to supply the gyrus rectus, olfactory bulb, and inferior frontal lobe.
  - The frontopolar artery: this arises just proximal to the genu of the corpus callosum to supply the frontal cortex.
- Variants:
  - Rarely, a single (or 'azygos') A2 is found following fusion of the A2 segments and can be associated with midline anomalies. This may be in the form of a single ACA or bihemispheric ACAs, one of which being dominant and supplying both hemispheres. There are often associated midline anomalies with dysgenesis of the corpus callosum, lobar holoprosencephaly, septo-optic dysplasia, aneurysms, and arteriovenous malformations (AVMs).
  - ACA trifurcations.
  - Early division of the ACA may result in the origin of a duplicated pericallosal or callosomarginal artery from the ACA–ACOM complex.

A3 (precallosal) segment

- The A3 segment extends around the genu of the corpus callosum.
- Segments inclusive of and distal to the A3 are generally called the pericallosal artery, although sometimes the A2 segment is also referred to as such. Small perforating branches supply the corpus callosum and the callosal arteries, and these traverse the corpus callosum to supply the septum, anterior pillars of the fornix, and anterior commissure. Distally, there are anastomoses with the posterior pericallosal branch of the PCA via perisplenial branches.
- The callosomarginal artery is the major branch of the A3 segment and runs parallel to the vessel inside the cingulate sulcus. It may be absent, with its branches arising directly from the pericallosal artery. It gives off four arteries that supply the medial frontal lobe: the anterior, middle, and posterior internal frontal arteries, and the paracentral artery.

A4 (supracallosal) and A5 (postcallosal) segments

- The A4 segment originates at the body of the corpus callosum and the A5 segment is the continuation of the vessel posterior to the coronal suture.
- Branches include:
  - Short callosal perforating arteries: supplying the pillars of the fornix and the anterior commissure.
  - Long callosal arteries: supplying adjacent cortex.
  - Dural branches: supplying the falx.
  - Parietal branches: supplying the medial parietal lobe. There may be distinct superior and inferior branches.

Further reading

Tahir RA, Haider S, Kole M, Griffith B, Marin H. Anterior cerebral artery: variant anatomy and pathology. J Vasc Interv Neurol. 2019;10(3):16–22.

Middle cerebral artery

The MCA (Figures 2.11 & 2.12) is the lateral terminal division of the ICA and supplies a broad region of the lateral cerebral hemisphere including regions of frontal, parietal, and temporal lobes and parts of the basal ganglia and internal capsule. Occlusion of the MCA results in variable neurological deficits depending on the affected branch and hemispheric dominance. Symptoms may include contralateral hemiparesis, sensory loss, hemianopia, and aphasia or neglect, contingent on whether the dominant or non-dominant hemisphere is involved.

M1 (horizontal) segment

- The M1 segment runs horizontally from the termination of the ICA to the limen insulae (the anteroinferior insular and lateral limit of the anterior perforated substance), along the sphenoid wing.
- Branches:
    - Lenticulostriate arteries (between 1 and 20, average 10) arise from the superior surface of this segment and perforate the anterior perforated substance. The medial group supplies the globus pallidus and lentiform nucleus. The lateral group supplies the anterior commissure, internal capsule, and upper head and body of the caudate nucleus, putamen, globus pallidus, and substantia innominata. They have an S-shape configuration on the right, and reverse S-shape on the left. The medial group may also arise from the A1 and the latter group may arise from the M2 segments.
    - Anterior temporal artery: this usually arises inferiorly from the middle of the M1 and supplies the anterior third of the superior, middle, and inferior temporal gyri.
- Variants: 'duplicated' and 'accessory' MCAs both refer to the presence of multiple apparent M1 trunks. The accessory variant is said to originate from the ACA and the duplicated from the ICA. Embryologically, however, the MCA develops from the fusion of lateral striate ACA perforators. Therefore, there is no true embryological distinction; it merely depends on the arbitrary definition of the ICA's bifurcation point. Both variants give off lenticulostriate perforators.

M2 (insular) segment

- There are different definitions of the start of the M2: either at the limen insulae as the vessel ascends vertically or at the M1 bifurcation. This inconsistency complicates applying principles derived from thrombectomy research, as studies use varying definitions. The most commonly accepted start point angiographically is probably the bifurcation, however.
- The artery usually divides into two trunks, although a single trunk, trifurcation, or quadrifurcation are all possible. Superior and inferior divisions are usually referred to. It is slightly more common for the inferior division to be dominant, covering the temporal and parietal lobes while the superior division tends to supply the frontal lobe. With superior dominance, its territory may extend to the angular gyrus and temporo-occipital regions.
- The branches angulate superiorly and course in the Sylvian fissure lateral to the insular cortex.

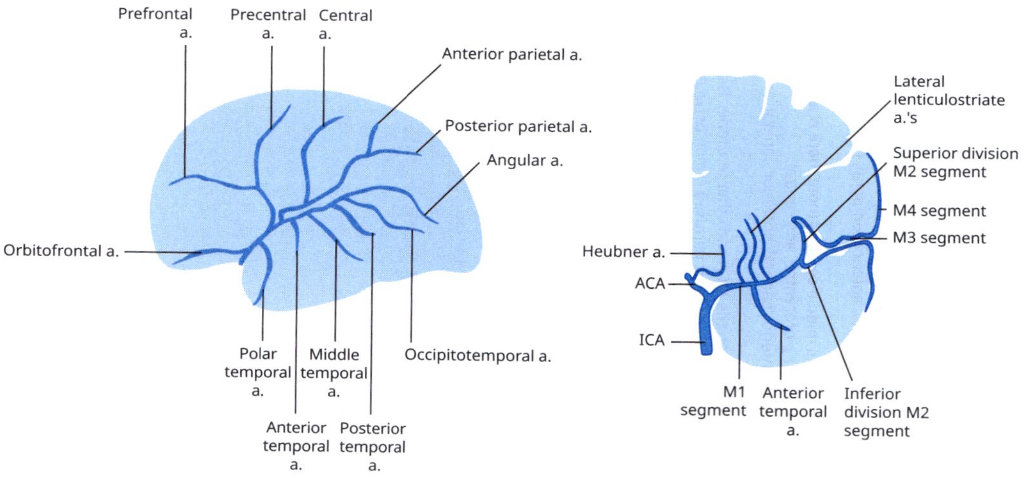

Figure 2.12 Middle cerebral artery.

M3 (opercular) segment

- The M3 starts at the circular sulcus of the insula and runs horizontally in the Sylvian fissure of the frontoparietal operculum.

M4 (cortical) segment

- The M4 (cortical) segments commence at the opercular turn and run on the surface of the cerebral convexity. The branches supply most of the lateral cerebral hemisphere, and the insular and opercular cortex.
- Branches are named after the regions they supply:
  - Temporal: polar temporal, anterior temporal, middle temporal, and posterior temporal.
  - Frontal: orbitofrontal middle cerebral (note there is also an ACA orbitofrontal branch), precentral, and central.
  - Parieto-occipital: anterior parietal, posterior parietal, angular, and occipitotemporal.
- The border zone between the MCA and other territories is called a *watershed* zone, meaning the least perfused region between territories. It is the most at risk of infarction in states of hypoperfusion, as with systemic hypotension or proximal occlusion. There may be a 'shift of the watershed' in situations where one territory expands to compensate for lack of perfusion in another territory, for example due to proximal stenosis.

Further reading

Fischer E. Die Lagenweichungen der vorderen Hirnarteie im Gefassbild. Zentralbl Neurochir. 1938;3:300–312.

Shapiro M, Raz E, Nossek E, Chancellor B, Ishida K, Nelson PK. Neuroanatomy of the middle cerebral artery: implications for thrombectomy. J Neurointerv Surg. 2020;12(8):768–773.

Vertebral artery

The vertebral artery can be divided into four segments (Figure 2.13).

V1 (preforaminal) segment

- This segment extends until the artery enters the foramen in the transverse process, typically at the C6 level (C4 if the vertebral artery arises from the aortic arch).

V2 (foraminal) segment

- The artery continues vertically upwards to the C2 transverse foramina, surrounded by the vertebral venous plexus.
- Branches:
  - C6–C1 segmental spinal arteries: spinal arteries supply structures including nerve roots, sheaths, bone, and the anterior and posterior spinal arterial systems. The C3 radicular spinal arteries participate in the odontoid arterial arcade (also formed from branches of the ascending pharyngeal and occipital arteries). The artery of cervical enlargement, or Lazorthes, is a prominent radiculomedullary branch arising from the lower cervical vertebral artery around C5–C6, although it may also originate from the deep cervical or supreme intercostal arteries.
  - Muscular branches to paraspinal arteries.
  - Anterior meningeal branch of the vertebral artery: this is a small branch of the distal vertebral artery that contributes to the dura of the anterior foramen magnum.
  - Anastomoses: there are extensive anastomoses with virtually any other artery in the neck, particularly the ascending cervical, deep cervical, ascending pharyngeal, contralateral vertebral, and occipital arteries.

V3 (extracranial) segment

- Starts at the foramen transversarium of the axis (C2). The artery turns laterally and ascends, passing through the transverse foramen of the atlas (C1). It then curves medially and is directed towards the foramen magnum. It imprints a groove on the posterior arch of the atlas, which may rarely form a bony ring called the arcuate foramen (a possible risk factor for paediatric ischaemic stroke).
- Branches:
  - Posterior meningeal artery: the posterior meningeal artery supplies the tentorium cerebelli and may originate from the extracranial vertebral artery, the occipital artery, the ascending pharyngeal artery, or the PICA.

V4 (intracranial) segment

- This segment pierces the atlanto-occipital membrane to become intradural (where it is focally smoothly narrowed), entering the cranial cavity via the foramen magnum. It continues medially until it joins its counterpart to form the basilar artery at the upper edge of the medulla oblongata.
- There is often hypoplasia of one of the intradural vertebral artery segments, and the artery may terminate in the PICA. In this case, a forceful injection during angiography risks rupturing this small terminal vessel.

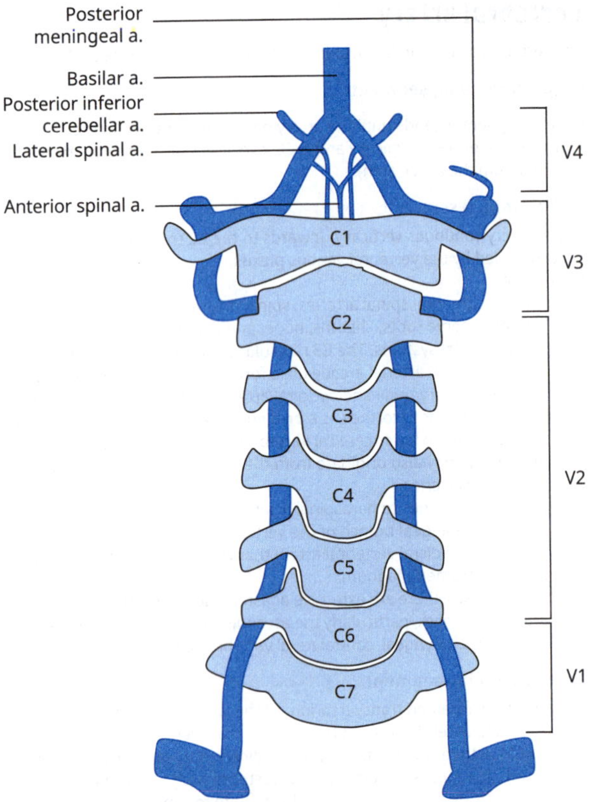

Figure 2.13 Vertebral artery.

Branches

- Perforators supplying the medulla and pyramids traverse the foramen caecum on the anterior medulla at the pontomedullary junction and penetrates all the way back to the tegmentum and floor of the fourth ventricle.
- Anterior spinal artery (ASA): the anterior spinal axis originates from the vertebral artery usually on the side with the dominant PICA, typically at the vertebrobasilar junction. Where there is no dominant PICA, it may arise symmetrically from both vertebral arteries, uniting to form a single vessel at C2–C4. There are anastomoses in the midline with other radiculomedullary arteries, particularly the artery of the cervical enlargement.

- Lateral spinal artery: the posterior cervical arterial pial network in its cranial portion is formed by the lateral spinal artery, which originates directly from the vertebral artery or the PICA. This runs caudally, anterior to the C1–C4 nerve rootlets and then joins the pial network of the spinal cord contributing to the posterolateral spinal arteries. Normally, the lateral spinal artery is small in calibre and is rarely visualised on angiography unless vascular malformations are present.
- PICA:
  - The artery most commonly originates from the intradural vertebral artery, however, its origin is variable. It may arise from the basilar artery, a joint AICA–PICA trunk, the extradural vertebral artery as low as C2, or the ascending cervical, occipital, and ascending pharyngeal arteries, or as a remnant of the trigeminal artery.
  - It may be duplicated or unilaterally or bilaterally absent, in which case its territory is served by another artery, usually the AICA.
  - It supplies the lower medulla, tonsils, vermis, and inferolateral cerebellar hemisphere.
  - The artery can be anatomically segmented into the following: anterior medullary (anterior to the apex of the inferior olive), lateral medullary (extends from the inferior olive), tonsillomedullary, telovelotonsillar, and cortical.
  - The first three segments emit perforators to the lateral medulla and anterior and lateral spinal arteries. The perforators may anastomose with those from the vertebral and basilar artery.
  - Conventionally, the apex of the cranial loop serves as the angiographic marker for the telovelotonsillar segment (Figure 2.14), which typically represents the distal limit for perforators originating from the PICA. Sacrificing the artery at or distal to this point is therefore unlikely to cause medullary infarction but will likely cause cerebellar infarction, depending on collateral blood supply to the region (usually from the AICA). Vermian branches may occasionally cross the midline and establish a bilateral supply.
  - The more distal the origin of the PICA, the greater the chances of medullary supply. In cases of extradural origin, the PICA is unlikely to supply the spinal cord or brainstem; instead, the supply is from perforators directly from the vertebral artery.
  - In addition to pial vessels, the posterior meningeal artery may arise from the PICA.
  - A proximal occlusion of the PICA can result in vertigo, nausea, vomiting, numbness on the same side of the face, Horner's syndrome, dysphagia, ataxia, and loss of sensation below the face on the opposite side.

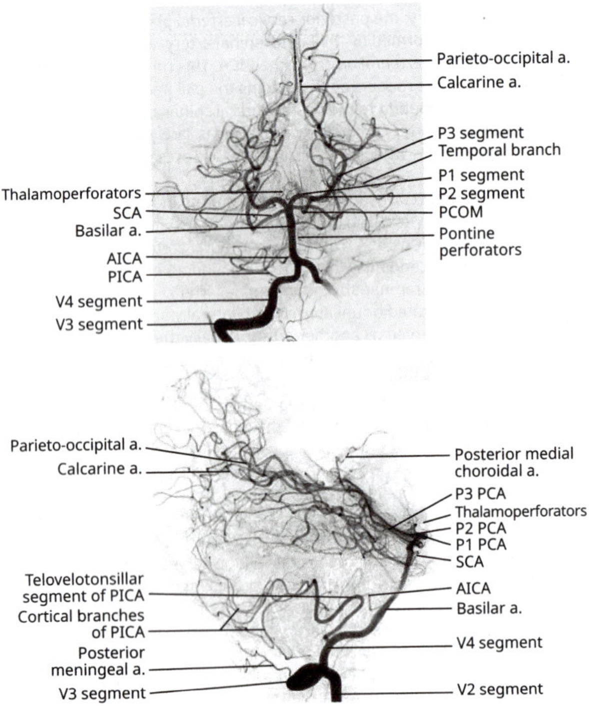

Figure 2.14 Posterior circulation angiogram.

Further reading

Krings T, Geibprasert S, Cruz JP, Ter Brugge K. Neurovascular Anatomy in Interventional Neuroradiology: A Case-Based Approach. Springer; 2015.

Santillan A, Nacarino V, Greenberg E, Riina HA, Gobin YP, Patsalides A. Vascular anatomy of the spinal cord. J Neurointerv Surg. 2012;4(1):67–74.

Basilar artery

The basilar artery arises at the pontomedullary junction. It runs over the surface of the pons and divides into the PCAs approximately at the level of the superior surface of the dorsum sella.

Basilar trunk perforating arteries

- Multiple perforators arise from the main trunk of the basilar artery. These do not opacify well on conventional angiography (they are better seen on high-resolution cone beam computed tomography angiography (CTA)). Their importance lies in the very eloquent brainstem structures that they supply, including white matter tracts (corticospinal and corticobulbar tracts, lemnisci, etc.) and the deep nuclei of the pons and midbrain. They typically do not supply structures across the midline. Their inadvertent occlusion is possible during stenting or flow diversion and there also is a tendency for the microguidewire to catch on them during navigation (use of a J-shaped wire tip, or leading with the microcatheter itself, can avoid this).
- The pontine perforators are classified into four main types:
  - Median branches penetrate the pons directly in the midline and are visible only when the basilar artery is retracted. They penetrate to the floor of the fourth ventricle.
  - Paramedian branches enter the pons off-centre.
  - Short circumflex branches partially encircle the pons.
  - Long circumflex branches fully encircle it and generally have fewer terminal branches.
- Anastomoses may be present between perforators on the same side mostly with those arising from the mid and lower basilar artery, and very infrequently from the more superiorly located perforators close to the bifurcation.
- The consequences of basilar artery occlusion or its branches depend on the level of occlusion:
  - Complete occlusion will usually lead to rapid loss of consciousness and impairment of normal homeostatic processes.
  - Proximal basilar: results in quadriplegia, horizontal gaze palsy, bifacial paralysis, contralateral limb weakness, hemibody loss of touch and proprioception, and ipsilateral tongue weakness.
  - Mid-basilar: leads to lateral and medial pontine symptoms including ipsilateral loss of facial sensation, ipsilateral dysmetria, contralateral arm and leg weakness, and gaze deviation.
  - Pontine paramedian perforators: causes ipsilateral nuclear facial palsy, horizontal gaze palsy, and contralateral arm and leg weakness.
  - Short pontine circumflex arteries: associated with ipsilateral intranuclear ophthalmoplegia, palatal/facial/pharyngeal/ocular myoclonus, dysmetria, and contralateral limb weakness.
  - Top of the basilar: associated with somnolence, nystagmus, skew deviation, oscillatory eye movements, and vertical gaze paralysis.

Anterior inferior cerebellar artery

- The AICA arises from the lower or mid-third of the basilar artery and runs over the anterolateral surface of the pons. It supplies the inferior and middle cerebellar peduncles, the inferior flocculus, the choroid plexus of the fourth ventricle, and the cerebellar hemisphere.
- It may be duplicated or arise from a common trunk with the PICA (AICA–PICA trunk).
- Occlusion leads to ipsilateral dysmetria, hearing loss, ipsilateral trigeminal loss, Horner's syndrome, dyskinesia, and contralateral loss of pain and temperature sensation.
- There are anastomoses with branches of the PICA and SCA.

Branches

- Medial branch: supplying the biventral lobule.
- Lateral branch: running in the hemispheric fissure and supplying the superior and inferior semilunar lobules.
- The internal auditory (labyrinthine) artery arises from the AICA or, less commonly, directly from the basilar artery. It divides into cochlear and anterior vestibular branches which are the main supply of the cochlea and vestibular apparatus. The internal auditory artery also supplies the facial nerve in the internal auditory canal.
- The subarcuate branch is dural, runs in the petromastoid canal, and anastomoses with the MMA and stylomastoid branches.

Superior cerebellar artery

- The SCA arises near the termination of the basilar artery and initially runs parallel and inferior to the PCA, separated by the oculomotor nerve. It deviates laterally in the ambient cistern, running over the middle cerebellar peduncle under the trochlear nerve, before continuing into the quadrigeminal cistern and veering towards the midline.
- It supplies the lower midbrain, upper pons, superior vermis, and superior cerebellar hemispheres.
- Occlusion results in ipsilateral limb ataxia, vertigo, nystagmus, dysarthria, and gait ataxia.
- The artery may share a common origin with the PCA or arise from the P1 segment, more common in caudal fusion types. It may be duplicated (in up to 28%), and this will correspond to separate origins of the medial and lateral divisions.

Branches

- Perforators from the proximal SCA to the pons, midbrain, and inferior colliculus.
- Medial (rostral) division: the artery further subdivides at the lateral pontomesencephalic level:
  - A further medial branch supplies the tectal anastomotic network that supplies the colliculi (occasionally anastomosing with collicular branches of the PCA) and superior cerebellar peduncle.
  - A lateral branch supplies the superomedial cerebellar hemisphere and superior vermis.
- Lateral (caudal marginal) division: this is usually the larger division and supplies the deep nuclei of the cerebellum including the dentate nucleus, and the superolateral cerebellar hemisphere.

- The artery of Wollschlaeger and Wollschlaeger: this dural branch arises from the lateral pontomesencephalic segment of the SCA. It runs through the ambient cistern to supply the medial tentorium.
- Superior vermian branch: the terminal branch supplying the vermis and anastomosing with the AICA and PICA.

Variants

- During embryonic development, the basilar artery is formed caudally by the fusion of the paired longitudinal neural arteries and cranially by the caudal divisions of the ICAs.
- Non-fused segments of the basilar artery are prone to aneurysm formation. As both limbs of non-fused segments may give off brainstem perforators, they must both be preserved during treatment.
- Three types of basilar termination architectures are recognised:
    - Cranial fusion type giving a 'T' shape caused by early fusion from the most cranial point at the pontomesencephalic sulcus.
    - Caudal fusion giving a 'V' shape caused by late fusion below the pontomesencephalic sulcus. The more caudal the fusion, the greater the likelihood of a P1 origin of the SCA.
    - Asymmetric fusion, with one side merging earlier than the other. In this situation, most of the midbrain and thalamic perforators arise from the more cranial P1 limb. The artery of Percheron is an extreme example of this type of situation, where a single trunk arises from the P1 segment and bilaterally supplies the thalami and midbrain.

Further reading

Krings T, Geibprasert S, Cruz JP, Ter Brugge K. Neurovascular Anatomy in Interventional Neuroradiology: A Case-Based Approach. Springer; 2015.

Kwiatkowska M, Rzepliński R, Ciszek B. Anatomy of the pontine arteries and perforators of the basilar artery in humans. J Anat. 2023;243(6):997–1006.

Posterior cerebral artery

- Consequences of occlusion of the PCA (Figure 2.15) depend upon the territory involved.
- The entire territory includes the occipital, posterior temporal and medial parietal lobes, thalamus, midbrain, and structures related to the third ventricular walls.
- Depending on the site of occlusion, a spectrum of debilitating deficits may develop. Many relate to vision, visual perception, integration of visual fields, and relay of information to visual association cortex:
  - Occipital lobe: homonymous hemianopsia.
  - Optic radiation or supracalcarine: inferior quadrantanopia.
  - Myers loop or infracalcarine: superior quadrantanopia.
- Injury to the thalamus and midbrain with involvement of the reticular activating formation affect arousal and consciousness. Memory and endocrine disturbance result from damage to the hippocampus and hypothalamus.

Posterior communicating artery

- In embryonic development the PCOM is the caudal division of the ICA. As the vertebrobasilar system develops and gives rise to the PCA, the PCOM regresses to a variable degree.
- Even a hypoplastic PCOM may be the sole supply of a significant thalamic territory via the 7–10 anterior thalamoperforating arteries. Sacrifice of a small, apparently insignificant, PCOM risks thalamic infarction. These thalamoperforators arise from the superolateral aspect and a particularly prominent one is the tuberothalamic artery, which supplies the anterior thalamus, reticular nucleus, and mammillothalamic tract. The anterior thalamoperforating group also supply the posterior optic chiasm, proximal optic radiations, posterior hypothalamus, and cerebral peduncle. They anastomose with choroidal arteries.

P1 segment

- Originating at the basilar bifurcation, the P1 segment runs within the interpeduncular cistern and terminates at the PCOM insertion.

Branches

- Posterior thalamoperforators (up to eight): these enter the posterior perforated substance, the interpeduncular cistern, and medial cerebral peduncles, and supply the posterior part of the thalamus, posterior part of the optic chiasm and tracts, posterior limb of the internal capsule, hypothalamus, subthalamus, substantia nigra, red nucleus, oculomotor and trochlear nuclei, rostral mesencephalon, and cerebral peduncles. The peduncular supply includes the corticospinal and corticobulbar tracts.
- Long and short circumflex arteries: these may arise from the P1 or P2 segments and supply the geniculate bodies, peduncle, and tegmentum. The long circumflex extends to the colliculi and additionally supplies the tectum.
- Collicular arteries sometimes arise distinctly from the P1 segment (running medial to P2) or P2 segment. They curve around and send branches to the cerebral peduncle, terminating at the collicular (quadrigeminal) plate. An anastomosis between the PCA and SCA can occur at this location.

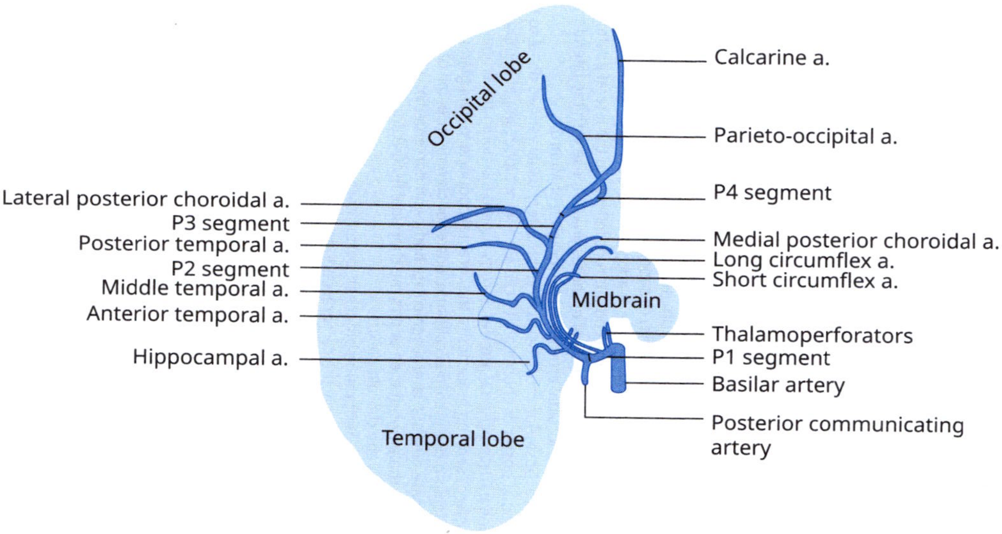

Figure 2.15 Posterior cerebral arteries.

- Artery of Percheron: this normal variant consists of a common trunk arising from one P1 segment giving off a bilateral supply to the medial thalami and sometimes rostral midbrain.

P2 segment

- This segment courses around the midbrain, under the thalamus, running in the crural and ambient cisterns. Branches supply the thalamus, cerebral peduncle, and quadrigeminal plate.

Branches

- Thalamogeniculate perforators (up to 12): these supply the optic tract, medial and lateral geniculate bodies, the lateral and inferior thalamus, and the posterior internal capsule.
- Medial posterior choroidal artery: this vessel usually arises from the medial P2 segment but may arise from the parieto-occipital, calcarine, or posterior pericallosal (splenial) branches. It runs medially and supplies the adjacent tectum, pineal gland, habenula and medial geniculate body, and posterior thalamus. It then enters the roof of the third ventricle within the velum interpositum (the small membrane just above and anterior to the pineal gland) to supply the choroid plexus. As it arches over the quadrigeminal plate, it adopts a characteristic '3' shape on a lateral angiographic projection. It runs inferior to the lateral posterior choroidal arteries. Terminal branches anastomose with the lateral posterior choroidal arteries at the foramen of Munro.
- Lateral posterior choroidal artery: this artery usually arises distal to the medial posterior choroidal but can arise from hippocampal, temporal, and parieto-occipital arteries. It runs superoanterior in the ambient cistern, sending branches to the cerebral peduncle, pineal gland, splenium of the corpus callosum, posterior commissure, tail of the caudate nucleus, lateral geniculate body, and dorsomedial and pulvinar of the thalamus. It then enters the choroidal fissure and lateral ventricle to supply the choroid plexus.
- Peduncular perforating branches: perforators arise from the P1 or P2 segment to supply the cerebral peduncles.

P3 and P4 segments

- The P3 segment runs posteromedially in the quadrigeminal cistern.
- The P4 segments are the cortical branches:
  - Anterior, middle, and posterior temporal: supplying the respective parts of the temporal lobes.
  - Hippocampal: supplying the hippocampus.
  - Parieto-occipital: usually the largest of the terminal branches, it runs initially superior and medial to the calcarine artery in the parieto-occipital fissure. The artery supplies the cuneus, precuneus, and superior occipital gyrus of the occipital lobe. It may also give branches to the precentral gyrus, superior parietal lobule, and an accessory calcarine branch to the visual cortex.
  - Calcarine: this runs initially inferior and lateral to the parieto-occipital artery within the calcarine fissure to supply the visual cortex, cuneus, and lingual gyrus. It occasionally originates from the parieto-occipital or posterior temporal arteries.

    - Posterior pericallosal (or splenial) branches: these small vessels originate from the P3 segment, parieto-occipital, calcarine, or posterior temporal arteries. They can form a common trunk with the medial posterior choroidal artery or can anastomose with the latter via a recurrent branch to the fornix. They are directed posteriorly initially and then turn abruptly anterosuperiorly to reach the corpus callosum. They anastomose with the terminal branches of the pericallosal artery.
    - Meningeal branch of Davidoff and Schechter: this eponymous branch is named after the mentors of those who first described it. It is a dural artery arising from the PCA near the falcotentorial junction to supply the falx cerebri. Often too small to be seen angiographically, it is more frequently seen in dural arteriovenous fistulas.
- There is extensive collateral supply to the P3 and P4 (and often P2) segments, such that parent vessel occlusion is often tolerated without adverse consequences. Nowadays, however, vessel reconstruction with flow diversion is probably the procedure of choice.

Variants

- The PCA annexes territory supplied earlier in development by the anterior choroidal artery. If this does not occur, the anterior choroidal may continue to supply large cortical regions of the temporal, parietal, and occipital lobes.

Further reading

Byrne JV. Tutorials in Endovascular Neurosurgery and Interventional Neuroradiology. Springer; 2012.

'Dangerous' cranial anastomoses

Embryological and phylogenetic development closely links extracranial arteries to intracranial arteries, forming common anastomotic routes. These anastomoses often do not appear on cerebral angiograms *but are always present* and may become evident during embolisation procedures due to haemodynamic changes, especially during prolonged injection of liquid embolic agents. Knowledge of these connections is crucial for avoiding embolic stroke and CN palsies. 'Ignorance is more expensive than education', to quote Richard Feynman. These anastomotic channels generally follow CNs through neural foramina and enlarge under certain conditions, particularly vascular skull base tumours, high-flow shunts, and major intracranial artery occlusions.

Three crucial skull base regions serve as key anastomotic pathways:

1 The petrous–cavernous region through the ILT, petrous branches of the ICA, and the MHT, connecting the distal IMA, MMA, accessory meningeal artery (AMA), and ascending pharyngeal circulation.
2 The orbital region via the ophthalmic artery, connecting maxillary and internal carotid territories.
3 The upper cervical region via connections from the ascending pharyngeal, occipital, and ascending and deep cervical arteries to the vertebral artery.

Petrous–cavernous region

Ascending pharyngeal artery collaterals

- The superior pharyngeal branch of the pharyngeal trunk contributes to the Eustachian tube anastomotic circle. It is connected to the petrous ICA's mandibular and vidian arteries and forms connections with the accessory meningeal artery and pterygovaginal artery (distal IMA). It also sends a branch through the foramen lacerum to the cavernous sinus, joining the recurrent artery of the foramen lacerum and the ILT from the cavernous ICA.
- The neuromeningeal trunk divides into jugular and hypoglossal branches, each giving off medial and lateral clival branches which anastomose with clival branches from the MHT from the cavernous ICA—important in the vascular supply to meningiomas.
- The inferior tympanic artery branch of the ascending pharyngeal artery travels with Jacobson's nerve through the inferior tympanic foramen, anastomosing with other tympanic (anterior tympanic, superior tympanic) and surrounding arteries within the middle ear including the caroticotympanic artery, a petrous ICA branch.
- In rare instances, cervical ICA agenesis and persistence of the embryological hyostapedial artery can lead to an 'aberrant ICA' where the ICA enters the skull base through the inferior tympanic canal, with the cervical ICA effectively being the ascending pharyngeal artery and its inferior tympanic branch, distally reconstructing as the caroticotympanic artery.

IMA collaterals

- After entering the foramen spinosum, the MMA has cavernous branches that connect with the superior or tentorial branch of the ILT, and orbital branches that anastomose within the superior orbital fissure with the anteromedial branch of the ILT.

- The superior division of the AMA enters the cavernous sinus through the foramen ovale to connect with the posteromedial branch of the ILT, which runs beneath the trigeminal ganglion and along the second branch of the trigeminal nerve (CN V2).
- Occasionally, the AMA supplies the entire territory normally served by the ILT. These connections are particularly significant in cases of cavernous dural arteriovenous fistulas.
- The AMA forms smaller anastomotic connections around the Eustachian tube with the superior pharyngeal branch of the ascending pharyngeal artery, the mandibular branch of the petrous ICA, and the pterygovaginal artery from the distal IMA.
- The MMA's petrosquamous or posterior branch also anastomoses with the marginal tentorial artery, which may originate from the ILT, ophthalmic artery, or the MHT of the ICA.
- The artery of the foramen rotundum from the IMA connects to the anterolateral branch of the ILT and, in rare instances, with the lateral clival artery.
- The vidian artery, running horizontally, arises from the distal IMA and runs through the vidian canal to the foramen lacerum, where it meets the vidian branch of the mandibulovidian artery from the petrous ICA.
- The pterygovaginal artery, typically adjacent to the vidian artery, follows a more inferior path through the pterygovaginal canal, terminating in an anastomotic circle around the Eustachian tube.

Orbital region

- The primary risk of embolisation in this region is occlusion of the central retinal artery, potentially causing blindness, or embolic stroke from retrograde flow into the ICA.
- The central retinal artery originates from the ophthalmic artery just distal to the posterior ciliary arteries. Although the retinal artery itself might be too small to see clearly, the choroidal blush (from the posterior ciliary arteries) acts as a helpful secondary indicator. When injecting an artery, if the choroidal blush is seen, one can deduce that there is a connection with the ophthalmic and retinal arteries.
- There are various collateral routes to the ophthalmic artery, with the meningo-ophthalmic artery being the most common. This variant, a remnant of the embryonic stapedial artery, consists of the entire orbital supply including the central retinal and ciliary arteries arising entirely from the MMA via the superior orbital fissure. Non-visualisation of the ophthalmic artery from the ICA and a choroidal blush on ECA injection suggest this configuration. You cannot occlude the MMA in this situation as it may be the sole supply of the retina.
- Additional collateral connections include the superficial recurrent meningeal branch of the lacrimal artery (where the middle meningeal arises from the ophthalmic artery) and the anterior falcine artery, a meningeal branch arising from the ethmoidal branches of the ophthalmic artery.
- The distal IMA has anastomoses with the inferior branch of the lacrimal artery via the anterior deep temporal and infraorbital arteries.
- The sphenopalatine artery connects with the ethmoidal branches of the ophthalmic artery. This should be considered in embolisation procedures

aimed at controlling epistaxis and for juvenile nasopharyngeal angiofibromas. Embolisation of branches is considered safe with larger particles (at least 100 µm, but safer with >200 µm) as their diameter usually exceeds the size of collateral pathways.

- Other anastomoses to the distal ophthalmic artery include the frontal branch of the STA and the distal facial artery via the dorsal nasal artery.

Upper cervical region

- The occipital artery, derived from embryological type I and II proatlantal arteries (C1 and C2 segmental arteries), maintains anastomotic pathways from the ECA to the vertebral artery via posterior radicular branches at the C1 and C2 levels. These connections serve as major collateral pathways from the vertebral artery to the carotid system, particularly visible in cases where the common carotid is ligated or occluded.
- The stylomastoid artery (from the posterior auricular or occipital artery) supplies the meninges in the posterior fossa and forms anastomoses with other meningeal branches from the MMA (via the facial arcade), ascending pharyngeal artery, ILT, MHT, and the posterior meningeal artery from the vertebral artery.
- The ascending pharyngeal artery, a remnant of the embryological hypoglossal artery, retains its connection to the vertebral artery through two proximal branches:
    - The musculospinal branch laterally anastomoses with the C3 radicular anastomotic artery from the vertebral artery.
    - The prevertebral branch, running along the ventral surface of the C1–C2 vertebrae and typically emerging from the neuromeningeal trunk, forms a U-shaped curve and anastomoses medially with C3 vertebral artery radicular arteries on the surface of the dens and also its contralateral counterpart (the odontoid arcade).
- The ascending cervical artery (from the thyrocervical trunk) and the deep cervical artery (costocervical trunk) are primary anastomotic channels with the vertebral artery at the C2–C4 levels.

Further reading

Byrne JV. Tutorials in Endovascular Neurosurgery and Interventional Neuroradiology. Springer; 2012.

Geibprasert S, Pongpech S, Armstrong D, Krings T. Dangerous extracranial-intracranial anastomoses and supply to the cranial nerves: vessels the neurointerventionalist needs to know. AJNR Am J Neuroradiol. 2009;30(8):1459–1468.

Cranial nerve supply

See Table 2.1.

Table 2.1 Arterial supply of the cranial nerves

Cranial nerve	Intraosseous and dural supply
CN I: olfactory	Sphenopalatine a. (IMA) & ethmoidal a. & ophthalmic a. (anastomose with each other; ethmoidals anastomose with anterior falcine branch of MMA) Cisternal and brainstem supply: vertebrobasilar a.
CN II: optic	Central a. of the retina: ophthalmic a. (sometimes arises from MMA; other anastomoses include MMA, IOA, FA, ADT, STA)
CN III: oculomotor	ILT, MHT (latter anastomoses with MMA, APA)
CN IV: trochlear	
CN V: trigeminal	ILT (anastomoses with IMA, AMA, MMA, APA), MHT Trigeminal (Gasserian) ganglion: ILT, MHT, petrosal MMA, Cav MMA, carotid APA V1: ILT, MHT V2: a. of the foramen rotundum (ILT) anastomoses with IMA V3: a. of the foramen ovale (AMA, MMA, APA)
CN VI: abducens	MHT, ILT, APA
CN VII: facial	Internal auditory artery, petrosal MMA, stylomastoid, AMA (+ middle ear anastomoses) Geniculate ganglion: petrosal MMA, STMA, superior tympanic a. (MMA)
CN VIII: vestibulocochlear	Internal auditory a. (branch of AICA)
CN IX: glossopharyngeal	Jugular division NMT APA (anastomoses with ILT, MHT)
CN X: vagus	
CN XI: accessory	Jugular division NMT APA (anastomoses with ILT, MHT) Spinal: musculospinal APA (anastomoses with VA, cervical arteries)
CN XII: hypoglossal	Hypoglossal division NMT APA (anastomoses with contralateral NMT, MHT, C3 radicular branch VA)

ADT: anterior deep temporal artery; AICA: anterior inferior cerebellar artery; AMA: accessory meningeal artery; APA: ascending pharyngeal artery; FA: facial artery; ILT: inferolateral trunk; IMA: internal maxillary artery; IOA: infraorbital artery; MHT: meningohypophyseal trunk; MMA: middle meningeal artery; NMT: neuromeningeal trunk; STA: superficial temporal artery; STMA: stylomastoid artery; VA: vertebral artery.

Extracranial veins

Face, scalp, and skull

- The extracranial drainage of the head and neck mirrors the arteries, e.g. the supratrochlear and supraorbital veins drain to the facial vein, and the superficial temporal, internal maxillary, posterior auricular, and occipital veins drain to the external jugular vein (EJV).
- There is bidirectional flow between veins that communicate with the diploë, emissary veins to the dural sinuses, and veins of the pericranium and meninges.

Internal jugular vein

- Together with the vertebral venous plexus, the IJV is the largest drainage pathway for the brain, face, and neck. It is the continuation of the sigmoid sinus in the jugular foramen, runs vertically in the carotid sheath in the neck, and joins the subclavian vein to form the brachiocephalic vein.
- Its tributaries, from cranial to caudal, are the inferior petrosal sinus, anterior condylar vein (vein of the hypoglossal canal), facial vein, lingual vein, pharyngeal vein, posterior EJV, superior thyroid vein, and middle thyroid vein.
- Incidental narrowing of the IJV between the lateral mass of C1 and the styloid process is common.
- The IJV has a valve just prior to its termination in the neck that may provide some resistance to cross with the guide catheter. Persistence usually pays off, however.

Pterygoid plexus

- The pterygoid plexus is a large venous network located between the temporalis and lateral pterygoid muscles. It drains into the maxillary vein and connects with the cavernous sinus via emissary veins. The plexus receives blood from numerous tributaries, including the sphenopalatine, middle meningeal, deep temporal (both anterior and posterior), pterygoid, masseteric, buccinator, alveolar, and some palatine veins (including the greater and lesser palatine veins). Additionally, it receives blood from the inferior ophthalmic vein, deep facial vein, and infraorbital vein.
- The plexus becomes the maxillary vein, which later converges with the superficial temporal vein to form the retromandibular vein.

External jugular vein

- The EJV drains the deep face, scalp, and posterolateral neck. It originates from the convergence of the retromandibular, posterior auricular, and the superficial temporal veins in front of the angle of the mandible. The vein runs caudally on top of the sternocleidomastoid to join the subclavian vein.
- Like the IJV, it has a valve just prior to its termination.

Anterior jugular veins

- This is a small network of veins in the anterior neck that receives tributaries from submental, muscular, and cutaneous veins. There are communications across the midline, and it ultimately drains into the EJV or subclavian vein.
- It may be injured during tracheostomy.

Vertebral venous system

- This system consists of internal and external vertebral plexuses.
- The internal vertebral venous plexus consists of epidural veins within the cervical canal.
- The external vertebral venous plexus consists of two systems:
  - The vertebral artery venous plexus: arises at C2 and receives blood from the suboccipital plexus, and the anterior, lateral, and posterior condylar veins. It continues as a solitary vertebral vein in the vertebral canal surrounding the vertebral artery, leaving at C6 via the foramen transversarium to join the brachiocephalic vein.
  - The deep cervical vein: receives tributaries of the suboccipital venous plexus. It follows the deep cervical artery to end in the IJV or brachiocephalic vein.
- There are connections between the internal and external systems via the intervertebral foramina. These are the sites of cerebrospinal fluid (CSF)–venous fistulas (see 'CSF–venous fistula embolisation', p. 483).
- The system has probably been somewhat overlooked due to the usual method of visualisation—angiography in the supine position. In this state, contrast drains via the IJV; however, in the erect position, the vertebral system most likely contributes a major, if not the most, important drainage pathway.

Subclavian and brachiocephalic veins

- The subclavian vein is the continuation of the axillary vein and follows the subclavian artery anteriorly, separated by the insertion of the anterior scalene muscle.
- The brachiocephalic (or innominate) veins originate behind the sternoclavicular joint from the internal jugular and subclavian veins and run inferomedially. They end to the right of midline (hence the left brachiocephalic is longer than the right) as the superior vena cava.
- The left receives the left vertebral, internal thoracic, inferior thyroid, superior intercostal, the thymic, and the pericardial veins.
- The right receives the right vertebral, the internal thoracic, and the thyroid veins, and occasionally the first right posterior intercostal veins.

Further reading

Byrne JV. Tutorials in Endovascular Neurosurgery and Interventional Neuroradiology. Springer; 2012.
Moore KL, Dalley AF, Agur AMR. Clinically Oriented Anatomy. 8th ed. Lippincott Williams & Wilkins; 2018.

Dural venous sinuses

The intracranial venous system is complex and exhibits significant individual variability. It is challenging to visualise on angiography and has generally been less extensively studied than the arterial system. There has been renewed interest recently because of transvenous embolisation of AVMs and venous stenting.

Dural sinuses

(See Figures 2.16 & 2.17).

- The dural venous sinuses are valveless, triangular trabeculated channels enclosed between dual layers of dura mater. Their walls do not contain smooth muscle.
- Larger sinuses contain arachnoid granulations, which are clumps of arachnoid villi that drain CSF into the venous system. These can be mistaken for sinus thrombosis (or vice versa) but are generally more discreet and rounded and return CSF signal on magnetic resonance imaging (MRI).

Superior sagittal sinus

- The superior sagittal sinus extends from the foramen caecum to the confluence of sinuses. It is located within the superior attachment of the falx to the calvarium.
- It receives the superficial cerebral veins from the medial and lateral cerebral hemispheres, the largest of which is the vein of Trolard. It drains into the confluence of sinuses.
- There are several variations which include high splitting at the torcula, anterior hypoplasia (where the frontal cortical veins take over), and absence of the posterior aspect with anterior drainage via a sinus pericranii.

Inferior sagittal sinus

- This lies in the inferior edge of the falx parallel to the superior sagittal sinus.
- It receives blood from the anterior corpus callosum, cingulate gyrus, medial cerebral hemispheres, and the falx.
- The sinus joins the internal cerebral veins to form the vein of Galen.

Straight sinus

- The straight sinus is an unpaired structure located at the junction between the falx and tentorium in the midline, and it follows a straight course posteriorly.
- It receives blood from the inferior sagittal sinus, vein of Galen, posterior cerebral veins, superior cerebellar veins, and falx cerebri, and drains into the confluence of sinuses.

Confluence of the sinuses (torcular Herophili)

- The confluence joins the superior sagittal, straight, and occipital sinuses and drains into the transverse sinuses.

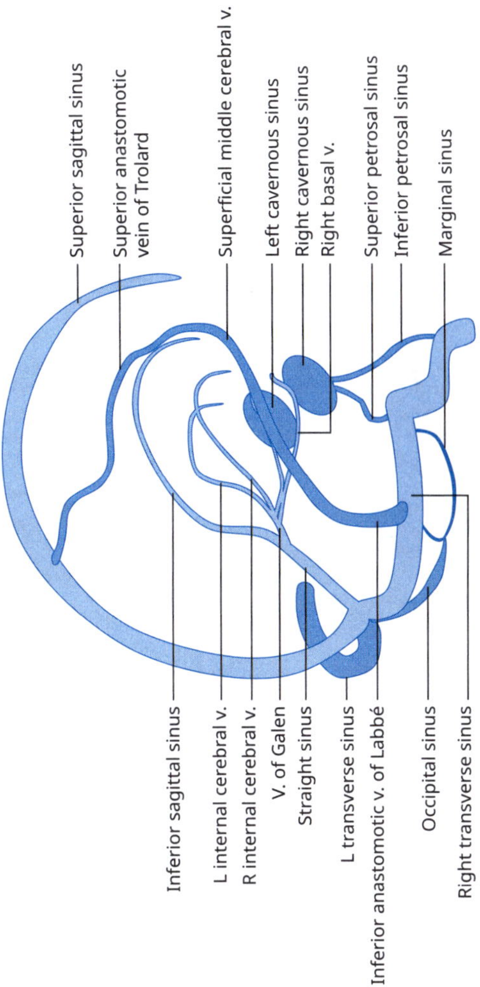

Figure 2.16 Dural venous sinuses.

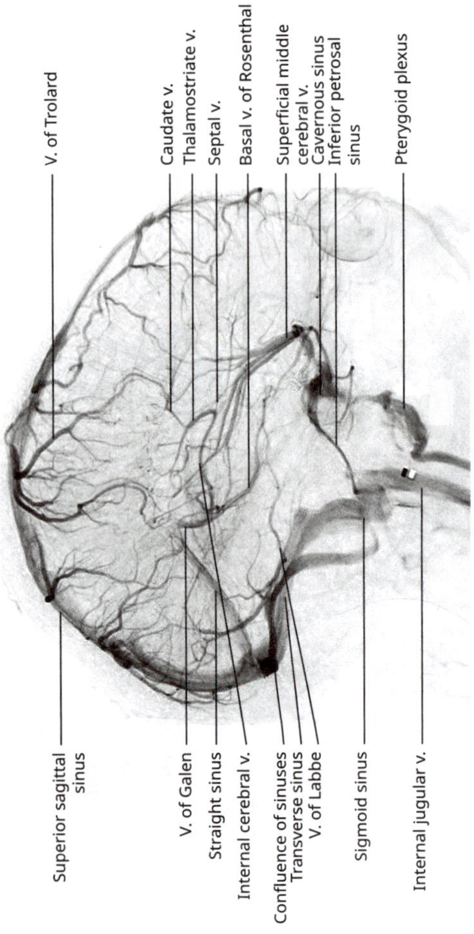

Figure 2.17 Venous phase angiogram of the internal carotid artery.

Occipital sinus

- The occipital sinus usually drains superiorly to the confluence but may drain inferiorly to the sigmoid or marginal sinuses.
- It is often hypoplastic or absent in adults.

Marginal sinus and anterior condylar confluence

- The marginal sinus encircles the foramen magnum and is connected to a network of adjacent venous structures including the clival plexus anteriorly, the vertebral venous plexus inferiorly, and sigmoid sinuses laterally.
- It is connected also to the IJV at the bulb via the anterior condylar vein in the hypoglossal canal, the lateral condylar vein, and the posterior condylar vein (which may also connect to the suboccipital plexus and internal vertebral venous plexus through the posterior condylar canal).
- The anterior condylar confluence is formed by the anterior and lateral condylar veins and tributaries of the clival plexus.

Transverse (lateral) sinuses

- The transverse sinuses arise at the confluence of sinuses and drain the superior and/or straight sinuses.
- They sweep around anterolaterally, confined by the tentorium, receiving veins from the temporal and occipital lobes, particularly the vein of Labbé, cerebellar veins, the superior petrosal sinuses, and accessory sinuses. They may connect with scalp veins via mastoid emissary veins.
- Hypoplasia of one or the other is common, usually the left.

Sigmoid sinuses

- This is the anteromedial inferior continuation of the transverse sinus and ends within the jugular fossa.
- It receives blood from the pons and medulla. It also connects to the scalp veins through the mastoid and condylar veins.

Superior petrosal sinuses

- These run in the petrosal ridge to connect the posterior aspect of the cavernous sinus to the junction of the transverse and sigmoid sinuses.
- They may receive blood from supra- or infratentorial structures.

Inferior petrosal sinuses

- These sinuses run inferiorly and laterally to connect the posterior aspect of the cavernous sinus to the jugular vein in the pars nervosa.
- They also receive blood from the internal auditory veins and infratentorial structures.

Sphenoparietal sinus

- This runs along the lesser sphenoid wing, receiving adjacent Sylvian, uncal, inferior frontal, meningeal, diploic, and, finally, orbital veins before draining into the cavernous sinus.
- A variant involves drainage not into the cavernous sinus, but instead into the transverse sinus, superior petrosal sinus, or tentorial sinuses.
- Occasionally it may drain to the pterygoid venous plexus rather than the cavernous sinus.

Cavernous sinuses

- The cavernous sinuses are located on each side of the pituitary fossa, on the greater sphenoid wing, bounded laterally by the free edge of the tentorium. They are an important bidirectional confluence of the intracranial and extracranial venous systems.
- They are compartmentalised by multiple fibrous strands that can obstruct the movement of a microcatheter and wire when attempts are made to navigate through them.
- The sinus contains the ICA, its sympathetic plexus, and the abducens nerve (CN VI).
- Within the lateral wall, from superior to inferior, are CN III, CN IV, CN V1, and CN V2.
- The cavernous sinuses are connected to multiple venous channels:
  - Superiorly and anteriorly to the ophthalmic veins, the middle cerebral vein, and the superficial Sylvian vein.
  - Superiorly and posteriorly to the deep middle cerebral (uncal) vein.
  - Inferiorly to the pterygoid plexus.
  - Posteriorly to the superior petrosal sinus, inferior petrosal sinus, and the basilar plexus.
  - Medially to the contralateral side through the intercavernous sinuses.
- It is the only location in which an artery, the ICA, is completely enclosed in a venous structure. Rupture of the cavernous segment of the ICA (or an aneurysm in this segment) can lead to direct carotid–cavernous fistulas. Indirect fistulas usually develop between meningeal branches of the ICA and/or ECA and the sinus, most commonly due to sinus thrombosis.

Further reading

Byrne JV. Tutorials in Endovascular Neurosurgery and Interventional Neuroradiology. Springer; 2012.
Krings T, Geibprasert S, Cruz JP, Ter Brugge K. Neurovascular Anatomy in Interventional Neuroradiology: A Case-Based Approach. Springer; 2015.

Supratentorial and medullary veins

Diploic, emissary, and meningeal veins

Diploic veins

- Diploic veins are located between the inner and outer tables of the skull. These have connections externally with the scalp venous system and internally with meningeal veins and dural sinuses.

Emissary veins

- Emissary veins are inconstant channels and serve as two-way connections linking extracranial veins, diploic veins, and intracranial meningeal veins and sinuses.
- Major emissary veins are the parietal (between the superior sagittal sinus and scalp), mastoid (between the sigmoid sinus and superficial occipital or posterior auricular veins), and condylar (between the inferior petrosal sinus, distal sigmoid sinus and vertebral venous and suboccipital plexuses).
- In addition, there are typically emissary veins passing through skull foramina: the foramen rotundum, ovale, Vesalius (sphenoid emissary vein), lacerum, hypoglossal (hypoglossal vein), and posterior condylar canals (the anterior and posterior condylar veins).
- Substantial venous outflow may occur through diploic and emissary veins. Anterior superior sagittal sinus hypoplasia may be compensated for by frontal diploic or emissary drainage. Sinus pericranii is an extreme form of emissary venous drainage. Great care and angiographic evaluation must be given before closure of larger lesions to avoid extensive venous infarction.
- Emissary veins are also potential routes of transmission of extracranial to intracranial infection.

Meningeal veins

- Meningeal veins exist in the outer layer of the dura.
- They accompany the arteries that supply the meninges and often follow similar paths and ultimately drain into the dural sinuses or directly into the venous system outside the skull.

Supratentorial veins

The supratentorial veins are a network of valveless veins in the sulci of the cerebral hemispheres and drain cortical grey matter and subcortical white matter. Bridging veins cross the subdural space and may fuse with meningeal veins before entering a major sinus.

Principal collectors

- The three principal venous collectors for cortical drainage are:
  - The superficial middle cerebral (Sylvian) vein (SMV): this arises in the Sylvian fissure and drains the adjacent operculum. It empties anteriorly into the cavernous sinus or pterygoid venous plexus.
  - The superior anastomotic vein of Trolard: this is the largest anastomotic vein connecting the SMV with the superior sagittal sinus.
  - The posterior anastomotic vein of Labbé: this is the largest anastomotic vein connecting the SMV with the transverse sinus.

- These veins are in haemodynamic balance such that either Trolard or Labbé may be absent. However, the SMV is almost always present. If the SMV is not visible, thrombosis must be suspected.

Cortical drainage

- Cortical veins drain regions of the cerebral cortex into nearby sinuses as follows:
    - Peripheral medial surfaces: superior sagittal sinus.
    - Central frontal and parietal regions: inferior sagittal sinus or posterior pericallosal vein.
    - Cingulate and paraterminal gyri: anterior pericallosal, paraterminal, and anterior cerebral veins drain to the basal vein of Rosenthal (BVR).
    - Medial occipital cortex: straight sinus, vein of Galen, and tentorial veins.
    - Inferior frontal lobes: superior sagittal sinus anteriorly or middle cerebral vein and cavernous sinus posteriorly.
    - Inferior temporal lobes: BVR medially, transverse sinus laterally.
    - Inferior occipital lobes: transverse sinus or BVR.

Medullary veins

(See Figure 2.18.)

- Medullary veins drain the cerebral deep white matter.
- Transmedullary veins transmit blood from the deep to superficial systems and drain to subependymal veins, running along the surface of the lateral ventricles.
- Developmental venous anomalies are benign deviations in venous drainage patterns, characterised by a single collector vein that receives blood from an extensive territory. These anomalies are typically discovered incidentally. Developmental venous anomalies contributing to the drainage system of an AVM increase the likelihood of rupture due to the increased fragility of the vascular system.

Medial subependymal veins

- These drain the inner corpus callosum, septum pellucidum, fornix, and hippocampus.
- The anterior septal vein starts in the frontal horn of the lateral ventricle, formed from the deep medullary veins of the anterior frontal lobe. It runs posteriorly to join the thalamostriate vein at the venous angle near the foramen of Munro. Not infrequently, the anterior septal vein may join the internal cerebral vein more posteriorly, passing within the lateral ventricle to the splenium.
- The medial caudate head is drained by the anterior caudate vein which drains to the thalamostriate vein. It also receives posterior frontal, anterior parietal, and internal capsular transmedullary veins.
- The posterior and middle septal veins, which are variable, drain the posterior frontal and parietal regions, and the corpus callosum, directly into the internal cerebral veins or via subependymal veins.
- The medial atrial vein, draining the posterior parietal and occipital lobes, joins the lateral atrial vein to form a common channel entering the posterior internal cerebral vein.

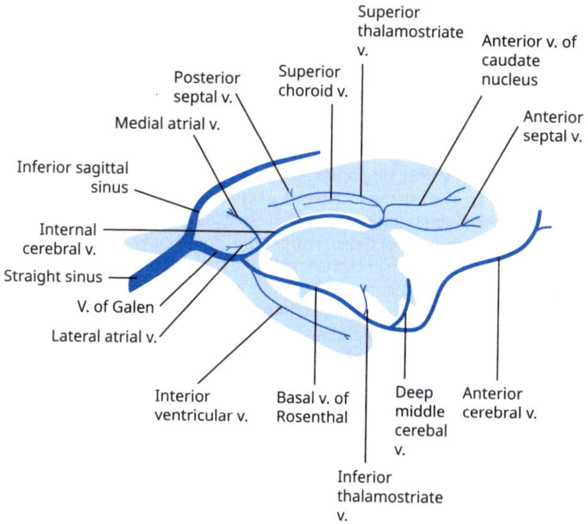

Figure 2.18 Deep venous drainage.

Lateral subependymal veins

- These drain the walls of the lateral ventricles and roof of temporal and occipital horns.
- The thalamostriate vein primarily drains the lateral subependymal, posterior frontal, and anterior parietal veins, as well as the caudate nucleus and internal capsule. It receives minimal drainage from the thalamus itself (despite the name) but does receive the superior choroidal vein. This vein is formed by the anterior caudate vein, which drains the medial caudate nucleus, and the terminal vein, starting in the atrium and running along the thalamocaudate groove.
- The lateral atrial vein primarily receives blood from the posterior temporal and parietal lobes. It runs anteroinferiorly along the lateral wall of the atrium and departs the choroidal fissure to join the BVR or connect with the medial atrial vein. This forms the common atrial vein that drains into the internal cerebral vein.
- The inferior ventricular vein, which drains the temporal lobe and receives the inferior choroidal vein, starts in the lateral ventricle, runs anteriorly, and turns medially to drain into the BVR.

Basal vein of Rosenthal

- The BVR originates under the anterior perforated substance in the chiasmatic cistern medial to the uncus of the temporal lobe, runs posteriorly, and terminates in either the vein of Galen or internal cerebral vein. It is formed by the confluence of the anterior cerebral vein (receiving olfactory, posterior orbitofrontal, and anterior pericallosal veins) and the deep middle cerebral vein (formed from insular and inferior striate veins). It therefore has a large venous territory.

- The first segment extends to the anterior margin of the cerebral peduncle.
- The second segment encircles the cerebral peduncle and extends to lateral aspect of the midbrain. It receives blood from the midbrain, hypothalamus, basal ganglia, and medial temporal lobe, including the inferior thalamic vein, hippocampal veins, and ventricular veins, and communicates across the midline via a communicating vein.
- The third segment is located behind the midbrain and ends at the junction with the vein of Galen. It drains the posterior fossa structures through the lateral mesencephalic vein and the precentral, tectal, and vermian veins. It connects to the superior petrosal sinus via the lateral mesencephalic vein and may drain into the straight sinus, internal cerebral veins, or a tentorial sinus, especially in cases associated with vein of Galen malformations.
- It may be discontinuous with the anterior aspect draining to the cavernous sinus or posteriorly to the superior petrosal sinus via the lateral mesencephalic vein.

Venous circle

- A venous circle (perhaps the venous equivalent of the arterial circle of Willis) connects the basal veins anteriorly in the suprasellar cistern and posteriorly in the interpeduncular cistern.
- The anterior cerebral veins are connected by the anterior communicating vein in half the population. The septal, callosal, anterior cerebral, chiasmatic, olfactory, inferior striate, insular, and uncal veins also contribute to the anterior venous circle.
- The posterior communicating vein is a constant vessel in the interpeduncular fossa. This, in addition to hypothalamic and ventral mesencephalic veins, contribute to the posterior aspect of the circle.
- The venous circle outflow is to deep Sylvian veins, the cavernous sinus, petrosal veins, the superior petrosal sinus, the lateral mesencephalic vein, and the medial pontine vein.

Internal cerebral veins

- The paired internal cerebral veins form at the foramen of Munro from the junction of the superior choroidal and the superior thalamostriate veins and drain the subependymal and choroid venous systems.
- They extend posteriorly along the roof of the third ventricle and the velum interpositum. Initially running parallel to the midline, they diverge laterally near the pineal recess, tracing the pineal body. They then join with the basal vein and converge under the splenium to form the vein of Galen.

Vein of Galen

- This short subarachnoid vessel is formed by the midline convergence of the internal cerebral veins, below the splenium, beneath which it curves. It ends at the tentorial hiatus apex, where it joins the inferior sagittal sinus to become the straight sinus.
- The vessel also receives blood from the posterior pericallosal veins, the internal occipital veins, and veins of the posterior fossa.

- It therefore connects multiple drainage pathways including the cerebellum and basal ganglia and can distribute drainage anteriorly to the cavernous sinus via the basal veins, laterally towards the inferior temporal vein, and posteriorly to the straight sinus.
- Note that the term vein of Galen malformation is a misnomer, as the disease involves persistence of the *precursor* to the vein of Galen, the median promesencephalic vein.

Further reading

Byrne JV. Tutorials in Endovascular Neurosurgery and Interventional Neuroradiology. Springer; 2012.

Krings T, Geibprasert S, Cruz JP, ter Brugge KG. Neurovascular Anatomy in Interventional Neuroradiology: A Case-Based Approach. Springer; 2015.

Morris P. Practical Neuroangiography. 3rd ed. Lippincott Williams & Wilkins; 2013.

Infratentorial veins

Veins of the brainstem

(See Figure 2.19.)

- These veins are often named depending on (i) whether they are orientated transversely or longitudinally and (ii) their relationship with the mesencephalon (midbrain), pons, or medulla.

Transversely orientated veins

- Peduncular veins: drain the cerebral peduncles. They arise in the interpeduncular fossa and run laterally around the cerebral peduncles beneath the optic tract. They link the anterior pontomesencephalic vein to the BVR and may also form an anastomosis with the lateral mesencephalic vein.
- Transverse pontine veins.
- Pontomedullary sulcal veins.
- Transverse medullary veins.

Longitudinally orientated veins

- Midline group: this is a continuous anastomotic venous channel comprised from cranial to caudal of the median anterior pontomesencephalic vein, the median anterior pontine vein, and the median anterior medullary vein. It continues inferiorly as the anterior spinal vein. Blood may flow cranially to the posterior communicating vein or peduncular veins, or caudally into the spinal veins.
- Lateral group: these anastomose with other veins of the brainstem and comprise:
  - Lateral mesencephalic veins: these connect the BVR to lateral brainstem and medullary fissure veins. They act as a crucial collateral drainage route, especially when the basal vein is discontinuous, draining posteriorly to infratentorial veins. In vein of Galen malformations, they facilitate venous drainage between deep venous and extracranial systems.
  - Lateral anterior pontomesencephalic veins.
  - Lateral medullary veins.

Veins of the cerebellum

(See Figure 2.19.)

- The venous drainage of the cerebellum can be grouped into superficial veins draining the cortical surfaces and deep veins within the fissures and adjacent to the peduncles.

Superficial group

- Tentorial surface drainage:
  - The precentral cerebellar vein, an unpaired vein, ascends in the quadrigeminal cistern behind the tectal plate to drain into the vein of Galen. It can merge with the superior vermian vein to form the superior cerebellar vein or drain directly into the vein of Galen independently.

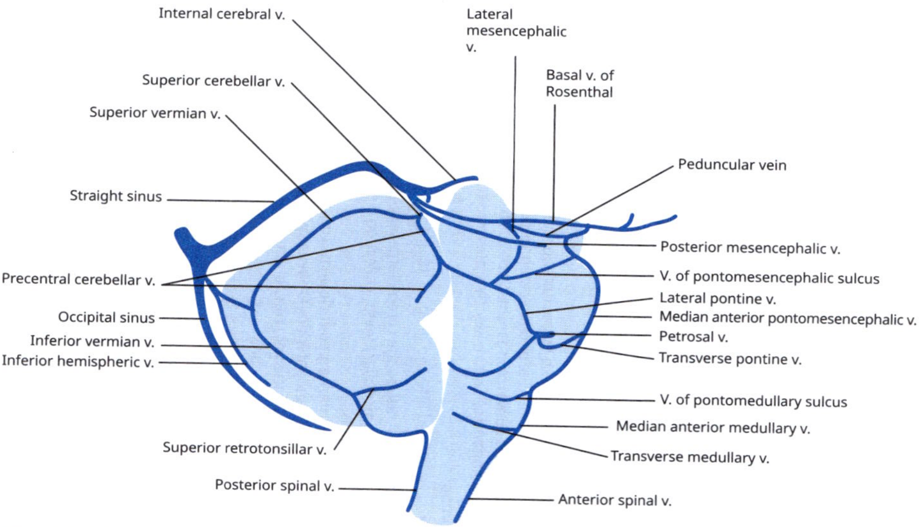

Figure 2.19 Infratentorial veins.

   - The superior vermian veins drain the superior vermis and the medial parts of the superior (tentorial) cerebellar hemispheres. The anterior veins drain into the vein of Galen, and the posterior veins drain into the confluence of sinuses.
   - The superior hemispheric veins can be subdivided into three groups. The anterior group drains via the cerebellomesencephalic fissure vein or the superior vermian vein. The posterior group drains into the confluence, superior petrosal, transverse, or tentorial sinuses via bridging veins. The smaller lateral group drains into the superior petrosal sinus.
- Suboccipital surface drainage:
   - The paired inferior vermian veins lie in the cerebellovermian fissure and drain the inferior vermis and medial suboccipital surface into the torcular or transverse sinus, directly or via a tentorial sinus.
   - Inferior hemispheric veins can run longitudinally or transversely. Longitudinal veins join superior hemispheric veins and drain into a dural or tentorial sinus, while transverse veins are associated with cerebellar fissures and drain into the inferior vermian vein.
   - Superficial tonsillar veins, divided into retrotonsillar, medial, and lateral groups, converge to form the inferior vermian veins.
- Petrosal surface drainage:
   - This surface is drained by the anterior hemispheric veins, subdivided into superior, middle, and inferior groups.
   - These veins converge near the flocculus to form the vein of the cerebellopontine fissure, which drains into the superior petrosal sinus.

Deep group

- These are divided into two groups: fissure veins and peduncle veins.
   - Fissure veins include the cerebellomesencephalic, cerebellopontine, and cerebellomedullary veins, collecting from hemispheric and peduncle veins.
   - Superior and inferior peduncle veins run along the posterior surfaces of the superior and inferior cerebellar peduncles, respectively. The middle peduncle vein runs on the lateral surface in the cerebellopontine fissure.

Superior petrosal vein

- The superior petrosal vein (or simply the petrosal vein) is the largest vein in the posterior cranial fossa. It drains the anterior cerebellum and brainstem into the superior petrosal sinus.
- It is usually formed by multiple smaller veins converging into one, but sometimes there are two or three. Major contributors include the vein of the cerebellopontine fissure, as well as groups of tributaries: the petrosal, posterior mesencephalic, anterior pontomesencephalic, and tentorial groups.

Further reading

Byrne JV. Tutorials in Endovascular Neurosurgery and Interventional Neuroradiology. Springer; 2012.

Krings T, Geibprasert S, Cruz JP, ter Brugge KG. Neurovascular Anatomy in Interventional Neuroradiology: A Case-Based Approach. Springer; 2015.

Summary of spinal vascular anatomy

While the blood supply to the spinal cord is often perceived as complex, it is actually quite straightforward. This chapter provides a summary of anatomy that should meet most needs. More detailed descriptions are then presented over the subsequent three chapters for those with a particular requirement or interest.

Arterial cord supply

See Figure 2.20.

- The main arterial networks are visible on conventional angiography, while the vitally important subsegmental arterial networks are generally beyond standard angiographic resolution. In clinical practice, visualisation of the arterial networks of the cord has been enhanced dramatically with the recent developments in microCT.
- During development, paired segmental arteries arise from the posterior descending aorta and great arteries at each bony segment of the spinal column and also from the median sacral artery from the aortic bifurcation:
  - Cervical cord: the cervical cord derives a supply from the vertebral artery and the deep and ascending cervical arteries (costocervical and thyrocervical trunks, respectively). A prominent contribution is from the artery of the cervical enlargement of Lazorthes, usually a branch of the vertebral or deep cervical arteries, accompanying one of the C4–C8 roots (most commonly C6).
  - Thoracic cord above T3: several segmental arteries may arise from a common origin, namely the supreme or superior intercostal artery, usually a branch of the costocervical trunk. There are extensive anastomoses between the segmental arteries with connections above and below and contralaterally.
  - Thoracic cord below T3: the thoracic segmental arteries include the nine pairs of posterior intercostal arteries and one pair of subcostal arteries.
  - Lumbar cord: there are four pairs of lumbar segmental arteries.
  - The iliolumbar artery, a branch of the posterior division of the internal iliac artery, gives off spinal branches.
  - The median sacral artery arises from the posterior aspect of the abdominal aorta at its bifurcation. It descends in the midline over the L4–L5 vertebrae, sacrum, and coccyx, giving off small spinal branches.
- Segmental arteries (Figure 2.21) are named by the level they supply, not where they originate from. They can be correctly identified angiographically by the vertebral body vascular blush. In the thoracic spine, the segmental artery is easily identified according to the rib under which it courses.
- Radicular (*Latin: belonging to or pertaining to roots*) arteries supply all the paraspinal tissues, including muscle, bone, and dura, and persist throughout life. Radiculomedullary arteries supply the central grey matter of the spinal cord, while radiculopial arteries provide the dominant vascular supply to the peripheral white matter tracts. During development, a process of summation occurs, resulting in only a few of the segmental arteries eventually supplying the cord.

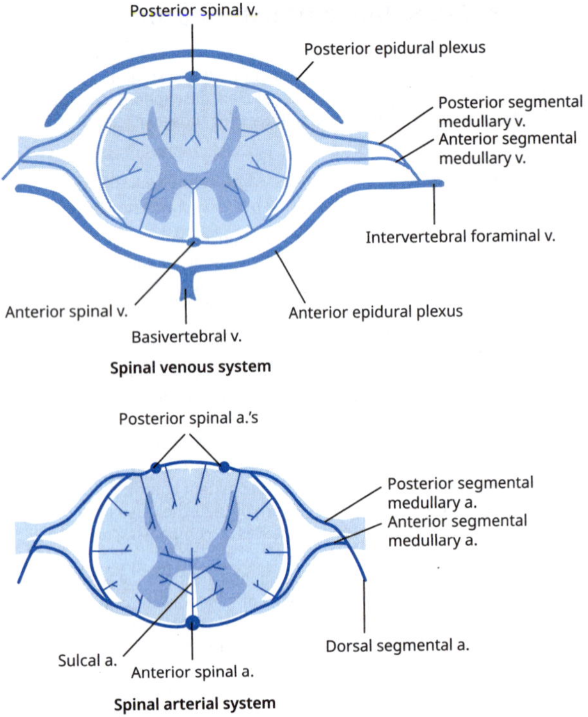

Figure 2.20 Organisation of spinal arterial and venous systems.

- Where an arterial branch to the cord is present, it travels alongside the exiting nerve root on an ascending trajectory. The angle of ascent depends on the level at which the artery arises from and is due to the cord being more fixed in length relative to the growing vertebral bodies. As such, the lower thoracic supplies are more vertical than their upper thoracic and cervical counterparts.
- There are more radiculopial arteries than radiculomedullary arteries, and, not unsurprisingly, the radiculopial arteries are smaller. Usually there are approximately 6–10 radiculomedullary, and 11–16 radiculopial arteries (although angiographic identification of these is sometimes very hard due to their size).

Radiculomedullary arteries

- The radiculomedullary arteries travel anterior to the cord, reaching the central sulcus in the midline. They then contribute to the midline arterial channel on the surface of the cord, the ASA. There is potential bidirectional flow within the ASA, i.e. blood can travel superior or inferior.

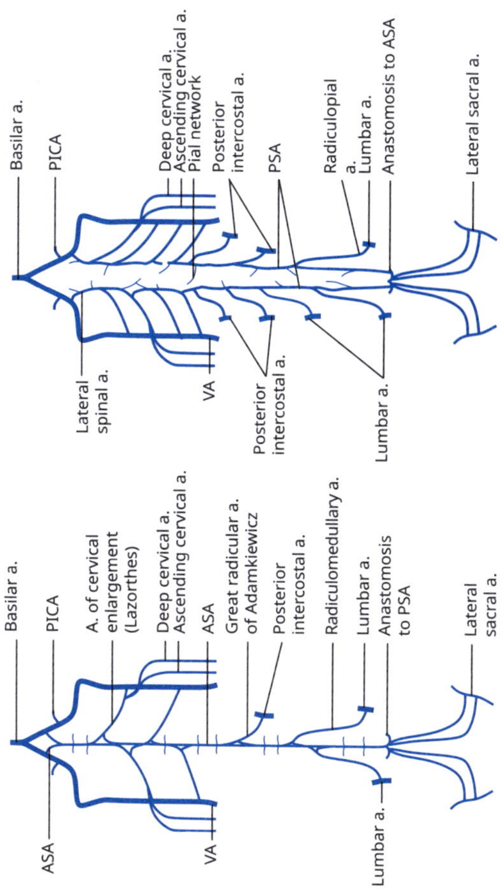

Figure 2.21 Spinal arterial anatomy.

- The cranial extent of the ASA arises at the foramen magnum from union of paired arteries from the intradural vertebral arteries. There is variation in this conventional anatomy, with asymmetry and absence encountered regularly.
- The ASA measures up to 0.8 mm in size, and receives contributions from 2–5 cervical sources, where it is richly vascularised.
- Within the thoracic region, there is a constant artery of thoracic enlargement, named eponymously as the artery of Adamkiewicz, diameter 0.5–1 mm. This characteristically arises between T8 and L2 in 75% of cases, and in 80% of cases on the left. It forms the classic hairpin loop when it reaches the ASA giving off a thin ascending branch and a larger descending branch.
- Between the cervical and mid-thoracic regions, there is a potential watershed area where the arterial supply to the spinal cord is believed to be more fragile. This is often cited as the reason why the upper thoracic spinal cord is a more common site for spinal cord strokes.
- The ASA terminates at the conus in a basket of arteries which anastomose with the posterior spinal arteries (PSAs). Occasionally, a small filum terminalis artery can persist, passing inferiorly.

Sulcal arteries

- Arising from the anterior spinal axis are innumerable sulcal arteries. These pass deeper into the central sulcus and then penetrate the anterior aspect of the cord in the midline (similar to the lenticulostriatal perforating arteries in the brain).
- In the non-pathological state (absence of arteriovenous shunting or tumour), these sulcal arteries are not seen angiographically. Their presence and location must be remembered when performing any treatment.
- Once penetrating the cord, the arteries divide and fan out centrifugally. They supply the majority of the grey matter (hence the term medullary) and also the anterior two-thirds of the cord including the anterior horn cells and spinothalamic and corticospinal tracts.
- Vitally important in the aetiology of spinal cord stroke is the absence of any cross communication between sulcal arteries at different levels. As such, a short occlusion of the ASA will give rise to an ischaemic stroke at the affected levels of sulcal arteries, even if thrombus (or embolic agent) does not penetrate into the sulcal artery itself.

Radiculopial arteries

- The radiculopial arteries also pass superiorly towards the cord, although their orientation is typically less vertical than those of the anterior radiculomedullary arteries. They pass more posteriorly, and join a network on the surface of the cord comprising of paired PSAs. An extensive arterial network on the entire surface of cord is formed by anastomoses between the ASA and PSA, known as the pial plexus or vaso corona. This supplies the periphery of the cord.
- The PSAs are positioned off midline, and hence identifiable on carefully performed true AP spinal angiography. They are sometimes visible arising from the intradural vertebral arteries or posterior inferior cerebellar arteries, particularly in the presence of cervical AVMs. In the non-pathological state, they are small and measure <0.5 mm.

- The PSAs and contributing radiculopial arteries create a network to supply the circumference of the periphery of the cord in a centripetal manner. In this instance, the network is analogous to the M2 perforators as they pass into the insular cortex from the Sylvian fissure.
- In contrast to the sulcal arteries, the PSAs communicate both around the cord linearly and also vertically between segments. Unfortunately, this does not make them immune from injury and PSA cord stroke complicating EVTs may occur, particularly when liquid embolic agents under wedged conditions are used. The PSAs principally supply the posterior third of the cord, including the dorsal columns, dorsal grey matter, and dorsal aspects of the lateral columns.

Venous drainage of the cord

See Figure 2.20.

- The venous drainage of the cord follows a similar pattern to that of the arterial system, with sulcal veins draining centrally (centripetal direction) as well as a radial system draining the periphery (centrifugally).
- However, a slight difference is that the sulcal veins only collect the medial aspects of the centre of the cord (rather than anterior two-thirds as the sulcal arteries supply). There is also extensive cross communication between the venous system. The sulcal veins drain into the anterior median spinal vein, which accompanies the ASA. The posterior venous system encompasses median and lateral channels and receives the radial venous drainage.
- Both the anterior and posterior median veins drain into the radiculomedullary veins which accompany the spinal nerve root. There are about 8–14 anterior radiculomedullary veins and about 5–10 posterior radiculomedullary veins.
- At the dural surface, the radiculomedullary veins take an oblique course which creates a valve-like effect. This prevents reflux from the epidural venous plexus into the spinal venous plexus. There is then drainage into the segmental veins and hence towards the ascending lumbar and azygos venous systems.

Further reading

Santillan A, Nacarino V, Greenberg E, Riina HA, Gobin YP, Patsalides A. Vascular anatomy of the spinal cord. J Neurointerv Surg. 2012;4(1):67–74.

Embryology of the spinal vascular system

- Thirty-one somites develop during the third week of embryological development. These mesodermal structures flank both sides of the neural tube and notochord, forming sequential embryological units along the embryo's AP axis.
- Segmentation initiates the formation of segments known as metameres. Each somite subsequently receives a pair of segmental arteries from the rostral and caudal ends of the embryo, originating from the dorsal aorta. These segmental arteries are responsible for vascularising the ipsilateral tissues developing from the corresponding metamere, such as muscles, skin, bones, nerves, and the spinal cord, establishing a metameric arrangement of the vascular structure.
- Metameric arteries play a crucial role in the development of the vertebral vascular system. Traditionally, each metameric artery is named after the nerve it accompanies within the transverse foramen. At each level, these arteries anastomose with both caudal and rostral metameric arteries, creating an extraspinal and extradural network, which further develops anastomoses crossing the midline. These connections give rise to multi-metameric longitudinal extraspinal common trunks.
- During embryogenesis, the peripheral nervous system matures before the central nervous system. The neural crest, which forms the peripheral nervous system, receives a dorsomedial branch from the ipsilateral segmental artery.
- The development of the two terminations of a spinal nerve serves two purposes: directing the dorsomedial artery towards the neural tube (central termination) and stimulating vascularisation of the distal segment (peripheral termination). A direct association between nerves and arteries exists: each artery is coupled with a nerve root that follows the same course to the cord. Therefore, the point where radicular arteries reach the spinal cord identifies the origin of the nerve root and its myelomeric origin. Any dysregulation in vascular development during this stage can affect the entire metamere, leading to conditions like Cobb syndrome or spinal arteriovenous metameric syndrome.
- Between the fourth and sixth weeks of embryological development, a definitive anatomical arrangement is established, following a distinct craniocaudal pattern. The two ventral longitudinal vessels migrate towards the midline and fuse, forming a single ventral longitudinal axis, the ASA.
- Duplications or fenestrations of this artery result from incomplete fusion along the midline, with each unfused segment perfusing the corresponding ipsilateral part of the spinal cord. During the first month of intrauterine life, the intrinsic vascularisation of the cord begins. Sulcal arteries appear on the dorsal surface of the ventral longitudinal axis, remaining lateralised after fusion. Each sulcal artery supplies the ipsilateral half of the spinal cord. Proximal fusions of these arteries, resulting in a common trunk, are exceptionally rare.

- Arteries following dorsal roots contribute to a superficial network on the posterior surface of the cord, known as the pial network. Corresponding arteries located ventrally help vascularise the anterior pial network. Subsequently, two longitudinal paramedian arteries develop on the posterior surface of the cord, corresponding to the dominant flow within the pial network, which later evolve into posterior or posterolateral spinal arteries.
- As fusion and de-segmentation progress, some radicular branches supplying the cord of both the anterior and posterior networks regress. Typically, 4–8 anterior radicular and 10–20 posterior radicular branches persist. Regression predominantly occurs in the caudal part of the cord, where only one radiculomedullary artery typically persists, known as the artery of the lumbar enlargement or artery of Adamkiewicz.
- Extraspinal arteries undergo minimal modifications. Longitudinal intersegmental anastomoses develop outside the spinal canal. At the cervical level, vertebral arteries arise from extraspinal longitudinal anastomoses. The ascending cervical artery forms and vascularises C3 and C4 nerves. At the thoracic and lumbar levels, the superior intercostal trunk develops, which can exhibit numerous multi-metameric variants. At the sacral level, these anastomoses give rise to the lateral sacral arteries originating from the internal iliac arteries, while the caudal portion of the dorsal aorta regresses to become the median sacral artery.

Spinal arterial anatomy

- Three distinct types of radicular arteries (Figure 2.22) can be distinguished: pure radicular, radiculopial, and radiculomedullary.
- They may arise from a common trunk or individually, with each of the 62 radicular arteries (31 left and 31 right) falling into one of these categories.
- A single segmental artery serves each nerve, dividing into ventral and dorsal branches. Radicular arteries follow trajectories with characteristic features evident in angiographic acquisitions on AP views: they exhibit an ascending course, mirroring the path of the nerve roots, with their obliquity varying according to the level of origin (almost horizontal at upper cervical levels and nearly vertical at lower lumbar levels).
- These arteries have fixed points in the transverse foramen and the origin of the nerve root from the spinal cord. They represent the smallest contribution of the segmental embryonic system to neural crest derivatives. A focal narrowing of the vessel is often observed as they penetrate the dura mater.

Supply of the spinal arteries

Pure radicular arteries

- These arteries solely vascularise the nerve without contributing to cord vasculature. They are typically small and infrequently visible on digital subtraction angiography (DSA) examinations.
- Pathological enlargement may be observed in the presence of a vascular lesion along the nerve route.

Radiculopial arteries

- Radiculopial arteries follow the corresponding nerve root to reach the anterior or, more commonly, posterior surface of the cord.
- These contribute to the respective pial networks but do not participate in the anterior spinal vascular axis.
- The dorsal pial arteries anastomose with their contralateral homologues and with the pial branches of the anterior spinal axis via circumferential coronal vessels.
- The lumbar 'basket' points to the caudal end of the cord, and links both PSAs with the ASA.

Radiculomedullary arteries

- These branches contribute to segmental and longitudinal vascularisation. They are the sole vascular supply to the anterior spinal axis, behaving as radicular arteries along their proximal tract where they vascularise the corresponding nerve root segment.
- These arteries follow the ventral surface of the nerve root. There, they reach the anterior surface of the cord where they may give rise to small pial branches contributing to the anterior pial network. Ultimately, they reach the anterior sulcus, dividing into ascending and descending branches which anastomose along the midline with corresponding arteries above and below to form the ASA.
- Two radiculomedullary arteries of particular relevance are the artery of the cervical enlargement (artery of Lazorthes) and the artery of the lumbar enlargement (artery of Adamkiewicz). The origin of the latter is highly variable, typically between T9 and T12 on the left side, with variations above T8 or below T12 accompanied then by additional associated radiculomedullary arteries arising caudally or cranially, respectively.

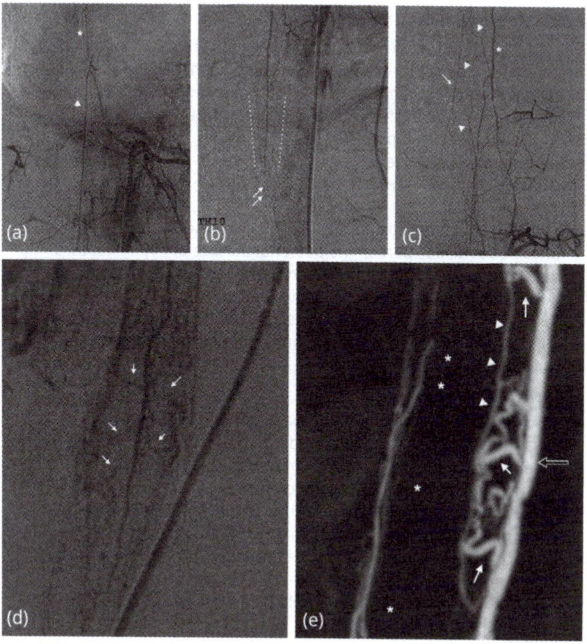

Figure 2.22 Spinal angiographic anatomy. (a) Selective injection in AP view of the radiculomedullary artery of the lumbar enlargement (artery of Adamkiewicz). The artery follows the nerve root and reaches the anterior portion of the cord above the ventral sulcus where it divides in a cranial (white asterisk) and caudal (white arrowhead) branch. (b) The latter anastomoses at the level of the conus medullaris with both pial posterior arteries, giving rise to the basket (white dotted lines). In the continuity of the anterior spinal artery below the basket is the artery of the filum terminalis (double arrow). (c) Selective injection in AP view of a dorsal left radiculopial artery. It is possible to clearly visualise the pial anastomoses (white arrowheads) between the left (white asterisk) and right (white arrow) pial channels at the posterior surface of the cord. (d) Magnified AP view of a selective injection of the artery of Adamkiewicz. From the continuity arise pial ventral arteries (white arrows) that leave the midline and run over the anterior funiculi, reaching the posterior spinal pial network. The cord is thus surrounded by a 'sleeve' of pial vessels. (e) Selective lateral view in cone beam CT of the anterior spinal artery (hollow arrow) at the cervical level in a case of spinal AVM (not shown). It is possible to observe the dilated sulcal arteries (white arrows) penetrating in the sulcus with longitudinal intrasulcal anastomoses (white arrowheads). The posterior spinal artery also fills: the centripetal perforating arteries (white asterisks) depending from this longitudinal channel are well depicted, penetrating in the posterior funiculi. Images courtesy of Prof Arturo Consoli and Prof Georges Rodesch.

Extrinsic vascularisation of the cord

- In the spinal cord, two primary arrangements prevail: longitudinal and transverse. Each of these systems receives distinct afferent arteries; the anterior longitudinal system (ASA) is supplied by radiculomedullary arteries, while the posterolateral longitudinal arterial systems (PSAs) are nourished by radiculopial arteries.
- Radiculomedullary arteries exhibit anastomoses at the midline (upper caudal branch and lower cranial branch), directly contributing to the continuity of the anterior spinal axis.
- Radiculopial arteries, being thinner and lateralised, display a similar longitudinal disposition on the posterior surface of the spinal cord. The posterior anastomosis between the two pial axes, left and right, aids in the development of the posterior pial network. These arteries possess a tighter, sharper 'hairpin' shape upon reaching the spinal cord surface, making them often identifiable compared to the homologous radiculomedullary anastomosis.

ASA (longitudinal ventral system)

- Described as a single continuous axis running superficially along the anterior sulcus in the subpial space, this artery extends from the vertebrobasilar junction to the filum terminalis.
- The morphology of the radiculomedullary junction varies across spinal cord segments, from a 'Y' shape at the cervical origin and to 'hairpin' shape typical at the thoracolumbar level.
- At the conus terminalis, the ASA anastomoses with branches of the posterior pial network, giving rise to the 'basket'.
- The caudal extension of the ASA below the basket (and the conus) is the artery of the filum terminalis.

Pial network (posterolateral longitudinal system)

- The spinal cord is wrapped in a plexiform pial vascular network, more prominent on the posterior surface. This network includes two dominant longitudinal vessels, the PSAs. Depending on PICA origin, the pial spinal vasculature may arise from the vertebral artery or the proximal part of PICA. Running anterior to dorsal roots, the dominant cervical dorsal network is represented by the lateral spinal artery. More caudally, this vessel connects with the posterior pial network at the C4 level. Radiculopial arteries contribute to the posterior pial network along the entire cord, with anterior radiculopial artery contributions being rare.
- Upon reaching the cord, radiculopial arteries exhibit a characteristic 'hairpin' curve shape, with sharper curves at lower levels. At the caudal cord, two dorsolateral arteries anastomose with the anterior axis, forming the characteristic tripod-shaped basket on angiographic imaging.
- The pial network, subdivided into dorsal, lateral, and anterior sectors, features anastomoses in the axial plane:
    - The dorsal pial network, which crosses the midline, vascularises the dorsal cord surface bilaterally and generates small-calibre perforating arteries ('centripetal arteries') that penetrate the posterior funiculi.
    - The lateral pial network, situated between dorsal and anterior nerve roots, receives small pial branches from radiculopial and radiculomedullary arteries, fostering axial dorsoventral anastomosis.
    - Short longitudinal anastomoses may also occur within the pial network, although they rarely effectively support a true lateral

longitudinal network. Vascularised by anterior radiculopial branches and collateral pial branches of radiculo-medullary arteries, the anterior pial network spans the entire spinal cord. Nonetheless, the pial network, though comprehensive, cannot adequately support collateral flow in the event of spinal artery occlusion.

Intrinsic vascularisation of the cord

- The intrinsic vascularisation of the spinal cord encompasses sulcal arteries ventrally, originating from the anterior spinal axis, and radial perforating arteries dorsally, arising from the circumferential pial network.
- Despite their axial plane positioning, both types of arteries exhibit longitudinal intrinsic or extrinsic anastomoses.

Sulcal arteries

- Sulcal arteries emerge from the anterior spinal axis.
- In embryogenesis, they originate from the dorsal surface of each anterior longitudinal axis. Upon fusion at the midline of these latter vessels, they remain laterally positioned, supplying either the left or right anterior half of the cord. When fusion fails to occur, each separated axis generates its own sulcal artery, nourishing its respective half of the spinal cord.
- While bilateral common trunks may rarely occur, no anastomoses cross the midline.
- Prior to penetrating the spinal cord, sulcal arteries traverse the anterior sulcus at a subpial level, giving rise to ascending and descending branches that anastomose with upper and lower sulcal arteries on the same side.
- Within the cord, sulcal arteries bifurcate in the grey matter, forming a centrifugal system. The density of sulcal arteries correlates with grey matter density and activity, varying in function at each spinal level.
- While sulcal arteries feed approximately 50% of the cord at cervical and lumbar enlargements, they supply up to 15–20% at the thoracic level. Nonetheless, a higher concentration of pial and intramedullary anastomoses at the thoracic level suggests a more effective arterial equilibrium between pial and anterior feeders. While radiculomedullary arteries anchor the spinal cord within the canal, sulcal arteries attach the anterior spinal arterial axis to the cord.

Radial perforating arteries

- Radial perforating arteries, originating from the pial network, form a centripetal system. These arteries penetrate the white matter, branching into numerous small-calibre branches predominantly on the axial plane but also longitudinally. Other blood vessels follow dorsal root nerve fibres, reaching the grey matter's posterior horns, primarily observed in the posterior columns but also in lateral and ventral columns.
- Intrinsic anastomoses encompass two main types: axial and longitudinal. Sulco-ventro-lateral or sulco-dorso-lateral anastomoses are more common at the thoracic level. Other anastomoses may involve sulcal and radial arteries marginally to the grey matter on the axial plane. Some precapillary anastomoses, larger than medullary capillaries, have been identified.

- Together, these arteries form an uninterrupted network inside the cord, traversing both grey and white matter, classified as terminal arteries. However, in spinal cord AVMs, shunted blood flow can maintain patent wide intrinsic anastomoses. Communication between normal and pathological vessels occurs, forming an intramedullary AVM comprising abnormal and dilated normal intrinsic vessels due to the shunt.
- The reported morbidity following surgical or endovascular treatments can be attributed to specific iatrogenic alterations of the normal intrinsic spinal cord vascularisation. Despite the fewer number of sulcal arteries observed at the thoracic level in comparison to the cervical and lumbar enlargements, the blood supply to this region is deemed adequate to sustain the volume of grey matter present at this level.
- The neuron cell, serving as the fundamental unit of the spinal cord's grey matter, acts as the focal point around which the development of blood vessels occurs.

Further reading

American Association of Neurological Surgeons/Neurosurgical Research and Education Foundation. The Rhoton Collection®. https://www.aans.org/education-publications/references/the-rhoton-collection/

Berenstein A, Lasjaunias P. Surgical Neuroangiography. Springer; 2012.

Spinal venous anatomy

- The understanding of spinal vascular malformations has contributed to an improved comprehension of the venous vascular anatomy and pathophysiology of symptoms associated with these malformations.
- Similar to the arterial system, it is possible to differentiate an intrinsic and an extrinsic venous circulation in the spinal cord.

Intrinsic spinal cord veins

- The intrinsic venous system of the spinal cord comprises a vast capillary network located within the spinal cord itself, symmetrically anastomosing on the axial plane.
- While an anterior dominance, akin to the arterial system, is partially observed at the thoracolumbar level, dorsal dominance is noted at the thoracic level. If a prominent intrinsic anastomotic network is seen predominantly at the thoracic level, it may extend throughout the entire spinal cord.
- Axial anastomoses connect sulcal veins with radial ventro-dorso-lateral and ventro-dorso-medial veins, with longitudinal anastomoses present within both grey and white matter.
- The significance of these anastomoses explains the spread of spinal cord alterations across multiple myelomeres even in the presence of small focal arteriovenous lesions, enabling venous congestion to propagate over multiple adjacent levels. Transmedullary veins, oriented obliquely and possessing a large calibre of up to 700 μm at the thoracic level, have been identified.
- Intrinsic veins may participate in the formation of a pathological intramedullary nidus, which may include abnormal vessels alongside normal dilated vessels represented by dilated intrinsic nutritional arteries or congested intrinsic venules.
- The term 'capillary neovascularisation', observed in patients with evolving vascular lesions, may denote either a dilated and congested intrinsic network or *de novo* intrinsic vascularisation due to repeated ischaemic damage and hypoxia related to chronic venous congestion. Complications reported following surgical curative treatment of intradural AVMs are likely due to iatrogenic damage to these normal vessels, which constitute part of the malformation and are not easily recognised.

Extrinsic medullary veins

- These comprise the venous pial network, longitudinal collectors, and radicular veins.
- The venous pial network is constituted by longitudinal venous arrangements connecting intrinsic perforating veins through large lateral and dorsoventral anastomoses. Drainage of venous blood from grey matter territories is facilitated by ventral sulcal and dorsal veins. Certain pial collectors merge to form common trunks, which are more prevalent than their arterial counterparts, particularly on the ventral aspect. Additionally, short intersegmental channels laterally serve as communication pathways between adjacent radial collectors; however, they are not sufficiently developed to establish a functional longitudinal venous network.

- Longitudinal collectors can be categorised into two primary systems: ventral and dorsal. Typically, only one collector is present along the midline at cervical and lumbar levels, whereas up to three distinct collectors have been identified at the thoracic level. The association between the number of transmedullary anastomoses and longitudinal collectors at this level may account for the tendency towards congestion and venous stasis.
- Lazorthes observed a vulnerability in the vascular arrangement of the thoracic spinal cord, which seems more linked to venous anatomical organisation than arterial. The thoracic venous draining system exhibits a bipolar disposition, collecting venous drainage cranially from the cervical level and caudally from the lumbar level, with a convergent aspect in both instances. This structural feature of the thoracic venous draining system can naturally impede blood drainage in conditions affecting thoracolumbar radicular veins.
- Dural fistulae draining into longitudinal veins can exacerbate this anatomical disposition's functionality, resulting in retrograde venous congestion and reflux into radial veins. Intracranial dural shunts draining caudally into medullary veins may encounter the convergent system of the thoracic level, potentially leading to symptoms associated with spinal cord pathologies.
- Slow flow in these lesions can precipitate irreversible haemodynamic conditions, culminating in stasis and venous thrombosis, even after complete occlusion of the shunt.
- Foix–Alajouanine myelopathy may represent the ultimate stage of venous myelopathy. At the cervical level, the cranial venous anastomoses of the spinal cord venous system create a favourable configuration for venous drainage. Ventral spinal veins reside in the subpial space, while dorsal veins are situated in the subarachnoid space. Moderate congestion of ventral veins due to an arteriovenous shunt may manifest on MRI only as signal hyperintensity indicative of spinal cord distress, even in the absence of visible venous dilatation, with the congested vein 'trapped' in the subpial space. In contrast, dorsal subarachnoid veins can dilate more rapidly and prominently, with a higher risk of rupture due to venous hypertension related to AVMs. Instances of subarachnoid haemorrhage (SAH) in spinal vascular malformations may result from the rupture of posterior subarachnoid veins, as anterior subpial vein rupture is more commonly associated with haematomyelia.
- A common finding during angiography is the presence of a thoracolumbar enlargement vein, which becomes apparent following proper injection of the radiculomedullary artery of the lumbar enlargement (artery of Adamkiewicz). However, the visualisation of the anterior venous axis is often inconsistent and varies. It is rare for the exit point of the radicular vein to coincide with the site of dural penetration by the artery. The quality of the phlebogram depends on the territory supplied by the injected artery.

Radicular veins

- Similar to radicular arteries, pure radicular veins can also be observed. These veins course along nerve roots exclusively in approximately 60%

of cases, while in the remaining 40%, they enter the dura mater through a different foramen between two distinct nerve roots, deviating from a segmental arrangement.

- The transdural segment of the radicular vein may extend up to 1 cm, and a constriction of the vessel is typically observed at the point of dural entry. This constriction has been proposed as an antireflux mechanism, safeguarding the spinal cord from alterations in intra-abdominal pressure. However, while intriguing, this theory cannot be definitively confirmed, as phlebography has permitted the visualisation of radicular veins.

The spinal and extraspinal venous system

- The epidural venous channels of the spine bear resemblance to those found at the base of the skull, with which they interconnect.
- Dorsal epidural veins typically exhibit a narrow diameter, while the ventral plexus is closely associated with the bone structure and primarily drains the vertebral body.
- Extradural venous channels adopt a hexagonal configuration and interconnect along the midline with both rostral and caudal systems, creating a continuous pathway from the sacrum to the skull base. These veins evenly drain the bony boundaries of the spinal canal, with both ventral and dorsal veins gathering venous blood from the vertebrae and merging into the extradural venous system, which lacks valves.
- Radicular veins may travel alongside nerve roots but do not exhibit the distinct metameric distribution observed in the arterial system. Typically, they converge with the perinervous foraminal venous plexus, although they may also extend to venous lacunae that feed into the extradural longitudinal ventral plexus.

Drugs and analgesia

Analgesia, sedation, and general anaesthesia *94*
Blood pressure control *97*
Antispasmodics *98*
Platelet aggregation and coagulation *101*
Aspirin *102*
P2Y12 inhibitors *103*
Glycoprotein IIb/IIIa receptor inhibitors *107*
Anticoagulation *108*

Analgesia, sedation, and general anaesthesia

Local anaesthesia

- A local anaesthetic (LA) drug temporarily prevents the transmission of nerve impulses from the site of administration to the brain without affecting consciousness.
- Common vascular access sites, including the femoral and radial arteries, are anaesthetised by localised LA injection.
- Ultrasound can more effectively achieve analgesia, as the tissues immediately adjacent to the artery can be visualised and infiltrated.
- Topical creams, particularly a eutectic mixture of local anaesthetics (EMLA®), a combination of prilocaine and lidocaine, may help reduce the pain of injection and initial arterial access. EMLA® is effective in 1 h.

Pharmacological properties

- Lidocaine and prilocaine are most commonly used in practice (Table 3.1).
- **Structure:** a lipophilic aromatic group and a hydrophilic amine group, with an amide linkage in between.
- **Mechanism of action:** they reversibly bind to and inactivate voltage-gated Na^+ channels on the neuronal cell membrane, so inhibiting further depolarisation and signal propagation. This process is concentration dependent.
- **Side effects:**
  - Nervous system: tingling lips, tinnitus, irritability, confusion, seizure, and reduced consciousness.
  - Cardiovascular: arrhythmias and reduced myocardial contractility.
  - Methaemoglobinaemia: LA metabolites can oxidise haemoglobin, affecting its oxygen-carrying capacity.
- **Notes:** LA enters cells in the unionised form. When tissues have an abnormal pH (e.g. in infection), the drug becomes more ionised and less effective.

Sedation and general anaesthesia

- Institutional guidelines for administration of sedation should be followed. Life support training is mandatory.

Table 3.1 Features of common local anaesthetic agents

	Lidocaine	Prilocaine
Onset	2–5 min	2–5 min
Duration	30–60 min	30–120 min
Maximum dose	3 mg/kg	6 mg/kg
Example in 70 kg patient using 1% solution	21 mL	42 mL
Maximum dose with adrenaline	7 mL/kg	9 mL/kg
Contraindications	Heart block, congestive heart failure, liver failure	Congenital or acquired methaemoglobinaemia, liver failure

- Sedation and general anaesthesia (GA) are both medically altered states of consciousness. The difference is in the level of consciousness, breathing depression, and drop in BP.
- Sedation should be given in small incremental doses to achieve the desired effect.
- Sedation is categorised as minimal, moderate, or deep.
  - Moderate (or conscious sedation) is a state of relaxation where patients are sleepy but easily rousable and can follow simple instructions. There should be minimal respiratory depression and no significant drop in BP. BP, oxygen saturation, and electrocardiogram (ECG) must be continually monitored and supplementary oxygen given.
  - Deep sedation and GA should be administered only by a qualified anaesthetist with provisions for airway and breathing support.

Common drugs in use

Sedative drugs may be used in combination to achieve a desired level of consciousness, and are frequently combined with opioid analgesia to obtund the response to noxious stimuli.

Midazolam

- Benzodiazepines have a dose-dependent effect mediated via interactions with gamma-aminobutyric acid (GABA) receptors. They produce both sedation and amnesia and also act as muscle relaxants and anticonvulsants.
- Midazolam is 2–4 times more potent than diazepam.
- **Dose:** midazolam is given in bolus doses of 0.01–0.05 mg/kg, titrated to response. Usually, 2 mg is given initially. Titrate in 1 mg increments.
- **Duration of action:** approximately 1 h.
- **Onset of action:** within 2–3 min.
- **Caution:** benzodiazepines can cause respiratory depression and the risk is increased if given with opioids. If given together, always give the opioid first.
- **Reversal:** the sedative effect can be reversed by flumazenil 0.2 mg repeated up to 1 mg. It acts by competitive inhibition of benzodiazepines. The peak effect is achieved in 6–10 min. The duration of action of flumazenil is only 30–60 min, so re-sedation can occur.

Morphine

- Morphine is a strong opioid, found naturally in opium, that binds to μ-opioid receptors in the central nervous system, producing analgesia.
- **Dose:** 0.05–0.1 mg/kg. Repeat as necessary.
- **Onset of action:** 5 min when given intravenously (IV). The duration of action is 3–7 h.
- **Caution:** opioids may cause nausea, vomiting, hypotension, and respiratory depression.
- **Reversal:** opioids can be reversed by naloxone which is a competitive opioid receptor antagonist with a high affinity for the μ-opioid receptor. Give 0.1–0.3 mg every 30–60 s. Onset of action is 2 min. Duration of action is 45 min.

Fentanyl

- Fentanyl is an analgesic and sedative that may cause profound respiratory depression. It is a potent synthetic piperidine opioid. It is 50–100 times more potent than morphine but with fewer side effects. It has no effect on BP.
- **Dose:** give in 25 mcg increments. Doses >100 mcg are seldom required.
- **Onset of action:** 1–2 min.
- **Duration:** short, its effects last around 20 min but with a further action peak at 40 min due to biliary excretion and reuptake into the bloodstream.
- **Caution:** it may rarely cause a 'stiff chest' syndrome, with rigid skeletal muscles including the intercostals. Treatment is with succinyl choline and airway management.

Ketamine

- Phencyclidine derivative with a dose-dependent effect, acting via antagonism of the *N*-methyl-D-aspartate (NMDA) receptor.
- **Dose:** sedation 0.5–1 mg/kg, GA 1.5–2 mg/kg.
- **Onset of action:** 30–60 s, with a duration from 5 to 15 min.
- **Notes:** it produces a state of dissociative anaesthesia and analgesia. It may induce emergence delirium.

Propofol

- A phenol derivative with a dose-dependent effect, acting predominantly on GABA receptors.
- **Dose:** induction of GA dose is 1–2.5 mg/kg. Maintenance of GA is achieved with a 50–150 mcg/kg/min infusion, whereas sedation dose ranges between 25 and 75 mcg/kg/min.
- **Onset:** it has a rapid onset, within 30 s. Patients wake after 10 min with a single injection.
- **Notes:**
  - It is usually administered as a target-controlled infusion (TCI) using specifically programmed pumps that estimate plasma levels. GA is achieved at plasma levels between 3 and 6 mcg/mL.
  - Pain on injection of propofol is common, this can be reduced by injecting in large veins, and mixing lidocaine with the propofol solution.
  - The level of consciousness can be monitored using a bispectral index monitor, which utilises processed electroencephalographic waveform analysis to produce an algorithmic value between 0 and 100, where 100 represents a fully awake individual, 60–80 indicates a moderate level of sedation, and 40–60 GA.

Inhalational anaesthetic agents

These are reserved for anaesthetists in most healthcare systems, so are beyond the scope of this handbook.

Further reading

Gropper MA, Cohen NH, Eriksson LI, Fleisher LA, Johnson-Akeju S, Leslie K, eds. Miller's Anesthesia. 10th ed. Elsevier; 2024.

Blood pressure control

- Control of BP may be necessary for a variety of clinical reasons during interventional procedures. Hypotensive agents are given to acute ischaemic stroke patients to treat hypertension >185/110 mmHg before initiating IV fibrinolytic therapy or mechanical thrombectomy (MT), and in a hypertensive crisis stimulated by angiographic contrast ± anaesthesia (e.g. secretory paragangliomas, previously undiagnosed phaeochromocytomas).
- Other agents may be used to treat hypotension induced by GA and to elevate BP in delayed cerebral ischaemia.

Drugs to treat hypertension

IV drugs are required for rapid and titratable responses and are given as bolus injections, followed by continuous infusions if required. They vasodilate and reduce peripheral vascular resistance.

Labetalol

- **Mechanism:** combined α- and β-adrenergic receptor blocker.
- **Dose:** 25–50 mg bolus injection (can be repeated every 5 min). Infusion at 1–2 mg/min.

Hydralazine

- **Mechanism:** direct action on vascular smooth muscle.
- **Dose:** 5–10 mg bolus (can be repeated every 20 min). Infusion at 0.05–0.15 mg/min.

Glyceryl trinitrate

- Glyceryl trinitrate (GTN) dermal patches can be used for a rapid hypotensive effect.

Drugs to treat hypotension

- A rapid and titratable response is achieved using the IV route.
- Commonly available drugs are predominantly α-adrenergic receptor agonists, causing vasoconstriction and increasing peripheral vascular resistance:
  - **Metaraminol:** 0.5–1 mg bolus, variable infusion 5–10 mg/h.
  - **Phenylephrine:** 0.05–0.1 mg bolus, variable infusion 0.03–0.18 mg/min.
  - **Noradrenaline:** infusion only, 0.05–1.5 mcg/kg/min.
  - **Ephedrine:** exerts direct α- and β-receptor effects, and an indirect effect by increasing the availability of noradrenaline in the receptor synapse. Ephedrine is less effective with repeated and prolonged use due to tachyphylaxis, and is therefore mainly used as a bolus (3–9 mg) and rarely as an infusion.

Antispasmodics

Antispasmodics are used in neurointervention to prevent or treat delayed cerebral ischaemia due to vasospasm, and to prevent or treat catheter-induced vasospasm during procedures.

Nimodipine

- **Mechanism:** nimodipine is a dihydropyridine calcium channel blocker that acts on smooth muscle cells causing reduced myocardial contractility and reduced coronary and systemic (including cerebral) vascular tone.
- **Use:** it is used to prevent or treat ischaemic neurological deficits after SAH.
- **Contraindications:** nimodipine is contraindicated in unstable angina and within 1 month of myocardial infarction.

Oral use

- It has been used in SAH after RCTs demonstrated an oral dose reduced the incidence of cerebral infarction and overall poor outcomes compared to placebo (Pickard et al., 1989).
- **Dose:** 60 mg every 4 h and must be started within 4 days of haemorrhage and continued for 21 days.

Intravenous use

- **Dose:** it can be given by IV infusion via a central catheter where it is started at 0.5 mg/h (for those <70 kg) or 1 mg/h (for those >70 kg) and titrated up to 2 mg/h if there is no severe drop in BP.
- **Maximum total duration:** 14 days, or up to 21 days if there is surgical intervention during treatment.

Intra-arterial use

- It can be given intra-arterially directly via the carotid or vertebral arteries (depending on the territory affected) for treatment of vasospasm following SAH.
- **Dose:** the nimodipine is diluted in 0.9% NaCl. Typically, up to 2 mg for each vessel in the affected territories is injected slowly. The rate is titrated against BP (if the injection is too fast then the BP will drop, which is undesirable in the presence of vasoconstriction).
- **Saline flush use:** nimodipine is also commonly diluted in the saline flush during neurointervention procedures to prevent catheter-induced vasospasm. 3 mg is diluted in 1 L of NaCl 0.9%. According to the protocol of the institution, heparin can also be added. Note that there is a theoretical risk of crystallisation of nimodipine in the flush bag (not observed by the authors in practice).

Verapamil

- **Mechanism:** verapamil is a calcium channel blocker and initiates reduction in vascular tone.
- **Dose for cerebral vasospasm:** verapamil is administered intra-arterially directly via the carotid or vertebral arteries. It is diluted in 0.9% NaCl and infused at a rate of about 0.5 mg/min. 5–10 mg can then be infused per vessel, titrating the rate against BP.

- **Dose for radial artery spasm:** the drug can also be used in the radial artery to reduce the chance of spasm. 2.5–5 mg is delivered.

Glyceryl trinitrate

- **Mechanism:** GTN is converted to nitric oxide in the body, ultimately leading to the synthesis of cyclic guanosine 3',5'-monophosphate (cGMP), which in turn activates protein kinase-dependent phosphorylation in smooth muscle cells, resulting in relaxation of the muscle fibres.
- **Dose for cerebral vasospasm:** typically used for catheter-induced vasospasm, GTN can be injected intra-arterially in 50 mcg boluses up to 200 mcg.
- **Dose for radial artery spasm:** the drug can be also used in the radial artery to reduce the chance of spasm. Usually, 200 mcg is delivered.

Milrinone

- **Mechanism:** milrinone is a phosphodiesterase-3 inhibitor, preventing the degradation of cyclic adenosine monophosphate in smooth muscle and thus increasing the activation of protein kinase A (PKA), ultimately leading to vasodilatation.
- It has been used IV and intra-arterially for the prevention and treatment of ischaemic neurological deficits after SAH.

The Nantes intravenous protocol

(See Lakhal et al., 2021.)

- 1 h after attaining a mean arterial BP of 100–120 mmHg, milrinone is infused IV initially at 0.5 mcg/kg/min and, if well tolerated and deemed necessary, is increased to a maximum of 1.5 mcg/kg/min. If the BP falls below 100 mmHg despite a high dose (1.5 mcg/kg/min) of IV noradrenaline, the IV milrinone infusion rate is first decreased to 0.5 mcg/kg/min, and then discontinued if even this level is not tolerated.
- A consecutive series demonstrated a lower rate of endovascular angioplasty and a lower likelihood of 6-month functional disability and vasospasm-related brain infarction in patients receiving IV milrinone in comparison to a historical cohort.
- **Contraindications:** aortic and pulmonary valve stenosis, hypertrophic obstructive cardiomyopathy, acute coronary syndrome, and arrhythmias causing cardiovascular stability.

Higher-dose intra-arterial protocol

(See Duman et al., 2017.)

- Administer through a catheter positioned in the cervical segment of the carotid or dominant vertebral artery.
- Milrinone is mixed with normal saline to a concentration of 0.1 mg/mL and administered over 4 min. Administer 6 mg for each territory, totalling 18 mg. After administration, perform control angiography.
- With refractory vasospasm, a higher dose of milrinone is usually given, totalling 24 mg.
- Observe for ECG changes, QT prolongation, hypotension, and cardiovascular instability.
- Intra-arterial nimodipine can be injected before or after milrinone.

Further reading

Duman E, Karakoç F, Pinar HU, Dogan R, Firat A, Yildirim E. Higher dose intra-arterial milrinone and intra-arterial combined milrinone-nimodipine infusion as a rescue therapy for refractory cerebral vasospasm. Interv Neuroradiol. 2017;23(6):636–643.

Joint Formulary Committee. British National Formulary. 90th ed. BMJ Group and Pharmaceutical Press; 2025.

Lakhal K, Hivert A, Alexandre PL, et al. Intravenous milrinone for cerebral vasospasm in subarachnoid hemorrhage: the MILRISPASM controlled before-after study. Neurocrit Care. 2021;35(3):669–679.

Pickard JD, Murray GD, Illingworth R, et al. Effect of oral nimodipine on cerebral infarction and outcome after subarachnoid haemorrhage: British aneurysm nimodipine trial. BMJ. 1989;298(6674):636–642.

Ritter JM, Flower R, Henderson G, et al. Rang and Dale's Pharmacology. 10th ed. Elsevier; 2023.

Platelet aggregation and coagulation

The aggregation/coagulation process

- A strong inflammatory/thromboembolic response is mounted in response to endovascular devices. Plasma proteins including fibrinogen, factor XII, immunoglobulins, complement, and von Willebrand factor (vWF) attach to surfaces within seconds. Coagulation is activated and platelets recruited and activated. These proteins have a lower affinity for hydrophilic surfaces because of the stronger binding of water molecules.
- Complement activation recruits inflammatory cells and platelets. Activated leucocytes produce tissue factor and activated neutrophils form neutrophil extracellular traps.
- Endothelial damage disrupts the protective glycocalyx and impairs endothelial release of nitric oxide, prostacyclin, and tissue-type plasminogen activator (tPA). There is local vasoconstriction because thromboxane-A2 (TxA2) and endothelin are released from the damaged endothelial cell. Local sheer stress is increased, facilitating platelet adherence to subendothelium. Subendothelial vWF and collagen activate platelets and collagen stimulates the intrinsic coagulation pathway. Damaged endothelial cells release tissue factor which stimulates the extrinsic coagulation pathway. Activated platelets release several vasoactive substances including adenosine diphosphate (ADP), TxA2, and some coagulation factors.
- Ultimately, the glycoprotein (GP) IIb/IIIa receptor is activated and binds fibrinogen bridges between aggregating platelets. Thrombin converts fibrinogen to fibrin.
- Antiplatelet medications are essential for certain procedures but precise use varies and there is a lack of evidence and guidelines.
- Diffusion-weighted imaging (DWI) lesions are frequently observed following endovascular procedures, with approximately half being symptomatic. Their occurrence increases with longer and more complex interventions, but can be mitigated through the use of anticoagulation and dual antiplatelet therapy (DAPT).

Aspirin

- **Mechanism:** aspirin (acetylsalicylic acid (ASA)) irreversibly acetylates cyclo-oxygenase-1 (COX-1), modifies the enzymatic activity of COX-2, and inhibits TxA2.
- **Use:** it is often used as monotherapy prophylactically reducing thromboembolic events in aneurysm coiling (ruptured and unruptured), together with P2Y12 inhibitors when stents/flow diverters are deployed, or with some intrasaccular devices. It may be given IV during procedures.
- **Oral use:**
  - **Dose:** 75–325 mg once daily (OD) orally. Note, dose is weight dependent and a 75 mg dose is likely less effective in those >70 kg.
  - **Onset of action:** within 30 min. Peak efficacy is within 1–2 h.
- **IV use:**
  - **Dose:** 250–500 mg IV may be given.
  - **Onset of action:** 30 s.
- **Half-life:** 2–3 h (however, the pharmacological action is much longer).
- **Duration of action:** aspirin acts on platelets for the remaining duration of their lifespan (typically 7–10 days in circulation).
- **Efficacy:** 10% of the platelet pool is replenished daily. 10–15% of normal platelets provide normal haemostasis.
- **Reduced efficacy:** aspirin is less effective in smokers, concomitant arthritis, surgical stress, and diabetes mellitus (insulin has antiplatelet action). Oxidative stress and elevated C-reactive protein can overcome the inhibitory effect on COX-1.
- **Aspirin resistance:** likely around 5%.
- **Duration of aspirin therapy:**
  - Varies between operator/centre. It is often given for 6–12 weeks after aneurysm coiling, 3–12 months after laser-cut stent placement, and 12 months to lifelong with flow diversion and braided stents.
  - There is a reported risk, around 5%, of thromboembolic events after stopping DAPT following stent placement. Risk factors include vasculopathy, incomplete aneurysm occlusion, neointimal hyperplasia, and poor apposition with the arterial wall. The risk is highest within the first 3 months.
- **Drug interactions:** non-steroidal anti-inflammatory drugs (NSAIDs), namely ibuprofen, naproxen, and indometacin, reduce the efficacy of aspirin by altering the structure of COX. Diclofenac and ketorolac do not interact with aspirin.
- **Anti-inflammatory effect:** this is an additional benefit via its action on COX-2. Inflammation is a key factor in aneurysm formation, enlargement, and rupture. Aspirin reduces aneurysmal wall inflammation and lessens risk of growth and rupture. Therefore, aspirin may have a role in the conservative management of unruptured intracranial aneurysms.
- **Side effects:** gastritis/gastric ulceration. Gastrointestinal bleeds occur in about 0.12% per year (given with clopidogrel it is 3–5% per year). Whether aspirin results in more cerebral microbleeds is controversial. The risk of major haemorrhage is around 1% per year.
- **Aspirin reversal:** consider desmopressin 0.3 mcg/kg in 0.9% NaCl solution over 15–30 min. Desmopressin can be used to reverse the effects of any antiplatelet because it increases plasma vWF and factor VIII, which enhances platelet adhesion.

P2Y12 inhibitors

- These are mainly used together with aspirin to minimise thromboembolic events and stent thrombosis in intracranial and cervical arterial stents by inhibiting the binding of ADP to platelets. Newer agents, such as prasugrel, are increasingly being used as monotherapy for stent and flow-diversion procedures.
- The P2Y12 receptor is the primary platelet receptor mediating ADP-induced platelet aggregation. Active metabolites of thienopyridine prodrugs, such as clopidogrel and prasugrel, bind covalently to the P2Y12 receptor, acting as indirect, irreversible inhibitors of platelet function. In contrast, direct-acting P2Y12 inhibitors like cangrelor and ticagrelor induce a conformational change in the receptor, leading to reversible, concentration-dependent inhibition.
- **Caution:** patients with renal or hepatic impairment are at an increased risk when using most antiplatelet medications.

Dual antiplatelet therapy for arterial stents

- **Stent-assisted coiling:** commonly 3–6 months for laser-cut stents and 6–9 months for braided stents/flow diverters.
- **Cervical carotid stenting:** the optimal regimen is not established (Sussman et al., 2021). It is reasonable to give DAPT pre-procedure and for at least 3 months after (Schirmer et al., 2023).
- **Intracranial atherosclerotic disease:** the WEAVE trial had positive results and following its protocol seems reasonable. It consisted of aspirin and clopidogrel for 7–10 days before stenting and 3 months post-procedure, at which point aspirin alone was continued.
- **Ruptured aneurysms (usually dissecting or blister type):** flow diversion is often necessary. DAPT or monotherapy with prasugrel or ticagrelor (but not aspirin monotherapy) with flow-diverters can be used. Often eptifibatide or tirofiban is given initially intravenously and stopped a couple of hours after loading with DAPT.
- **Patients with atrial fibrillation on anticoagulants:** it is necessary to refer to cardiology guidelines. The risk of major haemorrhage is high with concomitant DAPT and anticoagulant usage. European Stroke Organisation 2020 guidelines recommend a direct-acting oral anticoagulant (DOAC) (not warfarin) + aspirin + clopidogrel for 1–4 weeks post-procedure and then a DOAC + single antiplatelet therapy (preferably clopidogrel) for 12 months, followed by a DOAC alone.

Clopidogrel

- **Mechanism:** a second-generation P2Y12 thienopyridine receptor antagonist. Clopidogrel is irreversible and competitive. Only 10–15% of the administered drug is converted to its active form, requiring two metabolic steps—which are dependent upon various alleles of *CYP2C19* genes.
- **Platelet function testing:** controversial but recommended by the authors due to genetic variation in pharmacological response.
- **Response:**
    - There is hyporesponse in 20–50% and hyperresponse in 15–40%, with ethnic variation.
    - If hyporesponse, some recommend doubling the dose of clopidogrel (but a significant number will still be hyporesponsive) or changing to prasugrel or ticagrelor.
    - If hyperresponse, lower dose as required after platelet function testing.

- **Dose:** load with 75 mg OD for 3–7 days before procedure or 300 mg the day before. For emergency procedures, load with 600 mg 2 h before usage.
- **Maintenance dose:** usually 75 mg OD. This can be titrated with platelet function testing.
- **Delivery:** orally, or crushed and delivered via nasogastric tubes.
- **Drug interactions:** the National Institute for Health and Care Excellence (NICE) advises an increased risk of bleeding if combined with other drugs that also increase the risk of bleeding, such as other antiplatelets, NSAIDs, anticoagulants, selective serotonin reuptake inhibitors (SSRIs), and serotonin and noradrenaline reuptake inhibitors (SNRIs). There is a theoretical risk of suppression of effect with omeprazole, ketoconazole, lipophilic statins, calcium channel blockers, and erythromycin; however, these are not considered clinically relevant. There are a range of other potential interactions.
- **Reversal:** there are no specific reversal agents. Consider cryoprecipitate, fresh frozen plasma, and desmopressin. Consult haematology.
- **Risks with external ventricular drain (EVD):** the risk of significant haemorrhage in EVD placement in patients with SAH on DAPT (aspirin + clopidogrel) is around 4%.

Prasugrel

- **Mechanism:** this is a third-generation thienopyridine P2Y12 receptor antagonist. Like clopidogrel, it is irreversible and competitive.
- **Response:** it has a faster onset and gives more powerful and consistent platelet inhibition compared to clopidogrel as it requires just one metabolic step for activation. Few, but not zero, are hyporesponsive.
- **Maximal platelet inhibition:** achieved within 4 h. Procedures can usually be commenced after 2 h.
- **Half-life:** 2–15 h (but the therapeutic effect is longer).
- **Duration of action:** platelet aggregation gradually returns to baseline 7–9 days after a single 60 mg loading dose, and 5 days following maintenance dosing.
- **Dose:** this is controversial. There is a suggestion that the standard cardiology dose (60 mg loading, 5–10 mg OD maintenance depending on if weight is under or over 60 kg) is too potent for interventional neuroradiology procedures. Some, therefore, give a half dose for loading (30 mg), and 5 mg OD maintenance (Cagnazzo et al., 2019). Alternatively, the dose can potentially be titrated with platelet function testing.
- **Drug interactions:** there is an increased risk of bleeding when combined with other antiplatelet agents, NSAIDs, anticoagulants, SSRIs, and SNRIs.
- **Contraindications:** not recommended in acute stroke.
- **Reversal:** there are no specific reversal agents. Consider cryoprecipitate, fresh frozen plasma, or desmopressin. Consult haematology for advice.

Ticagrelor

- **Mechanism:** this is a non-competitive, reversible, selective P2Y12 inhibitor. It is an ATP analogue that induces conformational change in the receptor, binding to a different site independent of ADP. No metabolic activation is required. There are no genetic influences. Its metabolite has equipotent antiplatelet activity.

- **Response:** like prasugrel, it is much faster, stronger, and more consistent than clopidogrel. Few, but not zero, are hyporesponsive.
- **Maximum platelet inhibition is achieved:** 2–4 h.
- **Half-life:** 4–6 h.
- **Dose:** 180 mg loading, 90 mg twice-daily (BD) maintenance. If too strong a response, consider a maintenance dose of 45 mg BD.
- **Duration of action:** it is undetectable in the blood after 20 h. After stopping, platelet function normalises in 72 h. Patient compliance is mandatory.
- **Reversal:** IV bentracimab.
- **Side effects:** increase in ventricular pauses, dyspnoea due to inhibition of adenosine uptake by red blood cells, elevation of uric acid (usually mild and self-limiting but caution with gout).
- **Cautions:** gout, asthma, and chronic obstructive pulmonary disease.
- **Contraindications:** previous intracranial haemorrhage (ICH); ketoconazole (which markedly increases ticagrelor levels).
- **Drug interactions:** high-dose simvastatin (statin retention causes rhabdomyolysis), verapamil (increases ticagrelor levels), phenytoin, carbamazepine (decreases ticagrelor levels), and opioids (may reduce its absorption).

Cangrelor

- **Mechanism:** this is an IV, non-thienopyridine ATP analogue, P2Y12 antagonist. It is non-competitive, reversible, and requires no metabolic activation.
- **Dose:** 5 mcg/kg bolus followed by an infusion of 0.75–2 mcg/kg/min (far lower than the cardiology dose).
- **Onset of action:** 2–6 min.
- **Half-life:** 3–5 min.
- **Duration of action:** 30–60 min. Normal platelet function resumes 60–90 min after cessation.
- **Use:** it has been used for bridging therapy following stent deployment.
- **Notes:** ticagrelor should be used subsequently rather than clopidogrel or prasugrel because cangrelor occupies the P2Y12 receptor. Load with ticagrelor 1 h before stopping the cangrelor infusion (after cranial CT excluding haemorrhage).

Platelet function testing

- There is genetic and physiological variability in bioavailability of these agents, particularly clopidogrel. Platelet function testing allows dose adjustment to maintain platelet inhibition within therapeutic range.
- The VerifyNow® PRU Test is a point-of-care test that uses ADP to stimulate platelets with prostaglandin E1 (PGE1) to inhibit activation of the P2Y1 receptor, making it sensitive and specific for P2Y12 receptor activity and drugs binding to the P2Y12 receptor. The greater the aggregation, the less the effect of the antiplatelets. The results are presented as P2Y12 Reaction Units (PRU). Ticagrelor can be tested but the machine is not validated for this and testing could be less accurate.
- VerifyNow®-P2Y12 Assay reference ranges (as of 2024):
  - 180–376 PRU: no drug action (significant hyporesponse to P2Y12 inhibitor).
  - 10–180: decreased platelet aggregation due to action of P2Y12 inhibitor.

- Notes:
  - >180: No drug effect present.
  - 10–180 PRU: Decreased platelet reactivity due to P2Y12 inhibitor.
  - Haemorrhagic complications are more common with PRU <70 and thromboembolic events more common with PRU >150.
  - If insufficient response, the agent should be substituted for another or give additional dose.
- For VerifyNow® P2Y12 testing, the suggested sample draw times are:
  - Clopidogrel: 7 days for 75 mg maintenance, 8 h for 300 mg post-bolus, and 6 h for 600 mg post-bolus.
  - Prasugrel: 5 days for 5 mg and 10 mg maintenance doses and 45 min for 60 mg post-bolus.
  - Ticagrelor: 1 day (within 8 h) for 90 mg maintenance and 2 h (within 8 h) for 180 mg post-bolus.
- Aspirin efficacy testing is also available and is reported in Aspirin Reaction Units (ARU):
  - ≥550 ARU: no evidence of platelet dysfunction due to aspirin.
  - <550 ARU: platelet dysfunction consistent with aspirin detected.

Further reading

Borchert RJ, Simonato D, Hickman CR, et al. P2Y12 inhibitors for the neurointerventionalist. Interv Neuroradiol. 2022;28(1):92–103.

Cagnazzo F, Perrini P, Lefevre PH, et al. Comparison of prasugrel and clopidogrel used as antiplatelet medication for endovascular treatment of unruptured intracranial aneurysms: a meta-analysis. AJNR Am J Neuroradiol. 2019;40(4):681–686.

Entezami P, Holden DN, Boulos AS, et al. Cangrelor dose titration using platelet function testing during cerebrovascular stent placement. Interv Neuroradiol. 2021;27(1):88–98.

Paul AR, Entezami P, Holden D, Field N, Dalfino J, Boulos A. Use of intravenous cangrelor and stenting in acute ischaemic stroke interventions: a new single centre analysis and pooled-analysis of current studies. Interv Neuroradiol. 2021;27(6):837–842.

Schirmer CM, Bulsara KR, Al-Mufti F, et al. Antiplatelets and antithrombotics in neurointerventional procedures: guideline update. J Neurointerv Surg. 2023;15(11):1155–1162.

Sussman ES, Jin M, Pendharkar AV, et al. Dual antiplatelet therapy after carotid artery stenting: trends and outcomes in a large national database. J Neurointerv Surg. 2021;13(1):8–13.

Glycoprotein IIb/IIIa receptor inhibitors

- These are useful either prophylactically as bridging therapy following stent deployment when the patient has not been loaded on P2Y12 inhibitors or to lyse acute thromboemboli.
- A meta-analysis has found some evidence that GP IIb/IIIa inhibitors namely abciximab, tirofiban, and eptifibatide are superior to thrombolytics with respect to rescue treatment of thromboembolic complications during EVT (Brinjikji et al., 2015).
- These agents are typically administered as IV boluses followed by continuous infusion. Once the patient can tolerate oral antiplatelet agents (such as clopidogrel, prasugrel, or ticagrelor), a loading dose of the oral agent is given, and the infusion is discontinued a few hours later to maintain adequate platelet inhibition during the transition period.
- The dosages referenced are based on cardiology practice. However, local protocols for neurointervention procedures may favour reduced dosing.

Eptifibatide (Integrilin®)

- **Mechanism:** this is a reversible GP IIb/IIIa reversible inhibitor.
- **Half-life:** 1.5–2.5 h.
- **Platelet function normalises:** 4–8 h after stopping.
- **IV bolus dose:** 90–180 mcg/kg (180 mcg/kg achieves >80% platelet inhibition in 15 min).
- **IV infusion dose:** 2 mcg/kg/min.

Tirofiban (Aggrastat®)

- **Mechanism:** this is a reversible GP IIb/IIIa inhibitor.
- **Half-life:** 2 h.
- **Platelet function normalises:** 4–8 h after stopping.
- **IV bolus:** 25 mcg/kg over 3 min.
- **IV infusion:** 150 nanograms/kg/min for 12–24 h, maximum duration of treatment 48 h.

Further reading

Brinjikji W, Morales-Valero SF, Murad MH, Cloft HJ, Kallmes DF. Rescue treatment of thromboembolic complications during endovascular treatment of cerebral aneurysms: a meta-analysis. AJNR Am J Neuroradiol. 2015;36(1):121–125.

Anticoagulation

- Endovascular devices induce a strong thromboinflammatory response. Heparin has been used for >30 years to reduce thromboembolic complications.
- Additionally, many patients needing EVT are on anticoagulants, and it may be necessary to modify periprocedural anticoagulation accordingly.
- Anticoagulation may also be used to treat arterial dissection, a potential complication of interventional neuroradiology procedures.
- The coagulation pathway is summarised in Figure 3.1.

Coagulation pathway

See Figure 3.1.

- Most clotting factors are produced by the liver, which also synthesises proteins C and S.
- Factor VII is also produced by the endothelium.
- Platelets produce factors I (fibrinogen), V, and VIII.
- The intrinsic pathway (IP) is activated via subendothelial collagen, exposed after endothelial damage, and enhanced by platelet release of coagulation factors.

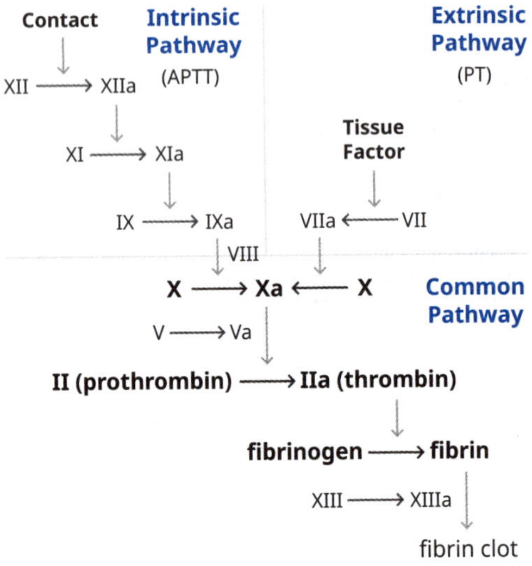

Figure 3.1 The coagulation cascade. Image courtesy of Dr Patrick Lawrence.

- The IP comprises factors I, II (prothrombin), IX, X, XI, and XII, and starts with activation of factor XII. Activated factor XII activates factor XI, activated factor XI activates factor IX, and activated factor IX activates factor X.
- The extrinsic pathway (EP) is activated by tissue factor (TF), released from damaged endothelial cells and activated leucocytes.
- The EP comprises factors I, II, VII, and activated factor X. TF activates VII to VIIa which then activates factor X to Xa (this requires factor III and calcium).
- Activated factor X requires activated factors IX, VIII, V, phospholipid (antiphospholipid syndrome, a risk factor for ischaemic stroke), and calcium.
- The common pathway (CP) begins with activated factor X which activates prothrombin (factor II) to thrombin (activated factor II). Thrombin converts fibrinogen to fibrin and activates factor XIII which reinforces the fibrin mesh and stabilises the platelet plug.
- Prothrombin can therefore be activated by either pathway and thrombin reinforces the IP, giving positive feedback to factors V, VII, VIII, XI, and XIII.
- To ensure that coagulation does not escalate, feedback loops regulate the process. Thrombin stimulates plasminogen (plasmin breaks down the fibrin mesh) and antithrombin (AT). AT inhibits formation of thrombin (and therefore the positive feedback on factors V, VIII, XI, and XIII) from prothrombin and decreases factor Xa.
- Thrombin additionally binds to thrombomodulin, activating protein C and S, which inactivate factors V and VIII. Deficiency of protein C and S therefore risk a hypercoagulable state. Factor V Leiden mutation also risks a hypercoagulable state because mutated factor V cannot be inactivated by proteins C and S.

Coagulation tests

- The activated partial thromboplastin time (APTT) is a measure of the time taken to generate fibrin from initiation of the IP (assessing the IP and CP, factors XII, IX, XI, VIII, X, V, prothrombin, fibrinogen). Normal is 25–53 s.
- Prothrombin time (PT) is a measure of the time taken to generate fibrin after activation of factor VII (assesses EP, CP, factors VII, V, and X, prothrombin, fibrinogen). Normal is 11–13.5 s.
- Thrombin time (TT) is the time to drive the conversion of fibrinogen to fibrin in the presence of thrombin. Normal is 15–19 s.
- Activated clotting time (ACT) is the time taken for blood to clot. Normal is 70–120 s.

Unfractionated heparin

- **Mechanism:** unfractionated heparin (UFH) is a negatively charged glycosaminoglycan. The agent binds to and activates ATIII. Activated ATIII inhibits thrombin (free, not clot-bound), as well as factors XIIa, XIa, Xa, IXa, and VIIa. Clot-bound UFH continues to inactivate factors V, VIII, XI, and XIII.

- **Use:** UFH is used to treat deep vein thrombosis, pulmonary embolism, cerebral venous sinus thrombosis (CVST), and arterial dissection and is used as a prophylactic anticoagulant agent in many endovascular procedures.
- **Dose in EVT:** generally 5000 IU bolus. Bolus doses are not recommended in MT because of the higher risk of symptomatic intracranial haemorrhage (sICH) (van der Steen et al., 2022).
- **Dose in arterial flushes:** the amount of heparin in flushes varies from none to 5000 IU/L but should not exceed 2500 IU/L in MT (van der Steen et al., 2022).
- **Caution:** do not use if your patient is already taking anticoagulants.
- **Half-life:** 60–90 min.
- **Monitor:** use APTT (≥2 times normal) or ACT (typically 200–300 s). The former is more reliable but requires laboratory analysis whereas ACT can be measured using point-of-care machines intraprocedurally.
- **Reversal:** protamine is used for urgent reversal. In non-urgent cases, stopping the infusion for 4–6 h results in near-complete reversal.

Immune-mediated thrombocytopenia

- The main serious side effect of UFH is immune-mediated thrombocytopenia, reported in 1–5%. Mortality approaches 30%.
- **Onset:** 5–14 days after starting heparin but sooner if the patient has had heparin in the previous 100 days.
- **Mechanism:** an immune complex forms between negatively charged heparin and positively charged platelet factor 4 which is released by activated platelets. Antibodies (IgG) form against the complex and the antibody/heparin/platelet factor complex bind to a platelet receptor. Further platelet activation is generated (clot formation) and/or the complex is removed by the reticuloendothelial system (RES) (resulting in thrombocytopenia).
- **Management:** stop heparin and switch to argatroban or bivalirudin (direct thrombin inhibitors) if necessary. Avoid platelet transfusions.
- **Notes:**
  - It is much less common with low-molecular-weight heparin (LMWH).
  - Non-immune thrombocytopenia occurs more frequently than immune-mediated. It is not harmful, generating only a mild decrease in platelet count, and occurs early, on day 1. This requires no action.

Reversal of unfractionated heparin

- Protamine, a protein derived from salmon sperm, reverses the anticoagulant effect of UFH.
- The positively charged protamine binds to the negatively charged arginine groups of UFH and dissociates the AT/heparin complex.
- **Dose:** 1 mg reverses 100 IU UFH, given within 2–4 h of the last UFH dose, acting within 5 min and lasting up to 2 h. Maximum dose is 50 mg. It should be given slowly over 10–15 min to avoid hypotension (due to release of nitric oxide), bradycardia, and pulmonary vasoconstriction (due to release of TxA2).
- **Half-life:** 10 min.
- **Side effects:** excess may cause anticoagulation by inhibition of factor V activation. It can also interact with vWF, having a negative effect on platelet function.

- **Allergic reactions:** 0.3–6% (mainly in those allergic to fish and in vasectomised, infertile men). Anaphylaxis is reported in 0.06–10.6%.
- **Contraindications:** fish or documented insulin-neutral protamine Hagedorn insulin allergy; vasectomised patients.

Low-molecular-weight heparin

- **Use:**
  - This is commonly used for treatment and prophylaxis of deep vein thrombosis, treatment of CVST. Consider venous thromboembolisim (VTE) prophylaxis after aneurysmal SAH when the ruptured aneurysm is secure (usually ≥24 h after coiling providing the aneurysm is secured). These patients are usually in bed and are hypercoagulable.
  - LMWH can be used to treat CVST and is considered to have a superior safety profile and probably greater efficacy than UFH.
- **Forms:** enoxaparin and dalteparin are derived from UFH and also bind to and activate ATIII, only inhibiting factor Xa (LMWH is about one-third of the size of UFH and has limited binding capacity). They are more predictable than UFH.
- **Dose:** Lower doses are used for VTE prophylaxis. Treatment doses vary according to agent, weight and renal function.
- **Onset of action subcutaneously:** 20–60 min.
- **Half-life:** 2–4 h.
- **Monitoring:** usually unnecessary but can be performed if required (bleeding, impaired renal function) by laboratory-based anti-Xa assay or prothrombinase ACT.
- **Reversal:** only partially (50%) reversed by protamine. 1 mg for every 100 IU dalteparin, 1 mg per mg enoxaparin. Consider prothrombin concentrate.
- **Side effects:** the incidence of immune-mediated thrombocytopenia is 10% that of UFH.

Warfarin

- **Mechanism:** warfarin competitively inhibits vitamin K epoxide reductase, which activates vitamin K. Vitamin K is necessary for the hepatic synthesis of factors II, VII, IX, and X, as well as proteins C and S. Consequently, warfarin may initially induce a hypercoagulable state, and its complete therapeutic anticoagulant effect may take around 5–7 days to be fully realised. During the initial loading period, it is essential to combine warfarin therapy with UFH.
- **Use:**
  - Oral anticoagulants are used to treat CVST and arterial dissection, as well as prophylactically, to reduce the incidence of embolic stroke in cardiac disease.
  - In cervical arterial dissection, although the European Stroke Organisation recommends either antiplatelet therapy or anticoagulation, a meta-analysis of the CADISS and TREAT-CAD RCTs indicates superior efficacy of warfarin in limiting thromboembolic events. More recently, the STOP-CAD study reported a non-significant lower risk of ischaemic stroke within 30 days with anticoagulation (vitamin K antagonists), but a definite benefit in cases of occlusive dissection.
- **Half-life:** 35–45 h.

- **Dose:** 10 mg oral for 2 days (or 5 mg if frail or elderly) and subsequent doses depending on international normalised ratio (INR).
- **Monitoring:** INR (PT).
- **Drug interactions:** many medications, including numerous antibiotics, NSAIDs, antiplatelets such as aspirin and P2Y12 inhibitors, steroids, paracetamol, and certain antiepileptic drugs, can have potential interactions.
- **Side effects:** high incidence of bleeding. DOACs have a lower risk of major haemorrhage.
- **Duration of action:** after discontinuing, INR levels can take 3–7 days to normalise.
- **Reversal:** if pharmacological intervention is required, consult haematology and consider fresh frozen plasma and prothrombin complex concentrate, both of which replace the clotting factors immediately and/or administer vitamin K, 5–10 mg IV. Combination therapy may be necessary. Major haemorrhage requires 5–10 mg of vitamin K. For minor haemorrhage, administer 2–5 mg. Vitamin K may lead to temporary warfarin resistance.
- **Intravenous thrombolysis (IVT):** in ischaemic stroke IVT may be given to those on warfarin/vitamin K antagonists if INR <1.7.
- **MT:** not contraindicated in large vessel occlusion (LVO), but some studies have reported an elevated risk of sICH and mortality. It is important to take into consideration the extent of infarcted brain tissue and the potential for salvageable brain tissue, as well as its eloquence. Reversal of anticoagulation therapy before MT is not commonly practised.

Direct oral anticoagulants

- **Mechanism:** these are either thrombin (free and clot-bound) inhibitors, including dabigatran (half-life 12–17 h), or factor Xa inhibitors such as rivaroxaban (half-life 7–11 h), apixaban (half-life 8–15 h), and edoxaban (half-life 10–14 h). DOACs have a significantly shorter half-life compared to warfarin.
- **Use:** they are more effective than warfarin in preventing strokes in non-valvular atrial fibrillation. They have a quicker onset of action than warfarin/vitamin K antagonists and fewer drug interactions. No monitoring is necessary. Meta-analyses report that DOACs significantly decrease the rate of sICH and mortality compared to warfarin, without a significant increase in functional outcome.
- **DOACs and IVT:**
  - The European Stroke Organisation recommends reversal of dabigatran before thrombolysis.
  - The American Heart Association recommends against thrombolysis unless the last dose of DOAC was >48 h earlier.
  - 28% of patients on DOACs are eligible for IVT within the time window.
- **DOACs and MT:** observational studies (with small patient numbers) suggest that there is no increased risk of sICH in MT in patients taking DOACs.
- **DOACs for deep vein thrombosis and aneurysm treatment:** the Society of NeuroInterventional Surgery (SNIS) Standards and Guidelines Committee states:

For patients being evaluated for neurointerventional brain aneurysm treatment who had venous thrombosis more than 3 months prior, discontinuation of oral anticoagulation (OAC) or vitamin K antagonists should be considered as weighed against the risk of delaying aneurysm treatment. For venous thrombosis less than 3 months in the past, delay of the neurointerventional procedure should be considered. If this is not possible, see atrial fibrillation recommendations (Class IIb, Level C-LD).

- **DOACs for atrial fibrillation and aneurysm treatment:** the SNIS Standards and Guidelines Committee states:

  For patients with atrial fibrillation receiving OAC and in need of a neuro-interventional procedure, the duration of TAT (triple antiplatelet/anticoagulation therapy=OAC plus DAPT) should be kept as short as possible or avoided in favour of OAC plus single antiplatelet therapy (SAPT) based on the individual's ischaemic and bleeding risk profile (Class IIa, Level B-NR).

Further reading

Aldhaeefi M, Badreldin HA, Alsuwayyid F, et al. Practical guide for anticoagulant and antiplatelet reversal in clinical practice. Pharmacy (Basel). 2023;11(1):34.
Van der Steen W, van de Graaf RA, Chalos V, et al. Safety and efficacy of aspirin, unfractionated heparin, both, or neither during endovascular stroke treatment (MR CLEAN-MED): an open-label, multicentre, randomised controlled trial. Lancet. 2022;399(10329):1059–1069.
Yaghi S, Shu L, Bakradze E, et al. Direct oral anticoagulants versus warfarin in the treatment of cerebral venous thrombosis (ACTION-CVT): a multicenter international study. Stroke. 2022;53(3):728–738.
Zhang H, Chen S, Zhu Q, Li Z, Lv T, Liu C. Mechanical thrombectomy in anticoagulated patients with acute ischaemic stroke: a meta-analysis. Neurologist. 2024;29(3):194–203.

Equipment and devices

Introduction *116*
Guidewires *117*
Sheaths and catheters *119*
Balloon devices *125*
Coils *129*
Carotid stents *131*
Aneurysm-bridging stents *132*
Flow diverters *133*
Stent retrievers *134*
Intrasaccular and neck-bridging devices *134*
Gelatin, particles, and sclerosants *135*
Cyanoacrylate glue *137*
Copolymer liquid embolics *140*

Introduction

The number of neurointerventional devices has increased dramatically in recent years due to advances in engineering and a widened scope of neurointerventional practice. Knowledge of the characteristics of specific devices is integral to the practice of neurointervention. Choice of one device over another in a particular situation may mean the difference between procedural success or failure. Information on compatibility and sizing these devices is available on the free non-commercial online resource www.neurotool.org (developed by one of the authors).

A note on units

By convention, different units are used in neurointervention for different purposes, mainly for historical reasons:

- **Inches (in, ")** are used for the inner luminal diameter of catheters and the diameter of wires.
- **French gauge (Fr)** (or just **French**) is generally used for the outer diameter of catheters and the inner diameter of sheaths. 1 French is 1/3 of a millimetre.
- **Centimetres** and **millimetres (cm, mm)** are generally used for length.
- **Birmingham gauge (G)** (or just **gauge**) is used for the outer diameter for hypodermic needles. Counterintuitively, the larger the gauge the smaller the diameter.

Guidewires

Guidewires are engineered to be flexible, pushable (capable of transmitting force to the tip), gentle on vessels, and torqueable (controlled rotation of the tip). To accomplish this, they feature soft, atraumatic tips and more rigid shafts. Guidewires can possess straight or angled tips, which are often shapeable. 'J'-angled tips, in particular, are less prone to dissection and perforation of vessels. Wires can be torqued by hand or by using torque devices screwed onto the end of the wire. Wires can be standard or exchange length. Exchange wires are over double the length of the catheter they are used with so that the catheter can be fully removed while keeping the wire in place, prior to introducing an alternate catheter.

"Standard" diameter wires

- Wires used in combination with angiographic or guide catheters are most commonly of 0.035" or 0.038" diameter.
- They must be flushed before withdrawal from packaging.

Commonly used wires for diagnostic angiography

- The Glidewire (Terumo) is probably the most commonly used guidewire for selecting the brachiocephalic, subclavian, carotid, and vertebral arteries. It is made of a nitinol alloy core with a tungsten-infused polyurethane jacket, which provides radiopacity, and a hydrophilic coating, which increases lubricity. The wire comes in various sizes but the 0.035" 180 cm wire is considered the most versatile, while the 260 cm version is used for catheter exchange. It typically has an angled tip, although straight shapeable and J-tip versions are also available. There is a stiff version that confers enhanced support. For navigating tortuous aortic arch vessels, the Glidewire Advantage is an option. This version is also available in 0.035" diameter with lengths of 180 cm and 260 cm and is designed to provide support and torqueability.
- The Amplatz wire (multiple manufacturers such as Boston Scientific and Cook Medical) is a stainless-steel wire with flat-wire coils and a polytetrafluoroethylene (PTFE) coating to improve lubricity. It is very supportive when navigating a catheter through tortuous vessels. 0.035" and 0.038" diameters are available and there are a range of lengths and stiffness variants. The wire comes with straight (shapeable) or J-tips and stiff and extra stiff variants are available.

Microwires

- Microwires are used inside small, fragile vessels, particularly the intracranial segments of vessels.
- To aid navigation, these wires are typically equipped with torquing devices and shapers.
- They must be flushed before withdrawal from packaging.
- Microwires have shapeable tips, which can be moulded using the supplied metal shapers. A gentle curve is ideal for selecting vessels, while a J curve is less traumatic but reduces vessel selection ability. For navigating acute-angled vessel bifurcations, a double curve consisting of a tight distal angled curve and a broader, more proximal angle is helpful.

- To achieve very tight distal curves (up to 1 mm), the wire can be threaded through the shaping device until a tiny length protrudes out. By gently tapping on the end of the protruding wire, a very tight curve can be formed.
- When a wire has a more tightly curved tip, it needs to be back-loaded for insertion into the microcatheter as the curve prohibits direct insertion. This process involves threading the supplied hollow introducer device via the stiff back-end of the wire all the way until it reaches the tip, straightening the wire tip for insertion into the hub. It is crucial to avoid shaving off the hydrophilic coating layer when threading wires with this type of coating as this substance may embolise if inadvertently inserted into the bloodstream. Introducers must be flushed with saline before use.

Commonly used microwires

- The Synchro (Stryker) is a general-purpose microwire. It is very torqueable. 0.014" and 0.010" diameter variants are available. The wire comes in 200 cm and 300 cm (exchange length) versions. The tip is shapeable and pre-shaped versions are available. There are 'support' versions that provide enhanced proximal support and 'select' variants that have improved torqueability.
- The Traxcess (Microvention) is a general-purpose microwire. It is 0.014" or 0.007" in diameter and approximately 200 cm in length. The 0.014" version can be used with an additional 115 cm docking wire that attaches on to the end of the wire for exchange manoeuvres. The tip is softer than the Synchro wire but the wire is less torqueable. The Traxcess shaft mid-portion is actually 0.012", allowing it to be inserted into microcatheters, usefully the 0.013" Marathon, despite the apparent size discrepancy.
- The Transend (Stryker Neurovascular) is a general-purpose microwire that comes in 0.010" and 0.014" diameters. The 0.014" version comes in 182 cm, 205 cm, and 300 cm lengths and the 0.010" version is 200 cm.
- The Hybrid (Balt) is a microwire that can be used for navigation into the very distal cerebral circulation in pathologies involving smaller vessels, for AVM/dural arteriovenous fistula (DAVF) embolisation. It is soft and available in diameters as small as 0.007". Other diameters include 0.008", 0.010", 0.012", and 0.014". It has a shapeable tip and comes in straight, angled, and double-angled varieties.
- The Mirage (Medtronic) is a 0.008" microwire used for similar purposes to the Hybrid. It is subjectively slightly stiffer, which might be useful when pushability is required. It is mainly used for small vessels in AVM/DAVF embolisation.
- The Chikai (Asahi) is available in 0.008", 0.010", 0.014", and 0.018" diameters. The smaller versions are mainly used in AVM/DAVF embolisation. The 'black' variant has greater radiopacity.
- Terumo also sells hydrophilic wires in sizes down to 0.014".

Sheaths and catheters

Catheters require certain characteristics: they should provide proximal support, maintaining a stable position without prolapsing or kinking, be gentle on vessels, easily navigate through tortuous vasculature, have a small outer diameter to access narrow vessels, and a large inner diameter for accommodating devices. Additionally, they should be non-thrombogenic and affordable. In practice, a balance between these desirable design features is necessary.

Sheaths and catheters must be flushed inside and outside before use.

A *coaxial* configuration refers to a smaller catheter being inserted into a guide catheter or a long sheath. A *triaxial* configuration refers to inserting a microcatheter into an intermediate (or 'distal access') catheter, which is then inserted into a guide catheter/long sheath.

Vascular sheaths

- Vascular sheaths are placed at the vascular access site to reduce friction between the catheter and the vessel wall.
- The size of the sheath is indicated by the largest device that can be inserted through it. For example, a 6 Fr guide catheter can be inserted into a 6 Fr sheath.
- The outer diameter of the sheath is usually about 2 Fr sizes larger than the inner diameter. However, newer sheaths are now available with an outer diameter of just 1 Fr larger than the inner, particularly advantageous for radial and paediatric access. These include the Prelude Ideal (Merit) and Glidesheath Slender (Terumo). These typically come with micropuncture needles and microwires for introduction into smaller, more delicate, vessels.
- Sheaths used in neurointervention typically range in size from 4 to 9 Fr. For adult interventional procedures, 5–8 Fr sheaths are generally used since most guide catheters are sized between 5 and 8 Fr.
- The larger the sheath, the greater the rate of puncture site complications.

Angiographic and select catheters

- Catheters used for cerebral angiography come in a range of sizes and shapes but usually range from 4 to 6 Fr. They typically have tip curves to aid in selective catheterisation. Different vessel angulations may favour specific curves. Occasionally, it is necessary to try different catheters to achieve success.
- 'Select' catheters are introduced inside the lumen of guide catheters/long sheaths and used to select the great arteries of the aortic arch. It is necessary that they are longer than the guide catheter/long sheath in which they are inserted.

Guide catheters and long sheaths

- A *guide catheter* is a flexible and relatively wide internal diameter catheter that is typically inserted through a short sheath in a peripheral artery, such as the common femoral or radial artery. The catheter's tip is typically placed in the carotid or vertebral artery to provide a stable platform for more distal intervention.

- 6 Fr guide catheters can generally accommodate two devices simultaneously, e.g. a microcatheter and balloon microcatheter, or an intermediate catheter large enough for a single microcatheter. 8 Fr catheters can accommodate a 6 Fr intermediate catheter.
- Depending on the stiffness of the catheter and the tortuosity of the vasculature, the tip is placed in different locations. In the ICA, guide catheters with soft tips like the Benchmark may be placed in the cavernous segment if the artery is relatively straight but generally not distal to the ophthalmic origin. In the vertebral artery, soft catheters can sometimes be brought into the V4 segment if the anatomy is favourable. Stiffer catheters should be kept more proximal to avoid vessel dissection.
- A *long sheath* serves the same purpose as a guide catheter, and in practice is often exactly the same device, the difference being it is sited directly in the vessel without an additional vascular sheath. The main advantage of a long sheath, therefore, is that it requires a smaller arteriotomy at the puncture site. For example, an 8 Fr guide catheter requires an 8 Fr vascular sheath which, in turn, requires a 10 Fr arteriotomy (the outer diameter of a short sheath is typically 2 Fr larger than the inner diameter). However, an identically proportioned 8 Fr long sheath creates just an 8 Fr arteriotomy as the additional vascular sheath is not used.
- In practice, many guide catheters can be used as long sheaths and vice versa. This can lead to confusion over size designations. Guide catheters are usually named after their inner diameter whereas long sheaths are named after their outer diameter (like other sheaths). Therefore, an identically proportioned device may be sold in two versions with a different labelled size. For example, the 8 Fr Fubuki (Asahi) guide catheter is also sold as the 6 Fr Fubuki long sheath. The only difference is that the latter is packaged with an obturator. The obturator is placed inside the long sheath and reduces the ledge between the wire and the catheter as it is introduced through the arteriotomy into the artery over a wire.
- The conventional vascular sheath is often placed first and then exchanged for the long sheath with the same outer diameter.

Commonly used devices

- The Neuron Max (Penumbra) is a general-purpose long sheath/catheter. It is useful when proximal support and a relatively large inner diameter (0.088") is required. The tip is usually positioned in the straight cervical segment of the internal carotid or the extracranial vertebral artery. The tip is not generally brought inside the skull to avoid vessel dissection. It is also not commonly used via the radial artery as the catheter may kink. The catheter comes in 80 or 90 cm lengths. It can be used with or without an 8 Fr femoral sheath. Like all long sheaths, it comes with an obturator.
- The AXS Infinity LS (Stryker) is a general-purpose long sheath/catheter similar to the Neuron Max with an identical inner diameter (0.088"), coming in 70, 80, and 90 cm lengths. It is supportive proximally (probably more so) and can be used via the radial artery without a sheath, providing the vessel is large enough. It provides a stable platform when used in tortuous vessels. The AXS Infinity LS Plus is a larger, more flexible, version with a 0.091" inner diameter but still retaining the 8 Fr outer diameter.

- The Benchmark (Penumbra) is a general-purpose catheter that is smaller and more flexible than the above-mentioned. It can be used via the femoral artery with a 6 Fr groin sheath and via the radial artery with or without a sheath. The inner diameter is 0.071" and it comes in 95, 105, and 115 cm lengths. It has a very flexible distal segment that may be taken intracranially, obviating the need for intermediate catheters. It does not provide as much proximal support as larger catheters. There are newer Benchmark BMX 81 and 96 versions with, respectively, 7 Fr outer diameter/0.081" inner lumens, and 8 Fr outer diameter/0.96" inner lumens.
- The Envoy (Cerenovus) is a relatively stiff, inexpensive, guide catheter that comes in 5, 6, and 7 Fr variants. Lengths vary from 90 to 105 cm.
- The RIST (Medtronic) is a guide catheter designed for radial use. The intention is to provide good proximal support but allow the tip to be placed distally, obviating the need for an intermediate catheter.
- A range of other modern guide catheters/long sheaths are available. These tend to be proximally supportive and distally atraumatic. The 0.090" Cerebase DA (Cerenovus) is available in 70–95 cm lengths and has a very soft tip that can be brought distally. It can be used radially. The 0.088" Ballast (Balt) is an 80–100 cm guide catheter/long sheath which is often used radially.

Intermediate, distal access, and reperfusion catheters

- *Intermediate* or *distal access* catheters are inserted within guide catheters/long sheaths and used to provide a more stable and distal position through even tortuous anatomy. They are of particular use when lots of proximal support is required, e.g. deploying a flow diverter.
- *Reperfusion* or *aspiration* catheters are inserted within guide/catheters and designed to be taken to the clot face during thrombectomy. Negative aspiration force is applied to retrieve the clot. These catheters tend to have large inner lumens, so they can apply the greatest negative pressure to the thrombus, and longer lengths to reach the clot.
- There is overlap between the design of intermediate and reperfusion catheters and many can perform both functions.

Commonly used devices

- The Navien (Medtronic) is an intermediate catheter that comes in 0.058" and 0.072" inner diameter variants. It is a very supportive catheter and a good choice for stent and flow-diverter deployment. The support comes at the cost of rigidity, meaning that it cannot be taken as far distally as some other devices. It is not used as a reperfusion device.
- The Sofia (Microvention) is a very flexible and trackable catheter that can be used as a reperfusion or intermediate catheter. It comes in 5 Fr (0.055" inner diameter), Ex (standing for 'eXtra support and eXtra stability' with an 0.058" inner diameter), 6 Fr (0.070" inner diameter), and Plus 6 Fr (0.070" inner diameter) versions. These are highly navigable but not as supportive as some other devices.
- The RED (Penumbra) family of reperfusion catheters include 0.043", 0.062", 0.068", and 0.072" inner diameter variants. They have a lubricious outer coating designed to be easily trackable. They can be steam-shaped with a supplied mandrel, to help avoid it catching on the ophthalmic origin.

- The REACT (Medtronic) family of reperfusion catheters comes in 0.068" and 0.071" inner diameters and is designed to be easily trackable.
- The Vectra (Stryker) family of reperfusion catheters include 0.043", 0.071", 0.074", and 0.078" inner diameters. The latter is one of the largest reperfusion catheters available.
- The 3MAX, 4MAX, and 5MAX (Penumbra), are smaller reperfusion catheters with lumen sizes of, respectively, 0.035", 0.041", and 0.054". The 3MAX is especially good for aspiration of clots in small vessels.
- There are multiple other reperfusion catheters such as the Emboglide (Cerenovus) and Zoom 71 (Imperative Care). The MIVI Q (MIVI Neuroscience) features a novel design consisting of a flexible catheter section mounted on a control wire, which is designed to result in a greater overall system radius.
- The Fargo Mini (Balt) is a small and highly flexible intermediate catheter with an inner diameter of 0.040" and available in lengths 120 and 135 cm. It is useful in providing support for a single microcatheter. For example, the Fargo Mini can be positioned in the internal maxillary artery when taking a distal microcatheter into the middle meningeal artery to perform a fistula embolisation.

Microcatheters

- Microcatheters are used to access the small, distal vasculature or vascular lesions lying more proximally. They can be used to deliver coils, stents, liquid embolics (LEs), particles, and other devices/substances. They generally have very soft tips.
- Microcatheter tips can be heat shaped using a supplied mandrel to enhance catheterisation of vessels or aneurysms. Some systems also come with various pre-shaped tip options. Heat shaping also softens the tip, potentially reducing vessel trauma.
- There is a radiopaque tip marker. Microcatheters used for coil embolisation additionally have a proximal coil detachment marker.

Commonly used microcatheters

- The SL-10 (Stryker) is a general-purpose microcatheter commonly used for coil embolisation. The inner diameter is 0.0165" and the length is 150 cm and there is a distal coil detachment marker. It can also be used to deliver low-profile stents such as the Atlas (Stryker), LEO+ Baby (Balt), and LVIS Junior/Evo (Microvention). The SL-10 is not dimethyl sulfoxide (DMSO) compatible but can deliver *n*-butyl-2-cyanoacrylate (n-BCA) glue. Officially, only the SL-10 is compatible with Stryker Target coils.
- The Echelon-10 and Echelon-14 (Medtronic) general-purpose microcatheters are commonly used for coil embolisation, low-profile stent placement, and LE use. They both have the same inner diameter of 0.017" but the outer diameter of the Echelon-14 is greater than the Echelon-10, providing more support. The outer diameter of the Echelon-10 is less than the SL-10. Both microcatheters are 150 cm in length and feature distal coil detachment markers. The Echelon-14 is better suited for situations where rigidity is necessary, providing support during coiling of an acutely angled aneurysm after steam-shaping the catheter. In contrast, the Echelon-10 is more useful when space within the guide catheter is limited. Both microcatheters are compatible with DMSO allowing Onyx (and other LE) embolisation.

- The Headway (Microvention) microcatheter comes in 0.017", 0.021", and 0.027" sizes. The 0.017" variant (called the Headway 17 Advanced) is another 150 cm microcatheter similar to the Echelon and SL-10 that has a distal coil detachment marker. The 0.017", 0.021", and 0.027" microcatheters are useful for delivering stents and flow diverters. The Headway catheters are DMSO compatible.
- The Headway Duo (Microvention) low-profile microcatheter comes in two sizes which are named after their lengths rather than their diameters. The Headway Duo 156 is 156 cm long and has an inner diameter of 0.0165". It has a coil detachment marker. It is one of the longest and narrowest of all the coiling microcatheters. The Headway Duo 167 is 167 cm long and has an inner diameter of 0.013". It is DMSO compatible and useful for LE delivery for AVF/AVM embolisation. While the 167-length version does not have a coil detachment marker, it can be used to deliver small coils if necessary (specifically the Barricade from Balt, and ED 10 from Kaneka). The Target Nano (Stryker) coils also usually fit into the catheter although not reliably (they may get stuck or not detach).
- The Magic (Balt) is a low-profile microcatheter with 1.2, 1.5, or 1.8 Fr outer distal tips. These may be used with wires of maximum sizes respectively of 0.008", 0.009", and 0.010". It is typically used for n-BCA glue embolisation and is *not* DMSO compatible. The Spif Flow coils (Balt) coils can be delivered through this microcatheter. Preparation and usage are slightly different than other microcatheters:
  - Flush the packaging of the microcatheter before removing it.
  - The Magic catheter comes with a supplied insertion mandrel that runs the length of the catheter to help push it through the guide catheter.
  - Slightly withdraw the insertion mandrel and steam-shape the tip between your fingers (this requires practice!).
  - Once the tip is shaped, fully reinsert the mandrel.
  - Load the Magic catheter into the guide catheter. Thread the catheter for a length but do not poke the tip beyond the end of the guide. Next, remove the mandrel and protrude the Magic catheter into the blood vessel. Wait for blood to drip back from the hub.
  - Flush the Magic catheter with a 3 mL syringe of saline. Attach to a rotating haemostatic valve (RHV).
  - The Magic catheter can be navigated in three ways: leading with a wire (conventional technique), keeping the wire just before the tip, or by injecting jets of saline from a syringe attached to the hub (flow-directed technique).
- The Sonic (Balt) microcatheter is available in 1.2 or 1.5 Fr outer distal tips with inner diameters of, respectively, 0.0090" or 0.012". Unlike the Magic it is DMSO compatible. The tip of the catheter is detachable which prevents the whole length of the device getting glued into the intracranial circulation or rupturing the vessel when removing the device. It is important to be careful not to prematurely detach the tip of microcatheters with detachable tips when navigating through tortuous vasculature by keeping the microwire close to or distal to the tip. There should not be reflux proximal to the detachment point (indicated by a marker) when injecting n-BCA. There is an additional, more proximal, marker that should not be refluxed beyond when injecting other LEs (you can reflux slightly more with non-glue LEs).

- The Marathon (Medtronic) is a DMSO-compatible microcatheter with a 1.5 Fr outer distal tip useful for embolisation. Similar to the Headway Duo 167 certain coils can be delivered through this microcatheter.
- The Apollo (Medtronic) is a DMSO-compatible microcatheter available with a 1.5 Fr outer distal tip similar to the Marathon, but it has a detachable tip (which comes in lengths of 1.5, 3, and 5 cm).
- In addition, several specialist microcatheters are available, each specifically designed for certain applications. For instance, the Via series of microcatheters (including Via-17, Via-27, and Via-33) from Microvention are engineered for WEB deployment, while the Phenom series (Phenom-17, Phenom-21, and Phenom-27) from Medtronic are designed for deploying the Pipeline flow diverter. The XT series (XT-17 and XT-27) from Stryker are created for deploying the Surpass Evolve flow diverter, and the Trevo Pro and Trak-21 microcatheters from Stryker are designed for the Trevo stent retrievers. Although these microcatheters are designed for specific purposes, many of them can also be used in a general-purpose fashion.

Balloon devices

Balloon guide catheters

- Balloon guide catheters (BGCs) are designed with a balloon near their tip, which, when inflated and combined with lumen aspiration, aim to achieve flow reversal during MT. This technique is intended to minimise the risk of distal thrombus embolisation into other territories during clot retrieval.
- The balloon has to be prepared before use to remove air in the system by replacing the dead space with at least 50% contrast:saline mixture (similar to angioplasty catheters, see 'Angioplasty balloon catheters', p. 127). A test inflation is typically performed prior to use.

Devices

- The Merci (Stryker) is an older BGC, available in 8 and 9 Fr sizes.
- Several newer devices with larger inner diameters are now available, such as the Bobby (Microvention) with a 0.086" inner diameter, the Emboguard (Cerenovus) with a 0.087" inner diameter, and the Walrus (Q'Apel) with a 0.087" inner lumen. These devices are compatible with larger reperfusion catheters and are designed to be more easily navigable and proximally supportive.

Remodelling balloon catheters

- Balloon remodelling is the process of temporarily inflating a balloon catheter across the neck of an aneurysm during coil embolization, e.g. to prevent prolapse of coils into the parent artery.
- Similar to BGCs, balloons used in these devices are soft and compliant and will mould to the shape of the vessel. Balloon inflation is accomplished using a small syringe containing a contrast:saline mixture. The higher the contrast percentage, the greater the visibility but the less the compliance.

Single-lumen balloon catheters

- The first devices had a single lumen, i.e. the same lumen where the wire is passed for navigation is also used to inflate the balloon. The seal on the balloon is created when the wire is in place, and hence it is important not to withdraw the wire proximal to the tip of the catheter during procedures, as the balloon may become filled with blood.
- Preparation:
  - Flush the plastic case containing the balloon catheter (the dispenser coil) with saline to activate the hydrophilic coating.
  - Prepare a contrast:saline mixture in a pot with about 50–70% contrast.
  - Attach a one-way stopcock or flow-switch to a RHV. Then, attach a 5 mL syringe filled with the contrast:saline mixture to the stopcock and flush the RHV with the mixture to remove any air. Tighten the RHV and attach it to the balloon catheter. Flush the balloon catheter forward to fully purge the system.
  - Insert the microwire into the balloon catheter lumen via the RHV, but keep it proximal to the distal seal so that it does not protrude from the end. Flush the system again. Advance the guidewire until it passes distal to the catheter tip. The wire acts as a seal on the balloon at this point. Form a curve on the wire tip if desired.

- Use the same 5 mL syringe to perform a test inflation of the balloon to its nominal pressure underwater. Inspect the balloon for any abnormalities or air bubbles. If satisfied, deflate the balloon by aspirating on the syringe with the catheter tip submerged underwater.
- Once satisfied, fill a 1 mL syringe with the contrast:saline mix to about two-thirds full and replace the 5 mL syringe.

Commonly used single-lumen balloon catheters

- The Hyperform (Medtronic) is a single-lumen balloon with 3, 4, and 7 mm diameter sizes. The Hyperform pouts well into the neck of aneurysms. It is used with the supplied X-Pedion 0.010" microwire (which is difficult to navigate). Other 0.010" wires risk spontaneous balloon deflation during use, but the Asahi Chikai 10X seems to work well with the device.
- The Hyperglide (Medtronic) is a similar single-lumen balloon available in 3, 4, and 5 mm diameters and longer balloon lengths. Hyperform and Hyperglide are DMSO compatible.
- The Transform (Stryker) is a single-lumen balloon available in C ('Compliant') and SC ('Super Compliant') versions. The C balloon ranges in diameter from 3 to 5 mm and the SC balloon ranges from 3 to 7 mm. One advantage of the Transform is that it can accommodate a 0.014" wire, such as the Synchro-14.
- The Eclipse (Balt) comes in single- and dual-lumen versions (see below), in 4–6 mm balloon diameters and 7, 9, 12, 15, and 20 mm lengths (same as the dual-lumen version). It requires an 0.014" wire.
- The Copernic (Balt) is another single-lumen balloon that comes in 3–5 mm diameters and 10, 15, 20, 30 lengths and requires the Traxcess 0.014", Hybrid 0.012", or Hybrid 0.014" wires. The Copernic RC, a larger, longer version with balloon diameters measuring up to 10 mm and lengths up to 80 mm is designed for venous sinus protection during embolisation of dural fistulas. It requires the Transend or Traxcess 0.014" wire for usage.

Dual-lumen balloons

- Dual-lumen balloons feature one lumen for wire insertion and a separate lumen for balloon inflation. This design allows for continuous irrigation of saline during use, permits the withdrawal of wires proximal to the tip, and even (compatible) coil/stent deployment.
- Preparation:
  - Prepare a contrast:saline mixture in a pot with about 50–70% contrast.
  - Attach the microwire introducer or a blunt needle to a 5 mL syringe filled with the contrast:saline mixture and insert it into the bottom of the inflation port. Fill the port from deep to superficial to purge any air.
  - Remove the needle and attach the syringe directly to the inflation port. Hold the balloon tip vertically and slowly inject the syringe over about 60 seconds. Initially, you may see the balloon inflate with air,

but eventually a fluid level will appear, the air will be expelled, and the balloon will fill with fluid. Sometimes, it fills immediately with fluid. Ensure that the balloon is fully inflated by holding it vertically to expel any remaining air.
- Hold the balloon tip in the contrast:saline mix and aspirate to empty the balloon, being careful not to introduce any air into it.
- After deflating the balloon, remove the balloon tip from the liquid. Fill a 1 mL syringe with the contrast:saline mix to about two-thirds full and attach a one-way tap or flow switch to it. Attach this to the inflation port while taking care not to introduce any air bubbles.
- Flush a RHV with saline and attach it to the catheter hub. Insert the microwire into the balloon catheter until the tip protrudes from the end.

Commonly used dual-lumen balloon catheters

- The Scepter (Microvention) comes in C ('Compliant') and XC ('eXtra Compliant') versions. They all have 4 mm balloon diameters but have different lengths ranging from 10 to 20 mm. The Scepter takes a 0.014" diameter wire. The Scepter is DMSO compatible and can be used to deliver coils and low-profile stents such as the Atlas, LVIS Junior, and LEO+ Baby.
- The Scepter Mini (Microvention) is a smaller balloon catheter designed for distal access and LE embolisation. Inflating the balloon prevents reflux of the LE. It has a 0.009" inner lumen to be used with a 0.008" wire. It should be used with a low-viscosity LE, typically Squid 12. There are some differences in comparison to the normal Scepter:
  - A mandrel is inside the main lumen of the device and needs to be replaced with a wire before use.
  - A 1 mL syringe (instead of a 5 mL syringe), 100% contrast, is used for the test inflation.
  - This is replaced with a 0.25 mL syringe filled with 0.1 mL 100% contrast for use in the body.
  - The balloon dilates from 1.7 to 2.7 mm in diameter depending on injection of 0.01–0.04 mL of fluid.
  - Usually 0.02 mL is injected, giving a diameter of 2.2 mm.
  - A stopcock rather than a flow-switch should be used to keep the balloon inflated.
  - The device is compatible with 0.008" or smaller wires.
- The Eclipse 2L (Balt) has a 6 mm balloon diameter, ranging from 7 to 20 mm in length. The Eclipse can be used with a 0.014" wire. The Eclipse is DMSO compatible and can also be used to deliver low-profile stents.

Angioplasty balloon catheters

- Angioplasty balloon catheters are non-compliant, of variable size, and used to mechanically expand vascular stenosis. Larger balloons are used for carotid stenosis and smaller balloons have been developed for intracranial stenosis.
- Balloons are used over a wire (usually a microwire). Angioplasty balloon catheters typically use a 'rapid exchange' system whereby the catheter can be exchanged with a carotid stent using conventional length wires.

- Inflation devices are utilised to inflate balloons during procedures, and are specifically designed to measure pressure during inflation, preventing vessel damage and rupture from over-inflation. Pressure can be accurately adjusted using a rotating handle, and the balloons can be rapidly and completely purged by withdrawing the handle.
- Preparation:
  - Prepare a contrast:saline mixture with a ratio of 50% contrast and 50% saline in a pot.
  - Fill a 5 mL syringe with the contrast:saline mixture and attach a blunt needle to it. Insert the needle into the inflation port and fill the port from deep to superficial to avoid creating any bubbles.
  - Fill a 20 mL syringe with the 50% solution.
  - Remove the air from the system by withdrawing the plunger of the syringe to replace it with the contrast:saline mix in the syringe while tapping on the hub. Repeat this process three times.
  - Prepare the inflation device by holding the tubing tip in the contrast solution and rotating the handle anticlockwise to fill up the device with solution.
  - Once sufficient solution is inside the device, attach it to a three-way stopcock and attach to the angioplasty balloon.
  - Insert the stiff back end of the wire through the tip of the balloon catheter until the wire's tip is just protruding. Then, shape the wire to the desired curve.
- Examples of these devices include the pITA (Phenox) which ranges in size from 1.25 to 4 mm and is licensed for intracranial use and the Trek and MiniTrek (Abbott) which are available from 1.2 to 5 mm and designed as coronary angioplasty balloons.
- The Neurospeed (Acandis) is an intracranial balloon angioplasty device that enables stenting directly through the same catheter, thereby eliminating the need for potentially risky exchange manoeuvres, and speeding up the procedure.

Further reading

Brinjikji W, Starke RM, Murad MH, et al. Impact of balloon guide catheter on technical and clinical outcomes: a systematic review and meta-analysis. J NeuroInterv Surg. 2018;10(4):335–339.

Coils

A coil is a metallic wire with a preformed shape that can be detached within an aneurysm or blood vessel to reduce blood flow and induce thrombosis. This process produces a chronic inflammatory response, which involves the organisation of thrombus and fibrosis and eventual healing and stable occlusion.

The first cerebral aneurysm 'wiring' and electrothermic coagulation of an ICA aneurysm was performed in 1938 via a direct puncture technique utilising 30 feet of silver-enamelled wire. The Guglielmi Detachable Coils were the first detachable coils used in humans for aneurysm embolisation in 1990.

Features of coils

- Almost all coils used in neurointervention are detachable, which allows for safe repositioning or complete removal if necessary. Coils are typically made from platinum because it is radiopaque and biologically inert. Platinum is also unaffected by electrolysis, utilised for coil detachment. Alternatively, other coils can also be detached using a mechanical system.
- A wide range of coils are available, including electrolytically detachable coils such as Target (Stryker), Galaxy (Cerenovus), the Cosmos, MicroPlex, Hypersoft, Hyperframe, and Hydrofill series (Microvention), Optima and Barricade (Balt), and Kaneka's ED coils. Mechanically detachable coils include Axium (Medtronic), Avenir (Wallaby Medical), and Smart/PC400/PAC400 (Penumbra). Although many different coils are available, their utility is roughly comparable. Some coils may have a slight advantage in specific circumstances depending on different factors, particularly aneurysm size and shape and access route.
- Coils are available in various wire diameters to suit different clinical applications. The Spif Flow coils (Balt) have the lowest profile and can fit through the Magic catheters. These are not detachable and therefore cannot be repositioned once inserted. The next smallest coils are the ED-10 (Kaneka) and Barricade (Balt) coils, which can be deployed through 0.013" microcatheters. The Target Nano and Tetra (Stryker) coils are soft coils deployed through standard 0.0165" and 0.017" microcatheters and are good for small aneurysms (at least 1 mm). The SL-10 is the only microcatheter formally compatible with the Stryker Target Nano coils (other microcatheters may occasionally have detachment problems with these coils). The Tetra coils are specifically designed for small, wide-necked, aneurysms. Target Nano and Tetra often work through 0.013" catheters but can be unreliable. The PC400 (Penumbra) are large 0.020" coils and require the PX Slim 0.025" microcatheter. These coils are particularly useful for occluding venous sinuses or large arteries.
- Within a single range of coils, the coil diameter reduces as the size of the coil decreases to increase the softness. Generally, coils are labelled either '10' or '18', implying 0.010" or 0.018"; however, this only approximates the true diameter.
- Coils within a given range are available in different lengths and sizes. The diameter of the loop of the coil is typically listed first, followed by its stretched-out length. The first loop of the coil is usually smaller than the labelled coil diameter as the microcatheter must be positioned inside the aneurysm during deployment.

- Coils are available in two main types: filling and framing. Helical coils have a spring-like shape and are ideal for filling space. Framing coils, on the other hand, create a stable 'basket' in which subsequent coils can be placed without protruding outside. The diameter of the basket is typically similar to the spherical aneurysm dome, excluding any irregularities. For an elongated aneurysm, slightly over-sizing the coil may be necessary to fill the entire aneurysm. Complex, three-dimensional (3D), or 360 coils have non-helical shapes and are better for framing the aneurysm and forming the basket.

Further reading

Guglielmi G. History of the genesis of detachable coils: a review. J Neurosurg. 2009;111(1): 1–8.

Carotid stents

- Carotid stents are used to treat stenosis occurring in the cervical section of the carotid artery, frequently in conjunction with angioplasty. They are typically designed with a high radial force.
- The Carotid Wallstent (Boston Scientific) is the only cobalt alloy carotid stent. It is made from a single wire woven into a tubular stent structure.
- The majority of other carotid stents are composed of nitinol (a nickel–titanium alloy). These are generally laser-cut to create a tubular mesh stent structure. They have sequentially aligned annular rings interconnected by bridges.
- Nitinol stents are available in both open and closed-cell configurations. Open-cell stents, such as Zilver (Cook Medical), have larger gaps between struts which result in larger free-cell areas. In contrast, closed-cell stents have smaller gaps between struts.
- Carotid stents may be used with distal embolic filter protection devices such as the SpiderFX (Medtronic) or Emboshield (Abbott) to catch clots thrown off during angioplasty and deployment.
- Usage of carotid stents is described in Chapter 10 (see 'Carotid artery stenting', p. 400).

Further reading

Bosiers M, Deloose K, Verbist J, Peeters P. Carotid artery stenting: which stent for which lesion? Vascular. 2005;13(4):205–10.

Aneurysm-bridging stents

- Aneurysm-bridging stents act as a scaffold by sitting across the neck of the aneurysm to prevent coil prolapse and promote aneurysmal thrombosis. Over time, an endothelialised arterial layer forms over the struts of the stent.
- Most stents used in neurointervention are self-expanding, i.e. they expand immediately after being pushed out of the microcatheter (using an attached pusher wire).
- Many stents are manufactured from nitinol and have radiopaque platinum markers. They come in a range of lengths and diameters. Low-profile versions are available that can fit through 0.0165" microcatheters: Neuroform Atlas (Stryker), LVIS Junior/Evo (Microvention), Atlas (Stryker), and LEO+ Baby (Balt), and Accero/Acclino/Credo (Acandis).
- Stents can be categorised by the method of manufacture:
  - Laser-cut stents generally have reduced metal surface coverage (around 7–10%) and so are theoretically less thrombogenic. They usually deploy easily without shortening. Examples include the Neuroform Atlas (Stryker), Acclino/Credo (Acandis), Enterprise (Cerenovus), and the Solitaire (Medtronic).
  - Braided stents generally have a greater metal surface coverage (around 18–23%) and may also provide some flow-diverting properties (theoretically improving occlusion of the aneurysm). Examples include the LVIS, LVIS Evo (Microvention), LEO+ (Balt), and Accero (Acandis). These can be deliberately 'bunched up' over the neck of the aneurysm to improve neck coverage, and may provide some flow-diversion effect.
- To prevent introducing air into the circulation, stents must be flushed prior to use. This is achieved by introducing the end of the stent sheath into the RHV chamber and slightly tightening the valve. Once saline is seen to drip out, the proximal end of the stent sheath flushing is completed.
- Resheathable stents have the advantage of allowing repositioning during deployment, which can be useful in achieving optimal stent placement. In terms of laser-cut stents, the Atlas stent is non-resheathable whereas the Acclino/Credo, Solitaire, and the Enterprise are resheathable. Unlike most others, the Solitaire AB is an electrolytically detachable and thus fully resheathable. Braided stents are generally resheathable to a certain point of deployment (typically 80–90%).
- Neurointervention stents are generally unsheathed on a pusher wire that becomes detached when the stent is unsheathed proximal to the proximal end of the stent. After deployment, it is usually possible to re-enter the lumen of the stent using this wire.
- In contrast to flow diverters, it is possible with most stents to cross through the struts with a microcatheter to enter the lumen of an aneurysm for coiling after the stent has been deployed. If the braid is fine, as with the LVIS Evo, this can be challenging. Smaller microcatheters (Headway duo 156 and 167) are useful in this situation or microcatheter placement in the aneurysm prior to stent deployment ('jailing' technique) may be employed.

Flow diverters

- Flow diverters are braided fine-mesh stents that are placed across the neck of the aneurysm within the parent vessel to facilitate the redirection of blood flow away from the aneurysmal sac. This induces thrombosis of the aneurysm and the formation of an endothelialised arterial layer within the artery over days to months, often without requiring coiling of the aneurysm.
- Adjunctive coil embolisation (usually loosely packed) may result in faster thrombosis and probably reduces the risk of early haemorrhage sometimes seen in the weeks or months following treatment in large and giant aneurysms.
- The two variables affecting device permeability are porosity and pore density. Porosity is the percentage ratio of metal-free surface area to the total surface area. Pore density is the number of pores per unit surface area. Lower porosity (i.e. greater area percentage of metal over the aneurysm neck) and increased pore density are associated with greater aneurysm occlusion. Flow diverters generally work better on side-wall rather than bifurcation aneurysms.
- Device construction is broadly similar between manufacturers although the alloy differs. Flow diverters are commonly manufactured from cobalt–chromium (e.g. the Stryker Surpass Evolve) or nitinol (e.g. Phenox P64/P48, Microvention FRED, and Balt Silk).
- Extruded wires are woven into a complex collapsible tubular structure that allows the wires to move against each other to adapt to vessel anatomy and curvature. Due to the presence of metallic components which activate the clotting system via the platelet pathway, patients conventionally require pretreatment with dual antiplatelet therapy.
- Many manufacturers have adapted their devices to lower the thrombotic and thromboembolic risk. This involves a combination of precision engineering and polishing the struts to reduce platelet adhesion. A further modification is surface coating (e.g. the Shield coating with Pipeline, and Heal with Derivo). The addition of these agents is not considered to interfere with the physical properties of the device.
- The struts of flow diverters are small and are impossible to cross with a microcatheter to enter the aneurysm to place further coils (as with laser-cut and braided stents). If coils are required, it is necessary to either coil the aneurysm first, i.e. 'jail' the microcatheter in the aneurysm while deploying the flow diverter and then remove the jailed microcatheter after coiling. Note that the flow diverter will not fully expand until the jailed microcatheter is removed.
- A description of devices available is given in 'Flow diversion', p. 286.

Further reading

Bageac DV, Gershon BS, De Leacy RA. The evolution of devices and techniques in endovascular stroke therapy. In: Dehkharghani S, ed. Stroke [Internet]. Exon Publications; 2021: Chapter 9. https://www.ncbi.nlm.nih.gov/books/NBK572010/

Biondi A, Primikiris P, Vitale G, Charbonnier G. Endosaccular flow disruption with the Contour Neurovascular System: angiographic and clinical results in a single-center study of 60 unruptured intracranial aneurysms. J Neurointerv Surg. 2023;15(9):838–843.

Dholakia R, Sadasivan C, Fiorella DJ, Woo HH, Lieber BB. Hemodynamics of flow diverters. J Biomech Eng. 2017;139(2):021002.

Stent retrievers

- Stent retrievers are used to retrieve thrombus from the intracranial circulation.
- Numerous stent retrievers are now available including the Solitaire (Medtronic), Trevo (Stryker), Embotrap (Cerenovus), CatchView (Balt), pRESET (Phenox), Aperio Hybrid (Acandis), and Tigertriever (Rapid Medical).
- Stent retrievers are generally laser-cut and made of nitinol.
- Typical labelled unconstrained diameters for stent retrievers are between 3 and 6 mm. Note that labelled size is usually larger than the vessel diameters they are to be used in (e.g. 3 mm stent retrievers can often be used in smaller vessels, such as 1.5 or even 1 mm).
- Larger stent retrievers are usually delivered through 0.027" or 0.021" microcatheters. The lowest profile device is currently the Tigertriever 13 which fits through 0.013" microcatheters like the Marathon. The Tigertriever devices also, uniquely, are not self-expanding but their expansion is controlled via a hand-adjustable lever. They can thus be adjusted to the vessel size. The device is therefore similar in design to the Comaneci device.
- Usefully, the Catchview Mini (Balt) can also be deployed through the 0.013" Headway Duo (despite the apparent labelled size discrepancy).
- The Nimbus (Cerenovus) is a specifically designed 'rescue' stent retriever for tough clots, intended to be used after failure of standard stent retrievers. After deploying the stent and waiting, the microcatheter is re-advanced into the clot to 'pinch' it against the stent retriever before retrieval.
- A description of devices available is given in Chapter 9 (see 'Mechanical thrombectomy principles', p. 344).

Intrasaccular and neck-bridging devices

- These sit inside (intrasaccular) or across the neck of (neck-bridging) aneurysms. They are designed to treat aneurysms that are difficult to embolise with simple coiling, especially wide-necked bifurcation aneurysms.
- A key advantage of intrasaccular devices is their placement within the aneurysm itself rather than in the parent artery, minimising the need for antiplatelet medication. Consequently, they can be used more safely in acutely ruptured aneurysms.
- In elective aneurysms, patients might still be given a loading dose of antiplatelets before the procedure in case bail-out stenting is required. If stenting is not performed, aspirin alone is often continued for several weeks afterwards to reduce the risk of delayed thromboembolic complications. However, these medications are usually not required in the long term.
- Descriptions of common devices are given in Chapter 8 (see 'Intrasaccular devices', p. 298).

Gelatin, particles, and sclerosants

Particles

- Particles function by lodging within and obstructing small blood vessels. This results in reduced blood flow, which induces an inflammatory response and thrombosis. Typically, particle embolisation is temporary.
- They are cost-effective and versatile, making them useful in a variety of procedures, including tumour embolisation, epistaxis, and middle meningeal artery embolisation.
- Particles are composed of either polyvinyl alcohol or spherical acrylic polymer (microspheres). The latter may have a reduced tendency to clump together (resulting in a lower chance of inadvertent catheter blockage).
- They come in sizes ranging from 50 to 1200 μm. In tumour embolization, the smaller the size, the greater the risk of penetrating intratumoural anastomoses or dangerous anastomoses and causing ischaemic stroke and/or cranial nerve palsy. 250–300 μm is often a good compromise of efficacy and safety. Particle sizes <100 μm are generally avoided in neurointervention.

How to use particles

- Particles may be injected with the patient awake as they are non-painful. The risk of non-target embolisation is higher if the patient moves, however.
- The particles are usually suspended in approximately 50% contrast:saline solution, mixed in a plastic pot prior to aspirating into the syringe. Use different colour or sized syringes for the particles so they can be readily identified.
- It is advisable to use larger microcatheters (e.g. 0.027") to prevent clumping of particles within the catheter. However, this may not always be possible in smaller, more distal, vessels.
- The microcatheter cannot be wedged. Forward blood flow is required to inject particles.
- Mixing must be performed continuously during injection as particles have the tendency to sediment and clump together, potentially blocking the catheter.
- A useful technique to prevent clumping is to connect a 20 mL syringe to a 5 mL syringe using a three-way stopcock, which in turn is connected to the guide catheter. By turning the stopcock to block flow into the guide, you can inject the particle solution back and forth between the 20 mL and the 5 mL syringes to mix the particles thoroughly between injections. Once mixed, the solution remains in the 5 mL syringe, ready for injection into the catheter, and the stopcock can be adjusted to allow for catheter injections again.
- Apply a new "glue" blank roadmap.
- Inject in gentle puffs while watching the screen for the increase and decrease in opacity over the target. Watch in particular for reflux into the parent vessel. Initially there will be none but this will develop over the course of the procedure as forward flow is reduced.

- When significant reflux occurs, the injection must be stopped. At this point slowly and continuously inject saline to wash out the particles inside the dead space of the microcatheter while screening and continuing to watch for reflux.
- If the catheter becomes blocked during use it must be removed.
- After removal of the microcatheter aspirate blood from the guide catheter before further use or removal.

Sclerosants

- High-concentration alcohol (96%) can be used as an embolisation agent and acts by hyperosmolar damage and as a chemical irritant, causing vessel wall ischaemia and anoxia, and hence thrombosis.
- Sclerosants can be injected endovascularly or via direct puncture. It is useful to mix with radiopaque contrast medium for visualisation.
- Alcohol is painful when injected and so GA is generally used. Complications include profound local vasospasm and intoxication. Very rarely, cardiac arrest and pulmonary oedema can occur.
- Sodium tetradecyl sulphate (STS) is a detergent that denatures the cell membrane causing thrombosis. The agent is less painful during injection than alcohol. Contrast agents can be added, but are is usually mixed with air to form foam.
- Bleomycin is a cytotoxic antibiotic used in oncology as a chemotherapeutic agent. It is often used for venolymphatic malformations of the head and neck where it is typically injected directly into the lesion (although it can also be delivered intravenously). Very rarely it may cause pulmonary pneumonitis. The agent can cause hyperpigmentation of the skin particularly at sites where sticky plasters and tape are applied (and so these are avoided perioperatively).

Further reading

De Maria L, De Sanctis P, Balakrishnan K, Tollefson M, Brinjikji W. Sclerotherapy for venous malformations of head and neck: systematic review and meta-analysis. Neurointervention. 2020;15(1):4–17.

Cyanoacrylate glue

- Cyanoacrylate glue rapidly polymerises into an adhesive, permanent solid cast upon contact with ionic substances like blood. This causes an exothermic reaction resulting in temperatures of 80–90°C. Cyanoacrylates contain the same active ingredient as household superglue and are relatively inexpensive.
- The agent causes permanent vessel occlusion. Glue is very thrombogenic in comparison to other LEs.
- A disadvantage with cyanoacrylate use is that the microcatheter may become glued inside the vasculature. The microcatheter therefore has to be removed rapidly after injection. A second disadvantage is that the injection must be performed rapidly, and it can be difficult to control where the agent infiltrates.
- Cyanoacrylate glue comes in different formulations:
  - n-BCA such as Histoacryl (Braun) or Trufill (Cerenovus).
  - n-BCA mixed with the proprietary monomer metacryloxysulfolane to extend the polymerisation time as with Glubran 2 (GEM).
  - n-hexyl cyanoacrylate which has a lower adhesive strength to extend injection time without gluing in the microcatheter such as Magic Glue (Balt).
- When used, glue is mixed with lipiodol. Lipiodol is an oil-based radiopaque liquid that provides radiopacity, slows polymerisation, and increases viscosity. Usually, concentrations of cyanoacrylate in the mixture vary from 16% to 90%. Determining the correct concentration is an art and varies depending on several factors, particularly blood vessel diameter, location of the microcatheter, and velocity of blood flow. To occlude rapid shunts and aneurysms, a 50% concentration is typically used. For AVM treatments where the microcatheter is relatively proximal, a 25% concentration might be used.
- The chemical element tantalum, which comes in powder form, can also be added to increase radiopacity. This is typically necessary at 50% or more concentrations of cyanoacrylate. Acetic acid is another substance that can be added to create an acidic solution to delay polymerisation.
- Glue can be injected through practically any microcatheter, in contrast to Onyx/Squid/PHIL, which require DMSO compatibility. Theoretically, some catheters are more resilient than others with the lipiodol component and there is a small risk of dissolving the inner lining of the device. In practice, glue injections are generally quite rapid and so the risk is low.
- Some syringes (such as the ones sold by Guerbet) are labelled as lipiodol compatible. These are probably more resilient than normal syringes where there is a theoretical risk of the substance damaging the syringes if left inside for a long time. Therefore, if non-lipiodol syringes are used, it is important to inject soon after drawing up the mixture.
- Very small catheters such as the 'flow-directed' Magic (Balt) and Sonic (Balt) may be used to navigate into very small, tortuous, or distal vessels.
- It is absolutely mandatory to thoroughly flush the microcatheter with a 5–10% glucose (dextrose) solution prior to use to prevent polymerisation of glue within the catheter lumen.
- The substance is versatile, although its use has been greatly superseded by copolymer LEs such as Onyx. Injecting glue takes experience and may produce unpredictable results. Glue may rapidly penetrate into the vein in high-flow shunts risking venous hypertension and haemorrhage.

In comparison to LEs, multiple injections via different pedicles are usually necessary. In comparison, however, glue is more thrombogenic and produces less artefact than copolymer LEs.

- Cyanoacrylates and lipiodol can damage balloons and should not be used with balloon catheters.

How to inject glue

(See Figure 4.1.)

- Equipment: two 3 mL syringes (it is suggested that the same size syringe is used every time to inject glue to increase familiarity with the feel of the injection), 2 mL of glue (usually two vials), 2 mL of lipiodol (usually two vials), and 5% glucose (or similar non-ionic solution).

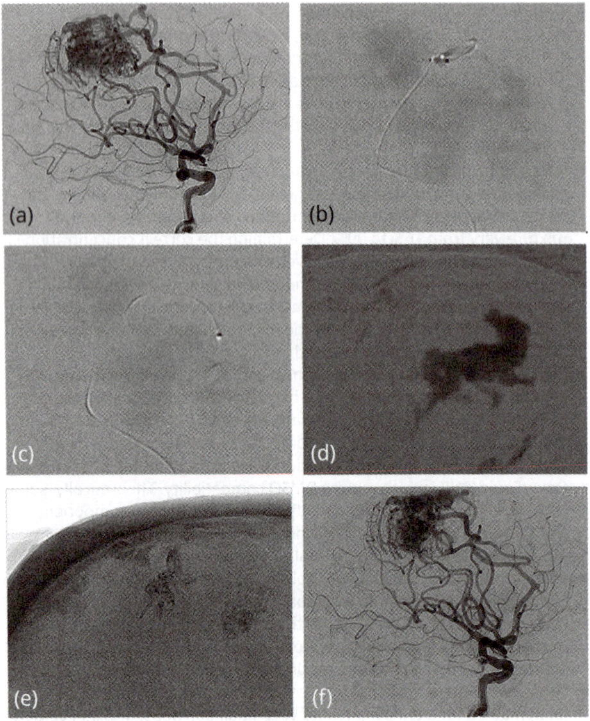

Figure 4.1 Glue partial embolisation of an AVM. (a) A large parietal AVM is identified, with multiple feeders. (b) A Magic 1.5 microcatheter was navigated into one of the feeders. Initial microangiography identifies the AVM, but the Magic is seen to be folded back on itself. (c) The microcatheter is straightened by tugging it gently with the wire in place. (d) Injection of glue under fluoroscopy roadmap. (e) Unsubtracted exposure showing final glue cast after a second injection. (f) Final angiography revealing reduction in the posterior compartment of the AVM.

- The glue and lipiodol is mixed in a Gallipot to the desired concentration. Mixing 2 mL of glue and 2 mL of lipiodol would be 50% concentration. Varying ratios of glue:lipiodol affect the rate of polymerisation. Polymerisation times can be increased from about 5 s to several minutes by decreasing the amount of glue in the mixture. High-flow shunts require higher polymerisation whereas low-flow shunts or the situation of flow-arrest requires lower concentrations. Tantalum must be added for radiopacity if 50% or more glue is added. Continue to mix the glue until just before injection so that it does not harden.
- The glucose is drawn up into a labelled 3 mL syringe.
- The anatomy of the target lesion is defined. A cone beam CT scan is often helpful. The desired working projection for navigation and injection can then be chosen.
- Often small, distal, arteries must be navigated first. The Magic (Balt) or Sonic (Balt) catheters are particularly useful as they have small diameter tips but supportive proximal shafts. It is often useful to use a triaxial system in these distal vessels, e.g. using the Fargo Mini (Balt) as an intermediate catheter.
- A wedged position is ideal for injection of glue to prevent reflux. If not wedged, make sure that the catheter is not abutting the wall of the vessel or curved back on itself.
- Perform microcatheter angiography to identify the specific anatomy of the injected vessels.
- Prepare a blank glue roadmap. Inject contrast into the dead space of the microcatheter.
- Irrigate the hub of the microcatheter with glucose and then inject through the microcatheter. Screen when injecting the glucose as contrast within the dead space of the microcatheter will be expelled from the syringe and you will appreciate what the glue injection will look like.
- Next, inject the glue while screening. Watch carefully for reflux while injecting. When you have achieved the desired result, aspirate on the syringe while rapidly pulling out the microcatheter. Let the guide catheter hub drip back with blood to ensure that no glue particles are within the guide catheter.
- Perform angiography to assess the result.

Complications

- Blocked catheter. If the injection is too slow or there has been insufficient glucose irrigation, the glue can polymerise inside and block the catheter. In addition to this being an annoyance, the build-up of pressure can potentially rupture the catheter, causing glue to leak at the rupture site (which may not be seen on the monitor).
- Catheter glued in. There is the risk of gluing the catheter tip in place. Try slowly pulling on the catheter, wait, and then repeat. Pulling on the catheter too hard risks rupturing the vessel. If the catheter cannot be removed without excessive force (risking haemorrhage), it may be necessary to leave it in place, cutting the end off at the access site. The patient is typically left on antiplatelet or anticoagulant for a period of time.
- Toxicity. Cyanoacrylates can cause toxic tissue damage due to the exothermic polymerisation reaction and release of compounds such as acryl acetate and formaldehyde. Perioperative corticosteroids are sometimes used to ameliorate these effects.

Copolymer liquid embolics

Onyx

- The Onyx Liquid Embolic System (Medtronic) is composed of the copolymer ethylene vinyl alcohol (EVOH) dissolved in DMSO together with suspended tantalum powder to provide contrast for visualisation under fluoroscopy. The name comes from the dark grey colour of the liquid. Unlike cyanoacrylate, Onyx is non-adhesive. It is particularly useful in DAVF and AVM treatment.
- Onyx requires shaking for 20 minutes prior to use.
- There are three formulations:
  - Onyx 18 is 6% EVOH and 94% DMSO. This is lower viscosity and will travel further and penetrate deeper. It is useful for low-flow situations.
  - Onyx 20 is 6.5% EVOH and 93.5% DMSO.
  - Onyx 34 is 8% EVOH and 92% DMSO. This is higher viscosity and is useful for embolisation of larger vessels and fistulas.
- In the packet is a 1.5 mL vial of Onyx, a 1.5 mL vial of DMSO, and three 1 mL Onyx delivery syringes.
- Onyx is delivered by controlled injection through a DMSO-compatible microcatheter. On contact with blood, the DMSO solvent dissipates, causing the EVOH copolymer to precipitate into a spongy cast. Unlike glue, it does not polymerise.

Squid

- Squid (Balt) is a non-adhesive LE with similar properties to Onyx. It has the same composition as Onyx: an EVOH copolymer dissolved in DMSO with tantalum powder (for radiopacity). The main difference is that the tantalum is micronised to decrease the powder grain size. This is intended to cause a slower precipitation of the radiopaque powder, reduce clumping (which can cause microcatheter blockage), to increase visibility and make the agent more homogeneous. Squid is also black (like squid ink).
- Squid requires shaking for 20 minutes prior to use.
- There are a range of formulas:
  - SQUID34: high-viscosity version.
  - SQUID34LD: 30% lower radiopacity ('Low Density') to avoid the oversaturated effect. Achieved by having a lower amount of tantalum.
  - SQUID18: the standard formulation for AVM embolisation.
  - SQUID 18LD: lower-opacity version.
  - SQUID12: lower viscosity to allow deeper penetration into the nidus and to reach smaller distal vessels.
  - SQUID 12LD: lower-opacity version.

Menox

- Menox (Meril Life Sciences) is another agent similar to Onyx composed of EVOH copolymer dissolved in DMSO with micronised tantalum powder.
- It comes in 18, 20, and 34 strengths (also similar to Onyx).

PHIL

- Precipitating Hydrophobic Injectable Liquid, or PHIL, is a non-adhesive LE with similar properties to Onyx but a different composition. It is composed of two copolymers (polylactide-co-glycolide and polyhydroxyethylmethacrylate) as its active components and triiodophenol (an iodine compound) covalently bound to the two copolymers to give radiopacity. This is then dissolved in DMSO.
- No shaking is required prior to use.
- The liquid is white after precipitating (yellow beforehand) so may be more suitable for subcutaneous vascular malformations. It is more homogeneous and has fewer artefacts on CT/MRI than Onyx.
- It is less radiopaque than Onyx and more difficult to see, particularly in small calibre vessels. The liquid has the potential for greater embolic capacity per volume due to a higher concentration of the copolymer. Due to the increased homogeneity, there is a lower risk of microcatheter blockage in comparison to Onyx. The substance overall tends to be less viscous than Onyx with improved forward flow. This brings with it, however, the increased possibility of non-target embolisation and early venous penetrance.
- PHIL comes with two prefilled 1.0 mL syringes of PHIL and DMSO, respectively.
- The following formulations are available: (i) 25%: low viscosity (the standard formulation); (ii) 30%: medium viscosity; and (iii) 45%: high viscosity.

Obtura

- Obtura is a novel, third-generation LE agent with promising utility in AVMs.
- It possesses the unique quality of losing its radiopacity after embolisation, enhancing the visualisation of AVM vasculature and helping to ensure that small, previously radiologically obscure shunts are indeed embolised. There may, therefore, be potential in improving embolised AVM occlusion rates.

How to inject copolymer liquid embolics

- Onyx and Squid (but not PHIL) require mechanical shaking 20 minutes prior to injection.
- Navigate the microcatheter to the pedicle to be injected and perform microcatheter angiography. This is usually as close to the point of fistulisation as possible.
- Identify the anatomical space that you want to fill with the LE, including other feeding pedicles. Ensure that you understand how far you can allow the LE to reflux and any dangerous anastomoses.
- Prepare a blank glue roadmap on the fluoroscopy machine.
- Fill the dead space of the microcatheter with DMSO, including the hub. DMSO often results in a pungent odour on the breath/skin for several hours after the procedure. Patients should be counselled about this beforehand. This is not related to toxicity.

- DMSO must be injected slowly because it can cause endothelial necrosis if injected too rapidly. In addition, bradycardia, hypotension, and even asystole can be induced during the injection of DMSO or LE. This is the trigeminocardiac reflex and is thought to be caused by chemical stimulation of the sensory nerve endings of the trigeminal nerve. Impulses are transmitted back to the motor nucleus of the vagus, via the reticular activating formation.
- Start screening and injecting the LE. Initially the LE will fill the dead space of the microcatheter and nothing will be seen on the monitor. It is useful to start a timer at this point.
- When the LE exits the microcatheter tip, it will become visible on the screen. Continue injecting if the LE is moving in the desired direction. However, if it begins to reflux excessively or enters unwanted areas, pause the injection and screening.
- LEs behave in a 'lava-like' fashion with a hard outer crust and liquid centre. The major advantage over glue is the slow precipitation times allowing for longer injections and greater control. This means that LE can often be injected through a single pedicle of a fistula/AVM as it can reflux into and occlude the other feeding pedicles through the fistula. It has good visibility which comes at the expense of some artefact on CT imaging.
- After a sufficient pause (30–40 s), start to inject again. If it again fills an undesirable space then repeat the pause. Eventually the undesirable space will become occluded with the LE, and it should fill the target space. It might be necessary to build up a plug of the agent proximal to the catheter tip to prevent reflux, and this can take some time.
- When you think you have achieved sufficient occlusion, perform an angiogram from the guide catheter to confirm.
- When removing the microcatheter, apply constant, gentle, slow, tension. If the tip is detachable, it will probably detach at some point, allowing the body of the microcatheter to be retrieved. It is obviously desirable to leave the microcatheter inside the body rather than avulsing a vessel by tugging too hard.

Tips

- The 'pressure cooker' technique addresses the issue of proximal reflux of LE into the injecting pedicle, a common challenge during injections. This involves using a second microcatheter to create a plug of coils and/or glue between the tip of the injecting microcatheter and the detachment zone. This method prevents reflux, establishes a 'wedge-flow' condition for the distal injecting microcatheter, reduces blood flow through fistulous compartments, and enhances the capability to push LE continuously into the nidus. It is beneficial to place the coils first before injecting glue, to avoid unintentionally occluding the feeding pedicle distal to the injecting microcatheter, thereby preserving the route to treat the fistula/AVM. Alternatively, coils alone can be used to form the plug without glue, but this is less effective. In addition, you can inject some LE prior to forming the glue plug, to avoid blocking the LE microcatheter tip.

- If the LE is not shaken for long enough, or there is a prolonged delay after removing from the shaker device, there may be aggregate formation (clumping) of tantalum. This can result in variable opacification and uneven resistance in the catheter. Microcatheter hub adaptors are provided and may also help with this clumping.
- Trigeminocardiac reflex. Bradycardia, hypotension, and even asystole can be induced during the injection of DMSO or LE (the 'trigeminocardiac reflex'). It is usually sufficient to stop injecting and wait to normalise the heart rate and blood pressure. Occasionally, vagolytics and sympathomimetics may be required.

Further reading

Chapot R, Stracke P, Velasco A, et al. The pressure cooker technique for the treatment of brain AVMs. J Neuroradiol. 2014;41(1):87–91.

Vollherbst DF, Chapot R, Bendszus M, Möhlenbruch MA. Glue, Onyx, Squid or PHIL? Liquid embolic agents for the embolization of cerebral arteriovenous malformations and dural arteriovenous fistulas. Clin Neuroradiol. 2022;32(1):25–38.

Non-vascular procedures

Periprocedural management *146*
Fluoroscopic-guided lumbar puncture *148*
Static myelography and cisternography *151*
Dynamic fluoroscopic myelography *153*
Fluoroscopic-guided lumbosacral nerve root injection and medial branch block *158*
CT-guided lumbosacral nerve root injection *162*
Fluoroscopic-guided transpedicular thoracolumbar spinal biopsy *164*
CT-guided thoracolumbar spinal biopsy *166*
Vertebroplasty and kyphoplasty *168*
Percutaneous venolymphatic malformations *172*

Periprocedural management

Standard management

- For all procedures described in this chapter, the following should be undertaken:
  - Review the referral and previous imaging.
  - Confirm the patient's anticoagulation and allergy status.
  - Check preprocedural full blood count and clotting screen, if required.
  - Confirm symptoms correlate with referral.
  - Obtain verbal and written consent.
  - Mark laterality if appropriate.
  - Perform the WHO Surgical Safety Checklist.

Equipment

- The following equipment is assumed for all sterile procedures and should be used unless otherwise stated:
  - Sterile gloves and gown.
  - Sterile drapes.
  - Cleaning solution (e.g. 0.5% chlorhexidine).
  - Sterile gauze.

Periprocedural anticoagulation/antiplatelets

- Anticoagulation guidance for spinal interventional procedures varies significantly according to both the level of procedural risk and the type of anticoagulation therapy.
- For comprehensive guidance relating to specific procedures and anticoagulants, refer to Goodman et al. (2017). The summary guidelines are reproduced in Table 5.1.

Table 5.1 The Modified SIS–ASRA antiplatelet and anticoagulant guideline of management prior to interventional spinal procedures

	High-risk Vertebral augmentation, intrathecal catheter, spinal cord stimulation	**Intermediate-high risk** Cervical/thoracic/sacral-1 transforaminal, cervical/thoracic disc stimulation, interlaminar epidural injection, caudal epidural injection, atlantoaxial joint block	**Intermediate-low risk** Transforaminal lumbar disc stimulation, lumbar sympathetic hypogastric plexus, ganglion impar radiofrequency neurotomy	**Low risk** Cervical/thoracic/lumbar medial branch block or zygapophyseal (facet) joint injection, posterior approach sacroiliac joint injection
Aspirin, including combinations	Shared decision-making*		Continue	
Non-aspirin NSAIDs	Consider off for 5 half-lives		Continue	
COX-2 inhibitors, SSRIs	Continue		Continue	

Table 5.1 (*Contd.*)

General anticoagulants		
Enoxaparin (LMWH)	Off 12–24h	Off 12–24h
Heparin, unfractionated	Continue if dose <5000 units twice daily	Continue
Warfarin	Off 4–5 days. INR ≤1.3 on day of procedure	INR at lowest recommended therapeutic range
Phosphodiesterase inhibitors		
Cilostazol, pentoxifylline	Off 2 days	Continue
Dipyridamole	Off 2–7 days	Continue
Novel oral anticoagulants (NOACs: direct thrombin and Xa inhibitors)		
Apixaban, edoxaban, rivaroxaban	Off 3 days	Continue
Dabigatran	Off 5 days or 6 days in renal impairment	Continue
Glycoprotein IIb/IIIa inhibitors		
Eptifibatide, tirofiban	Off 8–24h	Off 8–24h
Abciximab	Off 3–5 days	Off 3–5 days
P2Y12 inhibitors		
Ticagrelor	Off 5 days	Continue
Clopidogrel, prasugrel	Off 7 days	Continue
Ticlopidine	Off 14 days	Continue
Fibrinolytic agents		
Fondaparinux	Off 4 days	Continue

Note: clinical judgement supersedes recommendations as each patient-procedure situation is different. Stopping antiplatelet/anticoagulant agents should occur in consultation with the prescribing provider. From left to right, risk of bleeding decreases based on firm evidence (far left and far right columns) and theoretical/mechanistic suggestions (middle two columns). Where vertebral level is not specified, all levels are implied.

*The indication for aspirin use should be assessed, and shared decision-making regarding procedural management should be coordinated between the prescribing physician and pain interventionalist.

ASRA, American Society of Regional Anesthesia and Pain Medicine; COX, cyclooxygenase; INR, international normalised ratio; LMWH, low-molecular-weight heparin; NSAID, non-steroidal anti-inflammatory drug; SIS, Spine Intervention Society; SSRI, selective serotonin reuptake inhibitor.

Further reading

Goodman BS, House LM, Vallabhaneni S, Mallempati S, Willey MR, Smith MT. Anticoagulant and antiplatelet management for spinal procedures: a prospective, descriptive study and interpretation of guidelines. Pain Med. 2017;18(7):1218–1224.

Scott M, Stones J, Payne N. Antiseptic solutions for central neuraxial blockade: which concentration of chlorhexidine in alcohol should we use? Br J Anaesthesia. 2009;103(3):456.

Fluoroscopic-guided lumbar puncture

Fluoroscopic-guided lumbar puncture (LP) is performed when previous non-guided attempts have failed or are not possible, e.g. due to extensive spinal metalwork or challenging anatomy.

Indications

- Diagnostic CSF sampling.
- Assessment of opening pressures.
- Diagnostic/therapeutic CSF taps.

Contraindications

- Uncorrected coagulopathy (INR >1.4 or anticoagulated patient).
- Suspected raised intracranial pressure (perform cranial imaging if unsure).
- Local or systemic infection.

Antiplatelet and anticoagulant usage

- LP specific recommendations are given in Dodd et al. (2018). In summary:
  - Aspirin 75 mg OD can be continued.
  - Other antiplatelet/anticoagulant medications should be withheld if safe to do so (the specific time depends on the agent).

Equipment

- 22 or 20 G spinal needle: lower gauge (larger bore size) encourages CSF flow.
- Manometer and three-way stopcock.
- Labelled specimen tubes according to indication.
- LA.
- Tubing to connect the spinal needle.

Technique

(See Figure 5.1.)

- The procedure can be performed with the patient in either a prone or lateral position. However, for accurate measurement of CSF pressure, the manometer must be at the same level as the needle tip, and hence it is easier if the patient is lateral.
- Single- or biplane fluoroscopy can be used. Ensuring that the detectors are aligned face-on and laterally to the spine (which is not always the same as the patient) is crucial. Failure to do so could result in significant discrepancies between the needle tip's actual and perceived locations.
  - In the AP monitor, examine the pedicles to ensure they are en face and symmetrical. Slightly angle the AP detector caudally to visualise a radiolucent window, which serves as the target for your needle path.
  - Align the lateral detector so that it is en face with the lateral aspect of the vertebral bodies and spinous processes, ensuring there is no overlap. This alignment should provide a clear view of the spinal canal. The pedicles should be aligned on top of each other. You should also be able to see the gap between adjacent spinous processes, indicating the needle path.

- Identify a suitable puncture level under fluoroscopic guidance. Normally the conus medullaris is at L1–L2 in adults. L2–L3 or below is therefore generally considered safe, but optimally confirm this on MRI if available.
- Sterilise and drape the area. Inject LA into the skin first by raising a bleb and then injecting more deeply in the estimated needle path. More anaesthetic can be injected via the spinal needle if required.
- Insert and advance the spinal needle slowly in the plane of the beam. Screen AP and lateral intermittently to ensure the needle is centred and to assess depth. Should you find yourself on an incorrect trajectory, you will need to withdraw the needle (usually more than anticipated) before estimating a more appropriate angle and proceeding forward once more.
- As the needle passes beyond the ligamentum flavum there is often a slight release of pressure. Remove the stylet and confirm CSF flow. If absent, advance 1 mm at a time and repeat.
- Measure opening pressure: connect the three-way tap and manometer to the needle. Take readings once the CSF meniscus stops rising.
- Collect samples as required (typically 2–3 mL per sample).
- Replace the stylet and remove the needle. Clean and dress the puncture site.
- The patient should lie on their back for approximately 30 min, after which they may return home.

Tips

- Spinal needles are bevelled with short and long ends (Figure 5.2). There is usually a notch in the stylet which aligns with the short end. As such, when directing the needle, it will steer away from the side with the notch towards the needle tip.
- Angling the bevel's short head cranially encourages CSF flow.
- Head elevation, cough, and Valsalva manoeuvres can improve CSF return.

Complication avoidance and management

- Post-LP headache risk increases with the number of attempts. It is managed with bed rest, analgesia, and caffeine.

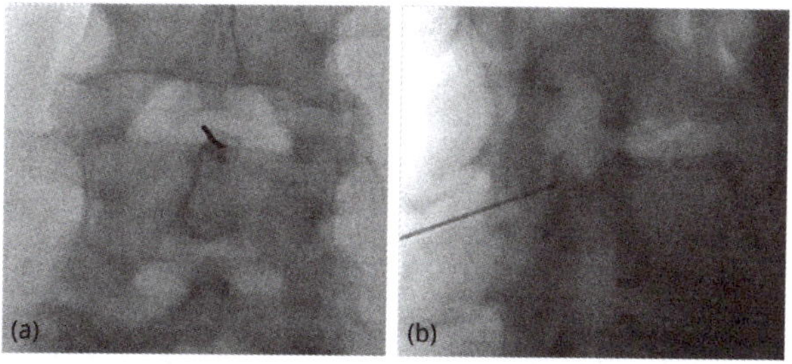

Figure 5.1 Lumbar puncture. (a) AP and (b) lateral images demonstrating final needle position. Images courtesy of Dr William Brown and Dr Steve Morgan.

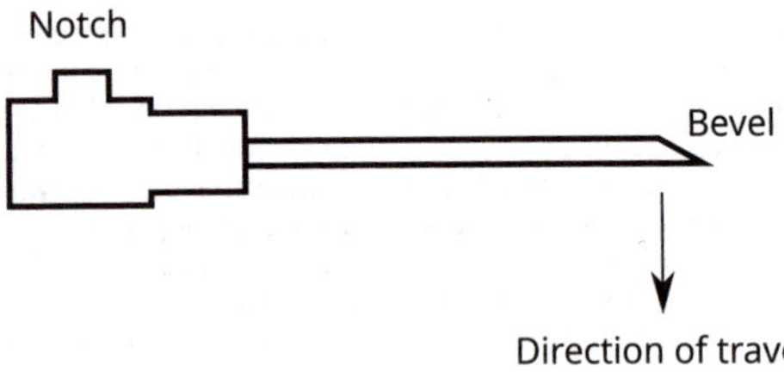

Figure 5.2 Spinal needle and direction of travel.

- A blood patch may be required in refractory cases of CSF leak.
- Epidural/subdural haematoma is rare but increased with coagulopathy or antiplatelet usage. It should be recognised by increasing pain and/or neurological deficit. MRI can be used for confirmation. Neurosurgical advice should be sought.

Further reading

Cauley KA. Fluoroscopically guided lumbar puncture. AJR Am J Roentgenol. 2015;205(4):W442–W450.

Dodd KC, Emsley HCA, Desborough MJR, Chhetri SK. Periprocedural antithrombotic management for lumbar puncture: Association of British Neurologists clinical guideline. Pract Neurol. 2018;18(6):436–446.

Karambelkar A, De Jesus O. Fluoroscopy lumbar puncture assessment, protocols, and interpretation. In: StatPearls [Internet]. StatPearls Publishing; 2023. https://www.ncbi.nlm.nih.gov/books/NBK570637/

Static myelography and cisternography

Static myelography and cisternography involve intrathecal administration of contrast into the spinal subarachnoid space and intracranial basal cisterns. They are useful for assessing compressive myelopathy and radiculopathy, particularly when MRI is contraindicated.

Occult CSF leakage is best assessed through a dynamic technique (see 'Dynamic fluoroscopic myelography', p. 153).

Contraindications

- *As for LP* (see 'Fluoroscopic-guided lumbar puncture', p. 148).
- Allergy to iodinated contrast media.

Equipment

- *As for LP*.
- Non-ionic iodinated contrast media approved for intrathecal injection (e.g. iohexol 240 mg/mL).
- 20 mL syringe and drawing-up quill.

Technique

- *Initial steps are as for LP.*
- Once free drainage of CSF is observed, connect tubing to the needle and conduct a test injection of 1–2 mL of contrast under fluoroscopy to verify the flow of contrast within the thecal sac and not in the epidural/ subdural space. If the contrast is in the thecal sac, the nerve roots become outlined. If epidural, a globular collection of contrast may be seen in the anterior or posterior epidural space.
- Administer the contrast injection gradually under fluoroscopy. The overall dosage of contrast should not exceed 3 g of iodine. Therefore, e.g. when using iohexol 240, do not exceed 12.5 mL.
- Remove the needle and encourage contrast flow to the relevant level via table tilting and patient rotation under fluoroscopic guidance.
- Obtain AP, oblique, and lateral images at relevant levels.
- Transfer the patient to the CT scanner to image the relevant levels. A single-slice acquisition at the level of interest is necessary to confirm contrast has entered this part of the canal. If necessary, further patient movement manoeuvres can be performed.
- Patients are observed for a short period of bed rest and should remain hydrated. The head should remain slightly elevated to avoid intracranial contrast accumulation.

Tips

- Tilting the couch head down by roughly 10° can help contrast flow to the thoracic spine.
- Flexion and extension views can help demonstrate dynamic cord or nerve root compression. Spinal flexion and extension can also help overcome extradural blocks to contrast passage.

Complication avoidance and management

- Globular collections of contrast on test injection indicate epidural or subdural injection. These can be aspirated out through the needle and then the needle repositioned.

- Post-myelographic seizures can occur within minutes to hours of the procedure. There have been reports of post-myelographic seizures in patients taking certain seizure threshold-lowering medications and some sites discontinue these prior to performing the procedure. There is no compelling evidence to support this practice, however (Shah et al., 2018). It is best to consult local protocols.

Further reading

American Society of Neuroradiology. ACR–ASNR–SPR Practice parameter for the performance of myelography and cisternography. Revised 2024. https://www.asnr.org/practice-guidelines/

Harreld JH, McMenamy JM, Toomay SM, Chason DP. Myelography: a primer. Curr Probl Diagn Radiol. 2011;40(4):149.

Shah LM, Kranz PG, Anzai Y, et al. Critical assessment of myelography practices: a call for rational guideline revision. AJNR Am J Neuroradiol. 2018;39(12):2378–2384.

Dynamic fluoroscopic myelography

- Spontaneous intracranial hypotension is caused by leakage of CSF from the thecal sac. Most commonly, it presents with an abrupt onset of persistent headache worsening in the upright position and subsiding after lying down. Other symptoms include tinnitus, decreased hearing, dementia, and decreased level of consciousness.
- A low opening CSF pressure (<6 cmH_2O) may be present but pressures in the normal range (6–20 cmH_2O) or even higher are possible. This suggests that the pathophysiology is not related to low pressure but rather low volume.
- Patients should optimally be diagnosed and treated within 12 weeks of symptom onset because compensatory mechanisms, increasing the rate of CSF production, take over, and treatment after 12 weeks may result in replacement of their low pressure/volume headache with a high-pressure headache.

Imaging

- The Bern score can be used to assess the likelihood of a spinal CSF leak based on cranial MRI:
    - Major signs (assigned 2 points) are: pachymeningeal enhancement, engorgement of the venous sinus, and effacement of the suprasellar cistern of ≤4 mm.
    - Minor signs (assigned 1 point) are: subdural fluid collections, effacement of the prepontine cistern of ≤5 mm, and a mamillopontine distance of ≤6.5 mm.
    - 2 or fewer points is classified as low probability, 3–4 as intermediate, and 5 or above as high probability. However, note that even a Bern score of 0 does not exclude a leak.
- Spinal imaging may reveal the presence of spinal longitudinal extradural collections (SLECs) (Figure 5.3), best seen on high-resolution sagittal T2 volumetric sequences. These help to determine the cause of the leak.

Causes

- May be categorised into the following four types:
    1. Mechanical tears in the ventral dura usually due to sharp degenerative discs or endplate osteophytes (Figure 5.4a,b). These are invariably SLEC positive.
    2. Lateral tears in the dura not associated with disc disease. These are also always SLEC positive. May be caused by thin or dehiscent dura (Figure 5.4c,d).
    3. CSF–venous fistulas between the spinal subarachnoid space and a paraspinal vein resulting in rapid shunting of CSF. The fistula is usually located in the nerve root sleeve. Perineural diverticula are commonly associated. These are SLEC negative (Figure 5.4e).
    4. Distal nerve root sleeve leaks into the adjacent fascial planes. These are SLEC negative.

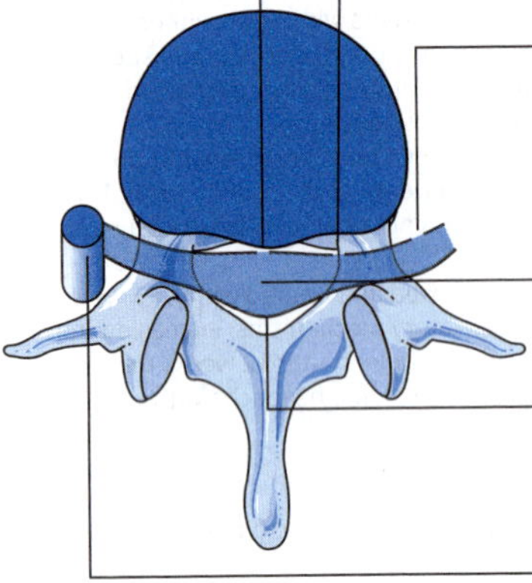

Figure 5.3 Locations of spinal CSF leaks. Adapted from Servier Medical art (Creative Commons License 3.0).

Contraindications

- As for static myelogram.

Equipment

- As for static myelogram.
- Bolsters for positioning under the pelvis and thighs.
- Two 20 mL syringes for contrast and saline administration (label these).
- Preservative-free normal saline.
- Tubing to connect syringe to needle (preferably with a low dead space volume).

Technique

- The procedure is performed with LA without sedation using fluoroscopy. GA can be used but is not essential.
- Patients positive for SLEC on MRI are positioned prone and patients negative for SLEC right- or left-side-down lateral decubitus position. Whichever position, the head is tilted down (to encourage CSF flow cranially) with bolsters placed under the pelvis and thighs with an additional 4–8° table tilt (Figure 5.5).
- A 22 G spinal needle is introduced into the thecal canal usually at L3–L4 under fluoroscopic guidance.
- In the lateral position, CSF opening pressures are recorded (rarely possible in the prone position as fluid may not ascend into the hub of the needle due to low pressures).
- A 20 mL syringe containing preservative-free saline and a second 20 mL syringe of contrast are prepared. Tubing is attached to the spinal needle.

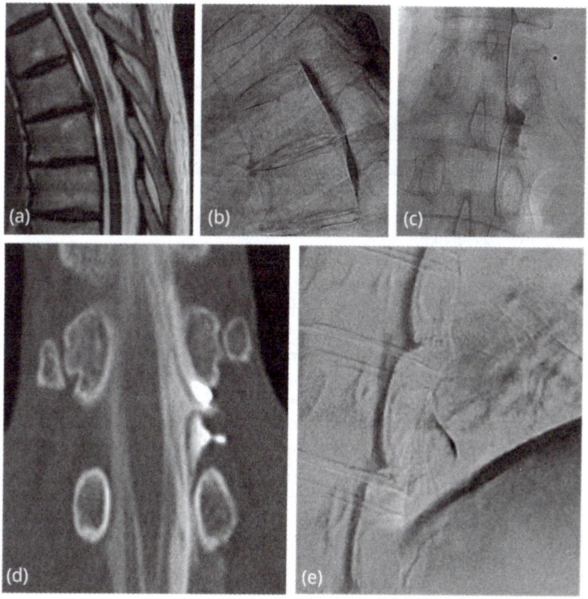

Figure 5.4 Types of CSF leak. (a) Sagittal T2 MRI demonstrating thoracic disc prolapse and adjacent SLEC. (b) Myelography in prone position demonstates a type 1 CSF leak from the ventral aspect of the thecal sac at the T7–T8 level. (c) Right-side-down myelogram demonstrates a type 2 lateral CSF leak below the right pedicle of the T12 vertebral body, with spread of contrast in the epidural fat. (d) CT myelography performed after the procedure of the same case. (e) Right-side-down digital subtraction myelography (DSM) demonstrates evidence of a CSF–venous fistula below the right pedicle of vertebral body T10. Images courtesy of Dr Eef Hendricks.

- A test injection of 0.5–1 mL injection of Iohexol (Omnipaque 300; GE Healthcare) is performed with fluoroscopic guidance to confirm needle tip position and adequate table tilt.
- 10 mL of saline is injected over 2–4 min to dilute and send the test dose down the spinal canal. This also pressurises the canal to encourage leaking. Intermittent screening is performed to ensure cranial flow.
- The detector is positioned initially to cover a field of view from C3–C4 to the mid thoracic level, positioned laterally.
- Dynamic myelography runs are performed using hand injection of initially 6 mL of contrast at a rate of 1 mL/s under breath-holding. After the injection, another 5–10 mL of saline are injected to push the contrast through the tubing and down the thecal sac. Image acquisition is performed at 1 frame per second for 15–25 s per run (screening is continued during this saline injection).

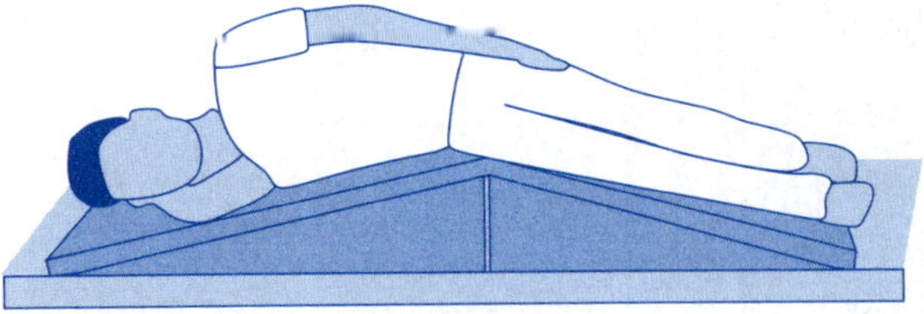

Figure 5.5 Positioning of patient for right-side-down lateral decubitus myelogram with bolsters under hips.

- The most common site for a CSF-venous leak in a series of 40 patients was the right T5–T12 level. The next most common sites in order were right T1–T4, followed by the left thoracic levels.
- If a leak is visualised on the first run, a second injection of 3–5 mL contrast with repeat myelography is performed with a smaller field of view to aid more precise localisation.
- If the first injection is negative, then the thoracic, lumbar, and sacral levels are imaged. The table tilt is reversed and for patients in the lateral decubitus position the patient is propped up on their elbow. Another 3–5 mL of contrast is injected followed by 5–10 mL of saline using the same technique.
- Following the procedure, a CT scan is performed with the patient maintaining the prone or decubitus position from C2 to S3. Alternatively, cone beam CT can be performed on the table itself if a suspicious level is seen.
- The presence of contrast within the renal collecting system on post-procedure CT within 1 h is highly suggestive of a CSF leak, more commonly a CSF–venous fistula where the renal collecting system contrast may be more concentrated on the side of the leak.
- Patients in whom a leak is not found return (after a minimum of 24 h) for repeat DSM. If the procedure was performed left side down, then right side down is employed. Prone patients are switched to lateral decubitus. DSM can be attempted on the other side in the same session providing the maximum amount of intrathecal contrast has not been exceeded.

Postprocedural care

- Standard post-LP care is instituted. Patients are discharged after lying flat on their back for 30–60 min.
- Post-procedure MRI may demonstrate improvement in the cranial and/ or spinal appearances.

Tips

- It is safe and useful to inject small columns of air (about 1 mL) in the tubing to demarcate columns of contrast and saline.
- It is necessary to study both the subtracted and un-subtracted runs as leaks may be subtle and obscured by movement.

Further reading

Dobrocky T, Grunder L, Breiding PS, et al. Assessing spinal cerebrospinal fluid leaks in spontaneous intracranial hypotension with a scoring system based on brain magnetic resonance imaging findings. JAMA Neurol. 2019;76(5):580–587.

Farb RI, Nicholson PJ, Peng PW, et al. Spontaneous intracranial hypotension: a systematic imaging approach for CSF leak localisation and management based on MRI and digital subtraction myelography. AJNR Am J Neuroradiol. 2019;40(4):745–753.

Kranz PG, Gray L, Malinzak MD, Amrhein TJ. Spontaneous intracranial hypotension: pathogenesis, diagnosis, and treatment. Neuroimaging Clin N Am. 2019;29(4):581–594.

Fluoroscopic-guided lumbosacral nerve root injection and medial branch block

- Fluoroscopic-guided nerve root block is used for diagnosis and treatment of radicular pain.
- Fluoroscopic-guided medial branch block serves as a diagnostic test to confirm facetogenic back pain and is used in selection of patients for consideration of rhizolysis or surgery.

Contraindications

- Uncorrected coagulopathy (INR >1.4).
- Local or systemic infection.
- Allergy to corticosteroids.
- Drug interactions (e.g. co-administration of ritonavir and cobicistat with triamcinolone).

Equipment

- 22 G spinal needle.
- 5, 10, and 20 mL syringes.
- Connecting tubing.
- Iodinated contrast media approved for intrathecal injection, e.g. iohexol 240 mg/mL.
- Nerve root block:
  - Injectable steroid: soluble/non-particulate steroids such as dexamethasone (6–9 mg) are increasingly favoured over insoluble/particulate alternatives such as methylprednisolone and triamcinolone due to the low but catastrophic risk of spinal cord infarction.
  - Nerve root block: long-acting LA (e.g. 0.25% levobupivacaine, but note use should be avoided if the patient is at high risk of falls due to risk of transient lower limb weakness).
- Medial branch block: only 1–2% lidocaine should be used.

Technique: nerve root block

- Obtain preprocedural Visual Analogue Scale pain score.
- Position the patient prone.
- Place the detector in the AP position. Adjust craniocaudally to minimise the lumbar lordosis. Oblique the projection approximately 15–25° to maximise visualisation of the affected neural foramen.
- Mark the site of entry (lateral to the targeted subpedicular space) and sterilise and drape the area.
- Inject LA into the subcutaneous tissues.
- Insert the spinal needle at the marked site, advancing slowly under fluoroscopic guidance:
  - The needle tip is seen as a single point on the obliqued AP projection. This should be directly supraneurally and thus visualised immediately below the pedicle lying above the targeted nerve root (within the 'safe triangle'; Figure 5.6).

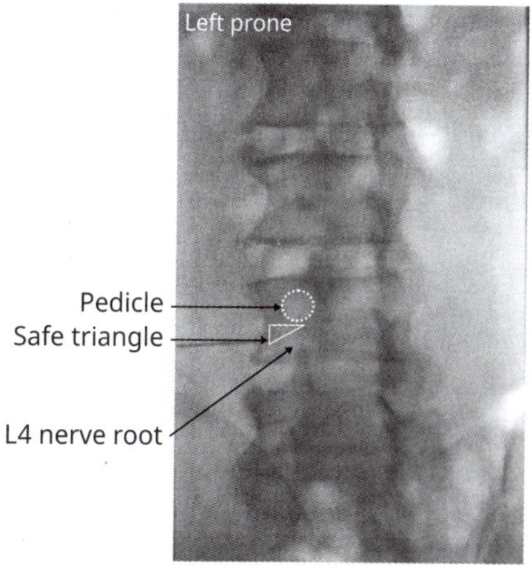

Figure 5.6 The 'safe triangle'. Images courtesy of Dr William Brown and Dr Steve Morgan.

- Alternative approaches targeting the dorsolateral disc ('Kambin's triangle') can be used, and may be preferable to a subpedicular approach in select cases.
- The lateral projection is used to assess needle depth relative to the foramen.

- Once needle depth is adequate (approximately 1 cm posterior to the vertebral body) or the patient reports radicular pain, remove the stylet and inject approximately 3 mL of contrast to confirm the needle tip is extravascular.
- Store the fluoroscopic images confirming needle position.
- Consider performing a test dose of a small volume of 1% lidocaine prior to steroid injection.
- Slowly inject long-acting anaesthetic and steroid along the targeted nerve root.
- Remove the needle and clean and dress the puncture site.

Technique: medial branch block

(See Figure 5.7.)

- Position the patient prone.
- Place the fluoroscopy unit in the AP position. Adjust craniocaudally to minimise the lumbar lordosis. Oblique the projection such that the facet joint is seen in profile.
- Identify target sites for injection: e.g. if targeting the L3–L4 facet joint, the ipsilateral L2 and L3 medial branches should be targeted as presumed innervation.
- Mark the sites of entry and sterilise and drape the area.
- Inject LA into the subcutaneous tissues.

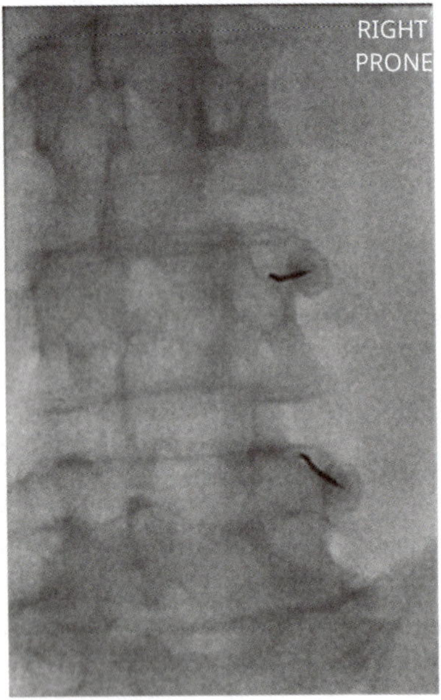

Figure 5.7 Right L3 and L4 medial branch block. Images courtesy of Dr William Brown and Dr Steve Morgan.

- Insert and advance the spinal needle under fluoroscopic guidance; direct the needle tip towards the junction of ipsilateral superior articular process and transverse process at the target level.
- Confirm needle position and depth on the lateral projection.
- Inject a small volume of LA (e.g. 0.5 mL 1% lidocaine).
- Remove the needle.
- Clean and dress the puncture site.

Tips

- While suboptimal, gadolinium-based agents are radiopaque, and represent a potential alternative contrast agent where there is a history of allergy/anaphylaxis to iodinated contrast.
- For fluoroscopic-guided nerve root blocks, curved needles may help navigation around obstructions such as degenerate facet joints.
- S1 nerve root blocks require a different approach to the other lumbar nerve roots; the fluoroscopy unit remains in the AP plane and is only adjusted cranially to view the S1 foramen.
- For fluoroscopic-guided medial branch blocks at the L5/S1 level, the L5 dorsal ramus is targeted instead of the medial branch, with the needle tip directed to the junction of the ipsilateral superior articular process and sacral ala.

Complication avoidance and management

- Systemic reaction to steroid injections may result in transient, self-limiting, facial flushing.
- Spinal cord infarction can occur secondary to intra-arterial injection of steroid into a feeding spinal artery. The aetiology is thought to be embolic secondary to particulate steroid use. Reduce risk by using non-particulate/soluble steroids and using contrast to confirm position before injection.

Postprocedural care

- Observe for 15–30 min post-procedure.
- Patients should be mobilised cautiously if LA has been injected into the perineural space due to the risk of leg weakness/paraesthesia.
- Review pain score post-procedure and provide pain diary.

Further reading

Bartleson JD, Maus TP. Diagnostic and therapeutic spinal interventions: facet joint interventions. Neurol Clin Pract. 2014;4(4):342–346.

Eckel TS, Bartynski WS. Epidural steroid injections and selective nerve root blocks. Tech Vasc Interv Radiol. 2009;12(1):11–21.

Mandell JC, Czuczman GJ, Gaviola GC, Ghazikhanian V, Cho CH. The lumbar neural foramen and transforaminal epidural steroid injections: an anatomic review with key safety considerations in planning the percutaneous approach. AJR Am J Roentgenol. 2017;209(1):W26–W35.

Palmer WE. Spinal injections for pain management. Radiology. 2016; 281(3):669–688.

Park JW, Nam HS, Cho SK, Jung HJ, Lee BJ, Park Y. Kambin's triangle approach of lumbar transforaminal epidural injection with spinal stenosis. Ann Rehabil Med. 2011;35(6):833–843.

CT-guided lumbosacral nerve root injection

As an alternative to performing nerve root blocks under fluoroscopic guidance, CT-guided techniques may help improve visualisation of both the needle tip and relevant anatomical structures.

This may also be the modality of choice in patients with a history of a known allergic reaction to iodinated contrast.

Indications

- Diagnostic confirmation of pain generator.
- Treatment of radicular pain.

Contraindications

- Uncorrected coagulopathy (INR >1.4 or anticoagulated patient).
- Systemic or local infection.

Equipment

- *As for fluoroscopic-guided injections* (see 'Fluoroscopic-guided lumbosacral nerve root injection and medial branch block', p. 158).
- Note, iodinated contrast media should be diluted to 10% to minimise streak artefact using the CT-guided technique.

Technique

(See Figure 5.8.)

- Obtain preprocedural Visual Analogue Scale pain score.
- Position the patient prone head-first on the CT table.
- Place a radiopaque grid on the patient's skin to help serve as a needle guide.
- Obtain a CT scanogram and limited CT slices at the level of the vertebral lesion.
- Plan the site of entry, angle of the needle, and required needle length on the CT console, and mark the skin with a pen.
- Sterilise and drape the proposed entry site, ensuring not to rub off your mark.
- Inject LA into the subcutaneous tissues.
- Insert the spinal needle at the marked site. Use the laser targeting to align your needle if the scanner has this facility. Advance through the tissues incrementally under CT guidance:
    - The needle should traverse the neural foramen, with the tip lying within the anterior epidural space, immediately below the pedicle and posterior to dorsal vertebral body.
    - Alternative approaches targeting the dorsolateral disc ('Kambin's triangle') can be used, and may be preferable to a subpedicular approach in select cases.
- Once needle depth is adequate (approximately 1 cm posterior to the vertebral body) or the patient reports radicular pain, remove the stylet and inject a small volume of dilute contrast medium, observing for contrast flow around the nerve root.
- Consider performing a test dose of a small volume of 1% lidocaine prior to steroid injection.

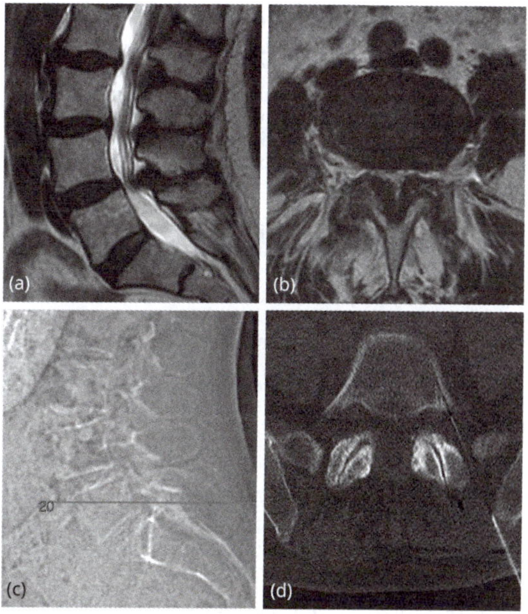

Figure 5.8 Female patient with left leg neuropathic pain. (a) Sagittal and (b) axial T2-weighted MRI scans demonstrating degenerative disc disease at L4/L5. (c) CT scanogram showing level to be imaged. (d) Left L5 nerve root injection through coaxially introduced 25 G needle. Images courtesy of Dr Ayman Qureshi.

- Slowly inject long-acting anaesthetic and steroid along the targeted nerve root.
- Remove the needle.
- Clean and dress the puncture site.

Tips

- Pre-curved needles are a more dexterous alternative to bevel-tipped, and may allow for easier steering and avoidance of obstacles.

Further reading

Amrhein TJ, Joshi AB, Kranz PG. Technique for CT fluoroscopy-guided lumbar medial branch blocks and radiofrequency ablation. AJR Am J Roentgenol. 2016;207(3):631–634.

Wagner AL. Selective lumbar nerve root blocks with CT fluoroscopic guidance: technique, results, procedure time, and radiation dose. AJNR Am J Neuroradiol. 2004;25(9):1592–1594.

Fluoroscopic-guided transpedicular thoracolumbar spinal biopsy

Fluoroscopic-guided biopsy samples the vertebrae and intervertebral discs, typically in the context of suspected malignancy or infection.

Fluoroscopy may have greater availability and shorter procedure times when compared with CT-guided approaches.

Indications

- Histological characterisation of suspected malignancy.
- Diagnosis of metastatic spinal disease in patients with a known primary malignancy.
- Differentiation between osteoporotic and malignant spinal compression fractures.
- Diagnosis of spinal osteomyelitis and identification of causative organisms.
- Investigation of diffuse spinal marrow abnormalities.

Contraindications

- Uncorrected coagulopathy.
- INR >1.4 or anticoagulated patient.
- Infection at proposed site of biopsy (unless an infectious lesion is specifically being targeted).

Equipment

- Biopsy needles (will vary according to lesion type).
- 22 G spinal needles: for LA placement onto periosteum/soft tissues.
- Coaxial biopsy system/needle: for bone biopsy.
- T-cut/cutting core biopsy needles: for soft tissue/lytic lesions.
- Surgical scalpel.
- Specimen pots for samples (histology and microbiology).
- Wound dressing.

Technique

- Review preoperative imaging with a view to identifying biopsy sites which are likely to be the highest yield; cystic and necrotic areas are unlikely to provide an adequate sample.
- Position the patient prone on the fluoroscopy table.
- Identify suitable puncture site under fluoroscopic guidance:
  - Adjust the craniocaudal projection to centre the pedicles within the vertebral bodies (essentially the same as vertebroplasty in Figure 5.10).
  - The spinous processes should be in the vertebral body midline on the AP view.
  - The pedicles should appear to overlap on the lateral view.
  - The typical site of approach is approximately 5 cm lateral to the spinous processes.
- Mark the site of entry and sterilise and drape the area.
- Inject LA into the subcutaneous tissues.
- Replace with the spinal needle and instil LA (i.e. 0.25% levobupivacaine) down to the pedicle.
- Make a skin incision.

- For a conventional transpedicular approach, insert a coaxial bone access needle into the skin at the marked site, advancing towards the ipsilateral pedicle in the plane of the beam. This is then used as the coaxial channel through which other needle types can be inserted (e.g. bone drill, needle, soft tissue needle).
- The position of the needle should be reviewed on AP and lateral imaging as it is advanced. A mallet is usually required.
- In the AP plane, the tip of the coaxial bone access needle should not breach the medial wall of the pedicle until safely within the vertebral body (i.e. tip has crossed the posterior cortex on the lateral).
- Advance the needle tip into the lesion and confirm final position on AP and lateral views.
- Obtain representative samples as required.
- Following biopsy, aspirates can be obtained (if required) by attaching a syringe to the bone access cannula.
- Remove the needle and clean and dress the puncture site.

Tips

- A standard oblique plane can be used in favour of a transpedicular approach when accessing the vertebral endplate or disc in the context of infection/spondylodiscitis. Targeting the superior endplate/lower disc helps avoid the exiting nerve root. Alternatively, an extra-pedicular trajectory may be considered when the pedicles are too small, or the lesion cannot be otherwise accessed.
- Generous injection of periosteal LA (e.g. 0.5% levobupivacaine) along with instillation into the soft tissue planes will reduce discomfort.

Complication avoidance and management

- Pneumothorax: in the context of a thoracic vertebral biopsy. Confirm with X-ray or CT and insert a chest drain if large or symptomatic.
- Bleeding and haematoma: due to direct vascular injury or biopsy of a hypervascular vertebral lesion. Spinal haematoma may require surgical decompression.
- Tumour seeding along biopsy tract: rare where coaxial systems are appropriately utilised.
- Neurological defect: typically secondary to nerve root traversal. Spinal cord injury is less common.
- Infection: can be seeded along the biopsy tract. Best avoided with proper sterile technique.

Postprocedural care

- Monitor the patient for 1–2 h post-procedure before discharge.
- Postprocedural chest radiographs should be considered where a thoracic biopsy has been performed.

Further reading

Dave BR, Nanda A, Anandjiwala JV. Transpedicular percutaneous biopsy of vertebral body lesions: a series of 71 cases. Spinal Cord. 2009;47(5):384–389.

Pierot L, Boulin A. Percutaneous biopsy of the thoracic and lumbar spine: transpedicular approach under fluoroscopic guidance. AJNR Am J Neuroradiol. 1999;20(1):23–25.

Ravikanth R. Diagnostic yield and technical aspects of fluoroscopy-guided percutaneous transpedicular biopsy of the spine: a single-center retrospective analysis of outcomes and review of the literature. J Craniovertebr Junction Spine. 2020;11(2):93–98.

CT-guided thoracolumbar spinal biopsy

Percutaneous needle biopsy of spinal lesions can be performed under CT guidance as an alternative to fluoroscopy. While more time and resource intensive, there is improved localisation of the needle tip, better delineation of surrounding anatomy, and superior access to smaller lesions.

Indications/contraindications/equipment

- *As for fluoroscopic-guided biopsy* (see 'Fluoroscopic transpedicular thoracolumbar spinal biopsy', p. 164).

Technique

(See Figure 5.9.)

- Review preoperative imaging with a view to identifying biopsy sites which are likely to produce the highest yield. Cystic and necrotic areas are unlikely to provide an adequate sample. CT-guided approaches may be particularly helpful for biopsy of anatomically complex areas (e.g. the sacrum).
- Position the patient prone on the CT table (alternative positions may be required for approaches other than conventional transpedicular).
- Place a radiopaque grid on the patient's skin.
- Obtain a CT scanogram and limited CT slices at the level of the vertebral lesion.
- Plan the path of the needle on the console and mark a suitable site of entry on the skin.
- Sterilise and drape the proposed entry site ensuring not to rub off your mark.
- Inject LA into the subcutaneous tissues.
- Replace with the spinal needle and instil LA (e.g. 0.25% levobupivacaine) down to the periosteum.
- Make a small cutaneous incision within the anaesthetised skin.
- Transpedicular approach:
  - A bone access needle is then used to gain hold/access, and is advanced under CT guidance towards the ipsilateral pedicle. This is then used as the coaxial channel through which other needle types can be inserted (e.g. bone drill, needle, soft tissue needle). A mallet is usually required to advance the needle into the bone.
  - Obtain a limited CT scan at the relevant level prior to periosteal breach to confirm the location and trajectory of the needle tip.
  - Advance the needle tip through the pedicle and into the lesion, performing a further limited CT scan to confirm final position.
  - Obtain representative samples as required.
- Paraspinal approach:
  - If the lesion exists/extends into the intervertebral disc or paraspinal tissues, it may not be necessary to enter the bone and a standard coaxial needle biopsy can be performed.
  - The needle is extended into the area of interest and the biopsy gun obtains multiple samples. It is important to ensure that there is sufficient safe distance beyond the coaxial needle as the biopsy needle will extend a variable length beyond (typically 5 or 10 mm).

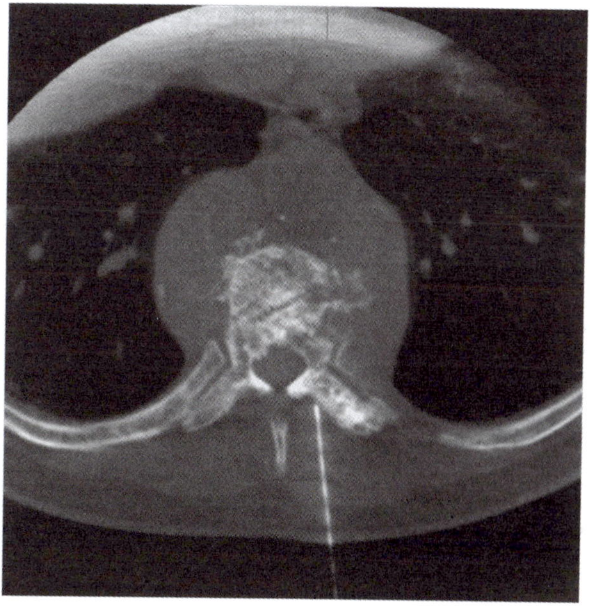

Figure 5.9 Left-sided transpedicular CT-guided spinal biopsy. Image courtesy of Dr William Brown and Dr Steve Morgan.

- Following biopsy, aspirates can be obtained (if required) by attaching a syringe to the bone access cannula.
- Remove the needle and clean and dress the puncture site.

Tips

- Generous injection of periosteal LA is advised (e.g. 0.5% levobupivacaine) to reduce discomfort/pain. Adequate anaesthesia of the periosteum is essential in minimising periprocedural patient movement.

Complication avoidance and management

- *As for fluoroscopic-guided biopsy* (see 'Fluoroscopic transpedicular thoracolumbar spinal biopsy', p. 164).

Further reading

Gala KB, Shetty NS, Janu AK, Shetty N, Kulkarni SS. Percutaneous CT-guided vertebral biopsy: anatomy and technical considerations. J Clin Interv Radiol ISVIR 2021;5(3):150–157.
Peh W. CT-guided percutaneous biopsy of spinal lesions. Biomed Imaging Interv J. 2006;2(3):e25.
Singh DK, Kumar N, Nayak BK, et al. Approach-based techniques of CT-guided percutaneous vertebral biopsy. Diagn Interv Radiol. 2020;26(2):143–146.

Vertebroplasty and kyphoplasty

Vertebroplasty and kyphoplasty are minimally invasive vertebral augmentation procedures involving percutaneous injection of bone cement into vertebral bodies. Kyphoplasty utilises balloons to create a cavity and attempts to restore vertebral body height, allowing cement to be injected more safely and reducing the risk of leakage. Several other vertebral implants are available as alternatives. Both procedures aim to provide pain relief and functional improvement. They are most commonly used for the treatment of osteoporotic fractures, but are increasingly used in combination with thermal ablation for the treatment of metastases and myeloma.

Contraindications

- Local or systemic infection.
- Uncorrected coagulopathy.
- Known allergy to bone cement or other injectate.
- Complex fracture with retropulsion.
- Tumour mass within the spinal canal.

Equipment

- 1% lidocaine.
- Scalpel.
- 22 G spinal needle.
- Vertebroplasty introducer needles.
- Injectable bone cement such as polymethacrylate.
- Kyphoplasty balloon/implant kit (kyphoplasty only).

Technique

(See Figures 5.10 & 5.11.)

- The procedure can be undertaken under conscious sedation or GA.
- IV antibiotics are administered to reduce infection risk.
- Ideally, a biplane fluoroscopy suite is used. Fixed fluoroscopic/CT imaging with supplementary C-arm, and alternating single-plane fluoroscopy are viable alternatives.
- Position the patient prone on the fluoroscopy table.
- Begin with AP fluoroscopy and confirm treatment levels. Next, adjust the cranio-caudal angle to align the beam with vertebral endplates. Then, centre the pedicle within the vertebral body using cranio-caudal angulation. Finally, oblique the detector laterally so that you are looking down the 'gun barrel' of the pedicle.

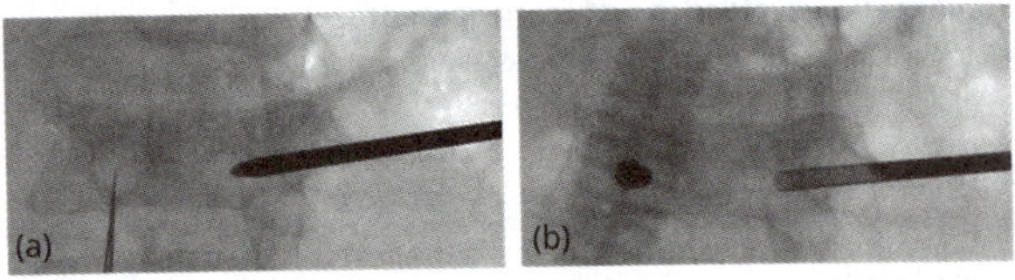

Figure 5.10 (a) AP fluoroscopic view with showing 'gun barrel' transpedicular approach (contralateral needle already in place). The needle should not cross the medial border of the pedicle. (b) Trocar has been inserted via the pedicle. Images courtesy of Dr William Brown and Dr Steve Morgan.

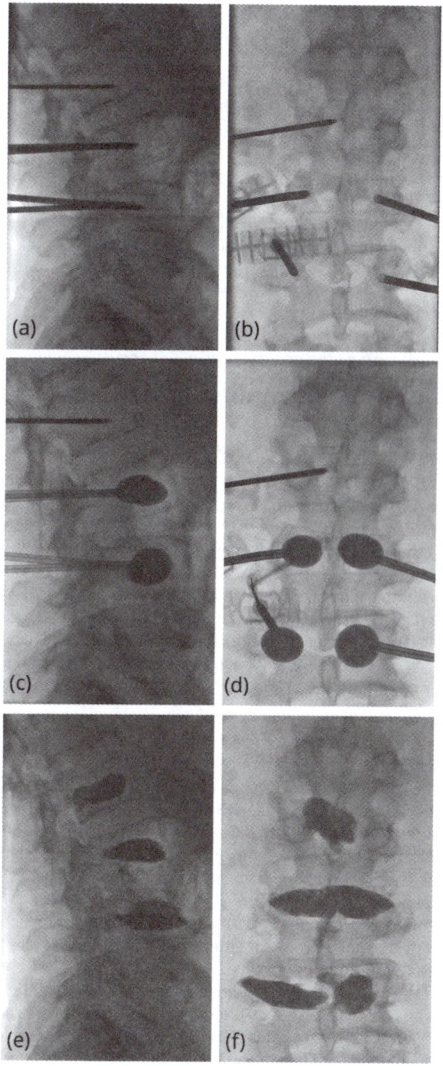

Figure 5.11 L2 vertebroplasty and L3 & L4 balloon kyphoplasty for a patient with vertebral metastases. (a) Lateral and (b) AP views showing needles inserted via the L2 (unilaterally) and L3/L4 levels (bilaterally). (c) Lateral and (d) AP views with the balloons inflated. (e) Lateral and (f) AP views showing final cement infiltration and needles removed. Images courtesy of Dr Ayman Qureshi.

- Plan the needle trajectory. For a transpedicular approach the needle entry site is at the lateral margin of the target pedicle.
- Mark the site/sites of entry and sterilise and drape the area.
- Inject LA into the skin.
- Replace with the spinal needle and instil LA (i.e. 0.25% levobupivacaine) down to the pedicle.
- Make an incision in the skin.
- Insert the bone access cannula (this is typically 10 or 11 G) and advance to the pedicle.
- Advance the bone access cannula through the pedicle using a mallet. The tip should not cross the medial wall of the pedicle until clearly within the vertebral body on a true lateral projection (needle tip past the posterior cortex). Alternate AP/lateral projections if using single-plane fluoroscopy.
- If required, a coaxial biopsy can be taken once the access cannula has been advanced past the posterior cortex (a hand drill could also be used to create a channel at this point).
- Advance bone access cannula into the anterior portion of the vertebral body and confirm needle position on AP and lateral views.
- Repeat on the contralateral side if a bilateral approach is required.

If balloon kyphoplasty is to be performed

- Remove the needle stylet and insert the kyphoplasty balloon via the bone access cannula.
- Position the balloon using radiopaque markers.
- Repeat this process on the contralateral side if using a bilateral approach (typically both balloons are inserted and then inflated together).
- Slowly inflate the balloon under fluoroscopic guidance. Inflation should be stopped once nominal pressure is obtained and vertebral height is maximally restored. The anterior and lateral cortex should not be breached.
- Deflate and remove the balloons.

Cement injection

- Prepare the bone cement for injection. It should have a paste-like consistency and matte appearance when ready.
- Insert the cement delivery cannula and connect the delivery system.
- Inject the cement slowly under continuous AP and lateral fluoroscopy (this process may be painful for the patient). The volume of cement injected varies (it is usually in the order of 3–10 mL per vertebra) and depends on several factors, such as the existing defect/cavity and size of vertebral body.
- Discontinue injection once cement has reached (but not breached) the posterior vertebral body or if it enters an epidural vein. Ideally, cement is seen to extend across the midline.
- Remove the cement cannula and reinsert the needle stylet (removing the risk of a cement spike/tail), prior to removing the access cannula in a controlled clockwise/counter-clockwise manner. It is advisable to wait 3–5 min, allowing the cement to set prior to removing the needles.
- Apply pressure over the needle site following removal for 5–10 min.
- Close the skin with adhesive strips or suture.

Tips

- Thoracic vertebral pedicles are smaller than those of lumbar vertebrae, with greater craniocaudal angulation. Access is more challenging and a more cranial approach is required.
- Bipedicular techniques typically deliver a more even distribution of cement than unipedicular, but an unipedicular approach may nonetheless be favourable in multi comorbid patients.
- Bevelled or diamond tip needles can be used depending on operator preference. The bevel helps steer the needle. Diamond tips are helpful if the needle keeps slipping initially before breaching the bone cortex.
- Waiting slightly longer than the recommended time after cement mixing will increase cement viscosity, and reduce risk of leakage.

Complication avoidance and management

- Pain is not uncommon after vertebroplasty but if it is more severe than usual after 2 h consider CT to exclude a complication.
- New lower extremity weakness or bladder/bowel incontinence is suggestive of cord or nerve injury.
- Cement leakage into the spinal canal is more common with vertebroplasty than kyphoplasty and can rarely lead to spinal cord damage or neural compression. Surgical decompression may be needed if there is significant mass effect.
- Cement embolus is also more common with vertebroplasty than kyphoplasty. There is a risk of pulmonary embolus and inferior vena cava syndrome. Typically managed with anticoagulation if symptomatic and supportive care such as oxygenation.
- Neurological deficit is usually due to nerve root irritation from cement leak. It is typically transient and can be treated with nerve block. Spinal cord injury is less common.
- Significant haemorrhage from the inferior vena cava/aorta can occur if the anterior cortex is penetrated. Epidural/paravertebral haematoma also rarely occur.
- Infection may be difficult to treat where bone cement has been injected. Procedures must be conducted under strict sterile technique to avoid this.
- Pneumothorax rarely occurs in cases of a very lateral thoracic approach.

Postprocedural care

- Postprocedural CT imaging may be used to confirm cement position and exclude complications.
- Patients may be discharged a few hours later after review to confirm a lack of any complications.

Further reading

Beale DP. Vertebral Augmentation: The Comprehensive Guide to Vertebroplasty, Kyphoplasty and Implant Augmentation. Thieme Medical Publishing; 2020.

National Institute for Health and Care Excellence (NICE). Radiofrequency ablation as an adjunct to balloon kyphoplasty or percutaneous vertebroplasty for palliation of painful spinal metastases [Internet]. Interventional procedures guidance [IPG759]. NICE; 2023. https://www.nice.org.uk/guidance/ipg759

Syed MI, Shaikh A. Vertebroplasty: a systematic approach. Pain Physician. 2007;10(2):367–380.

Vanni D, Galzio R, Kazakova A, et al. Third-generation percutaneous vertebral augmentation systems. J Spine Surg. 2016;2(1):13–20.

Percutaneous venolymphatic malformations

- Venolymphatic malformations are rare, congenital, slow-flow lesions which are commonly located in the head and neck region.
- Although congenital, they often manifest later in life as diffuse bluish cutaneous masses which are soft, compressible, and non-pulsatile. They may increase in size in dependent positions or during the Valsalva manoeuvre.
- The lesions may be present intraorally where, if large, they can cause dysphagia, difficulty speaking, or airway obstruction. In the orbital or periocular region, they may cause ocular issues, particularly exophthalmos.
- MRI appearances typically demonstrate T2/short tau inversion recovery (STIR) hyperintensity and T1 iso- or hypointensity with rounded signal voids representing phleboliths. The lesions enhance after IV gadolinium contrast administration and usually have well-circumscribed margins. There may be signs of recent or previous haemorrhage.
- Sclerosants act on the dysmorphic endothelium lining the venolymphatic malformation. Many types are available including ethyl alcohol, bleomycin, and STS. In general, alcohol is more efficacious but more toxic than other agents. Bleomycin is a cytotoxic antitumour agent that is less toxic but slightly less efficacious. It is not as painful to inject. STS 3% is a synthetic surfactant that is commonly used as a sclerosing agent in a similar fashion to bleomycin.
- Surgery is generally reserved for lesions that fail to resolve after several sessions or as an adjunct to sclerotherapy.
- Patients must be managed within an appropriate multidisciplinary team (MDT)—typically including interventional neuroradiology, plastic/reconstructive surgery, maxillofacial surgery, and dermatology.

Contraindications

- Allergy to contrast or sclerosing agent.
- Systemic or local infection.

Equipment

- 22 G Angiocath (Becton, Dickinson and Company, NJ, USA) needles.
- Syringes and tubing set.
- Water-soluble iodinated contrast media.
- Sclerosant agent.
- Wooden spatula (for transoral approach).

Technique

(See Figure 5.12.)

- The procedure is performed with or without conscious sedation using single-plane fluoroscopy. GA is used when treating intraorbital, tongue, or pharyngeal lesions or when injecting ethanol.
- The skin is made sterile and drapes are applied.
- A 22 G Angiocath is inserted into the lesion under ultrasound guidance. Typically, blood can be seen slowly filling the needle hub, which confirms its position.
- If the lesion is thought to be lymphatic, it may be worth trying to aspirate as much as possible to avoid diluting the sclerosant.
- Mini-tubing is flushed with contrast and then attached to the needle.

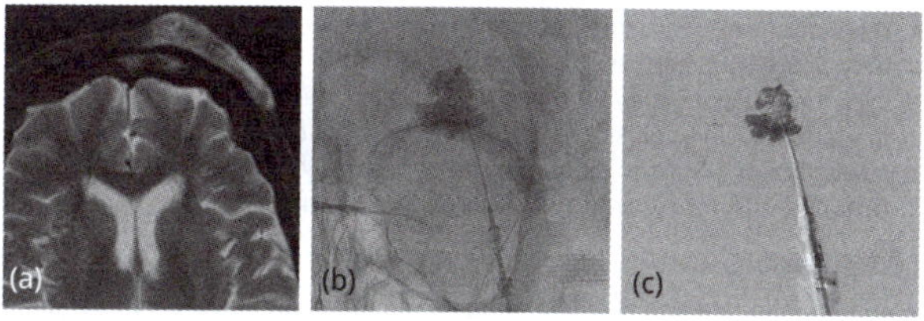

Figure 5.12 Percutaneous injection of bleomycin into a forehead venous malformation. (a) T2WI MRI of the forehead lesion. (b) Unsubtracted AP fluoroscopy showing needle in lesion after contrast injection. (c) Subtracted fluoroscopy image. Images courtesy of Dr Ronit Agid.

- The correct position of the needle is confirmed by injecting 1–2 mL of water-soluble iodinated contrast under digital subtraction fluoroscopy at a slow rate of one image every 2 s to produce a venogram. This is useful for confirming the diagnosis and identifying draining veins. This run can also now be set as a mask for further angiography. Do not inject too much contrast to avoid diluting the sclerosant.
- Injection of the sclerosant is next performed under fluoroscopy. The non-radiopaque sclerosant displaces the contrast material and appears as white ('negative' contrast).
- Further Angiocaths may be inserted in the same manner into different compartments of the lesion. It is advisable to wait until after the final injection before removing all the Angiocaths to facilitate haemostasis.
- If the injection is transoral, then the tongue is displaced with a wooden spatula.
- Upper limits for sclerosant per session are as follows: ethyl alcohol 100% 1 mL/kg (but typically not more than 20 mL), bleomycin 15 mg.
- For lesions resistant to therapy despite multiple treatments, the sclerosant can be mixed with albumin and air (ratio of 1:1:1) and injected as foam. Foam stays longer in the malformation and thus has a more significant effect.

Postprocedural care

- Needles are removed and haemostasis is achieved using light manual pressure. The patient is monitored and then allowed to go home later the same day.
- Tongue lesions can swell significantly after treatment and tend to get infected more often. Therefore, it is advised to provide all tongue sclerotherapy patients with a prescription for clindamycin, nystatin suspension (mouth wash), and tapering steroids.
- Further sessions may be required at recommended intervals of 4–6 weeks.
- MRI imaging should occur 6 months after the last sclerotherapy session.

Tips

- Medical photography is useful for objective assessment of treatment efficacy over several treatment sessions.
- Veins draining the lesion visualised during phlebography may be compressed during injection of sclerosant to concentrate the agent at the desired site and prevent systemic distribution or dangerous drainage pathways (such as via the cavernous sinus).

- It is important not to inject too much contrast during venography as this may dilute the sclerosing agent.
- Lymphatic lesions may be more resistant to treatment especially when presenting as a large single cyst. A higher-efficacy sclerosant, such as alcohol or albumin foam, might be considered if this is the case. Drainage of lymph from the cyst prior to sclerotherapy is recommended.

Complications

- Infection is rare and avoided using sterile technique. There may be some oozing after the procedure which generally settles with pressure.
- General complications with sclerosants include swelling, cellulitis, skin necrosis, and nerve injury (more common and severe with alcohol). The latter may be temporary or permanent and manifests as palsy or numbness. Nausea/vomiting or flu-like symptoms may be experienced in the days following the treatment.
- Ethanol is efficacious but relatively toxic with a narrow therapeutic window and can rarely result in systemic complications including cardiopulmonary collapse. It can also cause severe swelling, skin ulceration, and nerve palsy and can even be lethal if it enters the intracranial veins. For these reasons, it should not be injected in the regions of the orbit, tongue, and airway. Alcohol usually causes marked but relatively painless swelling for 3–7 days.
- The cytotoxicity of bleomycin necessitates strict precautions that must be followed during use and disposal. Skin discolouration can manifest at the injection site or at distal sites of minor pressure or trauma and so sticky substances, such as tape, are avoided periprocedurally (this includes the adhesive on the drapes, ECG stickers, etc.). Patients should be cautioned to avoid applying pressure to their skin in the weeks following treatment and to use sunscreen. Pulmonary toxicity resulting in pneumonitis and pulmonary fibrosis is rare. However, patients should be advised to seek medical advice if they develop any respiratory symptom in the following weeks. Steroids will prevent pneumonitis from progressing to irreversible fibrosis.
- STS is an anionic surfactant that is also less toxic but less efficacious than alcohol. In high doses, it can result in urticaria, anaphylaxis, and haematuria.

Further reading

Agid R, Burvin R, Gomori JM. Sclerotherapy for venous malformations using a 'negative subtraction' technique. Neuroradiology. 2006;48(2):127–129.

Legiehn GM, Heran MK. Venous malformations: classification, development, diagnosis, and interventional radiologic management. Radiol Clin North Am. 2008;46(3):545–597, vi.

Shigematsu T, Sorscher M, Dier EC, Berenstein A. Bleomycin sclerotherapy for eyelid venous malformations as an alternative to surgery or laser therapy. J Neurointerv Surg. 2019;11(1):57–61.

Spence J, Krings T, TerBrugge KG, Agid R. Percutaneous treatment of facial venous malformations: a matched comparison of alcohol and bleomycin sclerotherapy. Head Neck. 2011;33(1):125–130.

Spence J, Krings T, terBrugge KG, da Costa LB, Agid R. Percutaneous sclerotherapy for facial venous malformations: subjective clinical and objective MR imaging follow-up results. AJNR Am J Neuroradiol. 2010;31(5):955–960.

Ul Haq F, Mitchell SE, Tekes A, Weiss CR. Bleomycin foam treatment of venous malformations: a promising agent for effective treatment with minimal swelling. J Vasc Interv Radiol. 2015;26(10):1484–1493.

Chapter 6

Vascular access

Femoral *176*
Radial *182*
Carotid *187*
Venous *189*
Paediatric *190*

Femoral

The common femoral artery is historically the most common access site for interventional neuroradiology procedures as it is relatively safe and accessible, with a direct route to the brain.

Disadvantages include the risks of groin haematoma, vessel dissection/occlusion resulting in limb ischaemia, and potentially life-threatening retroperitoneal haematoma (RPH).

Cautions

- Peripheral artery disease: severe atherosclerosis, stenosis, occlusion in the femoral or iliac arteries, dissection, or aneurysmal dilatation can render catheterisation difficult or high risk. Disease is often indicated by a weak or absent femoral pulse and can be directly assessed with ultrasound.
- Prior surgery or procedures: insertion of aortofemoral bypass grafts or endovascular stents are contraindications.
- While not a contraindication, if there has been a recent femoral catheterisation, it is probably worth choosing another site, perhaps the contralateral side.
- Severe bleeding disorders: coagulopathies, as well as the use of antiplatelet or anticoagulant medications, increase the risk of bleeding complications. Consider radial access, which is inherently less risky for haemorrhage.
- Infection: local infection is a contraindication to puncture.

Puncture technique

Femoral puncture and sheath insertion

- Prepare and drape the area. The right side is usual, being closest to the operator.
- Puncture must be made with postoperative haemostasis in mind. The common femoral artery, located just above the bifurcation and below the inguinal ligament, is the target because the common femoral artery can be compressed at the level of the femoral head to achieve haemostasis. Puncturing above the inguinal ligament risks RPH. Puncturing the superficial femoral artery is higher risk for pseudoaneurysm formation or stenosis/occlusion.
- Ultrasound is strongly advised as evidence suggests it improves technical success and reduces complications. Both transverse and longitudinal visualisations of the vessel are acceptable. Locate the bifurcation first, then scan approximately 1 cm upwards. The femoral head is typically visible on ultrasound and serves as a useful landmark. Confirm with fluoroscopic visualisation of the femoral head (especially useful in obese patients as the tendency is to puncture too low).
- A radiopaque marker can be left at the site and used as the landmark for the puncture site.
- Infiltrate 10 mL of 1% lidocaine. First, create a bleb under the skin, then infiltrate using ultrasound guidance in the tissues around the vessel. The better the infiltration, the less the procedural discomfort.

- While stretching the skin, make a small incision. Avoid inserting the blade directly down; instead, angle it flat against the skin to mitigate the risk of injuring deeper structures.
- Insert the 18 G puncture needle with your right hand while scanning with your left. Insert at an angle of approximately 45°. Some ultrasound and needle combinations do not permit direct visualisation of the needle; instead, the tissues can be observed being deflected around it. Gentle tapping motions can help to indicate the location of the needle tip.
- Using ultrasound guidance, place the tip of the needle on the surface of the outside wall of the vessel. Next puncture the anterior wall until you reach the lumen. Rotating the needle might encourage entry through the wall.
- A successful first-attempt single-wall puncture carries the lowest risk. Double-wall puncture (anterior and posterior wall puncture, followed by withdrawal until back inside the vessel lumen) carries greater risk but occasionally may be necessary.
- Entry into the lumen is indicated by pulsatile blood spurts.
- Insert the introducer wire slowly, ensuring there is no resistance. A J-shaped wire (usually in the same packet as the sheath) reduces the risk of dissection. Flattening the angle of the needle to the skin, while ensuring the tip remains in the lumen, avoids the wire catching on the vessel as it enters. The more wire 'purchase', the easier it will be to subsequently introduce the sheath (occasionally longer wires can be helpful).
- Once the wire is in the vessel, remove the needle over the wire, pressing on the skin entry point with your left hand to ensure haemostasis.
- Insert the sheath/introducer over the wire until it is up to the hilt, fixing the wire to the skin. Ensure not to kink the wire which can happen when the wire and sheath are pushed together.
- Finally, remove the wire and the introducer together. Aspirate blood from the sheath to ensure it is in the right place. It is generally unnecessary to place the sheath on a heparinised flush.
- The sheath can be secured in position using medical dressings such as Tegaderm® (3M) or sutured in position (preferable if tortuous anatomy is anticipated as there is a risk it can be pushed out during the procedure).
- A femoral angiogram should be performed through the sheath (Figure 6.1). This helps ensure that there is no vessel damage or disease that could impede the passage of a catheter and allows for the assessment of vessel calibre if a closure device is to be inserted at the end of the procedure.

Tips for vascular access

Difficulty inserting the introducer wire

- If you encounter resistance, stop and retrieve the wire. If blood continues to spurt from the needle, the wire may be hitting the back wall of the vessel. Try flattening the needle against the skin or retracting it by 1–2 mm under ultrasound guidance before attempting again.
- If blood no longer spurts upon removing the wire, it is likely that the needle shifted during the wire insertion. It may be positioned in or beyond the wall of the vessel. Recentring under ultrasound may be required.

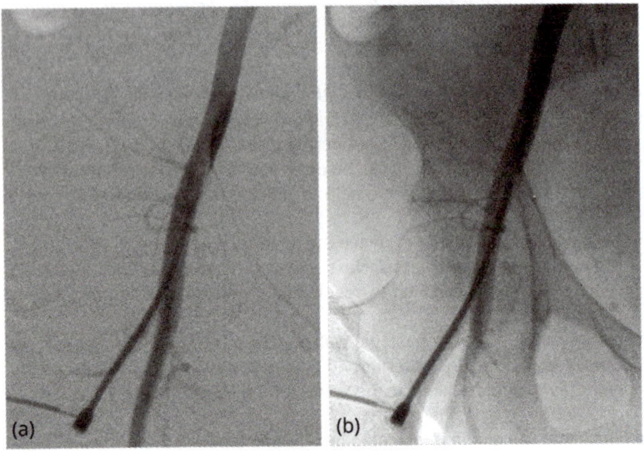

Figure 6.1 (a) Subtracted and (b) unsubtracted angiography via a femoral sheath. Note the entry site of the sheath over the femoral head.

- Advancing the needle slightly and then pulling it back (double-wall puncture) may, alternatively, successfully draw it into the vessel lumen. Note, however, that this technique may cause haemorrhage from the posterior vessel wall.
- If difficulty is encountered puncturing, it is important to perform a femoral angiogram as soon as the sheath is in place (this is our general recommendation).

Difficulty inserting the sheath

- This may be due to the wire becoming kinked or a thick, calcified vessel wall. In the former case, it may be necessary to retract the wire slightly to prevent the kink from being at the vessel entry site.
- In the latter situation, attempt to dilate the vessel using the dilator from the sheath before trying again with the assembled sheath. If the dilator can be inserted, but the sheath still will not pass, consider using a smaller sheath. Another suggestion is to use a longer wire, such as a Berenstein wire with a J-tip, which can be inserted via the dilator to achieve better distal purchase.

Haemostasis technique

Manual compression for haemostasis

- Manual pressure, achieved by applying both hands over the arteriotomy site for 10 min, is generally effective in achieving haemostasis for 5 Fr sheaths.
- Ensure the patient is in a supine position and clean the puncture site. Lower the bed if necessary so you can press comfortably and effectively.
- Slowly withdraw the sheath while applying firm pressure just above and below the puncture site.

- Maintain direct, steady pressure for 10 min with both hands over the site of the pulse. Do not obliterate the pulse completely. Blood should still flow into the lower limb to avoid ischaemic damage.
- Periodically check distal pulses and saturations to ensure adequate blood flow during compression.
- Gradually reduce the pressure while monitoring for any signs of bleeding. If bleeding recurs, reapply pressure for 5–10 min.
- Once haemostasis is achieved, apply a sterile pressure dressing over the site and monitor the site for signs of bleeding or haematoma formation for several hours after the procedure.

Closure devices for haemostasis

- For arteriotomies of 6 Fr or larger, or if the patient has a bleeding tendency due to antiplatelet therapy, anticoagulation, or haemophilia or other coagulopathy, a closure device is recommended.
- Some evidence suggests that vascular closure devices reduce the rates of haematomas and the time to mobilisation. However, a 2016 Cochrane review did not find 'robust' evidence that closure devices decrease the incidence of serious puncture site complications, nor did it demonstrate the superiority of any particular device.
- Several closure devices are available. The two most commonly used in our experience are as follows:
  - The Angio-Seal device is available in two sizes: 6 Fr (capable of closing up to 8 Fr arteriotomies) and 8 Fr (capable of closing up to 10 Fr arteriotomies). Note that a 6 Fr sheath creates an 8 Fr arteriotomy, while an 8 Fr sheath creates a 10 Fr arteriotomy.
  - The Perclose (Abbott) device is an alternative, utilising a suture to close arteriotomies and venotomies of larger size than the Angio-Seal.

Complications

Vessel dissection

- This may happen during the insertion of the sheath or wire. It can go unnoticed and is another reason to routinely conduct angiography via the femoral sheath. If non-flow-limiting, it is often well tolerated and resolves over time. The true lumen should be navigated carefully under roadmap fluoroscopy using the catheter. It is advisable to perform a delayed CTA after a few weeks to confirm the resolution of the dissection.
- If flow-limiting, it is advisable to seek vascular surgical and interventional help as the artery might require stenting (more commonly) or surgery (rarely).

Leg ischaemia

- Signs of ischaemia are paraesthesia, paralysis, pallor, absence of pulses, pain, and 'perishing' cold—the 'six Ps'.
- The arteries can be assessed using arterial Doppler during the procedure and followed by CTA afterwards. Anticoagulation, interventional radiology, or surgery may be necessary for resolution.

Groin haematoma

- While typically small and self-resolving, these can, rarely, be large and even fatal.

- If bleeding is observed during the procedure, on the initial femoral angiogram, apply pressure for 5–10 min and then repeat the angiogram to determine if the bleeding has stopped. Bleeding may also occur immediately after the procedure or in a delayed fashion several hours later due to movement or failure of the closure device. Special care should be taken with very obese patients, as even large collections of blood may go unnoticed for some time. Compartment syndrome can also, rarely, occur due to large collections.
- If the patient is stable, a Doppler ultrasound or CTA should be arranged to exclude a pseudoaneurysm and confirm distal arterial flow. If no pseudoaneurysm is detected, these conditions typically resolve on their own. The patient should be counselled to expect a large, sometimes dramatic, bruise that will change in colour over time.
- If the bleeding is large and unremitting, vascular surgeons and/or interventional radiologists should be called urgently. Press firmly on the area. The patient may enter haemorrhagic shock and require resuscitation with fluids and blood.

Pseudoaneurysm

- This may be identified immediately after the procedure or at a later time. The patient typically notices a pulsatile lump the size of a golf ball.
- The leg should be examined for limb ischaemia. The patient should be placed on bed rest, and a Doppler ultrasound or CTA should be arranged.
- It may resolve with direct pressure under ultrasound guidance.
- Ultrasound-guided thrombin injections are typically successful. A repeat ultrasound scan should be conducted 24 h after treatment. Further injections can be administered if the first attempt is unsuccessful.
- If a repeat thrombin injection fails, covered stenting or surgical repair may be necessary.

Retroperitoneal haemorrhage

- This should be suspected if the patient complains of abdominal/pelvic/back pain or exhibits any signs of haemorrhagic shock, e.g. tachycardia, hypotension, increased respiratory rate, decreased urine volume, or falling haemoglobin levels. Risk factors include puncture above the inguinal ligament, larger arteriotomies, antiplatelet or anticoagulation therapy, thrombocytopenia, malignant hypertension, and obesity.
- If there is any suspicion of RPH, consider the following measures:
  - Place the patient nil by mouth.
  - Resuscitate the patient, which may include administering oxygen, delivering IV fluid or blood, increasing the frequency of observations, and performing urinary catheterisation.
  - Examine the groins, abdomen, and flanks carefully for signs of haematoma.
  - If there is a large, obvious groin haematoma, apply firm manual pressure to the site.
  - Examine any available angiographic procedural imaging for evidence of vessel injury.
  - Draw blood and send it off for a full blood count and lactate assessment. If the haemoglobin or platelets are low, the patient may require a transfusion.

- If the patient is on antiplatelet therapy due to stent placement, exercise caution when stopping antiplatelets or transfusing platelets in patients with stents, as this may lead to stent thrombosis. Haematologists may need consultation if reversal of agents is needed.
- Request a triple-phase aortic CT scan (non-contrast, arterial, delayed) from the abdomen to the thighs.
- If the CT scan reveals evidence of RPH *without* active extravasation, the patient may only require resuscitation and observation, possibly along with packed red cell transfusion. Consider withholding prophylactic heparin. The patient may require transfer to a higher level of care in the intensive care unit (ICU).
- If there is evidence of active extravasation, action must be taken to stop it urgently. These include endovascular covered stent placement or open vascular repair.

Further reading

Gedikoglu M, Oguzkurt L, Gur S, Andic C, Sariturk C, Ozkan U. Comparison of ultrasound guidance with the traditional palpation and fluoroscopy method for the common femoral artery puncture: ultrasound-guided common femoral artery puncture. Catheter Cardiovasc Interv. 2013;82(7):1187–1192.

Robertson L, Andras A, Colgan F, Jackson R. Vascular closure devices for femoral arterial puncture site haemostasis. Cochrane Database Syst Rev. 2016;3(3):CD009541.

Radial

There has been growing acceptance of transradial access due to evidence, initially from cardiology, suggesting increased safety in comparison with transfemoral access.

The ulnar artery may be used as an alternative to the radial artery if it is larger and more suitable. All the following advice applies equally, and the word 'radial' can essentially be substituted for 'ulnar' below.

Procedures via the radial artery usually take slightly more time, and if time is critical, this may not be the best route.

Radial artery size

- The radial artery's limitation is that the larger the catheter, the greater the risk of radial artery spasm and occlusion.
- The outer diameter of the sheath should not exceed the diameter of the patient's radial artery. For this reason, thin-walled sheaths of 7 Fr or smaller are typically used and 8 Fr short sheaths are generally avoided. A 6 Fr sheath requires approximately a 2.0 mm diameter artery. If an 8 Fr guide catheter is necessary, the artery should have a minimum diameter >2.5 mm, and the catheter is used without a sheath. Not all catheters are suitable for radial access.
- Radial access is relatively contraindicated for patients with safe transfemoral access options whose radial artery diameter measures <2.0 mm.

Technique for radial access

- Specific radial support equipment, such as arm boards, are highly recommended.
- Traditionally, the collateral circulation of the hand has been assessed using Allen's and Barbeau's tests. However, evidence suggests that these tests are not predictive of ischaemic sequelae, and the 2020 guidelines from the SNIS do not recommend them.
- Most radial access is currently performed with the right wrist in supination approximately 1–2 cm proximal to the palmar wrist crease.
- An alternative site is via the anatomical snuffbox. This site theoretically has a lower rate of ischaemic complications and does not require the wrist to be in a supine position, making left wrist access easier with the arm crossed over the body.
- Left wrist access is useful if the left vertebral artery is to be cannulated, as this can be difficult via a right-sided approach.
- Ultrasound guidance is strongly recommended.
- The skin should be infiltrated with LA, usually 1% lidocaine.
- A micropuncture set, often packaged with radial sheaths, is used to puncture the radial artery. Single-wall puncture is preferred.
- A microwire is then introduced into the vessel, and the needle is removed.
- While applying pressure proximally to prevent any bleeding, a small nick can be made with a blade at the skin entry point.
- Insert the vascular sheath. The risk of kinking the wire is lower compared to transfemoral sheath insertion. Aspirate blood from the sheath to confirm successful entry.

- A radial 'cocktail' should be prepared, consisting of 2000–5000 IU of heparin to reduce radial artery occlusion, 1–5 mg of verapamil, and 200–500 mcg of glyceryl trinitrate for spasm. This mixture can be put in a 20 mL syringe and mixed with blood aspirated from the sheath before reinjection over a couple of minutes, thus avoiding the discomfort associated with initial saline injections through the sheath.
- The biplane table is swung to facilitate elbow imaging, and an angiogram is generated via the sheath (Figure 6.2). The artery is assessed for suitability of catheterisation. If there are loops, severe stenosis, or variants such as high take-off, it may be better to abandon radial artery access as even though it may be possible, there will be a high risk of spasm.
- The catheter is then navigated through the radial artery into the right subclavian artery over a wire. Once the catheter tip reaches the subclavian artery then the biplane table can be swung back to its normal position.
- The right vertebral artery (and sometimes the right and left carotid arteries) usually has a favourable angle for catheterisation with the wire and can be entered directly.
- To enter the other great vessels, it is often necessary to utilise a Simmons catheter which must be formed before use:
    - If the right vertebral has already been catheterised, then this can be attempted by positioning the catheter such that its bend is at the vertebral origin with the tip of the Terumo wire also at this level. Then push forward and rotate the catheter, and it will sometimes form in the aortic arch.

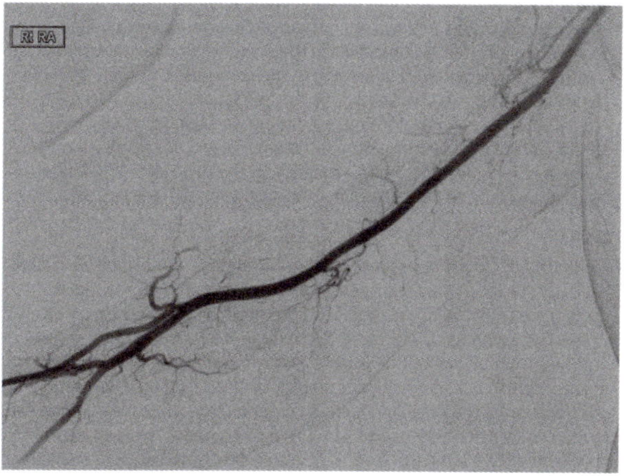

Figure 6.2 Digital subtraction angiography via radial sheath. The artery appears wide, with no loops that would impede catheter advancement. Note the small branches located proximal and distal to the elbow into which the wire can inadvertently enter.

    - Alternatively, pass the wire into the descending aorta and use it to position the catheter with its tip against the descending aorta wall. Then withdraw the wire to the angle in the catheter. Next, push forward and twist the catheter, forming the shape.
    - Another method is by deflecting the wire on the aortic valve such that its tip comes back and sits in the subclavian or carotid artery. Next, advance the catheter over the wire until it is directed upwards. Pull back the wire to align it with the curve of the catheter. Finally, twist the catheter to complete the formation. This method is probably the most reliable, but occasionally the catheter will flip into the heart and cause arrhythmias.
- At the end of the procedure, the diagnostic catheter should be removed over a wire from the right subclavian artery to prevent a shearing injury to the radial artery.

Closure

- Mechanical compression is employed after radial access, utilising a dedicated radial balloon compression bracelet such as the TR-band (Terumo).
- Initially, the radial band should be positioned at the arteriotomy site (indicated by a marker on the band) and inflated while the sheath is removed. Subsequently, slowly deflate the device until oozing is observed at the site. At this point, reintroduce a couple of millilitres of air into the band to restore haemostasis while ensuring flow in the artery (the 'patent haemostasis' technique).
- The orientation of the band should be such that the inflation port is directed towards the hand for radial arteries, and towards the elbow for ulnar arteries.
- Ulnar compression can also encourage radial artery patency. After applying the compression device in the standard manner, attach a pulse oximeter to the patient's index finger and compress the ulnar artery. If a normal waveform is observed, no further action is required (i.e. the radial artery remains patent). If not, under- and reinflation of the TR band, utilising the compression of the ulnar artery, for up to 1 h may help to re-establish the vessel's patency. In the PROPHET-II RCT, this technique reduced 30-day radial artery occlusion to 0.9% vs 3.0%.

Tips

- Radial artery loops: these rare congenital variants can complicate radial access. The loop characteristically occurs at the origin of the radial artery, just after its bifurcation from the brachial artery. They are often associated with recurrent radial artery branches arising from the apex of the loop and joining the brachial artery more proximally. Inadvertent catheterisation of the recurrent branch can lead to spasm, dissection, or perforation of the vessel. In fact, the wire will track more readily into the recurrent radial artery due to its more direct course. The loop may be navigated with a microcatheter and microwire; however, conversion to a transfemoral approach may be the better option as this manoeuvre can cause spasm.

- High take-off radial artery: in this variant, the radial artery starts from the brachial artery higher up the arm instead of at the elbow. Catheterisation is associated with an increased risk of spasm, and it might be best to convert to transfemoral access.
- Radial artery occlusion, a common complication, occurring in approximately 5%. Due to the dual blood supply of the hand from the radial and ulnar arteries via the palmar arch, radial artery occlusion is commonly asymptomatic; however, up to 10% do report symptoms.

Complications

Spasm and catheter entrapment

- Spasm is more likely with multiple puncture techniques, smaller arteries, larger catheters, more catheter manipulation, and variants described above. Use the smallest possible sheath that allows for the intended procedure. Try to minimise manipulation.
- Spasmolytics mentioned above should be routinely used to reduce the risk. Ultrasound-guided puncture also reduces the risk of spasm.
- Spasm can be mild, or so severe that the catheter is entrapped. This can be a dangerous situation, leading to limb ischaemia. Tugging too hard on the catheter can additionally result in vessel avulsion.
- The following measures can be employed:
  - Give the artery time to relax and proceed with the procedure from another access point (e.g. femoral). At the end of the procedure gently tug on the catheter for a slow retrieval under fluoroscopy.
  - Infiltration of additional spasmolytic agents through the radial sheath (if used) or guide catheter if the tip is within the radial, brachial, or axillary arteries.
  - The arm can be warmed (e.g. using a warming blanket) to encourage vasodilatation.
  - Flow-mediated dilatation via reactive hyperaemia may be performed using a sphygmomanometer placed on the upper arm and inflated 30–50 mmHg above systolic BP for 3 min.
  - Continuous infusion of ViperSlide or Rotaglide lubricants through the catheter/sheath.
  - Deep sedation with propofol or GA.
  - Ultrasound-guided axillary brachial plexus or radial nerve block may be attempted.
  - Ultimately, if the catheter cannot be removed, then surgical removal might be necessary.

Access site haematoma

- These are almost always resolved by appropriately positioning the inflation device or by manual compression.

Radial artery perforation

- This can arise from perforation of the radial artery or a side branch. The risk is of progression to compartment syndrome and limb ischaemia.
- If it occurs at the start of the procedure, an angiogram can confirm the bleed. Often, passing the guide catheter beyond the bleed site is enough to achieve haemostasis by the end of the procedure. If not, heparin can be reversed. Standard techniques such as inflating an

intraluminal compliant balloon at the site of the bleed, inflating the sphygmomanometer cuff distal to the artery, or placing a covered stent can be performed.

- After the procedure, bleeding can be difficult to spot in the early stages. Pain, pallor, or paraesthesia should prompt the palpation of a firm, growing, haematoma.
- Compression bandages utilising gauze balls along the radial artery can be used. In addition, a sphygmomanometer cuff can achieve haemostasis by inflating above systolic pressure and intermittently deflating or by gradual deflation over 1–2 h, monitoring with colour Doppler.
- Early surgical involvement is recommended if compartment syndrome is suspected.

Radial artery occlusion

- In PROPHET-II, the rate of occlusion was 3.0% in those randomised to standard haemostasis and 0.9% in those randomised to haemostasis with ulnar compression.
- Radial artery occlusion is most commonly asymptomatic. Symptomatic occlusion requiring medical attention occurs in approximately 0.2%.
- It is recommended to minimise the number of punctures (utilising ultrasound), employ procedural anticoagulation, avoid spasm, use smaller sheaths/catheters, employ patent haemostasis techniques, and use ulnar compression to encourage radial patency.
- If the patient become symptomatic a vascular consultation is recommended. Anticoagulation may be beneficial.

Further reading

Bhatia K, Guest W, Lee H, et al. Radial vs. femoral artery access for procedural success in diagnostic cerebral angiography: a randomized clinical trial. Clin Neuroradiol. 2021;31(4):1083–1091.

Li Y, Chen SH, Spiotta AM, et al. Lower complication rates associated with transradial versus transfemoral flow diverting stent placement. J Neurointerv Surg. 2021;13(1):91–95.

Pancholy SB, Bernat I, Bertrand OF, Patel TM. Prevention of radial artery occlusion after transradial catheterization: the PROPHET-II randomized trial. JACC Cardiovasc Interv. 2016;9(19):1992–1999.

Sandoval Y, Bell MR, Gulati R. Transradial artery access complications. Circ Cardiovasc Interv. 2019;12(11):e007386.

Snelling BM, Sur S, Shah SS, et al. Transradial cerebral angiography: techniques and outcomes. J Neurointerv Surg. 2018;10(9):874–881.

Starke RM, Snelling B, Al-Mufti F, et al. Transarterial and transvenous access for neurointerventional surgery: report of the SNIS Standards and Guidelines Committee. J Neurointerv Surg. 2020;12(8):733–741.

Carotid

Direct carotid puncture is usually employed as a last resort, generally during thrombectomy.

IVT is not a contraindication, but increased caution should be exercised.

Technique

- GA is advised.
- The patient is positioned supine, with a pillow placed under the neck to enhance stability.
- Prepare and drape the appropriate side of the neck to the level of the clavicle.
- A vascular sheath able to be inserted using a micropuncture set should ideally be used to minimise potential trauma to the artery.
- A guide catheter is not necessary. A 6 Fr sheath can accommodate most aspiration/intermediate catheters. Sheaths designed for radial access utilising micropuncture needles/wires may be preferable.
- The carotid should be punctured about 2–3 cm above the clavicle, at an angle of about 45°. The puncture should be performed as a single anterior wall puncture, medial to the sternocleidomastoid. Ultrasound guidance is recommended.
- Insert a guidewire through the needle while screening under fluoroscopy (ensuring the wire does not go too far cranial), and remove the needle.
- Make a small incision at the wire entry site with the blade flat to the skin, ensuring that the artery is not injured.
- Insert the vascular sheath. Where there is a loop in the carotid artery, it may not be possible to insert the full length of the sheath as this may cause spasm or dissection.
- The sheath should be connected to a heparinised flush, ensuring that no bubbles enter during the connection process.
- It is best to suture the sheath in place during the procedure.
- Insert a RHV on the end of the sheath if it allows (not all do), ensuring no air is introduced.
- An angiogram should be performed for navigation (Figure 6.3).

Closure

- Closure can be achieved utilising:
    - Manual compression for 20 min.
    - A closure device such as Angio-Seal (*NB: unlicensed application*).
    - Surgically utilising direct closure with sutures.

Complications

- Carotid injury can occur during insertion of the needle, wire, or sheath.
- Postprocedural neck haematoma can develop. The major risk of this is tracheal compression. For this reason, it may be advisable to keep the patient intubated for up to 6 h following the procedure.

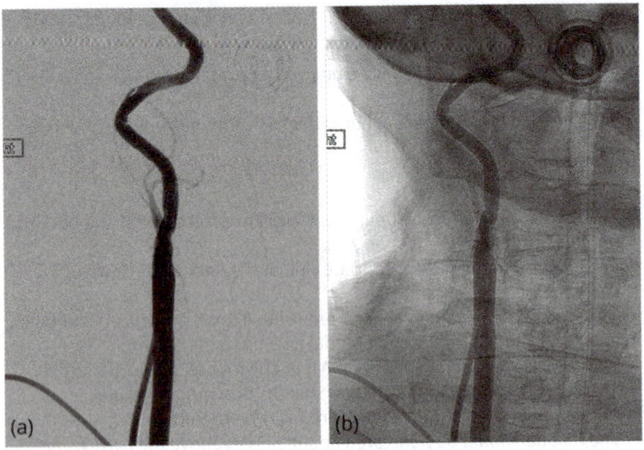

Figure 6.3 (a) Subtracted and (b) unsubtracted angiograms show a sheath placed inside the common carotid artery. A small internal carotid artery dissection is visible distally, which occurred during wire insertion. Images courtesy of Dr Tufail Patankar.

Further reading

Colombo E, Rinaldo L, Lanzino G. Direct carotid puncture in acute ischaemic stroke intervention. Stroke Vasc Neurol. 2020;5(1):71–79.

Karas PJ, Srinivasan VM, Burkhardt JK, Kan P; ENRG Endovascular Group. Direct carotid puncture for emergent thrombectomy: 2-dimensional operative video. Oper Neurosurg. 2021;20(2):E126–E127.

Venous

Venous access is used in for procedures such as DAVF and AVM embolisation, cerebral venous sinus stenting, and inferior petrosal sinus sampling (IPSS).

It is relatively safe in comparison to arterial access, the main risk being inadvertent arterial injury.

Technique

- With the patient supine, the leg is draped and prepared in a sterile manner.
- The femoral vein is located medial to the femoral artery, approximately 1–1.5 cm below the inguinal ligament (remember the NAVY mnemonic for the anatomical order of structures from lateral to medial: Nerve, Artery, Vein, and 'Y-fronts').
- Ultrasound guidance is advised.
- Make a nick in the skin at the puncture site.
- Attach a syringe with saline to an 18 G needle; insert the needle at a 45° angle towards the femoral vein. Follow the needle tip into the vein on the ultrasound probe.
- Aspirate gently when you think you are in the vessel. Venous blood return confirms entry (darker than arterial blood and less pulsatile).
- Replace the syringe with a wire.
- Insert the vascular sheath over the wire. If you are unsure whether the artery or vein has been cannulated, a sheath venogram can be performed. Alternatively, visualise the wire fluoroscopically, which should lie on the right side of midline in the inferior vena cava.
- Once venous access is confirmed, insert a guidewire and catheter as needed for the procedure.
- To enter the superior vena cava, it is necessary to traverse the heart. This is achieved by advancing the wire a few centimetres ahead of the catheter and then following with the catheter, ensuring that the wire does not get stuck or curl up in the heart. Some resistance may be encountered due to the heart valves, and occasional, usually temporary, arrhythmias may be induced.

Closure

- 5 min of manual pressure at the puncture site, medial to the femoral pulse, is all that is usually required for haemostasis.
- The site should be monitored for 2 h post-procedure for bleeding and haematoma formation.

Complications

- Haematoma can occur due to arterial puncture or inadequate post-procedure compression.
- Deep vein thrombosis is a rare potential complication.

Paediatric

The choice of vascular access is dependent on the age group of the patient: neonates, small children, or teenagers.

Transfemoral

- Ultrasound-guided transfemoral access is recommended for all age groups, and it is good practice to confirm femoral artery patency using colour and Doppler ultrasound.
- In neonates and small children, access can be achieved using a 22 G Angiocath (Becton, Dickinson and Company, NJ, USA) or micropuncture set.
- The femoral artery is quite mobile in children. Therefore, engage the surface of the vessel with the needle tip to stabilise it, then employ a short stabbing motion to enter the lumen.
- A 5 mL syringe filled with 2 mL of saline can be used to allow for aspiration of arterial blood to confirm an intraluminal position. Since only the tip of the Angiocath is echogenic, adjust the tip profile to the centre of the lumen as you advance the Angiocath. Remove the metal stylet and advance an 0.014/0.018" wire into the vessel.
- Once the wire is advanced, confirm position under fluoroscopy. Lack of free moment of the wire tip suggests subintimal dissection.
- In paediatric patients, the wire has the tendency to inadvertently enter the lateral superficial circumflex branch of the femoral artery. If this occurs, retract the wire and re-navigate towards the aorta under fluoroscopy.
- For diagnostic angiography, a 4 Fr slender sheath will suffice to allow for a 4 Fr Berenstein diagnostic catheter. In teenagers approaching adult size, arterial puncture can be achieved using standard 18–21 G arteriotomy needles.
- In neonates and small children, a femoral 'cocktail' consisting of GTN and heparin can be administered directly through the sheath to prevent thrombosis of the vessel. The sheath should then be attached to continuous pressurised heparinised flush. NB: verapamil is contraindicated in neonates.

Haemostasis

- Following completion of angiography, it is good practice to inject LA into the subcutaneous tissues of the groin prior to removal of the sheath.
- Closure devices are not licensed for children and so manual compression is necessary to achieve femoral haemostasis following removal of the sheath. Compression should be performed for 10 min via the non-dominant hand with two fingers above the arteriotomy, with an aim to feel the femoral 'thrill' beneath your fingers.
- It is important not to press too hard on the vessel during compression. Thrombosis of the femoral artery is a common complication which can be avoided, especially in neonates and small children. Occlusion not only limits access for future procedures, but in extreme circumstances can cause ischaemia and leg length discrepancy.
- An oxygen saturation probe can be attached to the ipsilateral toe during the postprocedural period in neonates to detect any potential evolving perfusion compromise.

Radial

(See also 'Radial', p. 182.)

- Radial access is increasingly used for cerebral angiography in older children who are eager to mobilise.
- For palmar radial access, a 22 G Angiocath can be used to gain access followed by a 0.014/0.018" wire.
- The sheath should be primed with a radial cocktail containing GTN, verapamil, and heparin. Do not attach a pressurised saline flush on the radial sheath as it may overwhelm the venous return of the hand and can cause severe oedema.
- As older children are generally those undergoing transradial access, a 5 Fr slender sheath is typically tolerated, allowing angiography to be performed with a 5 Fr Simmons catheter.
- The diagnostic catheter should be taken up over a hydrophilic 'Baby J' wire under roadmap guidance.
- Haemostasis is achieved with dedicated compression devices (small sizes are utilised).

Umbilical

- Umbilical access may be required in the neonatal group.
- If an existing umbilical artery catheter is already in place, it can be exchanged for a 4 Fr pre-shaped sheath over an 0.018/0.014" wire.

Further reading

Chaudhary N, Elijovich L, Martinez M, et al. Pediatric diagnostic cerebral angiography: practice recommendations from the SNIS Pediatric Committee. J Neurointerv Surg. 2021;13(8):762–766.

Chapter 7

Diagnostic angiography

Periprocedural details 194
Usage of the catheter and wire 198
Angiographic technique 203
Cerebral angiography 206
Spinal angiography 212
Paediatric angiography 216
Specific diseases 217
Complication management 220

Periprocedural details

Pre-procedure

- Review the patient's records and imaging to:
  - Assess the appropriateness of the indication.
  - Anticipate potential challenges, such as difficulty with arterial puncture or catheterisation of tortuous arch arteries due to atherosclerosis.
  - Determine which vessel(s) require evaluation.

History

- Purpose of study: enquire as to the patient's understanding of the procedure. What previous studies and procedures have already been undertaken?
- Medication: especially anticoagulants, antiplatelets, and metformin.
- Allergies: especially to contrast and local anaesthetic.
- Previous medical history: peripheral vascular, cardiovascular, renal diseases, hypertension, diabetes, sickle cell disease, connective tissue diseases, and coagulopathy.

Examination

- Baseline neurological examination: noting if there are pre-existing deficits (important for comparison post-procedure). If the patient cannot stay still or follow instructions due to a reduced level of consciousness or confusion, the study may require GA or postponement if not clinically urgent.
- Pulses: select the most suitable puncture site (radial vs femoral, left vs right), and assess overall perfusion.
- BP and respiratory rate: elevated BP increases risk, particularly at the puncture site. Rapid respiratory rate can negatively impact image quality.

Consent

- Obtain consent in a private environment where patients do not feel pressured to undergo the examination. In non-emergency situations, patients should receive information in advance and be given the opportunity to reflect and ask questions.
- Patients may be anxious and this is an opportunity to address and alleviate concerns. A comprehensive explanation of the procedure and postprocedural care should be provided, including information on the benefits and risks of various options, as well as the option to not undergo the procedure.
- Patients should be informed that they must remain still throughout and hold their breath when instructed. Warn about possible temporary visual sensations, a metallic taste, and the sensation of pressure in the head. Prepare them for a sharp pain at the site of the LA injection.
- Commonly quoted risks for cerebral angiography:
  - Neurological deficit: 0.7% transient and 0.1–0.5% permanent.
  - Damage to the puncture site vessel (including consequences such as haemorrhage, haematoma, and the need for further procedures to repair the vessel).
  - Allergy and renal dysfunction related to contrast.

    - Small long-term risks of cancer and hair loss due to radiation usage. Radiation risk is very low for DSA but higher for long procedures such as AVM embolisation. The risks for radiation doses are: 0.5 Gy transient hair loss, cataract with a single dose of 2 Gy; permanent hair loss with 7 Gy, skin necrosis with 12 Gy. In children, a 1% overall increase in the lifetime attributable risk of cancer has been estimated for DSA.
- Inform that observation is required post-procedure and a femoral puncture would necessitate lying flat for a period of time.
- If the patient does not have capacity for consent, it is important to discuss with the next of kin (even if legally in your country of practice they do not sign procedural assent).

Preparation

- The WHO Surgical Safety Checklist is performed pre- and post-procedure.
- If under LA without sedation, fasting is unnecessary unless local protocol dictates otherwise. Patients should be adequately hydrated.
- The patient is dressed in a gown. Radiopaque objects are removed from the head and neck.
- IV access may be obtained (based on local protocols).
- A BP cuff and a pulse oximeter are attached.
- Antibiotic prophylaxis is not required.
- Urinary catheters are generally not placed for diagnostic angiography but may be required for longer procedures.

Specific considerations

Contrast adverse reaction

- Risk factors include a previous reaction to iodinated contrast media, family history, atopy and allergic diseases such as asthma, renal insufficiency, cardiac disease, and anxiety. Seafood allergy as a risk factor for iodinated contrast is a myth (allergies to shellfish do not confer an increased risk any more than that of other allergies).
- Anaphylaxis may occur even after first exposure.
- If previous allergy:
    - Consider an alternative imaging modality.
    - Prophylaxis: 50 mg prednisolone orally at 13 h, 7 h, and 1 h before contrast administration, plus 50 mg diphenhydramine IV, intramuscularly (IM), or orally 1 h before contrast administration.
    - Anaesthetic presence during examinations is advisable.
- Treatment of contrast allergy is discussed in 'Complication management', p. 223.

Uncontrolled hypertension

- The diastolic BP should be <90 mmHg and systolic BP <180.
- Non-emergency setting: delay the procedure until the BP is controlled.
- In emergencies: consider GA and radial access.

Warfarin

- Many centres discontinue warfarin and require INR to normalise. Adhere to local protocols.
- LMWH bridging should be considered.
- If warfarin is continued, consider radial artery access to minimise haemorrhagic femoral complications.

Thrombocytopenia

- Thrombocytopenia increases the risk of haemorrhagic complications, especially at levels of <75,000 platelets/μL.
- Consult a haematologist regarding possible supplementation.

Metformin

- Metformin-associated lactic acidosis is rare but may be fatal. If acute kidney injury is caused by iodinated contrast media, accumulation of metformin could occur, with resultant lactate build-up.
- The American College of Radiology recommends:

> In patients taking metformin who are known to have acute or chronic kidney injury (eGFR [estimated glomerular filtration rate] <30 mL/min/1.73m^2) or who are undergoing arterial catheter studies that might result in renal artery emboli, metformin should be temporarily discontinued at the time of or prior to the procedure, and withheld for 48 h after the procedure and reinstituted only after renal function has been re-evaluated and found to be normal.

Chronic kidney disease

- Consult the nephrology team.
- Patients undergoing regular dialysis should ideally be dialysed the day before the procedure.
- Minimise contrast usage. 50% dilute contrast may suffice for roadmaps.
- Adequately hydrate patients before and after.
- Large RCTs demonstrate no benefit for IV sodium bicarbonate or oral acetylcysteine over placebo for the prevention of contrast-associated acute kidney injury.
- Post-procedure, closely monitor renal function. Consider high dependency unit (HDU) or intensive therapy unit (ITU) admission. Haemofiltration may be required if renal function deteriorates.

Pregnancy

- Radiation and iodinated contrast both carry risks during pregnancy. The highest risk from X-rays is in the first trimester. Transplacental passage of iodinated contrast media can pass to the foetus.
- In non-emergency settings, consider delaying the angiogram until after the baby is born.
- Should cerebral angiography be necessary urgently, minimise the radiation and contrast dose. Lead gowns can be placed under and over the abdomen and pelvis for added protection; however, this is no longer standard practice in many units as it may increase the automatic exposure control and actually increase the dose to the foetus.

Breastfeeding

- Iodinated contrast enters breast milk, but the dose is extremely low. The systemic dose absorbed by the infant from breast milk is <0.01% of the maternal intravascular dose (<1% of the recommended dose for an infant).
- If there is maternal concern, she may abstain from breastfeeding for 12–24 h and express and discard milk in this time period.

Post-procedure

- Complete the WHO Surgical Safety Checklist.
- Document the procedure in the patient's records including details of angiography technique, equipment used, medications delivered, vessels injected, puncture site haemostasis, and any complications. This should be completed immediately after the procedure.
- Documented postprocedural instructions should include puncture site monitoring for groin haemorrhage, awareness of the risk of retroperitoneal haemorrhage, palpation of distal pulses, vital observations, and regular neurological assessment. Necessary patient positioning (supine position with leg straight for groin punctures) should be described.
- Prescribe analgesia as needed.
- Before discharge, patients should receive verbal instructions and an information leaflet with contact details of the treating team:
  - Someone must accompany the patient home and stay with them for 24 h. They require telephone access.
  - The puncture site should remain dry until healed or be covered with a waterproof dressing when washing or showering.
  - For groin punctures, patients should avoid bending over, straining, exercising, or lifting heavy objects for at least 72 h. If bleeding occurs, the patient should lie down, keep their legs straight and someone apply pressure for 10 min. If bleeding persists, they should call an ambulance.
  - They should visit the emergency department if they notice a tender lump, or experience pain, redness, or discharge at the puncture site, or develop symptoms of limb ischaemia or stroke.

Further reading

Cha MJ, Kang DY, Lee W, et al. Hypersensitivity reactions to iodinated contrast media: a multicenter study of 196 081 patients. Radiology. 2019;293(1):117–124.

Health Protection Agency, Royal College of Radiologists, College of Radiographers. Protection of Pregnant Patients during Diagnostic Medical Exposures to Ionising Radiation [Internet]. Health Protection Agency; 2009. https://www.rcr.ac.uk/our-services/all-our-publications/clinical-radiology-publications/protection-of-pregnant-patients-during-diagnostic-medical-exposures-to-ionising-radiation/

Raelson CA, Kanal KM, Vavilala MS, et al. Radiation dose and excess risk of cancer in children undergoing neuroangiography. AJR Am J Roentgenol. 2009;193(6):1621–1628.

Shen J, Karki M, Jiang T, Zhao B. Complications associated with diagnostic cerebral angiography: a retrospective analysis of 644 consecutive cerebral angiographic cases. Neurol India. 2018;66(4):1154–1158.

Willinsky RA, Taylor SM, TerBrugge K, Farb RI, Tomlinson G, Montanera W. Neurologic complications of cerebral angiography: prospective analysis of 2,899 procedures and review of the literature. Radiology. 2003;227(2):522–528.

Usage of the catheter and wire

Catheter and wire manipulation requires practice. Strongly consider simulator training as the first step. Then start with lower-risk non-cerebral procedures under direct supervision.

Meticulous technique is always necessary to avoid complications. If appropriate handling of devices and flushing is not adhered to, a complication will inevitably develop, especially in patients with an unrecognised additional risk factor such as dehydration or prothrombotic tendency.

Catheters

- Catheters used for cerebral angiography are around 90 to 100 cm long and 4–6 Fr diameter.
- Catheters come in a range of tip shapes (Figure 7.1). Initially, it is best to become familiar with a small range of devices.
- The vertebral ('vert'), Berenstein, JB2, and Mani tip shapes are all good first-line catheters, suitable for selecting vessels in those with normal anatomy (Figure 7.1).
- The Simmons catheter is useful for accessing vessels that are angulated or tortuous, especially the left CCA when it shares its origin with the right brachiocephalic, or where the artery has a sharp leftward or posterior angulation. The tip shape must be reformed in the body before use:
    - The catheter has a preformed tip shape which must be straightened when passed through the vascular sheath and then reformed in the aorta. Various techniques are used to perform this manoeuvre (Figure 7.2).
    - Once formed, the Simmons is brought to the approximate position of the vessel of interest by keeping the tip inferiorly directed (so it does not catch on non-relevant vessels). Next, the tip is rotated superiorly to catch the origin of the vessel. Once the vessel has been selected, it is advanced distally, counterintuitively, by pulling (rather than pushing) to gain a stable position in the vessel, straightening the catheter. A wire is passed through the catheter, and then the catheter can then be advanced over the wire distally into the vessel.
- When a catheter has entered a new vessel, it is recommended to gently puff a small amount of contrast under fluoroscopy to ensure forward flow and confirm the vessel has not been damaged during catheterisation.
- The tip of the catheter should be free in the middle of the vessel, not lodged against the wall and not at the site of atheromatous plaque. Injections of contrast, or pushing the wire tip in when the catheter is against the wall, risks dissection. Ideally the curve of the catheter should roughly conform to the vessel curvature.
- Catheters can be navigated with or without wires. When a wire is not used, puffing saline or contrast when advancing the catheter forward provides a soft buffer between the vessel wall. Further, using contrast outlines the vessel of interest creating a temporary roadmap.

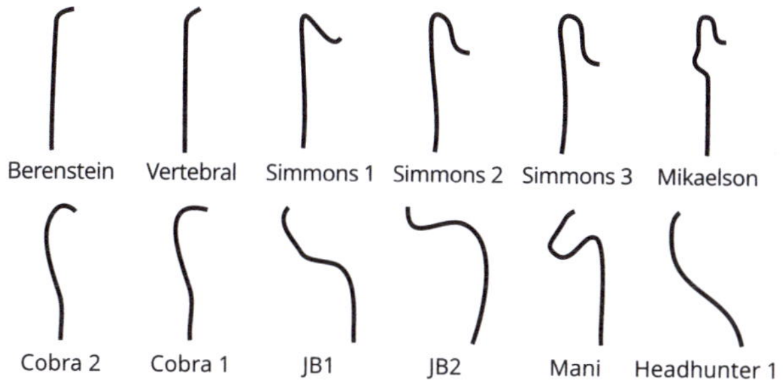

Figure 7.1 Common angiographic catheter shapes.

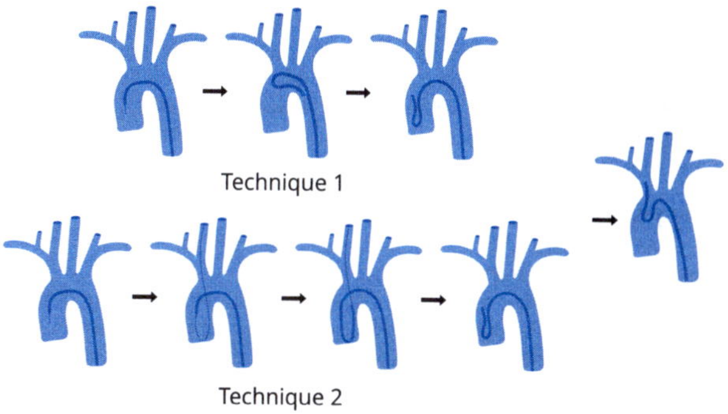

Figure 7.2 Reforming the Simmons tip via transfemoral approach. Technique 1: bring the catheter tip into the ascending aorta. Withdraw the wire tip so it is proximal to the secondary curve within the catheter. Pull the catheter back over the aortic arch while rotating it anticlockwise. When the desired tip shape forms, push the catheter back over the aortic arch. Technique 2: bring the catheter tip into the ascending aorta and insert a wire. Deflect the wire off the aortic valve until it moves superiorly, often into the right common carotid artery. Advance the catheter over the wire so it also deflects off the aortic valve, directing it upwards. Withdraw the wire while simultaneously rotating and pulling the catheter. For both techniques, once the shape is formed, the catheter is pulled (counterintuitively) to advance it forwards into the vessels.

Wires

- Wires are passed through catheters to help with vessel selection and advancing the catheter.
- The 0.035" and 0.038" Glidewires (Terumo) are soft, steerable wires widely used in cerebral angiography. They come in a range in lengths, but 180 cm is probably optimal for cerebral angiography. The wire has a hydrophilic coating and requires wetting before use.

- Wires can be advanced, withdrawn, and rotated (torqued). Torquing may be aided using a damp piece of gauze or a torque device screwed on to the end. Continuously torquing the wire while advancing reduces the likelihood of inadvertently entering small branches and reduces friction.
- Insertion of the wire into the catheter: first aspirate blood (if inside a vessel) and flush with saline. Insert and screen under fluoroscopy when the wire is close to the catheter tip to avoid inadvertent vessel injury.
- The catheter/wire assembly should never be advanced together with less than a few centimetres of wire extending from the catheter tip as short lengths of wire can act as a 'spear' (or 'roman sword') and damage the intima.
- Similarly, do not advance the catheter all the way to the tip of the wire.
- Advancement of both catheter and wire must be smooth and without force.
- When advancing a catheter over a wire in tortuous arteries, the wire may be insufficiently supportive, resulting in both catheter and wire prolapsing out of the vessel. This can be mitigated by placing the wire more distally (achieving more 'purchase') or using a stiffer wire.
- When withdrawing the wire from the catheter, irrigate the hub with saline to prevent air from entering into the vacuum created. Damp gauze is used to wipe and collect clots from the wire as it is withdrawn. Soak the wire in a bowl of saline in between use.

Syringes

- Use different size syringes for contrast and saline to minimise confusion (often 10 mL for contrast and 20 mL for saline).
- Just before attaching syringes to catheters, expel a small amount of fluid from the syringe so that the fluid is in contact with the fluid in the hub of the catheter or in the RHV ("drip to drip").
- After attaching, aspirate a small amount of blood to ensure there are no air bubbles. Flicking the syringe and holding it vertically up can help to release adherent bubbles which then ascend to the back/top of the syringe.
- There are often tiny bubbles at the back/top of the syringe. During injection leave 1–2 mL in the syringe to prevent injecting air. Inject hub down.

Flushing

- Catheters must be flushed with heparinised saline solution to prevent clot formation, either using continuous irrigation (often preferable for novice) or by hand and syringe.

Hand flushing

- Hand flushing is performed approximately every 90 s to prevent the formation of thrombi.
- When using an eccentric tip syringe, ensure the tip is positioned at the top. This orientation allows blood to naturally settle at the bottom of the syringe due to gravity, while saline or other fluids can be injected and remain at the top.

- The 'double flush' technique, utilising two syringes helps ensure all clots are aspirated before injecting fresh saline:
  - The wire is removed followed by gentle aspiration of blood into a syringe. Aspirating too hard will collapse the vessel.
  - This syringe is then discarded.
  - A fresh syringe of heparinised saline is attached and used to flush the catheter.

Continuous heparinised saline irrigation

- Continuous heparinised saline irrigation is used during interventional procedures and may also be used routinely for cerebral angiography.
- Preparation: begin by flushing the RHV with a syringe of saline through the side port while holding your finger on the Luer lock connector with the rotating cap open. Next, fully close the cap and flush the saline forward through the Luer lock. While keeping your finger on the Luer lock remove the syringe and connect the RHV to a pressurised bag of saline. Finally, screw the Luer lock onto the end of the catheter.
- The RHV rotating cap is unscrewed to insert wires, catheters, and other devices. During this manoeuvre, blood usually rushes back and leaks out and must be flushed away either with a syringe or by transiently speeding up the drip (it is essential to prevent stagnant blood forming thrombi which could embolise into the vessel).
- Note that even with a continuous flush, it is sometimes necessary to aspirate blood or air bubbles and reflush manually. Also, the rate of the saline infusion must be periodically checked to ensure it is not too fast or too slow. If too slow, insufficient flushing occurs. Too rapid risks fluid overload.

Exchange technique

- The exchange technique allows one catheter to be substituted for another (such as a guide catheter), over a long wire. It involves inserting a wire more than double the length of the catheter being exchanged. The first catheter is then removed keeping the wire in place.
- Avoid inadvertently allowing the wire tip to slip back by screening with fluoroscopy.
- After catheter removal, the exposed wire is wiped with a damp cloth to remove clots. Note that the wire inside the body may still have adherent clots; unfortunately, nothing can be done about these.
- The new catheter is then threaded onto the back of the wire until it is in the target vessel.
- The wire is then removed, and the catheter aspirated and flushed with saline.
- Avoid exchanges unless absolutely necessary as there is a risk of thromboembolism. In addition, the wire tip can actually dissect or perforate the vessel while the exchange is taking place. As a more modern alternative, the usage of 'select' catheters inserted inside a guide catheter can help to select the vessel of interest.

Microcatheter angiography

- Microcatheters are inserted through larger catheters for navigation into smaller vessels, distal angiography, coiling, stent-deployment, etc.
- A guide catheter is first positioned in the relevant vessel and an RHV and continuous saline irrigation system is attached.
- Microcatheters are also normally connected to an RHV and continuous irrigation.
- Microguidewires (microwires) are used with microcatheters. In neurointervention these typically range from 0.007" to 0.018" in diameter. The wire is inserted through the microcatheter RHV and the tip is shaped, and then pulled back proximal to the tip.
- The RHV cap attached to the guide catheter is then unscrewed and the microcatheter is threaded into the guide catheter for use. Once inside, the wire is extended a short distance beyond the tip.
- The microcatheter may be held within the palm of the right hand facing up with the index and thumb pinching the wire or torquing device, and the microcatheter between the little and ring finger. The microcatheter is tracked by fixing the wire against the table between the fingers and pushing the shaft of the microcatheter into the guide catheter with the left hand.
- The cerebral vessels are very delicate and have numerous tiny perforators that are often not seen on angiography but in which the microwire can catch. It is necessary to navigate gently, carefully torquing and following the shape of the vessel, with the utmost care to avoid dissection or perforation. A safe technique is to form the wire into a 'J' shape, while advancing the microcatheter and wire together. This is very atraumatic on the vessels but makes it difficult to select vessels at branch points.
- Microcatheter angiography is performed using smaller syringes (2–3 mL). The RHV is removed and the syringe containing contrast attached, ensuring no air bubbles are trapped in the hub. Aspirate gently so that blood enters the syringe. DSA is then performed by careful (not overly forceful) hand injection using the thumb, not palm, to press the syringe plunger.

Angiographic technique

Contrast injection

- Low-osmolality iodinated contrast agents are used. Common agents include: iohexol, iopamidol, iopromide, ioversol, and ioxilan. Iodixol is an iso-osmolar agent (the same osmolality as serum). Iodixol has a higher concentration of iodine atoms per osmole allowing angiography at lower levels of toxic osmolality.
- Contrast injections can be performed through hand injection or using a pump injector.
- Hand injections:
  - A 5–10 mL syringe is utilised with the plunger against the palm of the hand.
  - Usually 3–6 mL of contrast is sufficient.
  - Rate and force can be tailored to the vessel and adjusted dynamically during injection.
- Pump injections:
  - Ensures more uniformity between operators and better distal opacification of vessels. The operator does not need to be in the room, minimising radiation exposure.
  - Involves connecting the pump for each injection or connecting the tubing to an RHV system.
  - If the pump syringe tubing is connected to the catheter when it is already in the blood vessel, it is important to aspirate blood into the tubing from the pump to ensure no air bubbles are injected. If bubbles are seen, disconnect and expel some contrast with the bubbles, then reconnect. Alternatively, the bubbles can be aspirated into the pump chamber syringe ensuring that they float to the top of the chamber.
  - The parameters that can be altered during pump injection are (i) the rate in mL/s, (ii) total volume in mL, (iii) linear or rate rise in seconds: this allows for initial linear acceleration of rate over a specified time period and helps to prevent catheter tip recoil.
  - Suggested rates are given as follows:

Vessel	Rate (s)	Rate rise (s)	Total volume (mL)
Common carotid	7–10	0.2–1	10–14
Internal carotid	6–8	0.5–1	8–10
External carotid	3	0–0.2	6–8
Vertebral	4–5	0.5–1	10–12

  - It might be worth slightly lowering rates and volumes when injecting into a vessel with a ruptured aneurysm to reduce the risk of re-rupture.
- Instruct patients ('Don't move, don't breathe, don't swallow') prior to angiography runs. Patients frequently inhale deeply before breath holding; therefore, give them a few seconds additional warning beforehand.

- Continue the exposure into the venous phase for a complete interrogation of the cerebral vasculature.
- Minimise contrast load (important in children or patients with renal dysfunction):
  - Use dilute solutions of contrast:saline in a 1:1 ratio for roadmaps. Only brief injections of small volumes of contrast are required.
  - Lower-strength contrast agents or Iodixol can be used.
  - Contrast can be aspirated from the dead space of the catheter after angiography.

Digital subtraction angiography

- DSA produces images of blood vessels by subtracting the image of overlapping structures (mostly bone):
  - First, a non-contrast mask is produced by holding down the exposure pedal.
  - As further exposures are taken and the foot remains on the pedal, the screen goes blank.
  - At this point, contrast injection should begin. Only the contrast within the vessel is then visible on the screen.
  - Initially, the contrast appears in the arteries and then progresses to the capillaries, parenchyma, and finally, the veins.
- Any movement of the patient or table can misregister the mask and subsequent exposures, resulting in artefacts. To some extent this can be reduced by pixel shifting afterwards, which aims to realign the mask.

Frame and pulse rate

- The frame rate, measured in exposures per second, determines how frequently the machine captures images during DSA. A frame rate of 2–5 exposures per second is standard. This can be increased to 6 or above to visualise fast shunts. Variable frame rates are now standard on modern machines to reduce radiation exposure. This results in a decrease in the rate of exposure over time as the capillary and venous phases are reached. The dose per second can be set independently.
- The pulse rate, measured in fluoroscopic images per second, determines how frequently images are captured during fluoroscopy. On older machines, X-rays were delivered continuously during fluoroscopy. Modern machines now use short pulses to decrease dose (fluoroscopy involves much lower radiation exposure compared to angiography and is mainly used for navigation purposes). Although the pulse rate for fluoroscopy can be adjusted, it is generally kept on the standard setting.

Roadmaps and masks

- 'Roadmaps' are created by performing a subtracted fluoroscopic angiogram. Live fluoroscopic images are superimposed on this mask and used for navigation.
- The operator uses the foot pedal in this mode to create roadmaps in either one or both planes. To prevent capillary or venous contamination of the map, it is recommended to use short injections of contrast.
- Standard diagnostic DSA images can also be used for the same purpose (masks during navigation).

- It is important not to move the table or allow the patient to move when the roadmap is activated as this will result in misregistration of the vessel and roadmap.
- The blank 'glue' roadmap mode is used during injection of n-BCA glue, LEs, or particles and shows only the injected agent.

Cone beam computed tomography

- A single rotation of at least 180° of one or both C-arms (depending on the machine) is made around the patient. Scans can be performed with or without contrast injections.
- Non-contrast cranial CT is useful for detecting acute ischaemia, measuring ventricular size, and visualising on-table haemorrhage. Images are inferior to those acquired on a dedicated CT scanner.
- 3D rotational angiography (RA) involves direct contrast injection into the target vessel and is helpful in characterising aneurysms, AVMs, and DAVFs. Full-strength or dilute strength contrast can be used. Full-strength contrast is ideal for characterising aneurysms. Dilute contrast (usually about 15–20%) is useful in demonstrating stent apposition and assessing detailed anatomy utilising special modes with longer rotation times. On some equipment, subtraction RA is standard (low-dose non-contrast rotation followed by 3D-RA with contrast).
- Modern angiography machines can perform IV CTA and perfusion imaging for acute ischaemic stroke, stent patency, and aneurysmal filling on follow-up as an alternative to DSA.

Cerebral angiography

Basic catheter navigation techniques are described below for normal anatomy. The technique may be modified in different patients. Radial artery navigation is described in Chapter 6, see 'Radial', p. 182.

Femoral artery to aortic arch

- After achieving femoral access, advance the catheter and wire via the iliac arteries and aorta initially to the lower diaphragm.
- Roadmap navigation for tortuous, atheromatous iliac arteries is occasionally helpful. The roadmap injection is against the arterial flow, so a relatively hard injection is necessary.
- If the iliac arteries are extremely tortuous, using a longer sheath can help by straightening them and providing additional support.
- Fluoroscopy is recommended from the femoral sheath upwards to avoid complications. Torquing the wire while navigating from the common femoral artery to the aortic arch is useful to avoid catching on aortic branches and prevents intimal dissection. Navigating the abdominal aorta, keeping the wire relatively close to the tip, say 5 cm, is best to avoid catching on aortic branches. Beware of keeping it too close to the tip to avoid the 'spear' effect.
- At the level of the diaphragm it is good practice to remove the wire and flush the catheter.

Selecting the great vessels

- Target the most relevant vessel first. If the study has to be abandoned early some useful information will still have been gained.
- The origins of the aortic arch great vessels are best selected by first bringing the catheter into the ascending aorta. This is usually easiest with the wire. The catheter is then dragged back with the tip pointing cranially until it catches on the origins of the vessels in order: brachiocephalic, left common carotid, left subclavian (in conventional anatomy).
- It is not usually necessary to perform arch angiography (Figure 7.3a) although if a particular vessel is difficult to catheterise it is occasionally useful to perform angiography at or near the vessel origin.
- Once inside the origin of a vessel, do not inject contrast too hard as forceful injections can push the catheter out as well as damaging the intima.

Brachiocephalic artery

(See Figure 7.3c.)

- From the ascending aorta, the brachiocephalic origin can usually be selected by turning the catheter so the tip is vertically upwards and then pulling back until it catches in the vessel.
- A roadmap can be performed in this position to visualise the right subclavian and its branches, the vertebral artery, and the carotid bifurcation.

Distal right subclavian branches

(See Figure 7.3b.)

- The right costocervical trunk and thyrocervical trunks can be injected to interrogate the ascending and deep cervical and supreme intercostal arteries.
- From the subclavian origin advance a wire into the distal subclavian (or even axillary or brachial) artery and advance the catheter over the wire

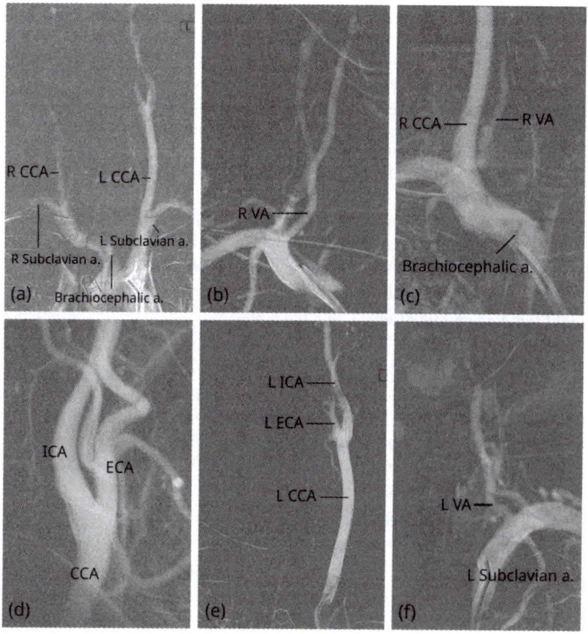

Figure 7.3 Fluoroscopic roadmaps for selection of the subclavian, carotid, and vertebral arteries. (a) Anteroposterior (AP) arch roadmap demonstrating the major branches. (b) AP roadmap via the right subclavian artery *distal* to the right common carotid artery (CCA) origin, to show the right vertebral artery (VA). (c) AP roadmap *proximal* to the right CCA origin. (d) Lateral roadmap via the CCA. (e) AP roadmap via the left CCA. (f) Roadmap via the left subclavian artery. ECA, external carotid artery; ICA, internal carotid artery. VA, vertebral artery.

distal to these vessel origins. Rotate the tip of the catheter so it is pointing upwards and then pull back until it catches on the desired vessel.

Right vertebral artery

(See Figure 7.3b.)

- From the subclavian origin it is usually possible to navigate a wire into the right vertebral artery under roadmap guidance and then advance the catheter into the vessel.
- The wire must first be advanced past the carotid origin, which it often has a predilection for. To optimally visualise this origin, it may be useful to oblique the C-arm to throw off the carotid origin, although this is usually unnecessary.
- If this is not possible, position the wire distal to the vertebral origin in the subclavian or axillary arteries and track the catheter distal to the vertebral origin. Perform a roadmap from this position. Next drag the catheter back until it catches on the vertebral origin.

- If there is proximal vertebral artery tortuosity, it is usually sufficient to perform angiography proximal in the vessel if a stable position can be reached (but don't inject too hard). Crossing the tortuous segment might straighten the vessel, resulting in spasm and vessel stasis. If the vessel is not tortuous, a more distal position can be obtained allowing better angiography and reflux of contrast down the contralateral vertebral artery (usefully imaging both intracranial vertebrals via one injection). 50% contrast solution facilitates reflux into the contralateral vertebral artery.
- Occasionally, a vertebral artery will end in the PICA. If so, the vertebral artery is invariably small/frankly hypoplastic. Beware of performing hard injections in this situation as this is a small end vessel that will rarely rupture due to the high pressure.

Right common carotid artery

(See Figure 7.3c.)

- From the brachiocephalic artery, a biplane roadmap can identify the common carotid origin (AP plane) as well as the bifurcation of the internal and external carotid arteries (usually lateral plane).
- A wire can is advanced into the CCA or even more distally into the internal or external carotid branches and used to advance the catheter to the desired location.

Right internal carotid artery

(See Figure 7.3d.)

- Under roadmap guidance, use the wire to advance the catheter into the ICA. The bifurcation is usually best seen on the lateral projection. There is typically a gentle curve in the proximal cervical ICA that approximately matches the Vert/Berenstein curve and is a good, stable, site for angiography.

Right external carotid artery

(See Figure 7.3d.)

- Under roadmap guidance, use the wire to catheterise this vessel. Finding a good position for the catheter in the external carotid artery can be tricky. Too distal and you will not opacify the proximal branches (such as the occipital and ascending pharyngeal arteries), too proximal and the catheter can flick out before, or during, injection.
- Positioned slightly distal to the occipital origin, the injection can be controlled such that contrast can reflux retrogradely into the occipital artery while maintaining a stable position.

Left common carotid artery

(See Figure 7.3e.)

- From the right brachiocephalic origin, pull back very slowly with the catheter tip pointing vertically upwards (you may need to dynamically rotate the catheter to keep it pointing upwards). At a certain point, the catheter usually flicks into the origin of the left CCA. Push very gently forwards on the catheter to obtain a slightly more stable position.
- Perform a roadmap and advance the wire and catheter into the CCA.
- If the angle of the vessel is directed acutely towards the left, or there is a common origin with the right brachiocephalic artery, a Simmons catheter may be required to catheterise the vessel.

Left internal and external carotid arteries

- These vessels may be catheterised in the same way as the right internal and external carotid arteries.

Left subclavian artery

(See Figure 7.3f.)

- From the left CCA origin, pull back slowly with the catheter tip angled cranially until the catheter flicks into the left subclavian origin. From this position, a roadmap may be performed to enter the subclavian branches.

Left vertebral artery

(See Figure 7.3f.)

- From the left subclavian origin, a roadmap identifies the course of the left vertebral artery. Often a wire passes straight up and the catheter will advance over it. If not, bring the catheter distal to the vertebral artery origin with the wire, remove the wire, and then pull back with the catheter until it catches on the vertebral origin.
- Occasionally (~1%) the left vertebral artery arises directly from the aortic arch between the left common carotid and left subclavian origins. It is relatively easy to advance a wire into it after catching the origin with the catheter.

Left distal subclavian branches

- From a roadmap at the origin of the left subclavian, the wire and catheter is advanced into the distal subclavian artery. The catheter is then dragged back until it catches on the costocervical or thyrocervical trunks.

Tips for vessel selection

- Preparation is key: study previous angiograms and CTAs of the aorta/neck/head. Evaluate which catheters might be best. Inspect for atheromatous disease, angulation, and tortuosity.
- Develop a preference and skill for a limited selection of angiographic catheters.
- Change strategies: try an alternate wire or catheter if a couple of attempts have been unsuccessful.
- Sometimes the wire can access the vessel of interest, but the catheter will not track as there is acute angulation. A stiffer wire can be used in this situation, such as a stiff Glidewire (Terumo) which provides more catheter support. Alternatively, a more flexible catheter can be tried such as the 'select' catheters.

Projections

(See Figure 7.4.)

- Biplane angiography enables simultaneous imaging in two planes, reducing contrast agent dose and procedure length/risks. The angiography table can be adjusted horizontally and vertically or swung or tilted to different angles. It is equipped with two hydraulic C-arms with X-ray sources and detectors that are rotated around the patient to capture images from different angles.

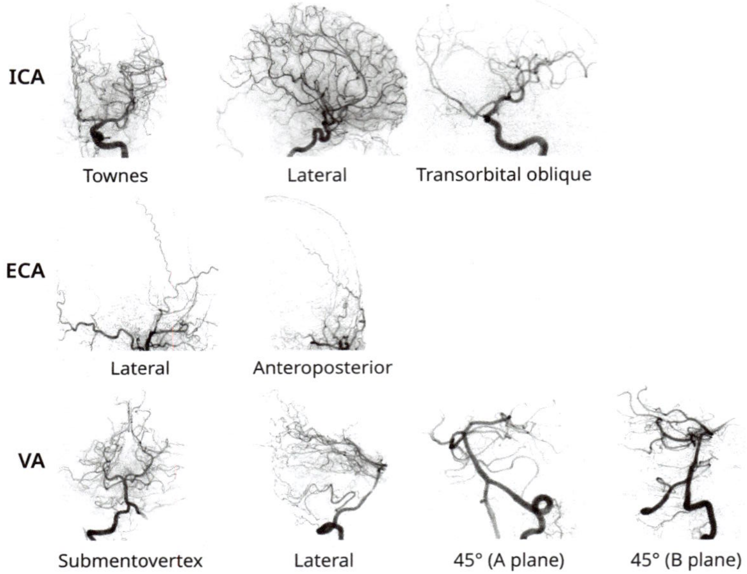

Figure 7.4 Common projections for cerebral angiography.

- Common standard projections of the AP detector:
  - Default position: the AP detector is parallel to the table. Differing projections will be produced depending on the angulation of the patient's head. This view is often used for the external carotid injection.
  - Townes view: the AP detector is angulated approximately 30° in the cephalad direction aligning the petrous ridges with the lower margin of the orbits (supraorbital ridge). There is improved visualisation of the M1 and A1 segments due to reduced subtraction artefact from the orbital rims.
  - Transorbital oblique: the AP detector is angled 30° caudal and with 30° ipsilateral obliquity. This visualises the middle cerebral artery bifurcation and ACOM.
  - Reverse transorbital oblique: the AP detector is angled 30° cephalad and with 30° contralateral obliquity. This view can also be useful for middle cerebral artery bifurcation visualisation.
  - Submentovertex: the AP detector is given steep caudal angulation revealing good views of the basilar artery bifurcation and ACOM.
  - Intermastoid oblique: ipsilateral oblique submentovertical. This is good for the posterior inferior cerebellar artery origins.
- There are variations in the 'standard' set of projections for a 'complete' six-vessel angiogram for SAH. One suggested regimen might consist of:
  - Townes and lateral projections of both ICAs.
  - Transorbital oblique projections of both ICAs.
  - Submentovertex, lateral, and 45° oblique ('windmill') projections of both vertebral arteries. Alternatively, in the investigation of SAH, only one vertebral artery is necessary if reflux is achieved via the contralateral vessel to enter the entire intradural segment.
  - AP and lateral projections of the ECAs.
- Alternatively, the transorbital oblique ICA projections and Townes vertebral artery projections can be omitted, and instead 3D-RA can be performed through both ICAs and at least one vertebral artery (with reflux into the other). This probably has increased sensitivity for subtle abnormalities. A pragmatic approach is to undertake 3D-RA only in vessel(s) where an abnormality is demonstrated/suspected from initial projections and/or earlier CT imaging.

Tips for projections

- If the ACOM is not opacified, try cross compression—manual compression of the contralateral ICA during injection by a colleague using a lead-lined glove (but be careful in patients with atheroma).
- Centre the detector to cover the vascular territory being imaged—on the AP detector this is usually not the entire skull.
- For the posterior circulation, the posterior fossa must be included down to the level of C2 for low posterior inferior cerebellar origins.
- For the external carotid injection, the whole cranium is included.
- For interventional procedures, optimal projections are chosen by studying 3D-RA.
- When repeating studies that have been conducted previously, take note of the projection used in the original study. This allows for direct comparisons.

Spinal angiography

A systematic approach is essential for a successful spinal angiogram. All relevant vessels must be injected, and documentation should follow an organised and consistent protocol.

Spinal angiography requires a comprehensive knowledge of spinal arterial and venous anatomy (see Chapter 2, 'Summary of spinal vascular anatomy', p. 77).

Indications

- Myelopathy or spinal haemorrhage: assess for, or rule out, spinal DAVF and AVM.
- Intracranial SAH where cerebral angiography is normal.
- Surgical/embolisation planning: map the vascular supply to the tumour site for surgical planning, identify preoperative embolisation targets, and localise the segmental artery that gives rise to the artery of Adamkiewicz.

Risks

- Standard risks associated with angiography: groin puncture, contrast, etc.; risks as for cerebral angiography.
- Radiation exposure: typically higher than for cerebral angiography, with attendant increased risk.
- Spinal cord infarction resulting in paraplegia and incontinence: the rate is difficult to quantify, nowadays likely somewhere between 0.05% and 0.1% (no cases were found in a series of 300 patients; Chen et al. 2011). When performing to demonstrate the anatomy of a spinal dural fistula, ensure that GA does not lead to hypotension, which may further compromise cord perfusion.
- Embolic stroke to the brain: rare.

Pre-procedure

- Consent the patient and perform a brief neurological examination of the lower limbs.
- Review patient documentation and study available imaging. Time-resolved magnetic resonance angiography (MRA) sequences (e.g. TRICKS/TWIST) are particularly useful prior to spinal angiography as they can sometimes identify the precise level that needs injection.
- Bowel preparation can additionally be used to reduce bowel artefact: IV hyoscine or glucagon.
- LA with breath holding is often sufficient if the patient is cooperative and the approximate level of pathology is known. GA with ventilation pauses during injection improves image quality and may be necessary if the level is not known and the whole spine is to be potentially interrogated.
- A radiopaque ruler can be used; however, be mindful that the markers may shift relative to the vertebrae due to the parallax effect when the table is repositioned.
- Alternatively, landmarks can be used, either bony (e.g. first thoracic vertebra, 12th ribs, count the number of 'lumbar type' vertebrae) or angiographic (e.g. superior mesenteric artery).

Technique

- Common femoral access is obtained and a 5 Fr sheath inserted.
- A single AP plane is usually sufficient.
- Many catheters are available. The Cobra C1 and the longer C2 (see Figure 7.1, p. 199) are good first-line catheters for spinal angiography. The Simmons 2 or 3 may also be used, particularly for the lumbar segments and the iliac arteries. 5 Fr catheters are usually appropriate, but 4 Fr may be required if the segmental vessel origins are small (however, they have poor shape retention and tolerance to repeated torquing). Pigtail catheters may be used for aortic runs.
- The lumbar/intercostal vessels are paired and arise from the posteromedial wall of the aorta. The catheter tip should be positioned posteriorly rather than anteriorly; however, the orientation is not always obvious. To find out, rotate the catheter clockwise; if the tip points to the patient's right on the screen, then it is correctly orientated.
- Next, select a level to be studied and position the catheter just below the pedicle, with the tip medial and right. Try to catch the origin of the vessel by brushing the tip superiorly and inferiorly, rotating it slightly as you do so. When a vessel is successfully selected, the catheter tip will catch in the vessel origin. If you think you have selected a vessel, apply a small amount of forward pressure to further engage, and carefully inject a small amount of contrast to confirm it.
- Before performing a run, if under LA ask the patient to hold their breath. If GA, the anaesthetist can pause the ventilation briefly.
- Perform an angiographic run. Beware that injecting too hard can cause the catheter to be pushed out of the vessel.
- Record the injected level, typically on a designated template where spinal levels are documented and the corresponding angiographic run number is filled in. It is crucial to ensure that all relevant levels are injected, that pathological levels are accurately noted, and that they can be correlated with MRI findings. Note that vessels are labelled based on the level *supplied* (indicated by the hemivertebral blush), not the vertebral body adjacent to the catheter tip.
- Lumbar and intercostal vessels are typically aligned approximately on the same vertical line, one vertebral level above or below each other. The contralateral vessel arises at the same craniocaudal level as its counterpart. Both vessels at a single level may arise from a common origin. If this is the case, small movements from right to left can preferentially opacify each side.
- If a level cannot be cannulated, an aortic run can be performed in the region to identify it.
- A 'complete' spinal angiogram requires injection of the following: subclavian arteries (including thyrocervical and costocervical trunks), vertebral, intercostal, and lumbar arteries, the median sacral artery, the lateral sacral and iliolumbar arteries (internal iliac). A cerebral angiogram may also be necessary. Ensure that the artery of Adamkiewicz has been identified. If the maximal radiation or contrast dose is reached before the examination is complete and a diagnosis not obtained, it is usual practice to complete spinal angiography on another occasion. This is not

uncommon, and so it is important to warn the patient in advance of this possibility.

- If the level supplying a vascular pathology is found, it is necessary to perform fast-frame-rate angiography in magnified views, potentially with different angulations. Cone beam CT with 20% contrast can also be helpful to delineate complex anatomy.
- It is necessary to inject regional levels (at minimum above, below, and on either side) in order to properly define the lesion, assess its relationship with the cord, identify the potential origin of each radiculopial and radiculomedullary artery, and plan the therapeutic strategies.

Tips

- Move the table as little as possible, as the parallax effect can make correct identification of levels confusing. Instead, select a field of view that covers the maximum possible levels, with an overlapping landmark that can be used to correspond with the imaging.
- Contrast and radiation dose can rise rapidly. Ensure that you have properly catheterised the vessel before injecting contrast and initiating angiographic runs. It is easy, if not careful, to waste whole syringes of contrast into the aorta.
- Appropriate X-ray beam collimation reduces dose and also improves image quality.
- Selective injections at each spinal level are essential. Non-selective aortic injections or injections that opacify a level through collateral vessels cannot definitively rule out pathologies.
- The use of cone beam CT with direct injections through the microcatheters or the diagnostic catheters enhances the visualisation of the extrinsic and intrinsic vascularisation of the spinal cord.

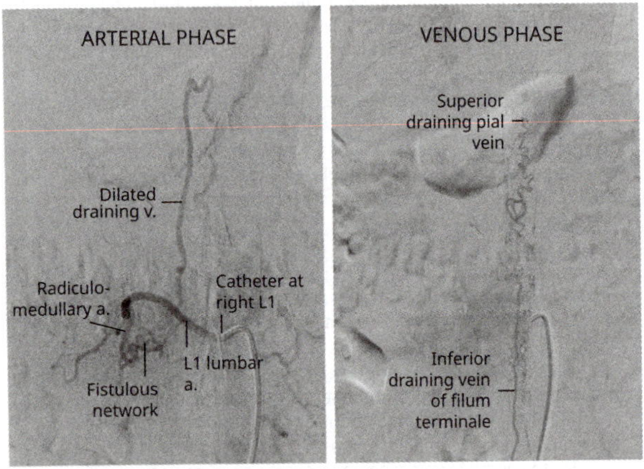

Figure 7.5 Spinal angiogram in the arterial and venous phases demonstrating a dural arteriovenous fistula. Image courtesy of Dr Eef Hendricks.

- A delayed or absent ASA suggests the presence of an AVM/AVF draining to perimedullary veins.
- It is crucial to visualise the lumbar basket enveloping the conus medullaris, facilitating recognition of the anastomosis between radiculomedullary arteries, radiculopial arteries, and the artery of filum terminalis (representing the continuity of the ASA). Injection of the radiculomedullary artery of the lumbar enlargement (artery of Adamkiewicz) aids in visualising the basket and cauda equina. If the basket is not visualised upon injection of the intercostal arteries, the iliolumbar arteries should be examined, as some radiculomedullary arteries may originate lower.
- To diagnose an epidural arteriovenous fistula, it may be necessary to extend imaging runs significantly (see Chapter 14, 'Spinal epidural arteriovenous fistula', p. 502).

Complications

In addition to the general complications of angiography, the following apply:

- Wrongly labelled or missing levels: this is probably one of the biggest risks, potentially leading to delayed diagnosis or wrong-site surgery. If surgery is to be performed, leaving a small, non-occlusive coil in the segmental vessel distal to the origin of the spinal branch (e.g. in the intercostal artery) can help align the level to be targeted in the operating theatre.
- Spinal cord infarction: caused by occlusion or embolism of a segmental vessel. Indicated by paraplegia and bladder or bowel dysfunction. MRI will reveal T2/STIR hyperintensity, and restricted diffusion, and sometimes haemorrhage. While the risk is lower than for cerebral angiography, meticulous technique is still the mainstay in preventing this complication, particularly in those with atherosclerotic disease.

Further reading

Berenstein A, Lasjaunias P. Surgical Neuroangiography. Springer; 2012.
Chen J, Gailloud P. Safety of spinal angiography: complication rate analysis in 302 diagnostic angiograms. Neurology. 2011;77(13):1235–1240.

Paediatric angiography

Consent

- A family-centred consent process is appropriate. The parents/guardians may have varying preferences for the degree to which they want to involve the child in the process.

Vascular access

- Refer to Chapter 6, 'Paediatric', p. 190.

Contrast agents

- The developing kidneys are more susceptible to nephrotoxicity than fully mature ones. The use of non-ionic low-osmolar contrast agents has reduced the risk of contrast-induced nephropathy.
- For diagnostic angiography, a limit of 6 mL/kg is acceptable.
- Contrast dose can be spared by prior planning of which vessels need to be injected. Contrast can also be diluted in saline 1:1 allowing the dose to be halved without compromising image quality.
- There should be consideration of oral or IV hydration pre- and post-procedure.

Radiation dose

- The paediatric population is more sensitive to stochastic radiation effects.
- Angiography should be performed using biplane flat panel detectors and operators should work closely with radiographers and radiation physicists to optimise dose-sparing practices.
- The delivered dose and fluoroscopy time should be recorded for audit after each case.

3D/4D rotational angiography

- RA is invaluable in the characterisation of vascular lesions and can be fused with cross-sectional imaging to view its relationship with the surrounding brain.
- A hand injection of 20 mL undiluted contrast is favoured over pump injection, delivered as a slow continuous bolus.

Complication avoidance

- ICAs in the paediatric population are prone to vasospasm. Due to the small calibre of vessels, vasospasm around a 4 Fr catheter can result in compromise of antegrade flow.
- To avoid this, angiography can be performed without a wire, with slow and controlled rotation of the catheter following the direction of the vessels to prevent 'over torquing'.
- Tonsillar loops occasionally occur in the paediatric age group. For diagnostic studies, the catheter should not traverse the loop.
- If severe vasospasm occurs, intra-arterial GTN may be administered.
- Thromboembolic complications are rarer due to the non-atheromatous nature of paediatric vessels.

Further reading

Chaudhary N, Elijovich L, Martinez M, et al. Pediatric diagnostic cerebral angiography: practice recommendations from the SNIS Pediatric Committee. J Neurointerv Surg. 2021;13(8):762–766.

Specific diseases

Subarachnoid haemorrhage

- If the source of bleeding is occult, all intracranial vessels must be interrogated with a six-vessel angiogram (both vertebrals, internal, and external carotid arteries). In some protocols, just one vertebral artery is acceptable if reflux down the entire intradural contralateral vertebral artery is achieved.
- It may be necessary to inject the costocervical and thyrocervical trunks if a cervical source is suspected. Spinal angiography is also occasionally necessary.
- If no lesion is found, but blood distribution is aneurysmal, repeat angiography after a few days. Aneurysms may be found in a small percentage of repeat DSAs after initial negative studies where diffuse SAH is present.

Perimesencephalic haemorrhage

- Subarachnoid blood is centred anterior to the midbrain but may extend minimally into the proximal Sylvian and interhemispheric fissures (see Figure 8.2d, p. 243). There may be small amounts of blood in the occipital horns but no significant intraventricular haemorrhage and no intraparenchymal haemorrhage.
- The clinical course is usually benign, with a low incidence of hydrocephalus and symptomatic vasospasm. A venous cause is postulated.
- If the clinical presentation and CT scan are entirely typical, good-quality CTA reviewed by interventional neuroradiologists is an acceptable substitute for DSA (depending on local protocols).

Aneurysms

- Angiography is performed for identification, characterisation, and follow-up after treatment of aneurysms.
- 3D-RA (with subtraction if previous treatment with coils or other devices) is useful to visualise the neck, dome, parent vessel, and adjacent vessels. This can also be used to select optimal projections for conventional biplane angiography.
- While the primary vessel to investigate is the one from which the aneurysm arises, it is valuable to assess other vessels in certain situations. The contralateral ICA might be injected for ACOM aneurysms to assess the contralateral A1 segment. The vertebral artery might be injected for PCOM aneurysms to assess the ipsilateral P1 segment.

Reversible cerebral vasoconstriction syndrome

- Patients present with thunderclap headaches, often recurrent, lasting a few hours. There is a female and middle-aged preponderance.
- Imaging may demonstrate convexity SAH, lobar haemorrhage, watershed infarcts, and vasogenic oedema.
- Angiography shows segmental narrowing and dilatation ('string of beads') of cerebral arteries (see Figure 8.2a,b, p. 243). There may be a latent period of 4–5 days before abnormalities are detected. Repeat angiography may reveal resolution in some vessels with new regions of narrowing, often migrating proximally.

- MRA is probably the better imaging modality in those with a typical history and radiographic features. Contrast can theoretically worsen endothelial dysfunction.
- The arterial irregularity normalises within 3 months.

Vasculitis

- May be primary (i.e. unknown triggering factor), or secondary to systemic disease.
- Angiography may reveal segmental narrowing or occlusions of cerebral vasculature (see Figure 8.2c, p. 243).

Intraparenchymal haemorrhage

- DSA identifies and characterises AVMs, DAVFs, and, more rarely, occult aneurysms. CTA/MRA will not exclude a small AVM.
- Patients with a known likely aetiology may not require DSA, particularly basal ganglia haemorrhage in those >50 years with vascular risk factors (such as hypertension), lobar or cerebellar haemorrhage in a patient with known or suspected cerebral amyloid angiopathy, cerebral venous sinus or cortical vein thrombosis, cavernous malformations, tumours, trauma, or infection. MRI may be the preferred initially imaging modality for these disorders.

Arteriovenous malformations

- Fast frame rates (≥5 frames/s) are helpful in high-flow lesions.
- All feeding arteries and draining veins must be identified—this usually requires six-vessel angiography; however, if the AVM is small and supratentorial, single-vessel angiography is sufficient.
- Cone beam CT is useful to characterise complex architecture.
- Identify associated aneurysms (proximal, perinidal, and intranidal), venous pouches, and stenoses.
- There are several different classification schemes for AVMs. Probably the most common is the Spetzler–Martin score for surgical risk (see Chapter 12, 'Classification of bAVMs', p. 451).

Dural arteriovenous fistulas

- Fast frame rates (≥5 frames/s) are useful as these are often high-flow lesions (see Figure 11.2, p. 429).
- A six-vessel angiogram is usually required. Identify all feeding arteries and draining veins. Documentation of normal cranial venous drainage pathways is crucial.
- Cone beam CT is useful to characterise complex architectures.
- Cortical venous reflux is especially important to visualise as this influences prognosis and management.
- The Cognard and Borden classifications are most commonly used (see Chapter 11, 'Classification of dural arteriovenous fistulas (DAVFs)', p. 421).

Moyamoya

- This is a progressive vascular occlusive disease initially involving the terminal supraclinoid internal carotid arteries. Tiny, abnormal, net-like lenticulostriate vessels proliferate distal to the ICA termination, giving a 'puff of smoke' appearance.

- A six-vessel angiogram characterises the pathology, assesses collateral flow, identifies areas of potential insufficiency, and images vessels required for surgical revascularisation (direct or indirect), e.g. the superficial temporal arteries.

Angiography for stereotactic radiosurgery

- Stereotactic radiosurgery delivers ionising radiation to a target in the brain, or, less commonly, the spine. For AVM treatment, this is typically gamma radiation from a cobalt-60 source.
- The target is defined by high-resolution stereotactic imaging. Stereotaxy accurately references the position of a target to a system of coordinate markers (fiducials).
- To achieve this, a rigid metal frame is securely attached to the skull. A plastic box with fiducial markers slides over this frame. An adapter allows attachment of the frame to the MRI/CT/angiography/Gamma Knife tables, keeping the head completely immobilised during imaging and treatment.
- With the frame attached, high-resolution cross-sectional imaging is performed (volume brain MRI or CTA) and DSA.
- Nine radiopaque fiducial markers are visible in each plane (AP and lateral) and are kept in the field of view during DSA. AP and lateral projections are acquired. All vessels supplying the AVM are injected to capture the entire nidus.
- The fiducial markers correspond to known positions on the Gamma Knife dose planning software, and therefore the AVM location can be cross-referenced between different imaging modalities. Using the software, a region of interest is drawn around the AVM nidus to create a target volume.
- A treatment dose is then prescribed (typically 20–25 Gy depending on lesion treatment volume and eloquence of adjacent brain).
- Once the treatment plan is approved, the patient is transferred to the Gamma Knife treatment room.

Further reading

Hou K, Yu J. Current status of perimesencephalic non-aneurysmal subarachnoid hemorrhage. Front Neurol. 2022;13:960702.

Miller TR, Shivashankar R, Mossa-Basha M, Gandhi D. Reversible cerebral vasoconstriction syndrome, part 2: diagnostic work-up, imaging evaluation, and differential diagnosis. AJNR Am J Neuroradiol. 2015;36(9):1580–1588.

Nesvick CL, Oushy S, Ravindran K, et al. Repeat catheter angiography in patients with aneurysmal-pattern angiographically negative subarachnoid hemorrhage. Neurocrit Care. 2022;36(1):52–60.

Complication management

Puncture site complications

- These are described in Chapter 6.

Catheter kinking and knotting

- Simmons tip catheters may rarely knot inside the aorta, making retrieval challenging. For this reason, avoid using the 4 Fr Simmons catheter as this issue tends to occur more frequently with this size.
- Other catheters might kink at sites of tortuosity or due to excessive torquing.

Prevention

- Keep the wire tip inside the catheter just proximal to the primary curve, to reduce the risk of kinking and knotting.

Management

- Kinks in a catheter can sometimes be resolved by gently reducing tension, which involves pulling back slightly and untwisting the catheter.
- If the catheter knots, try to pass the guidewire through it to straighten it.
- If the knot persists, a strong but cautious tug on the catheter as it enters the sheath may be necessary. If these techniques prove unsuccessful, involvement of a vascular surgeon may be required.

Iatrogenic vessel dissection

- Arterial dissection may be caused by the catheter, wire, or by intramural contrast injection.

Prevention

- Carefully study available imaging beforehand to identify pre-existing segments of dissection.
- The more distal the vessel, the easier it is to dissect. Always consider whether a more proximal injection might suffice.
- Perform angiography or roadmaps before entering new vessels.
- The wire tip can cause endothelial damage and must always be visualised fluoroscopically when navigating the catheter. It is dangerous to advance the catheter with the wire too close to the tip as this creates a 'spear' that may perforate or dissect vessels.
- Avoid snagging of the wire tip on the vessel wall. Instead, keep it free in the vessel lumen. This is especially important when advancing the catheter over the wire as more force is applied to the wire tip.
- Keep the catheter tip in the centre of the vessel, not against the wall, important when performing strong contrast injections or protruding the wire beyond the tip.

Identification

- After navigating into a new vessel, gently puff contrast under fluoroscopy. If it appears stagnant, then there may be dissection or spasm.
- A flap in the vessel may be directly imaged on DSA: contrast is stagnant and there may be a linear filling defect. If in doubt, cone beam CT is more sensitive.

Management

- If suspected, pull back the vessel until it is in a safe part of the vessel and perform gentle angiography.
- With a small dissection, without flow restriction, a course of aspirin and/or other antiplatelet may reduce the risk of thromboembolic events. Interval imaging over 6–12 weeks is required to demonstrate improvement.
- If there is flow restriction, it may be necessary to stent the vessel.

Vasospasm

- Vasospasm can be induced by the catheter or wire and manifests as stagnant flow in the vessel. This can mimic dissection if severe.
- Similarly, when a catheter straightens a normally tortuous vessel, it can cause stagnant flow by obstructing the lumen with intimal folds. It is necessary to withdraw the catheter proximal to the bend.

Prevention

- For interventional procedures, nimodipine can be added to a heparin-saline bag attached to the guide catheter (e.g. 3 mg of nimodipine in 1 L of heparin-saline) or injected directly.
- A 'radial cocktail' is given to prevent spasm in the radial artery (see Chapter 6, 'Radial', p. 182).

Identification

- The vessel becomes immediately stagnant after placement of the catheter.

Management

- The catheter is gently withdrawn until normal flow is restored.
- A softer intermediate catheter can be used to cross the segment without straightening the vessel.
- Nimodipine (up to about 2 mg per vessel) can be injected directly into the vessel to reduce spasm. It is necessary to titrate against BP as it induces hypotension. GTN can also be directly injected in 50 mcg boluses up to 200 mcg.

Microemboli

- MRI post-procedure often shows tiny DWI hyperintensities despite no clinical symptoms (17% in one study).
- These probably represent procedural microemboli and are seen more frequently in the elderly and those with vascular risk factors.
- Although seemingly clinically silent, a thorough neurological examination may reveal subtle neurological deficits.
- Meticulous technique is recommended to minimise these lesions.

Thromboembolism

- Risk factors include: age, history of cerebrovascular accident/transient ischaemic attack (TIA), sickle cell disease, and long/complex procedures.

Prevention

- Meticulous technique.
- Avoid dehydration pre-procedure.

- Systemic heparinisation is necessary during interventional procedures other than thrombectomy (where it has shown a higher incidence of haemorrhage).

Identification
- Angiographic signs may be subtle and include slowly filling vessels, absent branches, and regional hypoperfusion.
- Clinical presentation depends on the territory and may include weakness, dysphasia in the anterior circulation, or nausea/vomiting, dizziness, visual field deficit, or reduced Glasgow Coma Scale (GCS) score in the posterior circulation.
- Symptoms and signs may only be apparent post-procedure.

Management
- Consider arterial territory and risk/benefit considering that studies are often performed in the context of cerebral haemorrhage.
- Initially, systemic heparinisation and raising the BP may help with smaller, more distal emboli.
- IV aspirin and GP IIb/IIIa receptor inhibitors may be considered, although these should generally be avoided with an unsecured ruptured aneurysm or other active bleeding source.
- If an iatrogenic LVO is identified, thrombectomy may be necessary.
- Post-procedure, IVT may be considered in the absence of contraindications.

Air embolism

- Air bubbles are easily trapped inside syringes, catheters, valves, stents, and tubing. They are adherent to surfaces and may be injected into the circulation. Small bubbles can be tolerated and pass through the pial capillary bed, but larger bubbles can become trapped and cause vessel occlusion.

Prevention
- Diligence in preventing the air bubble formation while attaching devices, and removing them when noticed.
- A vacuum may be created within the catheter when removing the wire if the catheter is completely obstructing a vessel. If this happens, there is sometimes the sound of air being drawn into the catheter. Aspirating will not help in this situation due to the vacuum. Slowly withdraw the catheter until blood is seen to exit out of the hub. Then aspirate and flush the catheter.

Identification
- Intravascular bubbles appear as filling defects on angiography.
- In situations of doubt, on-table cone beam CT is sensitive.

Management
- If the patient is symptomatic, give high-flow 100% oxygen. Oxygen is many times more soluble than nitrogen in blood and oxygen saturated in blood helps displace the nitrogen in the air emboli.
- Aspiration and breaking up of air bubbles can be achieved with aspiration catheters or microcatheters.
- Flow reversal with a BGC may be successful if the bubble is in a large vessel.

- Systemic heparinisation to prevent clot forming in stagnant vessels.
- Hyperbaric oxygen chambers have been used and achieve better results if started within 6 h.

Aneurysm rupture

(See Figure 7.6.)

- Aneurysm rupture rarely occurs due to forceful injections during cerebral angiography.
- Manage as for any aneurysmal rupture: i.e. reverse heparinisation (if given), inform the anaesthetist, lower the BP if acute hypertension develops (Cushing reflex), inflate a balloon across the aneurysm neck, and occlude the aneurysm (e.g. coiling). Perform an on-table CT when the situation is controlled and in case of raised intracranial pressure (ICP), consider insertion of ventricular drain or performing a decompressive craniotomy.

Acute contrast reaction

- Hypersensitivity may be induced by contrast or other procedural medications.
- Risk factors: refer to 'Periprocedural details', p. 194.

Prevention

- Premedication: refer to 'Periprocedural details', p. 195.
- Anaesthetic presence during the procedure might be advisable if there is anticipation of allergy.

Identification

- Mild reactions: tachycardia, hypertension, nausea/vomiting.
- Severe reactions: skin rash, oedema, bronchospasm, hypotension, tachycardia, bradycardia, loss of consciousness.

Management in adults

(See Table 7.1.)

- In general: if severe, treat as a medical emergency. Call the emergency response team, assessment with airway, breathing circulation and oxygen, monitor vitals, gain IV access (if not already *in situ*) and consider IV fluids, attach pulse oximeter, consider oxygen supplementation.

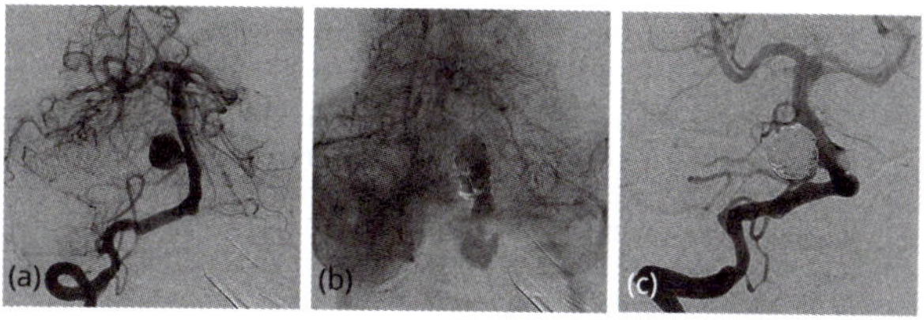

Figure 7.6 Aneurysm rupture during angiography. (a) A right vertebral artery angiogram shows the large right anterior inferior cerebellar artery aneurysm. (b) A second angiogram caused rupture of the aneurysm with extravasation of contrast. (c) A microcatheter was quickly used to catheterise and coil the aneurysm while a compliant balloon was inflated across the neck.

Table 7.1 Doses for emergency medications

Treatment	Indication	Dose
Diphenhydramine	Mild hives	25–50 mg orally (PO)
Fexofenadine	Mild hives	180 mg PO
Diphenhydramine PO, IM, or IV	Moderate hives	25–50 mg (if IV administer dose slowly over 1–2 min)
IV fluids (normal saline or lactated Ringer's)	Diffuse erythema or hypotension	1000 mL rapidly
Epinephrine IV	Diffuse erythema Hypotension with tachycardia Laryngeal oedema Bronchospasm (moderate, severe)	1 mL of 0.1 mg/mL (1:10,000) dilution (0.1 mg); administer slowly into a running IV infusion of fluids; can repeat every few minutes as needed up to 10 mL (1 mg) total
Epinephrine IM	Diffuse erythema	0.3 mL of 1.0 mg/mL (1:1,000) dilution (0.3 mg); can repeat every 5–15 min up to 1 mL (1 mg) total
Lorazepam IV	Seizures/convulsions	2–4 mg IV
Furosemide	Pulmonary oedema Hypertensive crisis	20–40 mg IV (administer slowly over 2 min)
Labetalol IV	Hypertensive crisis	20 mg IV; administer slowly over 2 min; can double the dose every 10 min
Glyceryl trinitrate tablet	Hypertensive crisis	0.4 mg tablet (can repeat 5–10 min)
Atropine	Hypotension with bradycardia	0.6–1.0 mg (administer into a running IV infusion of fluids); can repeat up to 3 mg total
Beta-agonist inhaler (salbutamol)	Bronchospasm (mild, moderate, severe)	2 puffs (100 mcg/puff) for a total of 200 mcg; can repeat up to 3 times

- Diffuse erythema:
  - Preserve IV access, monitor vitals, pulse oximeter, oxygen by mask, consider calling the emergency response team.
  - If normotensive: no other treatment usually needed.
  - If hypotensive: treatment with IV fluids (e.g. 0.9% normal saline).
  - If profound or unresponsive to fluids, consider epinephrine (IV or IM, IV preferred for hypotensive patients).
- Hives (urticaria):
  - Mild: no treatment often needed; however, if symptomatic, consider diphenhydramine or fexofenadine.

    - Moderate: monitor vitals, preserve IV access, consider diphenhydramine or fexofenadine.
    - Severe: monitor vitals, preserve IV access, diphenhydramine.
- Seizures/convulsions:
    - Turn patient on side to avoid aspiration, suction airway as needed, preserve IV access, monitor vitals, pulse oximeter, oxygen by mask.
    - If unremitting: call emergency response team and use lorazepam (IV).
- Pulmonary oedema:
    - Preserve IV access, monitor vitals, oxygen by mask, pulse oximeter, elevate head of bed if possible, use furosemide, call emergency response team.
- Hypertensive crisis:
    - Preserve IV access, monitor vitals, pulse oximeter, oxygen by mask.
    - Use labetalol (IV), or if not available, glyceryl trinitrate tablet (sublingually) and furosemide. Call emergency response team.
- Hypotension:
    - Preserve IV access, monitor vitals, pulse oximeter, oxygen by mask, elevate legs at least 60°, use IV fluids (0.9% normal saline or lactated ringers).
    - Hypotension with bradycardia: if mild and resolving no other treatment usually necessary. If severe, use atropine (IV) and call emergency response team.
    - Hypotension with tachycardia: use epinephrine (IV preferred), and call emergency response team.
- Laryngeal oedema:
    - Preserve IV access, monitor vitals, pulse oximeter, oxygen by mask. Use epinephrine (IM, IV if hypotensive).
    - Call the emergency response team.
- Bronchospasm:
    - Preserve IV access, monitor vitals, pulse oximeter, oxygen by mask.
    - Mild: beta-agonist inhaler (salbutamol (known as albuterol in the US/ Canada)), Consider sending patient to the emergency department or calling emergency response team.
    - Moderate: beta-agonist inhaler (salbutamol), consider adding epinephrine (IM).
    - Severe: epinephrine (IV or IM), beta-agonist inhaler (salbutamol), and call emergency response team.

Contrast-induced acute kidney injury

- This is impairment of renal function with a 25% rise in baseline serum creatinine or an increase of 0.5 mg/dL (44 µmol/L) in absolute serum creatinine value 48–72 h following IV contrast administration.
- Risk factors: raised serum creatinine, metformin, chronic kidney disease (especially with glomerular filtration rate <30 mL/min/1.73m^2), hypertension, diabetes mellitus, multiple myeloma, cardiovascular disease, sepsis, advanced age, dehydration, hyperuricaemia, and paraproteinaemia.

Prevention

- IV fluids: 0.9% normal saline 6–12 h before the procedure and continuing post-procedure.

- Consider stopping metformin 48 h pre-procedure.
- If the patient undergoes regular dialysis, this should be on the day before the procedure.
- Consider admission to HDU/ITU after the procedure.
- Minimise procedural contrast.
- There is no benefit in giving N-acetylcysteine or sodium bicarbonate.

Identification

- Renal function should be carefully monitored post-procedure.

Management

- Most acute kidney injury is self-resolving with adequate hydration, but if severe, dialysis might be required.

Contrast-induced encephalopathy

- This rare complication relates to endothelial injury and breakdown of the blood–brain barrier (BBB) and usually manifests 2–12 h post-procedure.
- Symptoms include headaches, seizures, transient cortical blindness, transient global amnesia, reduced consciousness, and other neurological deficits.
- Risk factors include larger doses of contrast, acute cerebral ischaemia, hypertension, kidney disease, and diabetes.

Identification

- CT reveals hyperdense cortical regions with mild swelling. MRI shows T2/ fluid-attenuated inversion recovery (FLAIR) hyperintensity without DWI hyperintensity.
- Exclusion of vessel occlusion is important with vascular imaging.

Management

- Most cases resolve spontaneously within 48–72 h. Persistent neurological deficit is rarely reported.
- Management is supportive. IV fluids and anticonvulsants may be required. Reassurance. Steroids may be given, although there is limited evidence for their efficacy.

Further reading

ACR Committee on Drugs and Contrast Media. ACR Manual on Contrast Media. American College of Radiology; 2023. https://www.acr.org/Clinical-Resources/Clinical-Tools-and-Reference/Contrast-Manual

Kesseler E, Tafelmeier S, Nikoubashman O, Iancu AM, Pinho J, Wiesmann M. Frequency and pattern of MRI diffusion restrictions after diagnostic catheter neuroangiography. Tomography. 2023;9(3):1010–1018.

Cerebral aneurysms

Patient information diagram *228*
Clinical presentation *229*
Investigations *231*
Pathophysiology *233*
Who to treat *234*
Subarachnoid haemorrhage grading *240*
Differential diagnosis of subarachnoid haemorrhage *242*
Coil embolisation of intracranial aneurysms *247*
Aneurysm types and locations *256*
Periprocedural complications *267*
Balloon test occlusion *273*
Parent vessel occlusion *275*
Paediatric aneurysms *277*
Stenting *280*
Flow diversion *286*
Intrasaccular devices *298*
Complications of subarachnoid haemorrhage *305*
Vasospasm and delayed cerebral ischaemia *310*

Patient information diagram

Patients are often unfamiliar with endovascular techniques and pathologies. A simple diagram of common aneurysm treatment techniques might help with explanations (Figure 8.1).

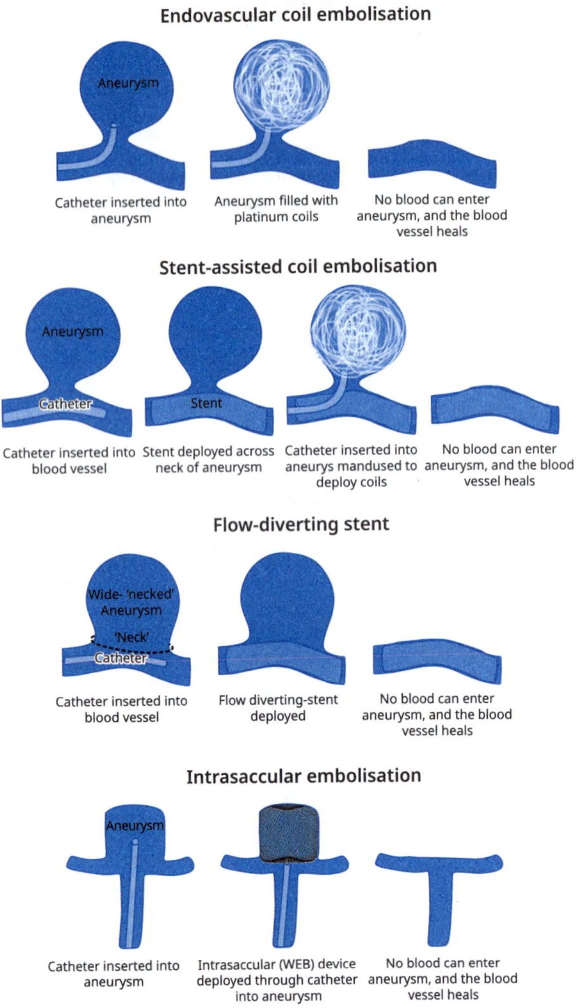

Figure 8.1 Patient information illustrating common aneurysm treatment techniques.

Clinical presentation

Epidemiology

- The incidence of spontaneous (i.e. non-traumatic) SAH is about 6–8 per 100,000 per year.
- In developed countries, the incidence is declining due to reduced smoking rates and superior control of vascular risk factors. Over the last 40 years, the mean age of SAH ictus has increased from around 50 to 60 years.
- 80–85% of spontaneous SAH is caused by the rupture of an intracranial aneurysm (aSAH). The prognosis remains poor; 27–44% of patients die and one-third of survivors are left dependent. Up to 20% die within the first 24 h, mostly from early rebleeding.
- There is excess risk of aSAH in post-menopausal females (protective effect of oestrogens) over males of around 1.4–1.9:1 but no sex difference in outcome.
- The main causes of non-aneurysmal spontaneous SAH are perimesencephalic SAH (idiopathic), reversible cerebral vasoconstriction syndrome, venous sinus thrombosis, amyloid angiopathy, and rupture of an intracranial vascular malformation (AVM or AVF) (see 'Differential diagnosis of subarachnoid haemorrhage', p. 242). More rarely, it is associated with other vasculitides, tumours, or dissection.
- Unruptured intracranial aneurysms (UIAs) are much more common than aSAH, occurring in approximately 3% of the adult population.
- UIAs <7 mm in maximum diameter are the most frequently detected but rarely cause symptoms.
- Given the difference between aneurysm prevalence and aSAH incidence, it is estimated that approximately 85% of intracranial aneurysms do not bleed.
- Conditions predisposing to UIA and/or SAH include:
  - Genetic factors: autosomal dominant polycystic kidney disease, connective tissue disorders (including neurofibromatosis type 1; Ehlers–Danlos syndrome, predominantly types III and IV; Loeys–Dietz syndrome; and possibly Marfan syndrome) and alpha-1 antitrypsin deficiency. They are more common in women and their prevalence is higher among Japanese individuals and some other ethnic subgroups such as black and Hispanic populations in the USA.
  - Acquired factors: cocaine or amphetamine abuse, hypertension, smoking, excessive alcohol consumption, and increasing age.
- Familial SAH is well recognised, but the risk is concentrated in those patients who have two or more first-degree relatives with aSAH and/or an intracranial aneurysm and even more so with coexisting hypertension and in those family members who smoke.
- 20–30% of patients have multiple aneurysms.

Symptoms and signs

- Patients with SAH usually present with:
  - Sudden onset of a severe headache, maximal immediately or within minutes, and lasting an hour or more (usually days).

  - Other symptoms of meningism: nausea, vomiting, photophobia, neck stiffness.
  - Loss of consciousness: transient at onset (around 50% of cases) or persisting.
  - Epileptic seizures: about 6% of cases.
  - Focal neurological symptoms: dysphasia and hemisensory or motor symptoms.
  - Sudden death: approximately 10% of cases of spontaneous aSAH.
- Sudden severe headache is the cardinal symptom and may be the only symptom in up to one-third of patients with aSAH.
- 40% will have benign thunderclap headache.
- The remainder have other primary and secondary headache syndromes.
- Most UIAs are asymptomatic until they cause mass effect or rupture. A large or growing aneurysm may press on adjacent structures causing:
  - Pain (especially behind the eye).
  - Cranial nerve palsy, usually oculomotor, optic, and abducens.

Further reading

Al-Shahi R, White PM, Davenport RJ, Lindsay KW. Subarachnoid haemorrhage. BMJ. 2006;333(7561):235–240.

de Rooij NK, Linn FH, van der Plas JA, Algra A, Rinkel GJ. Incidence of subarachnoid haemorrhage: a systematic review with emphasis on region, age, gender and time trends. J Neurol Neurosurg Psychiatry. 2007;78(12):1365–1372.

Huang J, van Gelder JM. The probability of sudden death from rupture of intracranial aneurysms: a meta-analysis. Neurosurgery. 2002;51(5):1101–1105.

Nieuwkamp DJ, Setz LE, Algra A, Linn FH, de Rooij NK, Rinkel GJ. Changes in case fatality of aneurysmal subarachnoid haemorrhage over time, according to age, sex, and region: a meta-analysis. Lancet Neurol. 2009;8(7):635–642.

Investigations

SAH must be excluded in patients presenting with a sudden severe headache, maximal within minutes, lasting >1 h, and without alternative explanation.

Initial

- Routine blood tests: full blood count, coagulation screen, group and save, urea and electrolytes, serum glucose, and serum magnesium (uncorrected disturbances are associated with poor outcomes in SAH).
- Unenhanced cranial CT as soon as possible after onset. The sensitivity of volumetric CT for SAH, when interpreted by an experienced neuroradiologist, is excellent (at least 99%) within 6 h of ictus, but it declines thereafter to 90–97% within 3 days and is <50% by 5–7 days post-ictus. The distribution of blood on CT can suggest the cause and aneurysm location.
- LP: CSF analysis is still indicated if cranial CT is normal. In patients with an acute headache and a normal head CT ≤6 h after ictus, there is no added value of CSF analysis.
    - The LP time window to reliably detect SAH is around 12 h to 2 weeks following ictus. If outside this window, MRI may be used to detect haemorrhagic breakdown products.
    - Care is required in handling CSF samples for orthochromatic analysis and local policy guidelines should be followed.
- CTA if SAH is confirmed (by CT or LP). This can confirm an aneurysmal cause. The sensitivity of CTA for identifying aneurysms >3 mm diameter is approximately 96%.
- Chest radiography to exclude aspiration or pulmonary oedema.
- 12-lead electrocardiography to exclude arrhythmia or myocardial ischaemia/stunning associated with SAH.

At neuroscience centre

- A diagnostic angiogram is warranted if (i) other pathology is suspected on CTA, (ii) no aneurysm on CTA when CT demonstrates diffuse SAH, or (iii) CT/CTA negative but LP positive.
- If an aneurysm is confirmed on CTA and endovascular management is planned, a separate diagnostic DSA is generally not required and can usually be performed during the EVT.
- If there is a perimesencephalic pattern of SAH ('perimesencephalic haemorrhage') with no aneurysm on neuroradiology review, good-quality CTA, and both clinical course and imaging correlate, then formal DSA may not be required (this is dictated by local policy). Note the CT scan must be within 3 days of ictus.

Screening for cerebral aneurysms

Who to screen

- A patient with two or more first-degree relatives with SAH. The prevalence of UIAs is around 8–10% of those screened. The risks are higher in siblings, females, smokers, and hypertensives.
- Autosomal dominant polycystic kidney disease: 10% prevalence of UIA rising to 20% in those with an additional family history of intracranial aneurysms or aSAH.
- Coarctation of the aorta: 10% prevalence of UIA (due to hypertension or other cause, as-yet undefined).

Who not to screen

- Widespread screening for cerebral aneurysm is not warranted as most aneurysms do not rupture. Every aSAH cannot be prevented by screening as many ruptured aneurysms probably rupture within a few months of formation, i.e. those in whom the aneurysm wall is not stabilised.
- Risk of *de novo* aneurysm formation after aSAH is 0.4–2.2% per year. However, the risk of future aSAH from *de novo* aneurysm was only 9 events in 16,579 patient-years of patient follow-up in the landmark ISAT trial. Screening is not recommended, because studies have shown that the quality of life is not enhanced (anxiety, treatment-related complications).

How to screen

- Thorough counselling is always recommended before screening.
- Begin screening at around 20 years old (conventional saccular aneurysms are extremely rare earlier).
- The goal is to increase the number of quality years of life.
- 3D time-of-flight MRA is the modality of choice. Its sensitivity in detecting aneurysms >2 mm is 87–100%.
- Repeat screening at 3–5-year intervals until 60–70 years, considering the patient's history, comorbidities, and treatment risks (and timing of any family history—e.g. if all familial SAH occurred <40 years, it is questionable to carry on screening after 50 years). Aneurysms can develop even after two negative screens.
- Screening studies should preferably be reported by neuroradiologists.

Pathophysiology

- Aneurysms are a disease of the arterial wall. Endothelial dysfunction triggers an inflammatory response, leading to the breakdown of the internal elastic lamina, a connective tissue layer that separates the intima (a single layer of endothelial cells lining the artery) from the media (composed mainly of smooth muscle and extracellular collagen type III).
- The media layer becomes disorganised as smooth muscle cells undergo a phenotypic switch from their normal contractile state to a form that promotes inflammation and tissue remodelling. This shift increases smooth muscle cell apoptosis, leading to a thinning and weakening of the media. The once tightly arranged smooth muscle bands become disrupted, and the media is eventually depleted of most smooth muscle cells.
- Inflammatory cells are frequently found in aneurysmal tissues where they are thought to contribute to the pathobiology. These include macrophages, neutrophils, T cells, and B cells.
- Aneurysms predominate at bifurcations, sites of turbulent flow and high arterial wall shear stress, both of which play a critical role in intracranial aneurysm formation and growth.
- Most intracranial aneurysms are polygenetic in origin with many possible candidate genes identified to date.
- Aneurysm stability depends upon the balance between wall repair, with vascular smooth muscle proliferation and regeneration of the extracellular matrix, and wall destruction, with degradation of the extracellular matrix.
- There are four broad categories of intracranial aneurysms: saccular, fusiform, dissecting, and infectious (colloquially, 'mycotic'). The saccular type accounts for >90%.
    - Saccular aneurysms are round, pouch-like dilations that arise at arterial bifurcations with a neck connecting the dome to the parent vessel.
    - Fusiform aneurysms are circumferential expansions that enlarge the entire vessel diameter along a segment.
    - Dissecting aneurysms result when blood enters through an intimal tear and separates the arterial wall layers, creating an intramural channel.
    - Infectious aneurysms are fragile, irregular outpouchings produced by infection of the arterial wall, typically from septic emboli.
- Additional subtypes include blister aneurysms—small, broad-based protrusions typically found at non-branching sites of the supraclinoid ICA—and pseudoaneurysms, which lack a true vessel wall and often follow trauma. Giant aneurysms, defined by a diameter >25 mm, may be saccular or fusiform and often partially thrombosed. Traumatic aneurysms, a subset of pseudoaneurysms, arise from blunt or penetrating injury. Rare neoplastic aneurysms can result from tumour emboli or vascular invasion by malignancy.

Who to treat

Acutely ruptured aneurysms

- The purpose of acute aneurysm treatment is to prevent rebleeding.
- Age, World Federation of Neurosurgical Societies (WFNS) grade, comorbidity, time from ictus, and vascular anatomy determine the most appropriate intervention.
- A ruptured aneurysm should be treated as soon as possible after admission to a neuroscience centre, ideally within 24 h (and within 48 h of the initial bleed, unless there is a delayed presentation or diagnosis). This necessitates daily availability of EVT for aSAH.
- The ISAT was a large, landmark, international, multicentre RCT that compared the safety and efficacy of endovascular coiling versus neurosurgical clipping in patients suitable for both treatments.
    - At 1 year, endovascular coiling resulted in significantly lower death and dependency compared with neurosurgical clipping.
    - At 10 years, patients in the EVT group were more likely to be alive and independent than patients in the neurosurgery group (68.2% endovascular coiling group vs 61.7% in the neurosurgical clipping group). The number needed to treat for one additional independent survivor was 15. The risk of developing epilepsy was significantly lower in coiling group patients.
    - At 18 years, despite aneurysm recurrences, retreatments, and rebleeding being slightly more common, the long-term clinical outcomes of EVT remained superior. Patients were significantly more likely (40 times) to die from another cause than from the treated aneurysm.
- Where aneurysm anatomy is amenable to EVT, the consensus recommendation, based on RCT evidence, is for coil embolisation as first line rather than neurosurgical clipping. Primary clipping is reserved for cases of aneurysm haematoma requiring immediate evacuation or anatomy unsuitable for EVT.
- A proposed exception is MCA bifurcation aneurysms, where the ISAT results were neutral (relative risk 1.01). However, a counterpoint by the ISAT authors was that dividing the data from any trial into subgroups makes it likely that the results in some subgroups (such as MCA) will become non-significant simply because of the reduction in the amount of data, and that there was no strong evidence that the benefit of EVT does not apply across all subgroups.
- The relevant NICE guidance is from section 1.2 ('Managing the culprit aneurysm') of guideline NG228:

> 1.2.4 An interventional neuroradiologist and a neurosurgeon should discuss the options for managing the culprit aneurysm, taking into account the person's clinical condition, the characteristics of the aneurysm, and the amount and location of subarachnoid blood. They should document a proposed treatment plan based on the following options: (i) endovascular coiling, (ii) neurosurgical clipping, (iii) no interventional procedure, with monitoring to check for clinical improvement and reassess the options for treatment.

1.2.5 Do not use a subarachnoid haemorrhage severity score in isolation to determine the suitability of any management option.
1.2.6 If interventional treatment to secure the aneurysm is an option, offer: (i) endovascular coiling or (ii) neurosurgical clipping if endovascular coiling is not suitable.
1.2.7 Discuss the proposed treatment plan and any alternative options with the person, and their family or carers if appropriate, then agree and document a final treatment plan (see recommendations 1.5.5 to 1.5.7).
1.2.8 If interventional treatment is planned, ensure that it is carried out at the earliest opportunity to prevent rebleeding. Be aware that the risk of rebleeding is highest within 24 hours of the onset of symptoms.

- Aneurysm coiling with or without balloon assistance is the mainstay but intrasaccular flow disruptors (e.g. WEB device, Neqstent, Nautilus) may be alternatives in some anatomical situations. Note that there is insufficient evidence that the Contour device without additional coiling provides sufficient immediate aneurysmal occlusion.
- Stent-assisted coiling or flow diversion requires DAPT and carries an appreciably higher risk of morbidity and mortality during the acute phase of SAH compared to other endovascular options. Therefore, these techniques are generally reserved for special cases (e.g. SAH from a blister aneurysm) or as a rescue option.

Unruptured intracranial aneurysms

- The International Study of Unruptured Intracranial Aneurysms (ISUIA), published in 2003, aimed to prospectively evaluate the natural history of unruptured aneurysms and assess the risks associated with their surgical or endovascular repair. The study involved centres in the USA, Canada, and Europe. It recorded the natural history of patients who did not undergo surgery and measured morbidity and mortality in those who had aneurysm repairs. Findings from 4060 patients showed that the 5-year cumulative rupture rates varied based on aneurysm size, location, and whether the patient had experienced the rupture of another intracranial aneurysm (Table 8.1).
- Most UIAs will never rupture (<0.25% annually). Furthermore, ruptured aneurysms may be biologically different from the majority of those discovered incidentally. Assuming an aneurysm prevalence of 3% and an annual incidence of aSAH of 6–10/100,000, only one UIA will rupture each year for every 300–500 persons harbouring an aneurysm.

Table 8.1 The 5-year risk of aneurysm rupture in ISUIA

Location	<7 mm		7–12 mm	13–24 mm	≥25 mm
	Group 1	Group 2			
Cavernous ICA	0%	0%	0%	3.0%	6.4%
ICA, ACOM/ACA, MCA	0%	1.5%	2.6%	14.5%	40%
PCOM/post circ	2.5%	3.4%	14.5%	18.4%	50%

- The benefit of treating an UIA must outweigh the potential risks related to treatment. The balance of risks is not always straightforward to determine.
- The decision to treat or not to treat a UIA depends on patient and aneurysm factors, and opinions will vary. Robust RCT data for UIAs are not available to enable definitive evidence-based judgements, and differences in approach between healthcare systems are apparent.
- Key patient factors include age, prior history of SAH, medical history (especially certain collagen vascular diseases or autosomal dominant polycystic kidney disease), smoking, hypertension, excessive alcohol intake, major life-limiting comorbidities, and family history of SAH/UIA.
- Key aneurysm factors include location, size, documented growth, neck width/dome-to-neck ratio, multiplicity, branch or incorporated vessels, and multilobulated (irregular) shape.
- The risk of neurosurgical complications is higher in older patients, those with larger aneurysms, and in cases of posterior circulation aneurysms. In these subgroups, EVT is the preferred therapeutic approach.
- The CURES trial (Darsaut et al., 2023) demonstrated that, for UIA, neurological deficits and hospital stays longer than 5 days were significantly more common in neurosurgical patients compared to those treated endovascularly. While neurosurgical clipping achieved a higher rate of aneurysm occlusion (predominantly the MCA location subgroup), there were no bleeds after treatment in the study for either surgical or endovascularly treated aneurysms and other studies have shown that the risk of bleeding after EVT for UIAs is extremely low (Rizvi et al., 2020). Additionally, the landscape of EVT has shifted significantly over the decade during which the CURES trial was conducted. Today, a much higher proportion of patients are treated with stents and flow diverters, which are associated with a lower rate of recurrence.
- It is recommended that cases of UIAs are reviewed in a formally constituted and properly minuted MDT meeting. MDT outcomes and advice should be communicated to the patient prior to any treatment planning.
- Sufficient time should be provided for the patient and their relatives to reflect on the often complex and substantial information relevant to UIA management decisions. Structured tools, such as PHASES (Table 8.2) or UIATS, can be used to support MDT decision-making.
- The range of EVT options is wider in the elective than acute setting, as antiplatelets can be administered more safely. Flow diversion (with or without adjunctive coiling) or laser-cut/braided stent-assisted coiling or Contour can be first-line options for UIAs, depending on aneurysm size and anatomy.
- Certain clinical situations are additionally worth considering:
  - If acutely symptomatic (usually due to enlargement or oedema): these should be regarded comparably to a ruptured aneurysm. Treat as soon as practicable, preferably within 48 h of presentation, to prevent imminent rupture.

Table 8.2 The PHASES risk prediction score

Category	Score	Criteria
Population (P)	0	North American, European (other than Finnish)
	4	Japanese
	5	Finnish
Hypertension (H)	0	No
	1	Yes
Age (A)	0	<70 years
	1	≥70 years
Size of aneurysm (S)	0	<7.0 mm
	3	7.0–9.9 mm
	6	10.0–19.9 mm
	10	≥20 mm
Earlier SAH from another aneurysm (E)	0	No
	1	Yes
Site of aneurysm (S)	0	ICA
	2	MCA
	4	ACA/PCOM/posterior circulation

Note: the 5-year absolute risk of rupture based on the score is estimated to be as follows: for ≤2 points, 0.4%; for 3 points, 0.7%; for 4 points, 0.9%; for 5 points, 1.3%; for 6 points, 1.7%; for 7 points, 2.4%; for 8 points, 3.2%; for 9 points, 4.3%; for 10 points, 5.3%; for 11 points, 7.2%; and for ≥12 points, 17.8%.

  - If chronically symptomatic or enlarging: these are semi-elective, but time should allow in most circumstances for thorough review prior to treatment, with an aim to treat within 2–4 weeks.
  - If asymptomatic and not enlarging: these cases are elective. A full MDT review of relevant imaging and history, along with an outpatient review to discuss management options, should all be undertaken and recorded before intervention.
- Conservative management should involve strict control of all vascular risk factors and interval imaging. CTA or MRA is recommended at 6–12 months, with subsequent imaging considered annually or biennially, or tailored based on the ELAPSS score (Table 8.3). The growth rate of UIAs smaller than 4 mm is very low. Some units choose not to follow up these patients, particularly if >70 years as the risk:benefit assessment is increasingly against intervention.
- Aspirin has been suggested to reduce wall inflammation and to decrease formation, growth, and rupture risk.

Table 8.3 The ELAPSS score for prediction of risk of aneurysm growth

Earlier Subarachnoid Hemorrhage	
Earlier SAH	
Yes	0
No	1
Location of the aneurysm	
ICA/ACA/ACOM	0
MCA	3
PCOM/posterior circulation	5
Age (years)	
≤60	0
61–65	1
66–70	2
71–75	3
76–80	4
81–85	5
86–90	6
91–95	7
>95	8
Population	
North America, China, Europe (other than Finland)	0
Japan	1
Finland	7
Size of the aneurysm (mm)	
1.0–2.9	0
3.0–4.9	4
5.0–6.9	10
7.0–9.9	13
≥10.0	22
Shape of the aneurysm	
Regular	0
Irregular	4

Note: summing the score stratifies the risk into low risk (0–9), intermediate risk (10–19), and high risk (≥20).

Further reading

Backes D, Rinkel GJE, Greving JP, et al. ELAPSS score for prediction of risk of growth of unruptured intracranial aneurysms. Neurology. 2017;88(17):1600–1606.

Darsaut TE, Findlay JM, Bojanowski MW, et al. A pragmatic randomized trial comparing surgical clipping and endovascular treatment of unruptured intracranial aneurysms. AJNR Am J Neuroradiol. 2023;44(6):634–640.

Etminan N, Brown RD Jr, Beseoglu K, et al. The unruptured intracranial aneurysm treatment score: a multidisciplinary consensus. Neurology. 2015;85(10):881–889.

Feghali J, Gami A, Caplan JM, Tamargo RJ, McDougall CG, Huang J. Management of unruptured intracranial aneurysms: correlation of UIATS, ELAPSS, and PHASES with referral centre practice. Neurosurg Rev. 2021;44(3):1625–1633.

Greving JP, Wermer MJ, Brown RD Jr, et al. Development of the PHASES score for prediction of risk of rupture of intracranial aneurysms: a pooled analysis of six prospective cohort studies. Lancet Neurol. 2014;13(1):59–66.

International Study of Unruptured Intracranial Aneurysms Investigators. Unruptured intracranial aneurysms—risk of rupture and risks of surgical intervention. N Engl J Med. 1998;339(24):1725–1733.

Molyneux AJ, Birks J, Clarke A, Sneade M, Kerr RS. The durability of endovascular coiling versus neurosurgical clipping of ruptured cerebral aneurysms: 18 year follow-up of the UK cohort of the International Subarachnoid Aneurysm Trial (ISAT). Lancet. 2015;385(9969):691–697.

National Institute for Health and Care Excellence (NICE). Subarachnoid haemorrhage caused by a ruptured aneurysm: diagnosis and management [Internet]. NICE guideline [NG228]. NICE; 2022. https://www.nice.org.uk/guidance/ng228

Rizvi A, Seyedsaadat M, Alzuabi MH, Kadirvel R, Brinjikji W, Kallmes DF. Long term rupture risk in patients with unruptured intracranial aneurysms treated with endovascular therapy: a systematic review and meta-analysis AJNR Am J Neuroradiol. 2020;41(6):1043–1048.

Wiebers DO, Whisnant JP, Huston J 3rd, et al. Unruptured intracranial aneurysms: natural history, clinical outcome, and risks of surgical and endovascular treatment. Lancet. 2003;362(9378):103–110.

Subarachnoid haemorrhage grading

World Federation of Neurological Surgeons grading scale

The original WFNS grading scale standardises clinical evaluation over time and helps estimate prognosis (Table 8.4). Frequent monitoring is important for the early detection of SAH complications.

The modified WFNS grading scale removes focal neurological deficit from the definition of grade II and III, and instead relies just on the GCS score (Table 8.5).

Hunt and Hess scale

This describes the clinical severity of aSAH and is used as a predictor of survival (Table 8.6).

Table 8.4 The WFNS grading scale

Original grade	Glasgow Coma Scale score	Motor deficit
1	15	Absent
2	13–14	Absent
3	13–14	Present
4	7–12	Present or absent
5	3–6	Present or absent

Table 8.5 The modified WFNS grading scale

Modified grade	Glasgow Coma Scale score
1	15
2	14
3	13
4	7–12
5	3–6

Table 8.6 The Hunt and Hess scale

Grade	Clinical presentation
1	Asymptomatic or minimal headache and slight neck stiffness. Asymptomatic, or minimal headache and slight nuchal rigidity
2	Moderate to severe headache, nuchal rigidity, no neurological deficit other than cranial nerve palsy
3	Drowsiness, confusion, or mild focal deficit
4	Stupor, moderate to severe hemiparesis, possibly early decerebrate rigidity and vegetative disturbances
5	Deep coma, decerebrate rigidity, moribund appearance.

Fisher scale

This scale classifies the amount of SAH on CT scans (Table 8.7).

There is some relationship to a greater likelihood of vasospasm. It is notable that Fisher groups 1–3 increase in severity of SAH in a stepwise manner. However, group 4 is not necessarily more severe than group 3.

A modified scale was devised in 2006 with five grades, starting at grade 0 (Table 8.8).

Table 8.7 The original Fisher scale

Original Fisher group	CT features
1	No blood detected
2	A diffuse deposition or thin layer with all vertical layers of blood <1 mm thick
3	Localised clots and/or vertical layers of blood ≥1 mm in thickness
4	Diffuse or no subarachnoid blood, but with intracerebral or intraventricular clots

Table 8.8 The modified Fisher scale

Modified Fisher group	CT features
0	No SAH or intraventricular haemorrhage (IVH)
1	Focal or diffuse thin SAH, no IVH
2	Focal or diffuse thin SAH, with IVH
3	Focal or diffuse thick SAH, no IVH
4	Focal or diffuse thick SAH, with IVH

Further reading

Frontera JA, Claassen J, Schmidt JM, et al. Prediction of symptomatic vasospasm after subarachnoid haemorrhage: the modified Fisher scale. Neurosurgery 2006;59(1):21–27.

Hunt WE, Hess RM. Surgical risk as related to time of intervention in the repair of intracranial aneurysms. J Neurosurg. 1968;28(1):14–20.

Sano H, Inamasu J, Kato Y, Satoh A, Murayama Y; WFNS Cerebrovascular Diseases and Treatment Committee. Modified World Federation of Neurosurgical Societies subarachnoid haemorrhage grading system. Surg Neurol Int. 2016;7(Suppl 18):S502–S503.

Differential diagnosis of subarachnoid haemorrhage

Traumatic

- Traumatic brain injury is the most common cause of SAH overall.
- A history of trauma and the presence of accompanying evidence on scans provide important diagnostic clues.
- However, patients who rupture a cerebral aneurysm and subsequently hit their head may exhibit similar histories and scan results, which can complicate the diagnosis.

Aneurysmal rupture

- The blood is often centred around the site of the ruptured aneurysm but if the presentation is delayed, this may not be the case. Additionally, if the volume of blood is extensive, then localisation may not be possible.
- If large, an aneurysm may be seen as a filling defect within the clot.

Arterial dissection

- The vertebral artery and branches of the posterior circulation are most commonly affected.
- There is typically a narrowing at the beginning of the dissection, followed more distally by aneurysmal dilatation. These changes may be subtle but often dynamically change on repeat imaging.
- There is a high acute rebleed rate for dissecting aneurysms and prompt treatment is required.

Reversible cerebral vasoconstriction syndrome

(See Figure 8.2a,b.)

- This is a disorder of cerebrovascular dysregulation (endothelial dysfunction and hypersympathetic stimulation) triggered by eclampsia, illicit drugs, anti-migraine medication, cough and cold suppressants, antidepressants, and chemotherapeutic and immune modulatory agents. Patients present with thunderclap headaches, often recurrent, lasting a few hours.
- Imaging may demonstrate convexity SAH, lobar haemorrhage, watershed infarcts, and vasogenic oedema.
- Angiography reveals segmental narrowing and dilatation ('string of beads') of the cerebral arteries. There may be a latent period of 4–5 days before abnormalities are detected. Repeat angiography may reveal resolution in some vessels with new regions of narrowing often migrating proximally.
- Intra-arterial infusion of verapamil has been described in the management of refractory reversible cerebral vasoconstriction syndrome (Ospel et al., 2020).

Vasculitis

(See Figure 8.2c.)

- May be primary (i.e. unknown triggering factor), or secondary to systemic disease.
- Angiography may reveal segmental narrowing or occlusions of cerebral vasculature.
- MRA has similar sensitivity to DSA. MRI vessel wall imaging may additionally be able to directly visualise the abnormalities of the vessel wall.

Perimesencephalic haemorrhage

(See Figure 8.2d.)

- Constitutes about 10% of spontaneous SAH. The initial clinical presentation may be very similar to an aneurysmal SAH, though it is often milder and usually without loss of consciousness. It is postulated that some of these haemorrhages are due to basilar perforator aneurysms, many of which spontaneously thrombose. A venous aetiology is an alternative theory.
- The clinical course is usually benign in comparison with aneurysmal SAH.
- The distribution of blood is relevant only when the CT scan is obtained *within 3 days* of the ictus.
- Blood is confined to the cisterns around the midbrain and usually centred anterior to the midbrain. There is sometimes a small amount of blood in the lateral ventricles. Blood should not extend into the lateral Sylvian fissure and only just reach the anterior interhemispheric fissure. Only a small amount of ventricular blood is acceptable. Note that approximately 10% of aSAH also has this distribution of blood.

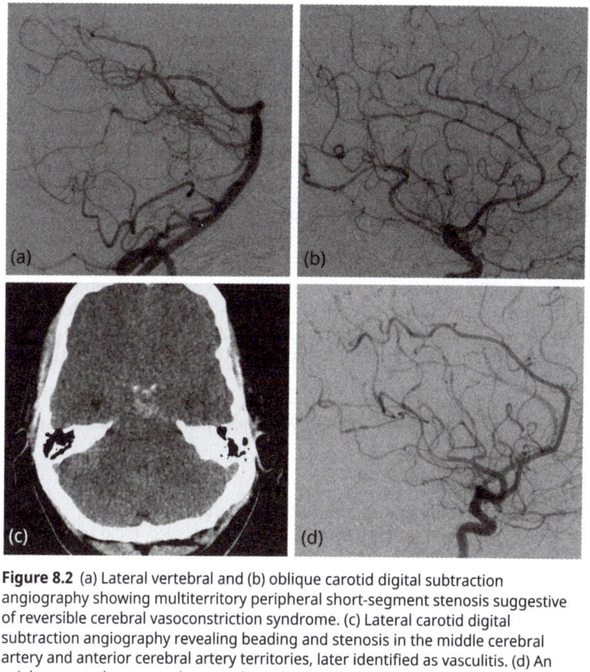

Figure 8.2 (a) Lateral vertebral and (b) oblique carotid digital subtraction angiography showing multiterritory peripheral short-segment stenosis suggestive of reversible cerebral vasoconstriction syndrome. (c) Lateral carotid digital subtraction angiography revealing beading and stenosis in the middle cerebral artery and anterior cerebral artery territories, later identified as vasculitis. (d) An axial computed tomography scan shows localised prepontine subarachnoid blood, consistent with perimesencephalic haemorrhage.

- The necessity for EVD insertion is rare, as is angiospasm.
- With a typical CT scan, good-quality negative CTA, and typical clinical course, some units do not perform catheter angiography.

Arteriovenous malformation

- AVMs most commonly rupture into the parenchyma, but about 5% of AVMs rupture solely into the subarachnoid space. Patients are usually younger than those presenting with aSAH.
- The risk of rebleed in the acute period is significantly lower than that of aSAH.
- The exception is the presence of prenidal or nidal flow aneurysms (present in 10–20% of AVMs) because these are more commonly the source of bleeding than the AVM itself. These aneurysms should be embolised if safe to do so acutely to avoid a rebleed (see Chapter 12, 'Targeted occlusion of perinidal/nidal aneurysms or pseudoaneurysms', p. 461).

Dural arteriovenous fistula

- DAVF can present solely with SAH (see Chapter 11). The major risk factor is the presence of cortical venous drainage or reflux, especially with venous ectasia.
- Clues to diagnosis include the presence of associated parenchymal oedema, enlarged vessels, curvilinear calcification in the subcortical white matter (venous ischaemia/hypertension), enlarged dural arteries, ectatic arterialised veins, and thrombosed sinuses.
- The risk of rebleed is relatively high, estimated at 35% within 2 weeks (Duffau et al., 1999). These should therefore be treated in the acute phase.

Spinal arteriovenous malformation

- About 10% of patients of spinal AVMs present with SAH (see Chapter 14, 'Spinal arteriovenous malformations', p. 504). These patients are younger than the aSAH population. Spinal AVM is an uncommon condition.
- The pain may start in the neck. Standard DSA should include injection of the subclavian branches and projections of the neck if a cranial cause is not found in the appropriate clinical context (definite/diffuse spontaneous SAH in younger patient).
- MRI spine, followed by time-resolved MRA, should be performed to exclude spinal AVMs after exhaustive cranial investigation, prior to spinal angiography.

Spinal aneurysms

- These are rare, but probably underdiagnosed (see Chapter 14, 'Spinal aneurysms', p. 511). There are often spinal motor and sensory symptoms.
- They may be seen on spinal CTA initially and subsequently confirmed on spinal angiography.
- Some of these small aneurysms will spontaneously thrombose, but there is a risk of acute rebleeding if they do not. Therefore, treatment (either endovascular or surgical) should be considered if safe/feasible to do so.

Cerebral amyloid angiopathy

- Cerebral amyloid angiopathy is caused by the deposition of cerebral amyloid β in the tunica media and adventitia of leptomeningeal and cortical blood vessels.
- The build-up leads to vascular fragility, typically presenting as lobar intracerebral haemorrhage in normotensive elderly patients. Convexity SAH may also be the presenting feature. It is usually limited to one or more adjacent cortical sulci at the brain's convexity.
- It is very uncommon in individuals younger than 60 years, except in cases of iatrogenic amyloid angiopathy caused by the transmission of amyloid β seeds, where onset may occur in the 20s to 40s.
- MRI often reveals prior lobar haemorrhage, peripheral microhaemorrhages, or old sulcal haemosiderin deposition.
- The Boston criteria version 2 may aid diagnosis.

Venous infarction

- Venous sinus or cortical vein thrombosis may result in SAH due to increased venous pressure and subsequent rupture of small, fragile veins.
- If angiography is performed, careful inspection of the venous phase may provide the diagnosis, but a high index of clinical suspicion with CT/CT venography and/or MRI/MR venography are the mainstays of diagnosis.

Tumours and cavernomas

- Tumours and cavernous malformations typically cause parenchymal haemorrhage, but if present at the surface of the brain may rarely present solely with SAH.

Drugs

- SAH may be associated with recreational (such as cocaine) or prescribed drugs.
- Nevertheless, patients who develop SAH while taking drugs may have an underlying aneurysm that must be treated. For those without an aneurysm, the cause may be drug-associated vasculitis. Rebleeds may occur even with a normal angiogram.
- SAH occurs with increased frequency in those taking anticoagulant medication, although, similarly, an alternative underlying cause is often discovered.

Sickle cell disease

- Sickle cell disease predisposes to the development of intracranial aneurysms, yet sickle-associated non-aneurysmal SAH may also occur. The latter is postulated to be due to rupture of hypertrophied leptomeningeal collaterals which develop due to intracranial arterial occlusive disease.
- Patients are typically young, presenting in childhood and young adulthood.

Idiopathic

- The source of bleeding may occasionally not be discovered even in the presence of extensive SAH.
- If the pattern of bleeding is non-perimesencephalic, at least two good-quality DSAs should be performed. Pump injections and 3D-RA may increase the sensitivity of the study.
- If these are negative, follow-up cranial and spinal MRI/MRA should be performed to rule out any serious pathology elsewhere.

Further reading

Duffau H, Lopes M, Janosevic V, et al. Early rebleeding from intracranial dural arteriovenous fistulas: report of 20 cases and review of the literature. J Neurosurg. 1999;90(1):78–84.

Ospel JM, Wright CH, Jung R, et al. Intra-arterial verapamil treatment in oral therapy-refractory reversible cerebral vasoconstriction syndrome. AJNR Am J Neuroradiol. 2020;41(2):293–299.

Sharma R, Dearaugo S, Infeld B, O'Sullivan R, Gerraty R. Cerebral amyloid angiopathy: review of clinico-radiological features and mimics. J Med Imaging Radiat Oncol. 2018;62(4):451–463.

van Gijn J, Rinkel GJ. Subarachnoid haemorrhage: diagnosis, causes and management. Brain. 2001;124 (Pt 2):249–278.

Coil embolisation of intracranial aneurysms

Preoperative assessment

- Obtain informed consent. Discuss the treatment plan and risks with the patient's family or next of kin (with the patient's consent).
- In cases of incapacity, procedures can be performed under country-specific legislation in the patient's best interest. Be familiar with those applicable in your hospital.
- Preoperative work-up should include full blood count, urea and electrolytes, clotting profile, and renal function studies at the very least.
- GA with paralysis is employed to keep the patient motionless and to enable greater physiological control of pulse, BP, temperature, respiration, etc. Uncorrected GA commonly lowers BP, so maintaining a desirable normotension should be discussed with the anaesthetist.
- Warming blankets and inflatable calf compression cuffs (e.g. Flowtrons) are advised.
- Urinary catheterisation should be considered for long procedures.
- Hold a team brief before each interventional procedure. This should include:
  - Confirmation of the patient's identity, the planned procedure, and that consent has been obtained.
  - Discussion of patient-specific risk factors and anticipated difficulties.
  - A local checklist template should be used; if one does not exist, adapt from the WHO Surgical Safety Checklist template. Pay particular attention to pretreatment medication, ensure the correct range of devices are available, check for any issues with imaging equipment, and make sure that arterial puncture closure devices are available.

Technique

(See Figure 8.3.)

Vascular access

- The right common femoral artery is traditionally the most common site. The puncture must be made with postoperative haemostasis in mind. A single-wall puncture technique is preferred. Sheaths up to 8–9 Fr can be safely used.
- A transradial (or transulnar) artery approach is increasingly utilised due to lower complication rates, particularly for less time-critical interventions. It is relatively contraindicated for patients with safe transfemoral access options whose radial artery diameter measures <2.0 mm due to the risk of spasm. When 8 Fr access is required, the catheter may be used sheath-less if the vessel diameter measures >2.5 mm.

Anticoagulation

- Most operators use heparinised saline for constant irrigation through catheters and/or sheaths (1000 IU heparin in 1 L of NaCl 0.9%). Some operators prefer to add antispasmodics such as 3 mg nimodipine or its equivalent in the guide catheter flush bag.
- Additional IV heparin is usually administered. Point-of-care testing may be used to monitor anticoagulation, and most centres use the activated clotting time (ACT). Doubling of ACT is usually adequate to prevent most thromboembolic complications. A starting dose of 50–100 IU/kg is recommended, but this is highly variable. In the absence of an ACT

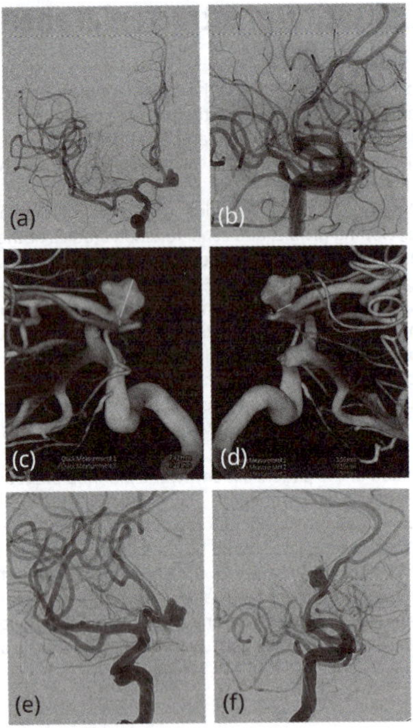

Figure 8.3 Stages of (balloon-assisted) coil embolisation of a ruptured cerebral aneurysm. (a) The procedure begins with the guide catheter placed in the internal carotid artery. Standard projection angiography is performed, identifying an anterior communicating artery aneurysm. (b, c) 3D rotational angiography is carried out to select two optimal projections that maximise the visibility of the parent vessel at the aneurysm neck and allowing for accurate measurement of the aneurysm. (d, e) The biplane detectors are configured according to these projections. A compliant balloon is first placed across the aneurysm neck, with the wire remaining inside, and a microcatheter is then used to catheterise the aneurysm. (f, g) Coils are inserted into the aneurysm, ensuring they do not prolapse into the parent artery. (h, i) The process continues until the aneurysm no longer fills with contrast, which required six coils in this case. Once the aneurysm is successfully treated, the microcatheter and balloon are removed, and final angiography is performed in standard projections to check for any thromboembolic complications.

machine, some units give an initial 5000 IU of heparin, followed by an additional 1000 IU every hour.

- The timing of anticoagulation varies among operators, ranging from immediately after sheath introduction, to after aneurysm cannulation, to after deployment of the first coil. Timing may differ depending on whether case is elective or emergent.

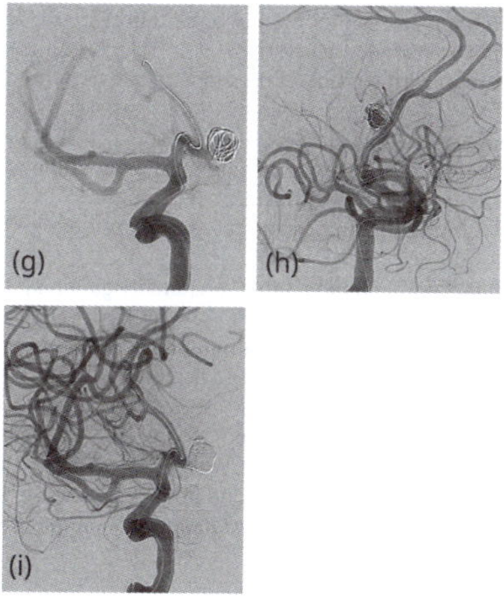

Figure 8.3 Continued

Antiplatelet usage

- In elective cases, single antiplatelet therapy or DAPT are frequently used, especially if either treatment with stents is planned or possible.
- If DAPT is necessary, it is useful to administer a single agent before the procedure (clopidogrel, prasugrel, or ticagrelor) and then administer IV aspirin only at the point in the procedure when it is required, such as immediately preceding/during stent deployment, to minimise haemorrhagic complications.
- IV aspirin can also be useful prophylactically if a coil protrusion occurs or even to treat a small thromboembolic event. Some use IV aspirin routinely.
- For urgent stenting procedures without prior antiplatelet loading, it is necessary to use a GP IIb/IIIa inhibitor (eptifibatide or tirofiban) or, alternatively, cangrelor. The former two potent antiplatelet agents can also be used for intraprocedural thromboembolism development, with or without stenting.
- Operators differ in the duration of antiplatelet use, but a common approach is 3 months of DAPT followed by a transition to aspirin monotherapy, except for flow-diverter stents, where 6–9 months of DAPT followed by aspirin is more usual. Traditionally, patients have been maintained on life-long aspirin therapy. However, for those with stents, and flow diverters placed in the ICA, there is a trend towards discontinuing aspirin after 1 or 2 years. This practice currently lacks a strong evidence base.
- Rebound thromboembolic events (5%) may occur following cessation of antiplatelet therapy, usually with aneurysms treated with stents, incomplete stent-wall apposition, incompletely occluded aneurysms, and in patients with vascular risk factors.

Guide catheter placement

- Typically, a 6, 7, or 8 Fr guide catheter, connected to a continuous heparinised flush, is navigated under fluoroscopic guidance over a 0.035" or 0.038" curved or J-shaped guidewire, from the puncture site to the aortic arch and into either the ICA or vertebral artery, depending on the location of the target aneurysm.

- A 'select' catheter with a range of tip shapes (such as Simmons or Berenstein) may be inserted within the guide catheter to aid in selection of the relevant vessel.
- The aim is to obtain the most distal safe position possible without causing vessel occlusion/vasospasm/dissection.
- Thoroughly aspirate the guide catheter after placement in the desired vessel.
- The guide catheter is connected to a constant irrigation system of heparinised saline via a RHV.
- An 'intermediate' or 'distal access' catheter can be placed within the guide catheter during the procedure to achieve more stable and distal access (also connected to an RHV).
- Multiplane and/or 3D-RA is performed to complete the planning process. The use of 3D-RA is strongly advised. Working projections can then be chosen for accessing the aneurysm and optimal coil delivery, with at least two projections on a biplane system, but sometimes more working projections are required.

Accessing the aneurysm

- If a balloon is to be used, then this is positioned first (see 'Balloon remodelling technique', p. 253).
- The aneurysm is then catheterised with a shaped microguidewire first, followed by the microcatheter, by sliding the latter over the former while maintaining the position of the wire.
- Pay attention to where microcatheter/wire lie in relation to parent vessel curves. The more stable position is to ensure outside wall (longer) curve apposition. This will reduce the risk of sudden tip movement.
- Note any tension that might build up on the microcatheter. It may be necessary to increase tension so that the catheter moves forward over the wire, but once the aneurysm is catheterised, it is prudent to remove this excess tension to avoid the catheter jumping forward.
- A good position for the catheter tip is one-third into the body of the aneurysm, not touching the aneurysm wall. The feasibility and suitability of such placement will depend on the aneurysm's size, location, and morphology. Catheter pre-shaping will assist both aneurysm entry and subsequent stability of position.
- Manufacturer-supplied pre-shapes can be used, but many neurointerventionalists prefer to steam-shape their own, according to the individual patient's anatomy. Steam-shaping can facilitate applying multiple curves as necessary.
- It is wise to choose the first coil before cannulating the aneurysm and have it ready in case of rupture during cannulation (although this is relatively rare).

Coiling

- Usually, the first coil is used to create a framework, crossing the aneurysm neck and lining the peripheral aneurysm wall, and can be filled, like a basket, with subsequent coils of reducing size and softness ('frame/fill/finish' technique).
- The size and shape of the first coil to be deployed is determined by the shape and measurements of the aneurysm. The coil diameter is usually

larger than the aneurysm neck and is approximately the size of the aneurysm (although for less experienced operators it is often best to slightly undersize the coil in ruptured aneurysms). If the aneurysm is not spherical, an average diameter may be calculated.

- The coil is introduced into the delivery microcatheter by positioning the introducer sheath at the microcatheter hub. The coil is pushed toward and ultimately into the aneurysm by a pusher wire, which is connected to the coil. It is important not to kink the delicate pusher wire as this may prohibit detachment.
- It is important to remove excess tension off the microcatheter before inserting the first coil (especially in small aneurysms). Take care not to pull the catheter completely out of the aneurysm, however.
- The coil is advanced into the aneurysm very slowly and carefully under fluoroscopy. Care must be taken not to push the leading edge of the coil into the aneurysm wall and thereby cause rupture. If positioning is difficult, or the aneurysm small, the coil can be 'unsheathed', withdrawing the microcatheter while advancing the coil rather than pushing it, to reduce pressure on the wall. During this manoeuvre, it is important to make sure that the catheter does not completely exit the aneurysm.
- Constant readjustment of the microcatheter may be required, and the coil often requires partial retrieval and repositioning at times to control its position within the aneurysm.
- If the microcatheter is pushed out of the aneurysm during coil deployment, it is usually possible to recannulate it over the coil, providing enough coil is in the aneurysm. If the microcatheter has prolapsed distal to aneurysm in the parent vessel, it is necessary to reduce tension on the catheter first to pull it to the aneurysm neck, and then advance over the coil.
- The coil is fully deployed once the proximal marker on the coil's pushing wire aligns with the proximal marker in the microcatheter. Once deployed in the desired position, the coil can be detached, pusher wire removed, and the next coil introduced, if required.
- Beware, although the system may register coil detachment, the coil may not be completely detached. Check detachment slowly and carefully under fluoroscopy when withdrawing the pusher wire. Rarely, on withdrawing the detached pusher wire, the coil comes back into the microcatheter (perhaps a pressure/suction effect). Push the displaced coil back into the aneurysm with a wire, the next coil, or the coil pusher.
- Intermittent angiography assesses residual aneurysm filling, exact position of coil loops, extravasation (in case of suspected rupture), thrombus formation at the neck, and to obtain fresh roadmaps (as a degree of drift and misregistration is inevitable).
- Judging when to stop coiling is an important skill, gained mostly through experience ('the enemy of good is better'). In general, the aneurysm should no longer fill with contrast. In ruptured wide-necked aneurysms, it is sometimes necessary to leave a small neck as the priority is aneurysm protection from rebleeding. In the elective aneurysms, delivering antiplatelets is safer and therefore stents may be used more readily to ensure complete aneurysm obliteration.
- Biofeedback during coil deployment (i.e. feeling how stiff it is to push), failure to deploy a small coil, packing density of the aneurysm, and filling of the aneurysm upon angiography are some of the aids used to determine whether further coils can/should be deployed.

- Once a decision is made to stop and the final coil is detached, the microcatheter may be removed. This should be done in a slow and controlled fashion to prevent the dislodgement of coils and the prolapse of a coil 'tail' into the vessel lumen. Before removal, reintroduce the microwire to the tip of the microcatheter to prevent coil tails 'sticking' to the microcatheter.

Check angiography

- Performing check angiography in working projections and standard angiographic projections at the end of a procedure provides a good baseline for follow-up angiography and should be scrutinised carefully to exclude thromboembolic vessel occlusion.
- The guide catheter can be removed once it is confirmed that the procedure is complete. Thoroughly aspirate the guide catheter during and after microcatheter removal before post-coiling angiograms, as clot formation around the tip of the guide/microcatheter interface may subsequently be dislodged.
- Since DSA is still more sensitive for detecting small aneurysms, consider angiography of the other vessels at this point (especially if MRA-only follow-up is their routine). Some operators prefer doing this at a later stage, during follow-up DSA.

Postoperative care

- Immediate postoperative care (after the theatre recovery suite) is often provided in a high-dependency nursing environment.
- Observations should include regular neurological assessments, standard monitoring (arterial BP, ECG, oxygen saturation), limb observations on the side of puncture, and access site checks.
- In ruptured aneurysms, BP control is of the utmost importance to prevent and treat delayed ischaemic injury. Maintenance of circulating blood volume is recommended to prevent delayed cerebral ischaemia (DCI). If vasospasm develops, it may be necessary to increase the BP provided the aneurysm is protected.
- Oral nimodipine should be continued as part of the standard management of aSAH, usually for 21 days.
- Daily transcranial Doppler ultrasound is optimal to monitor for the development of arterial angiospasm but is often not available.
- These patients are hypercoagulable and LMWH to prevent deep venous thrombosis is recommended after the ruptured aneurysm is secure.
- In some cases, further anticoagulation with heparin may be required, which in turn requires regular clotting profiles for adjustment of infusion rates.
- Mobilisation depends on the patient's general condition, but should be commenced as soon as the closure method of the puncture site allows, preventing complications of prolonged bed rest, e.g. deep venous thrombosis, chest infections, and urinary tract infections.

Adjunctive embolisation techniques

- The morphology of some aneurysms is inappropriate for simple, unassisted coiling using a microcatheter only. Adverse features include a wide aneurysm neck, complex anatomy of the parent artery/aneurysm interface, and branch arteries incorporated in the neck.

- In elective cases, stents and flow diverters are valuable tools. However, in aSAH, antiplatelet agents are generally avoided where possible. Instead, balloon-assisted or double-microcatheter techniques may be employed. Alternatively, intrasaccular devices can be considered.

Balloon remodelling technique

(See Figure 8.4.)

- All operators should be familiar with this technique. It involves deploying coils in an aneurysm through one microcatheter, while a compliant balloon is positioned across the aneurysm neck and intermittently inflated, keeping the coils within the aneurysm. It also provides protection in case of rupture.
- The technique is inexpensive, provides parent artery protection, facilitates unambiguous parent artery visualisation, adds to microcatheter stability, and being temporary does not require additional antiplatelet therapy.
- It is useful particularly for:
  - Wide-necked aneurysms (either >4 mm or relative to maximum width).
  - Small aneurysms or other aneurysms with a high risk of rupture.
  - Aneurysms at an acute angle to the parent vessel, making access difficult and unstable.
  - Branch vessels originating from the aneurysm neck.
  - Any aneurysm in which the catheter position is unstable.
- Disadvantages:
  - Increased procedural complexity.
  - Possibly increased risk of aneurysm rupture and small chance of parent vessel rupture or dissection by the balloon.
  - Possibly increased risk of thromboembolism.
  - Using the traditional approach (inflation–deflation cycle with each coil introduction), the method consumes more time as the inflation–deflation times for the balloons is 15–30 s.
  - However, in experienced hands, alternative approaches to balloon remodelling can be used, e.g. occasional balloon inflation only or multiple coils deployed during a single, longer balloon inflation.

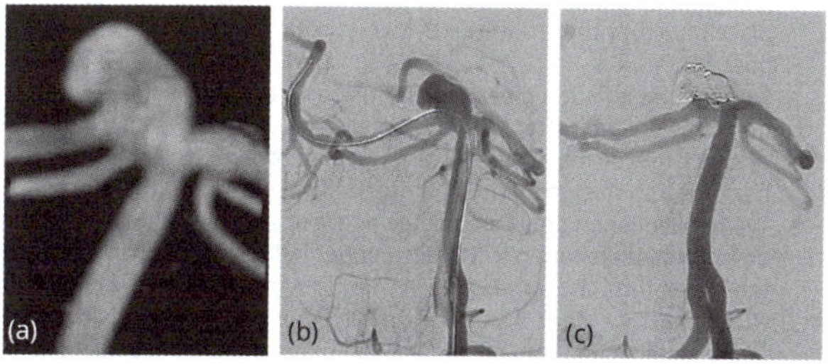

Figure 8.4 Balloon-assisted coil embolisation of wide-necked basilar tip aneurysm. (a) 3D rotational angiography. (b) Balloon placed first across aneurysm neck. (c) Coiling of the aneurysm has been performed.

- Complete occlusion of the parent vessel in the presence of poor collateral supply can cause ischaemic damage in the downstream territory. It is important to carefully study the collateral supply and ensure the balloon does not occlude these vessels as well.
- Contrast toxicity is greater in ischaemic brain tissue. If a balloon is inflated for a prolonged period (e.g. >2 min), it is advisable to wait >30 s after deflation before injecting contrast.
- Choosing a balloon:
    - A variety of balloons with different lengths, calibres, configurations, and compliances are available. Some double-lumen balloons, such as Scepter (Microvention) and Eclipse (Balt), also allow for 'bail out' coiling or stent deployment through the balloon.
    - More compliant balloons (Hyperform, Eclipse) offer greater neck branch vessel protection.
    - Larger-calibre balloons are necessary for larger vessels, and vice versa.
    - Longer balloons provide more stability, especially in inherently unstable positions within the vascular tree, particularly the apex of a curve or the carotid siphon.
    - Lower-profile balloons (e.g. single lumen) will cause less distortion/ straightening of branch points.
- Technique:
    - Balloons require meticulous preparation, including purging with diluted radiographic contrast, to ensure accurate inflation and optimal visibility during inflation. Carefully follow the instructions for use (see Chapter 4, 'Remodelling balloon catheters', p. 125).
    - Systemic heparinisation must be achieved before deploying the balloon microcatheter.
    - The balloon is positioned using a microwire across the neck of the aneurysm positioned in the branch where coil prolapse is most likely. This is achieved *before* the aneurysm is cannulated. Trying to do this after risks moving the coiling catheter within the aneurysm.
    - A test inflation can be performed once the balloon is in place, but it is not mandatory.
    - Some operators use a balloon routinely, while others deploy one routinely but only inflate and remodel when necessary.
    - While inflated, the balloon offers temporary support to keep coils in place until they mesh sufficiently to retain each other in the desired position.
    - To minimise inflation times and perfusion arrest, the balloon is generally deflated after the deployment of 1–2 coils. It is important to check for coil movement or dislodgement during deflation and to perform a shorter reinflation before the final detachment of the coil.
    - Typically, inflation times are limited to about 2–3 min, although some operators inflate for up to 10 min. Longer inflation times will increase the risk of thromboembolism.
- The Comaneci is a stent-like device that is temporarily expanded during coil embolisation and retrieved at the end to protect the parent artery. It is used similarly to balloons to prevent coil prolapse during coiling, but without the drawback of occluding the vessel in use. Care must be taken not to catch coils *inside* the device, as the whole coil mass might be pulled out when retrieving the Comaneci.

- When using multiple microcatheters or balloon catheters, cover the microcatheters not currently being manipulated with a drape to avoid confusing them. Consider using different coloured catheters to minimise any risk of confusion.

Double microcatheter technique

- Two microcatheters are used to catheterise the aneurysm. Coils are inserted through each microcatheter, and they intertwine with each other, forming a stable larger frame, covering and not herniating through the neck. Their stability is assessed before either is detached. Following detachment, of one of the coils (preferably the more stable looking one first), additional coils are deployed. The two microcatheters should have different tip shapes to reach different portions of the aneurysm.
- In small, wide-necked, shallow ruptured aneurysms, this technique enables framing and then the placement of a single filling coil to achieve occlusion or near occlusion of the aneurysm before anything needs to be detached. This approach avoids the risk of displacing the entire coil mass associated with dense packing using multiple small coils.
- It is a useful technique for wide-necked aneurysms. It is generally cheaper and simpler than alternative assist approaches and avoids any periods of distal ischaemia of balloon remodelling. Occasionally, there may be good reason not to use a balloon, e.g. a dissected segment, poor collateral reserve, or small vessel.
- It has been suggested that this enables a more proportional distribution of coils within an aneurysm, resulting in more complete occlusion with denser packing.

Aneurysm recurrence and re-haemorrhage

- MRA can be used to reliably to follow up coiled saccular aneurysms.
- Early identification of significant recurrences (in 10–20% of ruptured aneurysms) with appropriate retreatment is extremely important.
- The rebleeding rate after EVT is extremely low (<1%) but is higher than for surgically clipped cases. This small excess risk of rebleeding after the initial ictus does not offset the overall superior clinical outcome of coiling compared with neurosurgical clipping.

Further reading

Molyneux AJ, Birks J, Clarke A, Sneade M, Kerr RS. The durability of endovascular coiling versus neurosurgical clipping of ruptured cerebral aneurysms: 18 year follow-up of the UK cohort of the International Subarachnoid Aneurysm Trial (ISAT). Lancet. 2015;385(9969):691–697.

Aneurysm types and locations

Types

Saccular

- Narrow-necked aneurysms are the easiest to treat and the least likely to recur as coils can be tightly packed within the aneurysm and there is less neck area for re-endothelialisation.
- Wide-necked saccular aneurysms can typically be treated using various techniques such as balloon/Comaneci-assisted coiling, stents, flow diverters, the dual microcatheter technique, and intrasaccular devices. However, wide necks are predictive of higher rates of recurrence and complications.

Small

(See Figure 8.5.)

- The treatment of small—particularly wide-necked—aneurysms, especially in aSAH, can be challenging because of the need for catheterisation and coil deployment without aneurysm rupture or coil prolapse in a small, confined space.
- Placing a balloon (but not necessarily inflating) is recommended to prevent/manage rupture during treatment and help avoid coil prolapse. Small, soft coils such as the ED 10 (Kaneka), and Target Nano and Tetra (Stryker), are suitable.

Fusiform

- Fusiform aneurysms may be the result of atherosclerosis due to the loss of mural elasticity or dissection.
- Symptoms typically result from mass effect and adjacent parenchymal oedema, cerebral ischaemia, or SAH. They may be discovered incidentally.
- Common sites are the vertebral and basilar arteries, often presenting with brainstem compression and sometimes hydrocephalus.
- Most fusiform aneurysms are stable. Size ≥7 mm and partial thrombosis are risk factors for growth with a significantly increased risk of mortality when symptomatic. The prognosis of large, partially thrombosed, vertebrobasilar aneurysms, in particular, is grim (with or without EVT).
- In the presence of SAH, occlusion of the dissected segment may be an option ('deconstructive' technique), providing no important branches are occluded. Alternatively, flow-diverting stents (FDSs) ± coiling are used in the presence of a discrete sac ('reconstructive' technique). If coiling is not

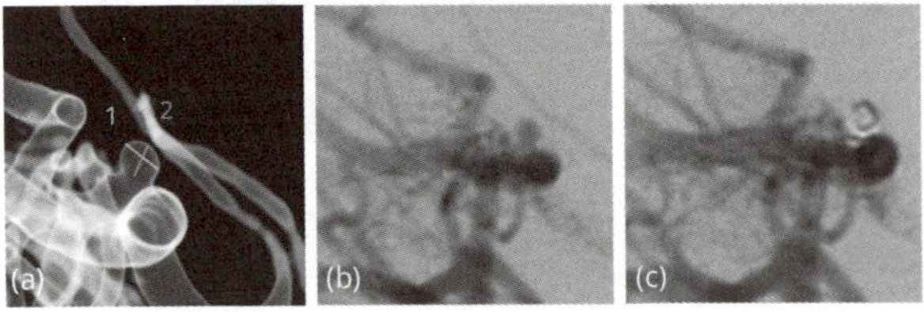

Figure 8.5 Treatment of a small aneurysm. (a) A 1.5 × 1.5 mm aneurysm was identified using rotational angiography in a patient with an aneurysmal subarachnoid haemorrhage. (b) The aneurysm was cannulated using an SL-10 microcatheter. (c) A 1.5 mm Target Tetra coil was deployed, successfully occluding the aneurysm.

performed, it may be best to implant two overlapping flow diverters, one shorter one inside the other at the location of the aneurysm, to increase the occlusion effect.
- Prophylactic insertion of an EVD might be considered prior to treatment and use of DAPT because the risk of hydrocephalus is high with the usually heavy blood load.

Dissecting

- Dissection occurs when blood enters the vessel wall deep to the internal elastic lamina, creating an alternative blood-filled channel. This weakens the arterial wall, making a rupture into the subarachnoid space possible.
- Large-volume haemorrhage is common and there is a high rate of rebleeding within the first 24 h.
- The vertebral arteries and posterior circulation are more frequently affected. Typically, there is a narrowed section at the point of the dissection, followed by fusiform dilatation of the weakened arterial segment. A 'pearl-and-string' sign is specific. Retention of contrast may be seen within the pseudoaneurysms. Rarely, a double lumen and dissection flap can be identified. Tapered occlusion may also be present and a mixture of ICH and infarction should alert one to the diagnosis.

Blister

(See Figure 8.6.)

- 'Blood blister'-like aneurysms (named after their appearance at surgery) manifest as broad-based bulges found at non-branch points.
- Suggested pathogenesis includes arterial dissection and atherosclerotic ulceration.
- They account for 0.3–1% of intracranial aneurysms and 0.9–6.5% of aSAHs.
- Initial angiography may be normal. A high index of suspicion is required. They typically appear as a shallow outpouching with a wide neck (mimicking an infundibulum but without a vessel arising from the dome).
- The most common site (>65%) is the dorsal wall of the supraclinoid ICA. Other sites reported include the ACOM, basilar trunk, and PICA.
- They may evolve rapidly in morphology on repeat angiography. The rebleeding rate is high and usually catastrophic.
- This type occurs in younger patients, usually women, often with a large volume of blood and the associated risk of vasospasm. WFNS grade is >3 in nearly 70%.
- These aneurysms are very friable and surgery carries a high risk of tearing the aneurysm, or causing post-treatment stenosis of the parent artery if the clip is inserted too deeply.
- EVT:
  - Sometimes the aneurysm can be coiled with balloon assistance. Note that complete occlusion of the aneurysm including its neck is probably necessary to avoid rebleeding. Early DSA follow up is recommended and definitive treatment (such as flow diversion) may be necessary.
  - However, most units have moved to treating these aneurysms using flow-diverter stenting at the outset. Consider prophylactic EVD placement as DAPT is required for FDS.
- Early angiographic follow-up is recommended to confirm stable occlusion (e.g. in a week, then a month).

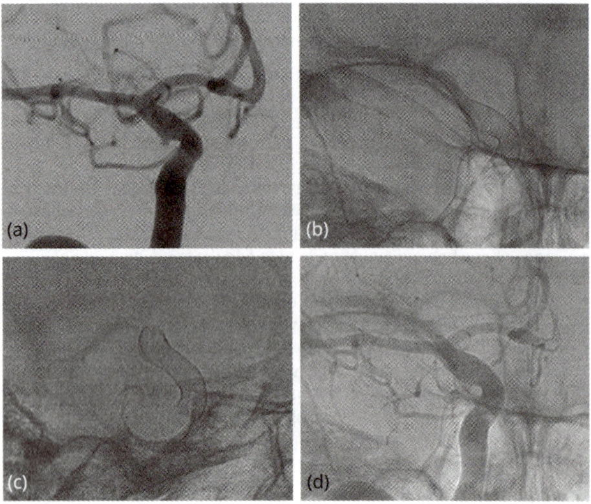

Figure 8.6 Flow diversion of a blister aneurysm. (a) Digital subtraction angiography revealing a typical internal carotid artery blister aneurysm in a patient presenting with subarachnoid haemorrhage, occurring at a non-branch site. (b, c) Orthogonal unsubtracted fluoroscopy and (d) unsubtracted angiography demonstrate the deployment of overlapping flow diverters over the neck. Stasis in the aneurysm sac was observed at the end of the procedure.

Giant

(See Figure 8.7.)

- Giant aneurysms are defined as ≥25 mm in size. They comprise about 5% of cerebral aneurysms.
- There is commonly mural thrombus formation. Growth occurs due to recurrent haemorrhage within the highly vascular wall.
- The most common presentation is mass effect-related symptoms (and thrombus may generate parenchymal oedema) followed by SAH. The haemorrhagic risk relates to lumen, rather than absolute, size.
- They have a high rupture risk and a poor prognosis after rupture.
- In acute aSAH, simple coiling may be sufficient to protect the aneurysm from rebleeding in the short term ('KISS': Keep It Safe and Simple, applicable to all of neurointervention). However, for large/giant aneurysms, particularly if wide-necked, the rate of major aneurysm remnants/recurrence is high for unassisted coiling, probably exceeding 50%. The presence of mural thrombus further increases this risk as coils migrate into the thrombus.
- Parent vessel sacrifice (PVS) offers the greatest chance among the endovascular options for providing permanent exclusion. The next most effective EVT is FDS and coiling. However, this carries a recurrence risk and a risk of early haemorrhage in rare cases that is not completely understood but may relate to rapid thrombosis of the aneurysm and breakdown of the wall from inflammatory proteolytic substances

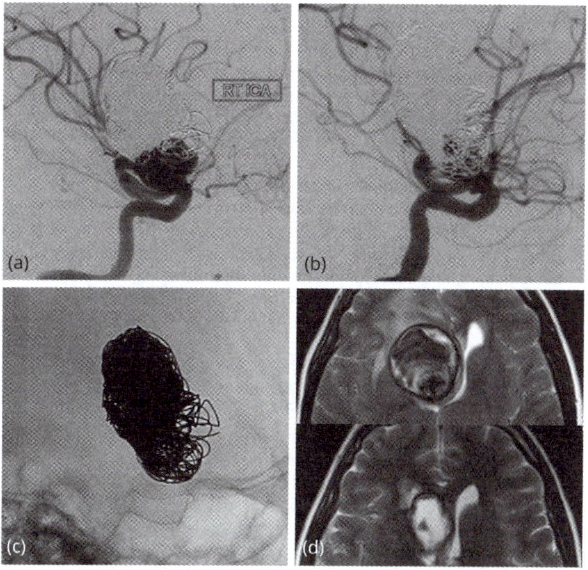

Figure 8.7 Retreating a previously coiled giant aneurysm. (a) Pre- and (b) post-coil embolisation and flow diversion of a recurrent, giant, and partially thrombosed supraclinoid internal carotid artery aneurysm. (c) Magnetic resonance imaging before retreatment showing surrounding oedema and mass effect. (d) After treatment, the aneurysm has shrunk, and the surrounding oedema has resolved, with an improved mass effect.

released by acute thrombus formation. This occurs despite (or perhaps because of) tight packing of the aneurysm.

- Surgery, including bypass, has a high rate of permanent occlusion but often carries significantly greater risks of morbidity.

Giant serpentine

- These are rare fusiform arterial dilatations resulting from repeated dissection of an abnormal arterial wall with thrombus formation. The thrombus contains non-endothelialised vascular channels containing slowly flowing blood.
- They predominantly involve the MCA and posterior circulation and present with mass effect, seizures, and ischaemia (due to emboli and/or side branch occlusion). There may be vasogenic oedema. Haemorrhage is uncommon.
- Untreated, their course is unpredictable. Some grow, others are stable.
- Flow diversion of the diseased segment or occlusion/resection ± bypass are treatment options. In acutely ruptured cases, parent vessel occlusion (PVO) feasibility may be assessed by temporary distal test occlusion (Scepter Mini is useful for this) and if the collateral supply is adequate then occlusion with coils is a quick, low-risk, and highly effective, procedure, avoiding the need for DAPT.

Infectious

(See Figure 8.8.)

- Infectious aneurysms (colloquially 'mycotic' aneurysms, although the infection is usually non-fungal) comprise 1–5% of intracranial aneurysms. They are more common in childhood.
- Two-thirds are associated with endocarditis (10% of patients with infective endocarditis will have an infectious aneurysm). Septic emboli generate acute inflammation in the arterial wall with neutrophil infiltration, degradation of the media and adventitia, and fragmentation of the internal elastic lamina. IV drug abuse is a risk factor.
- Other causes include meningitis, venous sinus thrombophlebitis, cranial osteomyelitis, and nasopharyngeal sinus infections.
- The most common causative organism is *Streptococcus*, followed by *Staphylococcus*. Blood cultures are often negative. Fungal causes are rare

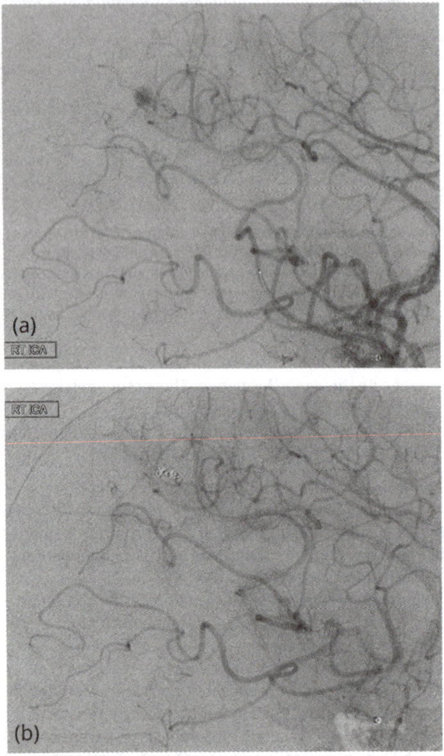

Figure 8.8 Mycotic aneurysm. (a) Distal middle cerebral artery mycotic aneurysm in a patient with endocarditis. (b) Target Nano (Stryker) coils were deployed into the aneurysm sac via a Marathon microcatheter and extended proximally into the parent vessel to occlude it.

and typically occur in immunocompromised patients. They have a worse prognosis.

- They are typically small and fusiform, with only 40% being saccular. They are multiple in 25% of cases, usually located distally, and may change in size on follow-up angiography. 50–80% involve distal branches of the MCA.
- Antibiotics tailored to the organism (usually found via blood cultures) are first line for unruptured aneurysms. A course lasting 6 weeks is often required. Repeated imaging during this treatment is necessary to ensure the aneurysm is shrinking in size.
- For ruptured aneurysms, those that do not resolve with antibiotics (e.g. after 1–2 weeks), or in cases where new aneurysms develop or an aneurysm enlarges, invasive treatment is recommended. This can be either endovascular or surgical. EVT offers particular advantages for patients with multiple aneurysms or those with coexisting cardiac morbidity.
- These aneurysms are often fragile, distally located, small, and fusiform, and care must be taken not to rupture them during treatment. PVO may be the safest option (test occlusion of sorts has already taken place as they are usually the result of embolic material!). n-BCA glue, LE agents, or coils can be employed.
- Bleeding and rebleeding have a high mortality rate.

Traumatic

- These comprise <1% of intracranial aneurysms, although are more common in childhood. They can arise from penetrating and non-penetrating head injury with either partial or total disruption of the arterial wall, with aneurysm and pseudoaneurysm, respectively.
- In non-penetrating head injury, the mechanism is rapid deceleration resulting in damage to vessels as they impinge on static intracranial structures (the pericallosal artery against the falx or the P2 PCA against the tentorium). Coexisting skull fractures are common.
- Iatrogenic cases also occur, e.g. post transsphenoidal pituitary surgery.
- Initial CTA may be normal and requires repeating after 1–2 weeks if the cranial CT is suspicious, demonstrating a callosal, parafalcine, or other haematoma in the region of an artery.
- The presentation may be of delayed SAH or other neurological symptoms 2–3 weeks after head injury.
- Treatment of the aneurysm is necessary to prevent the high mortality associated with acute rebleeding. This may involve simple coiling, test occlusion and vessel sacrifice, flow diversion, or surgery.

AVM-associated 'flow'

- AVM-associated aneurysms are haemodynamically related to the AVM ('flow-related') and may be intra- or extranidal:
  - Intranidal aneurysms exist within the boundaries of the nidus and appear opacified before substantial venous filling occurs. They are a risk factor for AVM-related haemorrhage.
  - Extranidal aneurysms occur on the feeding arteries ('prenidal'). Prenidal aneurysms may be quite distant from the AVM (e.g. in the circle of Willis), or just adjacent.
  - Dilatations distal ('postnidal') to the AVM nidus are sometimes called 'venous aneurysms'. These are histologically distinct from aneurysms but may also bleed.

- AVM-associated aneurysms have been shown to increase the risk of a haemorrhagic presentation in some studies.
- Management depends on presentation:
  - With haemorrhage, if the aneurysm is thought to be the site of the bleed rather than the AVM nidus itself, this is an indication for early treatment. SAH without associated intraparenchymal haemorrhage, or a focal haematoma immediately adjacent to the aneurysm, implicate the aneurysm. Flow-related aneurysms may be embolised via coiling, n-BCA glue, or LEs, depending on the morphology. The AVM can then be treated at a later date if considered necessary.
  - In the absence of haemorrhage, the treatment of associated aneurysms follows similar principles to other unruptured incidental aneurysms. Aneurysms in proximity to the nidus tend to regress after stereotactic radiosurgery (up to 80%), but those distant from nidus are much less likely to do so (just 4.3% obliterated in one study) (Rammos et al., 2016). Flow aneurysms in the circle of Willis increase the rate of rebleeding after stereotactic radiosurgery (6.4% compared to 1.0%), and so independent treatment of these aneurysms should be considered to decrease the risk of haemorrhage.

Locations

ICA cavernous segment

- Presentation is typically due to mass effect on the adjacent cranial nerves resulting in pain, diplopia, pupillary constriction, and compressive optic neuropathy. Some of this effect is probably inflammatory and, in some, symptoms may resolve spontaneously (Stiebel-Kalish et al., 2005).
- The rupture risk for small cavernous aneurysms is particularly low. In the ISUIA study, there were no ruptures for those aneurysms <13 mm over 5 years, for those 13–24 mm the risk was 3.0%, and for >24 mm 6.4%.
- One caveat is the carotid cave aneurysm. These are medially directed arising from the distal cavernous ICA segment but extend intradurally and therefore even small cavernous aneurysms with this orientation may present with rupture and aSAH.
- For ruptured or symptomatic small, narrow-necked, cavernous aneurysms, coil embolisation is sufficient. For large unruptured aneurysms, PVO (if balloon test occlusion (BTO) is tolerated), or flow diversion without coils (or loosely packed) is advocated. Packing tightly with coils risks worsening mass effect.

ICA PCOM segment

- The communicating ICA segment is a common site for aneurysms. Presentation may be with SAH or mass effect on the oculomotor nerve.
- For ruptured aneurysms, coil embolisation is first line. It is often necessary to have a sharply curved microcatheter tip (either steam-shaped or preformed) to catheterise the aneurysm and prevent it from prolapsing out during coiling. Use of a balloon is recommended, in particular if the neck is wide or to protect the PCOM origin (the balloon can even be positioned in the PCOM artery for this purpose if the vessel is large). The balloon is also helpful for stabilising the microcatheter in the aneurysm. The balloon has a tendency to jump forward when inflated in the ICA and so controlled back tension/withdrawal during inflation might be necessary.

- Large, wide-necked PCOM segment aneurysms have a high rate of recurrence. Flow diversion is an excellent option in unruptured or recurrent aneurysms. Jailing the microcatheter and loosely packing the aneurysm is often performed if large. BTO and parent artery sacrifice is also an option as may be surgery.
- Intrasaccular devices can also be used effectively for PCOM aneurysms. Shaped microcatheters may be necessary to facilitate catheterisation and deployment.

ICA choroidal segment

- ICA choroidal segment aneurysms are often small and tend to present with SAH.
- Despite its small size, the anterior choroidal artery supplies very eloquent brain (see Chapter 2, 'Internal carotid artery', p. 30). Occlusion may cause significant neurological deficits, including contralateral hemiplegia, contralateral hemisensory loss, and contralateral homonymous hemianopia. The artery usually has little collateral circulation and so should not be occluded.
- In acute aSAH, coil embolisation ± balloon assistance is first line. In the elective aneurysms, flow diversion is often a good option if the parent artery is difficult to protect.

ICA ophthalmic segment

- Presentation may be with SAH or visual symptoms due to distortion of the optic nerve.
- Coil embolisation ± balloon assistance is first line for ruptured aneurysms.
- These aneurysms are prone to recurrence after EVT and flow diversion is usually effective at preventing this. However, placing an FDS across the ophthalmic artery origin is not without risk. In one series, in-depth examination by an ophthalmologist identified complications in 39.3% of patients. In particular, when the ophthalmic artery originated from the aneurysm sac, there was a high risk for retinal emboli, and where the ophthalmic artery originated from the inner curve of the carotid siphon, there was a high risk for optic nerve ischaemic atrophy (Rouchaud et al., 2015).
- The ophthalmic artery has extensive collateral supply, from the sphenopalatine and middle meningeal arteries. Test occlusion is usually tolerated, in which case PVO may be undertaken.

ACOM

- ACOM aneurysms have been found to be the most common site for SAH in several series.
- Coil embolisation with or without balloon assistance, or intrasaccular device placement, is first line for ruptured aneurysms. Occasionally, the ACAs are of small calibre, hence inserting a balloon prevents sufficient flow, precluding usage. The Comaneci device (Rapid Medical) or simply withdrawing the balloon more proximally back into the ICA, are good options.
- Performing bilateral ICA runs to delineate the ACA and ACOM anatomy is often informative. If both ACAs are solely supplied by a single A1 segment, caution is required to avoid occluding the ACOM during treatment. Even when this is not the case, perforators frequently originate from the ACOM, making preservation important.

- For large, wide-necked, or recurrent ACOM aneurysms, stent or flow-diverter-assisted coiling may be required. Careful consideration must be made when placing a stent jailing the origin of an A2 vessel that has an hypoplastic or aplastic A1 segment. Well-sized intrasaccular devices are a promising alternative in these anatomical configurations.

Distal ACA aneurysms

- There is a strong association with azygos ACAs.
- Similar to the ACOM, the ACAs may be of small calibre, prohibiting balloon usage alongside the coiling microcatheter.
- In unruptured aneurysms, stent or flow-diverter coiling is usually an option.

MCA bifurcation

- Coil embolisation is the first-line treatment option for ruptured aneurysms in many units. A systematic review of EVT found comparable results to other intracranial sites (Brinjikji et al., 2011).
- It may be difficult to obtain a good angiographic projection due to multiple vessels in this region. Study the 3D angiography carefully to understand the anatomy and plan a good projection.
- In EVT treatment of elective aneurysms, stent-coiling or intrasaccular devices are a good option after neurovascular MDT discussion. Flow diversion across the MCA bifurcation is generally safe and feasible, but there is a small risk of ischaemia in the jailed branch. Generally, it is preferable to flow divert into the larger M2 branch, in this situation.

Vertebrobasilar

- If saccular and ruptured then EVT (techniques as above) is indicated. However, aneurysms in this location are more commonly of the fusiform dissecting type than other locations and these are often not amenable to simple coil embolisation. Surgery is also difficult in this location.
- There is a high rebleed rate within the first 24 h for fusiform/dissecting types of aneurysms. The recommendation is to treat as soon as the patient is admitted to the hospital. If there is a high blood load in the posterior fossa, decompression should also be considered.
- If there is a reasonably sized contralateral vertebral artery, and the PICA and ASAs can be preserved, vessel occlusion is a viable option for fusiform vertebral aneurysms.
- If the PICA, ASA, or other large perforators are at risk, consideration should be given to flow diversion (necessitating DAPT).
- Bypass surgery to preserve the PICA is also an option. This approach avoids the need for flow diversion and antiplatelet therapy but is technically challenging and may be unsuccessful, especially in aSAH.

PICA

- In aSAH, coil embolisation of the aneurysm is possible if the aneurysm is saccular. Fusiform aneurysms and more distal aneurysms are more challenging to manage.
- If the aneurysm cannot be coiled without compromising the parent artery, then PVO or flow diversion may be considered. Generally, vessel occlusion is safer if: (i) the level of occlusion is distal to the brainstem perforators, conventionally described as the telovelotonsillar segment

(the angiographic marker for which is the apex of the cranial loop) (see Chapter 2, 'Vertebral artery', p. 47), and (ii) there is a large ipsilateral collateralising vessel, usually the AICA.
- Flow diversion can be impossible if the vessel is overly tortuous, and involves the use of antiplatelets. Flow diversion of the vertebral artery adjacent to the PICA origin (with or without coil embolisation) may decrease the flow into the aneurysm enough to cause occlusion, or at least reduce the risk of rupture.
- A final option may be distal surgical bypass followed by coiling of the segment of the artery incorporating the aneurysm with risks as outlined above.

Basilar trunk

- Aneurysms of the basilar and vertebrobasilar junction trunk are often large, fusiform, thrombosed, and slowly enlarging, exerting mass effect on the brainstem. These have a poor natural history (Church et al., 2020).
- Flow diversion may be attempted but is not always successful in preventing growth. Other strategies include occluding one or both vertebral arteries in the presence of large PCOMs, potentially reversing the flow in the basilar artery.
- Basilar non-fusion is associated with saccular aneurysm development (Srinivasan et al., 2023). These may occur from one of the limbs, or from the cranial or caudal junction. If narrow-necked, coil embolisation is generally successful. Beware of inflating a balloon in a limb, as the lumen may be very narrow, risking rupture. Brainstem perforators may arise from either limb, and so both must be preserved. Flow diversion of both limbs may be necessary to prevent recurrence.

Basilar tip

- The basilar tip is a common aneurysmal site. It is generally accessible endovascularly, although it may incorporate the PCA origins. In ruptured aneurysms, coil embolisation with or without balloon assistance, or an intrasaccular device (especially if wide necked), is the first-line treatment.
- Probably due to the vector of flow along the basilar artery, recurrence is common (24% in one series; Henkes et al., 2005), particularly if the aneurysm is large and wide-necked. In elective aneurysms, stent-assisted coiling, flow diversion, or intrasaccular devices are recommended over simple coiling.

PCA

- These aneurysms are uncommon.
- Treatment options include coil embolisation for saccular aneurysms, and flow diversion or PVO for fusiform cases.
- Beyond the P1 segment, PVO is often well tolerated due to collateral circulation (Halacq et al., 2002). However, with the advent of low-profile flow diverters, many operators favour this approach.

Further reading

Benoit BG, Wortzman G. Traumatic cerebral aneurysms. Clinical features and natural history. J Neurol Neurosurg Psychiatry. 1973;36:127–138.

Brinjikji WBS, Lanzino GMD, Cloft HJMDP, Rabinstein AMD, Kallmes DFMD. Endovascular treatment of middle cerebral artery aneurysms: a systematic review and single-center series. Neurosurgery. 2011;68(2):397–402.

Chun JY, Smith W, Halbach VV, Higashida RT, Wilson CB, Lawton MT. Current multimodality management of infectious intracranial aneurysms. Neurosurgery. 2001;48:1203–1213.

Church EW, Bigder MG, Sussman ES, et al. Treatment of posterior circulation fusiform aneurysms. J Neurosurg. 2020;134(6):1894–1900.

Gross BA, Du R. Natural history of cerebral arteriovenous malformations: a meta-analysis. J Neurosurg. 2013;118(2):437–443.

Hallacq P, Piotin M, Moret J. Endovascular occlusion of the posterior cerebral artery for the treatment of P2 segment aneurysms: retrospective review of a 10-year series. AJNR Am J Neuroradiol. 2002;23:1128–1136.

Henkes H, Fischer S, Mariushi W, et al. Angiographic and clinical results in 316 coil-treated basilar artery bifurcation aneurysms. J Neurosurg. 2005;103(6):990–999.

Kano H, Kondziolka D, Flickinger JC, et al. Aneurysms increase the risk of rebleeding after stereotactic radiosurgery for hemorrhagic arteriovenous malformations. Stroke. 2012;43(10):2586–2591.

Korja M, Kivisaari R, Rezai Jahromi B, Lehto H. Size and location of ruptured intracranial aneurysms: consecutive series of 1993 hospital-admitted patients. J Neurosurg. 2017;127(4):748–753.

Liao L, Derelle AL, Merlot I, et al. Endovascular treatment of distal anterior cerebral artery aneurysms: long-term results. J Neuroradiol. 2020;47(1):33–37.

Piotin M, Mounayer C, Spelle L, Williams MT, Moret J. Endovascular treatment of anterior choroidal artery aneurysms. AJNR Am J Neuroradiol. 2004;25(2):314–318.

Rammos SK, Gardenghi B, Bortolotti C, Cloft HJ, Lanzino G. Aneurysms associated with brain arteriovenous malformations. AJNR Am J Neuroradiol. 2016;37(11):1966–1971.

Redekop G, TerBrugge K, Montanera W, et al. Arterial aneurysms associated with cerebral arteriovenous malformations: classification, incidence, and risk of hemorrhage. J Neurosurg. 1998;89(4):539–546.

Rouchaud A, Leclerc O, Benayoun Y, et al. Visual outcomes with flow-diverter stents covering the ophthalmic artery for treatment of internal carotid artery aneurysms. AJNR Am J Neuroradiol. 2015;36(2):330–336.

Santoro A, Armocida D, Paglia F, et al. Treatment of giant intracranial aneurysms: long-term outcomes in surgical versus endovascular management. Neurosurg Rev. 2022;45(6):3759–3770.

Srinivasan VM, Singh R, Karahalios K, et al. Endovascular embolization of basilar artery fenestration aneurysms: a 21-year institutional case series. Oper Neurosurg (Hagerstown). 2023;25(6):521–528.

Stiebel-Kalish H, Kalish Y, Bar-On RH, et al. Presentation, natural history, and management of carotid cavernous aneurysms. Neurosurgery. 2005;57(5):850–857.

Thermistoklis IP, Thermistoklis KM, Korfias SI, Sakas DE. Blister aneurysms. In Gurer B, Bektasoglu PK, eds. Vascular Malformations of the Central Nervous System [Internet]. IntechOpen; 2020: Chapter 6. https://www.intechopen.com/chapters/69198

Uzan M, Cantasdemir M, Seckin MS, et al. Traumatic intracranial carotid tree aneurysms. Neurosurgery. 1998;43(6):1314–1320.

Ventureyra EC, Higgins MJ. Traumatic intracranial aneurysms in childhood and adolescence. Case reports and review of the literature. Childs Nerv Syst. 1994;10(6):361–379.

Wiebers DO, Whisnant JP, Huston J 3rd, et al. Unruptured intracranial aneurysms: natural history, clinical outcome, and risks of surgical and endovascular treatment. Lancet. 2003;362(9378):103–110.

Periprocedural complications

Treating both ruptured and unruptured aneurysms has inherent risks. Overall risks of procedure-related morbidity–mortality are 3–5% for unruptured and 5–8% for acutely ruptured aneurysms. Please also refer to the general risks of angiography (see Chapter 7, 'Complication management', p. 220).

Thromboembolic

(See Figure 8.9.)

- This is the commonest cause of procedure-related morbidity. If unresolved, it results in stroke. Thromboembolic events are more common in large aneurysms with a greater volume of thrombus, with some residual flow in the coil mass, and in the presence of angiospasm.

Recognition

- Patients with aSAH are hypercoagulable. Clot formation may occur in the guide catheter during initial placement if flushing is inadequate, during coiling at the aneurysm neck (often due to coil protrusion), within the coil mesh, on the balloon used for remodelling, or due to insufficient heparinisation.
- Observe closely for clots. They are often missed if the eye as drawn to the aneurysm. Look particularly:
  - On initial cerebral angiography for embolic vessel occlusion.
  - At branches of aneurysms you are treating, showing up as insidious filling defects.
  - On final angiography. Check against the first run.
- Baseline angiography and regular check angiography should be performed throughout the procedure. Vigilance is of the utmost importance to recognise the complication.

Management

- If the embolism involves a branch not involving the aneurysm MT is usually successful in resolving it. If performed soon after recognition there may be no ischaemic sequelae.
- If the thrombus is at a branch coming from the neck of the aneurysm, the following measures may be helpful:
  - Raising the BP.
  - Infusing more heparin IV.
  - 300–500 mg IV aspirin.
  - GP IIb/IIIa inhibitors: a bolus dose is often successful in resolving or at least stopping the propagation of the thrombus. Often given in combination with a loading dose of aspirin, followed by a course of 6 weeks.
  - Rescue stenting may be necessary if the thrombus cannot be resolved by other means, preferably with low-metal laser-cut stents. Keeping a microwire in the branch that is at risk may be helpful in recatheterising if a clot completely occludes it.
  - MT may be attempted in certain circumstances but can be dangerous if performed adjacent to aneurysms leading to rupture. It is recommended to resheath any stent retrievers before pulling them across the neck of the aneurysm as the exposed stent can cause aneurysm rupture or coil ball dislodgement. Aspiration catheters can

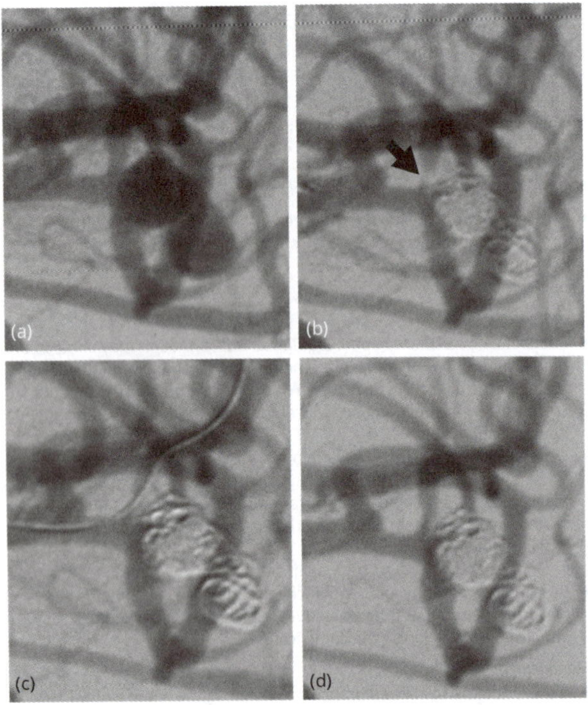

Figure 8.9 Intraprocedural thrombus formation. (a) Shows a ruptured multilocular middle cerebral artery aneurysm. (b) Coiling was successfully performed using balloon remodelling, but a thrombus was observed in one of the branches at the neck on the final imaging run, likely related to a coil tail. (c) A microwire was used to re-access the branch. Blood pressure was increased, additional heparin was administered, and 10 mg of eptifibatide was infused intravenously. (d) This approach resolved the majority of the thrombus, and the patient awoke without deficit. They were additionally given a loading dose of 300 mg aspirin and continued for 6 weeks on 75 mg a day.

be attempted, but similarly they can flick into the aneurysm as they are retrieved.

- Thrombolytic agents are not as efficacious as GP IIb/IIIa inhibitors and must be avoided in acutely ruptured aneurysms.

Intraprocedural aneurysmal rupture

(See Figure 8.10.)

- This complicates <2% of elective cases and <5% of procedures for ruptured aneurysms. Most patients survive if managed correctly.

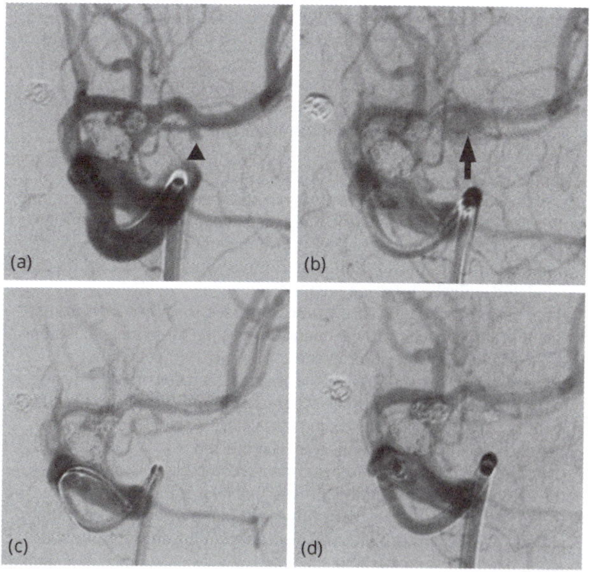

Figure 8.10 Managing a ruptured aneurysm during coiling. (a) Digital subtraction angiography demonstrating a small left middle cerebral artery aneurysm in a patient with subarachnoid haemorrhage (arrowhead). (b) During catheterisation, angiography detected extravasation from the aneurysm (arrow). (c) Heparin was reversed with protamine, a balloon was inflated over the aneurysm's neck for 3 min (after confirming temporary vessel blockage with gentle angiography), and the anaesthetist was instructed to lower the blood pressure. Repeat angiography showed that the bleeding had stopped. (d) The aneurysm was successfully re-cannulated and coiled. The patient recovered well, experiencing only a headache.

Recognition

- Rupture can occur due to coil/wire/microcatheter protrusion through the aneurysm wall, coil oversizing or overpacking, manipulation of the microcatheter or microwire, or overinflation of the remodelling balloon.
- The key risk points for rupture are initial aneurysm entry, first coil, and 'last' coil (i.e. when approaching to near end of coiling take care).

Management

- Stay calm. If suspected rupture/perforation but unsure, perform gentle angiography to confirm contrast extravasation. Keep your foot on the pedal as it may only been seen in the late phase.
- If you are certain that rupture has occurred, perhaps due to obvious microcatheter protrusion beyond the aneurysm wall, and/or a haemodynamic response, angiography is not required. Note that BP can also increase if a device stimulates the endothelium and this does not necessarily indicate rupture.

- Inform the anaesthetist. Raised ICP may cause bradycardia and hypertension and so instruct the anaesthetist to pre-emptively lower the BP.
- Reverse heparin with protamine (1 mg per 100 IU of heparin) and confirm with ACT monitoring.
- If a balloon is across the neck of the aneurysm (or even just proximal in the vascular tree) it should be immediately inflated, and gentle angiography performed to check that this has stopped the extravasation. If no balloon is prepared and there is a second operator, they can prepare and deploy it. Keep the balloon inflated until the leak is thought to be sealed or at least 3 min (longer if no aneurysm coils are *in situ*). Once the balloon is inflated, perform angiography to confirm that it is inflated sufficiently to halt the bleed.
- If the perforation is with wire or microcatheter, the objective is to seal the hole and get coils into the aneurysm as soon as possible to minimise extravasation. Do *not* withdraw the coil or microcatheter catheter responsible for the rupture initially. Instead, start coiling with the first loops potentially going into the subarachnoid space and then gradually withdraw the catheter until coiling takes place within the aneurysm. Continue coiling until the aneurysm is protected.
- Once the aneurysm is secured, perform an on-table CT scan to assess the extent of bleeding and the presence of hydrocephalus.
- Inform the neurosurgical team. An urgent EVD may be required if not already placed. This can often be placed within the angiography suite.

Coil dislodgment and/or migration

(See Figure 8.11.)

- The main risk of coil dislodgement and migration is thromboembolic stroke.
- A coil tail or single loop protrusion is not uncommon and is usually well tolerated. A few weeks of aspirin is advisable.
- Minor prolapse into a large vessel is usually inconsequential, but larger prolapses may require anticoagulation or platelet inhibition. If a large loop protrusion is felt to be at risk of downstream migration, stent pinning of the prolapsed coil may be required. A low-thrombogenicity laser-cut stent (e.g. Atlas or Acclino) is preferred.
- Small coils are often well tolerated in the distal vasculature if not occlusive. A period of observation and a course of antiplatelets is advisable.
- Potentially catastrophic complete dislodgement of the whole coil/coil ball with risk of occlusion of the parent vessel or migration into the more distal vascular tree is rare. If this does occur, it may be necessary to perform retrieval with rescue devices, e.g. a gooseneck snare or stent retriever. Once the coil is captured, pull the device completely back into the microcatheter, with just the coil protruding from the end to secure it during retrieval (pulling an unsheathed stent retriever across the neck of an aneurysm risks rupture).
- If retrieval is not safely possible, stenting may be required.

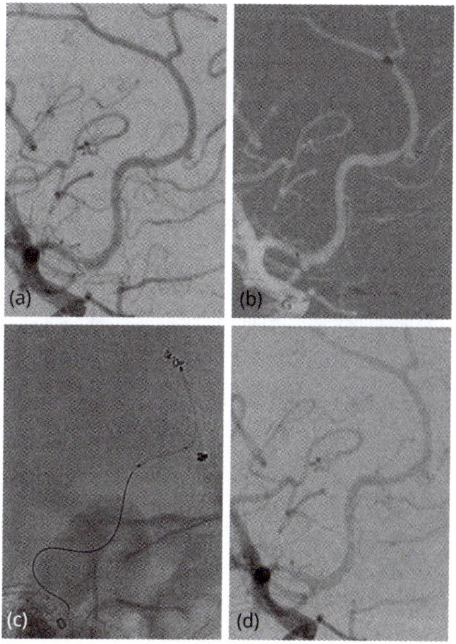

Figure 8.11 Migration of coil during procedure. (a) A coil was deployed in a small, wide-necked anterior communicating artery aneurysm. (b) After detachment, the coil migrated into the parent artery and embolised distally. (c) A stent retriever was deployed over the coil and completely resheathed within the microcatheter, trapping the coil at the tip of the microcatheter. (d) The coil, stent retriever, and microcatheter were then retrieved together.

Stretching a coil

- Coils may become prematurely detached from the pusher wire with the detachment zone still inside the microcatheter. This can be detected when the coil can be pushed forwards but not pulled back anymore ('one-to-one' is lost). Control over placement of the coil is limited, as while you can push it, you cannot retrieve it if it settles in an unwanted position (e.g. in the parent artery).
- If there is a sufficient length of coil within the microcatheter, then it may be possible to simply retrieve the microcatheter with the coil dangling out the end.
- If the coil remains in place when the microcatheter is tugged, then it may still be retrieved by threading a small gooseneck snare over the microcatheter (you will have to cut off the microcatheter hub first) and threading it along the microcatheter and thence over the coil—so-called railroading (Figure 8.12). After tightening the snare on the coil, the microcatheter and coil can be retrieved together.

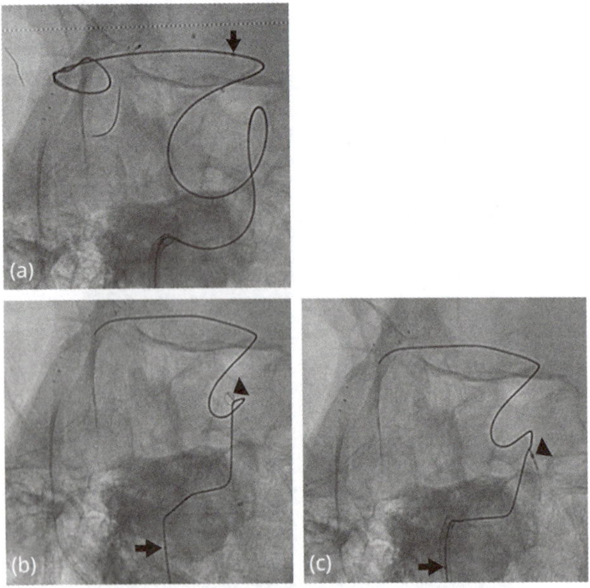

Figure 8.12 Snaring a stretched coil. (a) Digital subtraction angiography during aneurysm coiling, showing a stretched coil that could not be retracted, making repositioning impossible (arrow indicates the microcatheter tip). (b) The microcatheter hub was cut to allow a snare (arrowhead) to pass along the entire microcatheter and encircle the coil wire. (c) The snare was tightened and the microcatheter and coil were then pulled out together.

- If the above manoeuvres do not work, it may be necessary to pin the coil against the vessel wall with a stent throughout its length to prevent thrombus formation.

Delayed leucoencephalopathy

- This is rare, occurring in <1% of cases. Parenchymal contrast-enhancing lesions, likely granulomatous lesions, are seen in the territory of intervention, most within 2 months but can be more delayed.
- They are possibly emboli from the polymer coating of the microcatheter which may peel off due to friction between tight-fitting catheters.
- The patient may be asymptomatic or suffer headache and/or focal deficits.
- Treatment is symptomatic with steroids but the optimal dose or duration is not known.

Further reading

Taussky P, Lanzino G, Cloft H, Kallmes D. A checklist in the event of aneurysm perforation during coiling. Am J Neuroradiol. 2010;31(7):E59

Balloon test occlusion

A BTO is performed to assess the consequences of potential parent vessel sacrifice (PVS).

Balloon test occlusion

- While commonly performed in the ICA, it can be performed in most vessels. With modern balloon technology, distal vessels can increasingly be accessed.
- Clinical testing alone has been replaced by combined clinical and careful angiographic assessment during prolonged (30 min) balloon inflation, often combined with hypotensive challenge.
- The risk of test occlusion in an elective patient with the use of appropriately sized compliant balloons and adjunctive heparinisation is extremely low. Angiographic testing can reliably detect patients in whom delayed ischaemia will develop.
- A wide range of additional adjunctive techniques to test cerebrovascular reserve have been reported including CT/MRI perfusion, xenon CT, single-photon emission computed tomography (SPECT), hypotensive challenge, positron emission tomography, transcranial Doppler ultrasound, and electroencephalography. None are perfect; all report false positives and false negatives. The most practically useful are venous delay, transcranial Doppler ultrasound, and SPECT.

Technique

(See Figure 8.13.)

- A bi-arterial approach is used (femoral or radial) for adjunctive angiography of all relevant collateral vessels during BTO. A diagnostic catheter on a saline flush is placed in the contralateral vessel for angiography at baseline and during testing (remember that the dominant vertebral artery as well as the contralateral ICA should be studied).
- The patient is systemically heparinised.
- A guide catheter is placed in the vessel of interest and a double-lumen compliant balloon is sited, sized to vessel to be occluded (balloon diameter ≥1 mm larger).
- The site of the balloon depends on the planned level of vessel sacrifice. Ideally, the balloon should be placed at that level to enable the impact of occlusion on the entire relevant collateral circulation to be assessed during BTO. However, if a long-segment ICA occlusion is planned, then the balloon may be placed in a comfortable segment of the ICA for the patient, e.g. distal cervical ICA just beneath the skull base. Avoid the carotid bulb because of reflex hypotension and bradycardia.
- Once the balloon is inflated, gentle angiography is performed via the guide catheter to confirm complete occlusion (NB: repeat this intermittently). Contrast stasis in the vessel should be seen.
- The BP may be reduced to two-thirds of the patient's baseline to further reduce the chance of a false-positive pass.
- A non-scrubbed clinician performs repeat neurological testing during balloon inflation.

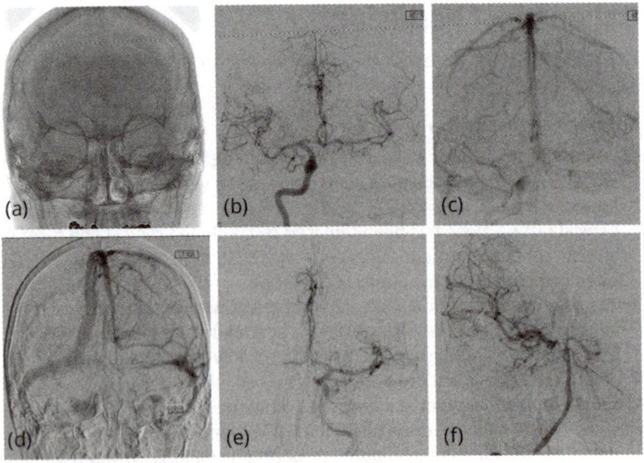

Figure 8.13 Images of balloon test occlusion. (a) A balloon is inflated in the laceral segment of the left internal carotid artery (ICA). (b) Arterial and (c) venous contralateral angiography shows no delay in arterial flow or venous return. (d) Venous angiograms of a second patient with a balloon inflated in the right ICA show a failed test, with a significant delay (>2 s) in venous return. (e) In a third patient, angiography demonstrates poor flow across the anterior communicating artery with a balloon inflated in the right ICA. (f) However, this is a false negative, as angiography via the right vertebral artery supplies the right anterior hemisphere through a large posterior communicating artery with no delay.

- In ICA occlusion testing, a delay in the start of the venous phase between the occluded and non-occluded hemispheres of >2 s represents a high risk of failure after PVO. A delay of <1 s is a clear pass.
- Thorough guide catheter aspiration is performed then flushing prior to balloon deflation.
- If the patient passes a well-conducted BTO, the risks of permanent PVO are low—but not zero—as a small percentage of patients may still suffer from ischaemia.

Further reading

Abud DG, Spelle L, Piotin M, Mounayer C, Vanzin JR, Moret J. Venous phase timing during balloon test occlusion as a criterion for permanent internal carotid artery sacrifice. AJNR Am J Neuroradiol. 2005;26(10):2602–2609.

Parent vessel occlusion

PVO involves deliberate occlusion of the main blood vessel supplying a diseased part of the vasculature, typically a large or otherwise complex aneurysm.

Risks

- The morbidity/mortality is low, ranging from 0% to 1.5%. A systematic review by van der Schaaf et al. found slightly higher complication rates for detachable balloon occlusion of 3.6% but 0% for PVO using coiling (the technique used currently). The overall permanent aneurysm occlusion rate was 98%.
- There is the risk of *de novo* aneurysm formation around the circle of Willis. The only prospective study to date found no increased aneurysm/SAH risk (de Gast et al. 2007) but there are multiple retrospective reports indicating a rate of around 4% in the decade following PVO (Arambepola et al., 2010) and nine cases occurred in 1644 patients (0.5%) in the ISAT trial with a mean 12 years of follow-up.
- Therefore, despite high efficacy and low procedural morbidity of PVO, reconstructive approaches preserving the parent vessel are often preferred where feasible, especially in younger patients.

Indications

- Aneurysms presenting with clinically significant mass effect.
- Large (>15 mm) and giant (≥25 mm) aneurysms.
- Symptomatic fusiform aneurysms.
- Ruptured fusiform/dissecting aneurysms.
- Other atypical aneurysms, including infectious.

Device

- Detachable balloons are the quickest and most cost-effective method for achieving vessel occlusion. However, controlled detachment can be difficult and there is the risk of deflation migration. In addition, the availability of detachable silicone balloons is currently limited in many countries. As a result, balloon PVO has been replaced by coil occlusion in most centres.
- Coiling has the advantage of precise placement with good control at the level of the aneurysm neck. The initial coil framework is more safely achieved with controlled detachment coils. Once in place, cheaper pushable coils may be used (if MRI compatible). Dual microcatheter or balloon assistance techniques may facilitate initial framework stability.
- Many coils may be required to achieve to complete occlusion, which can be time-consuming and expensive. Large, thick coils, are recommended, such as POD400 and PAC400 (Penumbra) (these coils are specifically designed for vessel sacrifice).

Technique

(See Figure 8.14.)

- Procedure preparation is as for simple coiling. GA is advisable as the procedure can be prolonged, but is not mandatory.
- Optimally, place coils in the aneurysm sac first and bring coil loops down through the neck into the parent artery once reasonable aneurysm coiling achieved (NB: loose packing if mass effect symptoms).

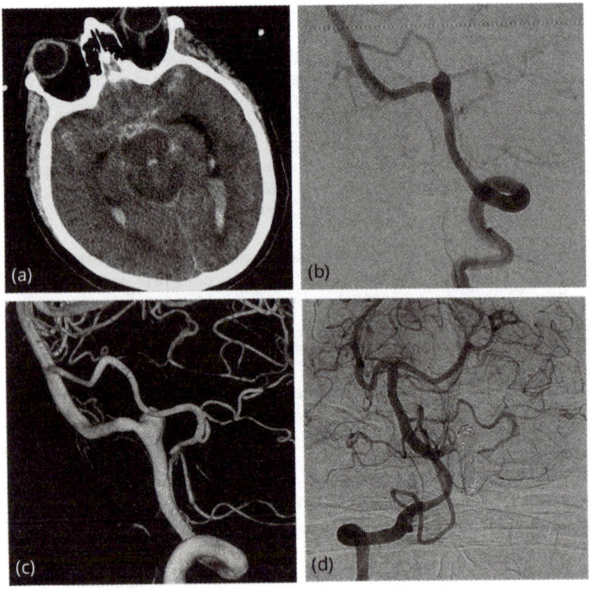

Figure 8.14 Management of a dissecting vertebral aneurysm. (a) Computed tomography shows large-volume subarachnoid haemorrhage caused by a dissecting vertebral aneurysm (b, c). (d) A large contralateral vertebral artery was present, and the posterior inferior cerebellar artery did not arise from this segment, so parent vessel occlusion was performed at the neck of the aneurysm using detachable coils.

Post-procedure

- It is important to monitor the patient closely after the procedure. Delayed infarction may occur if the BP drops sharply in the immediate postoperative period.
- Low-dose IV heparin (1000 IU/h for 24 h) and aspirin 75 mg per day for 1 month may be considered to reduce the risk of thromboembolic events.

Further reading

Arambepola PK, McEvoy SD, Bulsara KR. De novo aneurysm formation after carotid artery occlusion for cerebral aneurysms. Skull Base. 2010;20(6):405–408.

de Gast AN, Sprengers ME, van Rooij WJ, et al. Long term 3T-MRA follow-up after therapeutic occlusion of the internal carotid artery to detect possible de novo aneurysm formation. Am J Neuroradiol. 2007;28(3):508–510.

Molyneux AJM, Birks J, Clarke A, Sneade M, Kerr RSC. The durability of endovascular coiling versus neurosurgical clipping of ruptured cerebral aneurysms: 18 year follow-up of the UK cohort of the International Subarachnoid Aneurysm Trial (ISAT). Lancet. 2014;384(9969):691–697.

van der Schaaf IC, Brilstra EH, Buskens E, Rinkel GJE. Endovascular treatment of aneurysms in the cavernous sinus: a systematic review on balloon occlusion of the parent vessel and embolisation with coils. Stroke. 2002;33(1):313–318.

Paediatric aneurysms

Less than 1% of UIAs occur in children. Ruptured aneurysms in the paediatric population are even rarer, comprising 0.6% of aSAHs. There are significant differences in aetiology and treatment strategy.

Differences from adults

- More common in males (vs females in adults).
- More commonly in the posterior circulation (25% vs 8% in adults), compared with the anterior circulation.
- Giant aneurysms and mirror aneurysms are more common.
- Trauma accounts for 25% of paediatric brain aneurysms (rare in adults).
- Younger children have a higher rate of dissecting aneurysms, and older children have more saccular aneurysms.
- Familial aneurysms account for 5–20% of cases in children and young adults but only 5% of cases pre-puberty.

Pathophysiology of aneurysm formation

- Adult risk factors (e.g. atherosclerosis, systemic hypertension, and smoking) are not associated with paediatric aneurysm development.
- Aneurysm formation in children requires accelerated wall damage (infection, inflammation, dissection, trauma) in association with enhanced wall fragility (arteriopathies, developmental, connective tissue disorders).
- Vascular dysplasias, poor reparative mechanisms, and chronic microtraumas lead to the development of aneurysms in several conditions including vascular Ehlers–Danlos syndrome (*COL3A1* mutation), Hutchins–Menkes disease (*ATP7A* mutation), microcephalic osteodysplastic primordial dwarfism type II (MOPDII; *PCNT* gene mutation), sickle cell disease, PHACES syndrome, and neurofibromatosis type 1.

Giant aneurysms

- Children are 2–4 times more likely to have giant aneurysms, suggesting an altered underlying pathophysiology, e.g. trauma, dissection, arteriopathy, and vascular syndromes.
- These are usually discovered due to mass effect, neurological deficit, or epilepsy.

Dissecting aneurysms

- A history of mild trauma often precedes a haemorrhagic or ischaemic presentation.
- These are often predisposed by anatomical substrates such as a variant course of a vessel or the differential growth rate of blood vessels with adjacent structures, e.g. the skull base, tentorium, or corpus callosum.

Management of incidental paediatric brain aneurysm

- With the advent of 3 T MRI, incidental aneurysms account for 25% of unruptured aneurysms in children.
- Infundibulae at the limits of spatial resolution are often mistaken for aneurysms in small children.

Treatment considerations

- A 4 or 5 Fr guide catheter and a single microcatheter are normally sufficient, especially for PVO.
- In older children, and where dual microcatheters are required, 0.070" access is preferred. This can be achieved with either 5 Fr long sheaths or 6 Fr guide catheters (with or without sheath).
- Accessing the carotid and vertebral arteries is usually straightforward as vessel tortuosity is uncommon.
- Intracranial arteries increase in size rapidly in the first year of life and then sharply plateau. Despite the small size of a child, the intracranial vasculature may be surprisingly similar to that of adulthood.

Saccular aneurysms

- Proximal saccular aneurysms can be treated with conventional adult techniques, e.g. unassisted or balloon-assisted coil embolisation using 0.013–0.0165" microcatheters.
- The vessels of the paediatric intracranial circulation will straighten more readily than adult vessels after placement of the microcatheter. Repeat a roadmap to ensure the anatomy is where you think it is!
- Distal saccular aneurysms are often due to infectious aetiologies, tumour emboli, vasculitic processes, or trauma and can be treated with coils or LEs. Due to distality, access to the aneurysm or parent vessel is usually via 1.2 Fr catheter and 0.007" microwire. n-BCA glue is often the embolic material of choice to allow for rapid occlusion of the aneurysm, although EVOH-based LEs can also be used.

Fusiform aneurysms

- Fusiform aneurysms are more common in children and deconstructive strategies should be considered. Factors to consider when undertaking vessel deconstruction include the location of the aneurysm (proximal vs distal), assessment of collateral supply to the territory, and cross circulation.
- Vessel deconstruction is favoured when there is no other vascular disease, antiplatelet agents are contraindicated, and where there is a focal dissection. It should be avoided where multiple vessels are affected, e.g. sickle cell disease, collagen vascular disorders, and if the aneurysm involves a perforator-dependent segment.
- Where possible, deconstruction should only be performed after a BTO especially in proximal aneurysms and uncertainty of collateral supply. If parent vessel deconstruction is not feasible, one should consider reconstruction with an FDS.

Flow diversion in children

- There is a reasonable body of evidence demonstrating the safety of flow diverters in children. Concerns about growth in size of the blood vessel relative to the stent appear unfounded.
- Low-profile flow diverters are preferred, e.g. Fred Jr (Microvention) and Silk Vista Baby (Balt). Newer coated devices can reduce platelet aggregation.
- Antiplatelet agents and their durations should be discussed with paediatric haematologists. Aspirin with clopidogrel or prasugrel is

usually favoured in children although ticagrelor is increasingly used for teenagers (compliance is a consideration, however).

- Given the possibility of underlying vasculopathy, cross-sectional vascular imaging is recommended before stopping DAPT, usually at 6 months to 1 year, followed by aspirin lifelong.
- Imaging follow-up can be either with CTA or MRA, according to age, local availability, and preference.

Further reading

Bisson DA, Dirks P, Amirabadi A, et al. Unruptured intracranial aneurysms in children: 18 years' experience in a tertiary care paediatric institution. J Neurosurg Pediatr. 2019;24(2):184–189.

Hetts SW, Narvid J, Sanai N, et al. Intracranial aneurysms in childhood: 27-year single-institution experience. AJNR Am J Neuroradiol. 2009;30(7):1315–1324.

Taylor JM, Chang M, Vaughan J, et al. Cerebral arterial growth in childhood. Pediatr Neurol. 2022;134:59–66.

Stenting

Aneurysm bridging stents act as a scaffold by sitting across the neck of the aneurysm. They prevent coil prolapse and promote aneurysmal thrombosis. Over time, an endothelialised arterial layer forms over the struts of the stent.

Indications

- Unruptured wide-necked aneurysms where there is a risk of coil prolapse with coil embolisation alone, or to reduce the risk of recurrence.
- During coil embolisation when thrombus forms in the parent artery that cannot be dispersed through medications such as aspirin or GP IIb/IIIa receptor inhibitors, or when a significant mass of coil protrudes into the vessel.
- For acutely ruptured aneurysms, practice varies, but it is acknowledged that the risks of stent usage are higher than with coil embolisation alone mainly due to the necessity of antiplatelet medication. Laser-cut stents are preferred as they are less thrombogenic than braided stents.

Stent design

- A comprehensive description of currently available stents is presented in Chapter 4 (see 'Aneurysm bridging stents', p. 132).

Antiplatelet therapy

- In elective aneurysms, dual antiplatelets (aspirin and clopidogrel, ticagrelor, or prasugrel) are initiated. There are different regimens depending on the urgency of the situation (see Chapter 3, P2Y12 inhibitors p. 103).
- Acutely, GP IIb/IIIa inhibitors (eptifibatide, tirofiban) or cangrelor are options.

Access

- If access to the aneurysm is straightforward, a 5, 6, or 7 Fr guide catheter, such as Benchmark, can be used with a delivery catheter. Nowadays, most stents can be delivered via 0.017" or 0.021" microcatheters, which can be inserted alongside the coiling catheter if 'jailing' the microcatheter.
- In smaller radial arteries (<2.5 mm), a 6 Fr system is less likely to cause problems with spasm.
- If access is likely to be difficult (e.g. tortuous anatomy), it is recommended to use a triaxial setup with an intermediate catheter, such as Navien 0.072". This setup typically requires 8 Fr vascular access.

Aneurysm and vessel assessment

- Biplane equipment is used. Once the guide/intermediate catheter is placed, perform whole head baseline 2D angiography in standard projections. 3D flat panel angiography is then performed.
- Study the 3D angiography on the console to obtain projections suitable for (i) measuring and deploying the stent in the parent artery across the neck of the aneurysm (there must be good views of the proximal and distal landing zones in particular), and (ii) catheterising the aneurysm (if coiling is utilised).

- Considerations for stent selection:
  - Size of the vessels and landing zones: the stent should be sized to the largest vessel diameter (usually the proximal segment). Stents require some anchorage distally and proximally. Most stents have a wide range of sizes; however, at the extremes (very small or very large) certain companies offer more suitable sizes.
  - Laser-cut versus braided: laser-cut stents are less thrombogenic and are easier to deploy as their length alters little during deployment. It is simple to predict where they will sit by looking at the proximal and distal markers. Braided stents will gain length if oversized (in terms of diameter) in smaller arteries. They may offer some degree of flow-diversion effect, which can be increased by 'bunching them up' at the aneurysm neck.
  - Occlusion rates: there is some evidence to support the theoretical greater occlusion rates of braided versus laser-cut stents (e.g. Mokin et al., 2020).
  - Personal experience with the device: each device behaves differently during deployment and may have certain 'quirks'. If you are unfamiliar with the device, bring an experienced colleague to oversee and a representative from the supplier who has technical expertise.
  - Antiplatelet therapy: laser-cut stents have less metal overall (7–10%) compared to braided stents (18–23%), making them less thrombogenic.
  - Visibility: it is easier to see the individual strands of braided stents, whereas only the markers (proximal, distal, and sometimes more in the middle) on laser-cut stents can be seen.
  - Resheathability: some stents are resheathable up to a certain percentage of stent deployment (including the laser-cut Acclino stent and most braided stents—check device instructions for use if unfamiliar), whereas some laser-cut stents such as the Atlas are not resheathable at all.

Adjunctive coil embolisation

(See Figure 8.15.)

- Coil embolisation is necessary after stent placement. Unless the aneurysm is fully occluded with coils it is likely that it will continue to fill, and possibly enlarge or rupture at some stage.
- The coiling catheter can be 'jailed' within the aneurysm. This involves catheterising the aneurysm before deploying the stent and either leaving the wire inside or deploying a length of coil, without detaching it. After stent deployment, coiling is resumed. The catheter is retrieved in the normal way when the aneurysm is occluded.
- Alternatively, the stent can be deployed and the coiling catheter (which may be the same one used to deliver the stent) is navigated through the struts of the stent into the aneurysm. This is usually possible. However, for certain stents which have tight braids (e.g. the LVIS Evo), and when a braided stent has been 'bunched up', it may be difficult, requiring smaller microcatheters.

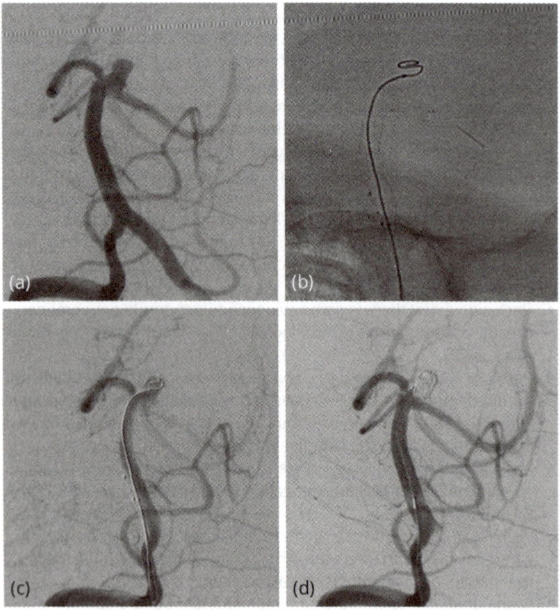

Figure 8.15 Stent-assisted coil embolisation of an unruptured aneurysm. (a) Digital subtraction angiography shows an unruptured wide-necked left P1 posterior cerebral artery aneurysm. (b) Unsubtracted and (c) subtracted angiography post deployment of LVIS Evo stent (note 'bunching' into neck of aneurysm), with coil loop and microcatheter 'jailed' in aneurysm sac. (d) Subsequent coil embolisation of aneurysm.

Deployment

- Navigate the stent delivery catheter further in the artery than where the distal end of the stent is required to be. Remove the wire.
- If the 'jailing' technique is employed, next catheterise the aneurysm with a second microcatheter and deploy some coil loops.
- Flush the stent in its sheath within the microcatheter hub, and load it into the microcatheter until the distal stent marker aligns with the microcatheter tip.
- Position the microcatheter tip just distal to where you desire the distal end of the stent. There may be a stent delivery wire which protrudes beyond the microcatheter.
- Start to unsheathe the stent. Once the distal end of the stent has emerged from the delivery catheter, the deployment must be gradual and controlled. The stent may fall back slightly during deployment, which must be anticipated.
- When deploying around tight bends, it may be necessary to pull back on the system (microcatheter and device together) to centre it in the middle of the vessel, as it tends to veer towards the outer curve.

- If using a braided stent, at the aneurysm neck you may choose to deploy with more forward pressure to alter the orientation of the strands to become more densely packed over the neck ('bunching up').
- Continue to unsheathe the stent until it is fully deployed. The delivery catheter and supporting delivery wire will now move independently of the device. You can re-enter the stent if required using the delivery wire. If not, the delivery wire is removed.
- If a coiling catheter has not been 'jailed', then one is then introduced through the struts of the stent into the aneurysm.
- The aneurysm is then fully coiled.

Y-stenting

(See Figure 8.16.)

- This technique is used for aneurysms with a wide neck and two branches that need protection, typically bifurcation aneurysms.
- The technique introduces complexity compared to a single stent. Nevertheless, morbidity and mortality have been found to be relatively low, with high occlusion rates (95.4%) (Cagnazzo et al., 2019).
- After deploying the first stent, the microcatheter then re-enters the stent over the stent delivery wire.

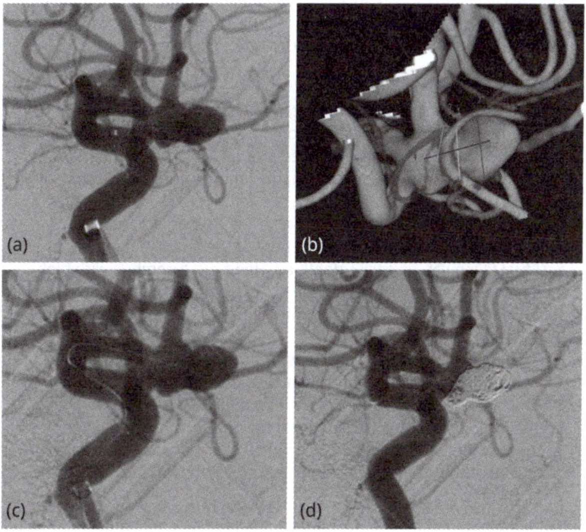

Figure 8.16 Y-stenting of a wide-necked middle cerebral artery aneurysm. (a) 2D and (b) 3D rotational angiography of unruptured wide-necked bifurcation aneurysm. (c) Microcatheter and coil loop 'jailed' within the aneurysm sac. (d) Two Atlas stents were deployed in a Y configuration across the neck of the aneurysm followed by coiling.

- It is pulled through the lumen of the stent until at the neck of the aneurysm.
- The stent delivery wire is removed and a microwire is inserted. This is used to navigate the microcatheter through the struts of the first stent into the second branch to be protected.
- The second stent is deployed in the usual manner. A short segment of the stent will be constrained as it passes through the struts of the first stent, after which it will expand and occupy the lumen of the proximal part of the first stent.
- Stents with wider braids, such as laser-cut stents, are typically used because they allow easier re-entry through the struts. However, braided stents have also been successfully utilised.

Patient aftercare and discharge

- Record in detail the procedure and post-procedure physician and nursing requirements, e.g. BP levels, regularity of access site observations, and neurological observations. This should be handed over directly to the receiving team but also documented on the electronic patient record or written into a care plan.
- Ensure there is a colleague who can review the patient in the morning and give instructions for mobilisation and discharge if not yourself.
- Ensure antiplatelet medication is prescribed prior to discharge.
- Ensure clinical follow-up (usually around 6 weeks) has been arranged.
- In addition, ensure there is a point of contact for the patient or family member should they have any queries once discharged home.

Imaging follow-up

- Some operators believe that angiography is necessary for a more detailed evaluation of device positioning, luminal patency, and aneurysm occlusion. This is typically performed around 6 months or later after treatment, following the discontinuation of one of the dual antiplatelet agents.
- MRI with time of flight, particularly at 3 T, is gaining acceptance for follow-up. It allows for clear assessment of the aneurysm lumen, as any residual filling can be easily identified. However, thrombus with high T1 signal within an occluded aneurysm can persist, potentially giving a false impression of flow if T1-weighted images are not performed and analysed in conjunction.
- IV cone beam CT has been used successfully for follow-up. This technique combines the high spatial resolution of angio CT with an IV contrast dose with additional metal artefact reduction software to create multiplanar reconstructions of the device. It has shown great promise in evaluating device placement, wall apposition, and vessel patency, without the risks/inconvenience/costs associated with catheter angiography.

Complications

Ischaemia

- This is the most common complication. It can occur acutely during or just after deployment, or in a delayed fashion.

- It can also occur at the time of stopping DAPT during conversion to aspirin only.
- Thrombus formation is more likely with Y-stenting and braided stents.
- Check heparinisation and increase if necessary.
- IV boluses of heparin and/or IV or intra-arterial aspirin 500 mg may resolve or stabilise the thrombus.
- Raising the mean arterial pressure can help increase perfusion.
- Eptifibatide or tirofiban bolus and infusion may be required to dissolve the clot (see Chapter 3, 'Glycoprotein (GP) IIb/IIIa receptor inhibitors', p. 103).
- Postprocedurally, CT/CTA and MRI/MRA are advised to assess in cases of ischaemia.

Late migration

- This can often be predicted if the device is not sized correctly to the vessel or positioned with insufficient anchorage. It can even drop into the aneurysm if it foreshortens (more likely with braided stents).
- If there is migration during the case, or it is visible on follow-up imaging (with continuing aneurysm filling), an option is to deploy a second device through the first to improve aneurysm coverage ('telescoping') and anchoring of the distal end of the deployed stent.

Failure to occlude the aneurysm

- The aneurysm should be coiled until there is no further filling on angiography. If there is residual filling at the end of the case, then this may progress over time.
- However, judgement and experience are required regarding when to stop coiling as over-packing carries risks. Remember: 'perfection is the enemy of good'.

Late ischaemic complications

- Delayed vessel occlusion.
- This may result from poor response to antiplatelet therapy, drug interactions, non-compliance with medication, or a lack of awareness among healthcare professionals regarding the importance of these agents, particularly discontinuation of antiplatelets for minor surgical procedures that could be delayed. It is crucial to clearly document and communicate the importance of these medications to both patients and medical practitioners.
- Traditionally, aspirin was continued lifelong. However, the necessary duration of antiplatelets is unknown and stopping antiplatelets after 1 or 2 years is an option, especially with low-metal laser-cut stents.

Further reading

Cagnazzo F, Limbucci N, Nappini S, et al. Y-stent-assisted coiling of wide-neck bifurcation intracranial aneurysms: a meta-analysis. AJNR Am J Neuroradiol. 2019;40(1):122–128.

Mokin M, Primiani CT, Ren Z, et al. Stent-assisted coiling of cerebral aneurysms: multicentre analysis of radiographic and clinical outcomes in 659 patients. J Neurointerv Surg. 2020;12(3):289–297.

Flow diversion

FDSs were developed to address limitations of coil embolisation. Their effect is to reduce the flow into the aneurysm to encourage thrombosis. They re-direct flow, reduce intra-aneurysmal flow velocity and shear stress, induce clot formation (although this may be a slow-delayed process), and provide a scaffold for endothelial growth.

Coatings and surface modifications have been developed to reduce thrombogenicity. Successful aneurysm occlusion depends on careful device sizing. The stent needs to be well apposed to the endothelium proximal and distal to the aneurysm to ensure maximum flow diversion away from the aneurysm. If achieved, the device causes progressive thrombosis, aneurysm shrinkage, and the promotion of endothelial growth across the neck.

A description of some of the design elements of FDSs is given in Chapter 4, 'Flow diverters', p. 133.

Devices

- Pipeline Embolisation device (PED; Medtronic): 48 wires of cobalt–chromium–nickel with 12 embedded platinum–tungsten wires. 'Shield' surface modification to reduce thrombogenicity. The latest-generation Pipeline Vantage is constructed from drawn filled tube wires and is compatible with the Phenom 0.021" microcatheter for diameters 3.5 mm and below. The larger Vantage sizes are currently not available at the time of writing, and the previous-generation PED device is used for larger sizes delivered with the Phenom 0.027" microcatheter.
- Surpass Evolve/Elite (Stryker): braided cobalt–chromium alloy with 12 wires of platinum–tungsten alloy. The number of wires depends on the size of the device and ranges from 48 mm in the 2.5 mm device to 64 for devices over 3.7 mm in diameter. Devices are deployable through 0.027" microcatheters (recommended XT-27).
- FRED (MicroVention): this is a dual-layer device with a 48-wire nitinol inner layer and a 16-wire nitinol outer layer. A radiopaque tantalum layer binds the two. The distal and proximal 10% of the device are single-layer only. FRED Junior (2.5–3 mm diameter) has 36- and 16-wire inner and outer layers, respectively, for smaller lesions.
- SILK Vista (Balt): 48 extruded nitinol wires with eight platinum wires and four platinum coils to enhance visibility. Tapered devices are available to accommodate differing distal and proximal parent artery diameters. The whole range (up to 5 mm diameter) is deployable through 0.021" microcatheters. Silk Vista Baby is constructed of 48 platinum-filled wires and intended for vessel sizes 1.5–3.5 mm. It is deliverable through 0.017" microcatheters.
- P64/P48 (Phenox): platinum-filled drawn filament nitinol tube with 64 (vessel size 3–5 mm) and 48 (vessel size 2–3 mm) wires. Deliverable through 0.021" microcatheters.
- Derivo 2 (Acandis): 48 nitinol wires with platinum core. Three markers at proximal and distal ends. This device has a large range of sizes, with the largest diameter of any currently available device, able to treat vessels up to 8 mm. Deliverable through 0.017" to 0.039" microcatheters dependent on the diameter of the device. It is available with or without Heal technology, an antithrombogenic coating.

- Turbridge (MicroPort): this is a braided nitinol device with 62 (vessel size 3.5–6.6 mm) and 46 (2.5–3 mm) wires. It requires a 0.029" microcatheter for delivery.

Indications for flow-diverting stents

- Recurrent aneurysms.
- Very large or giant aneurysms.
- Wide neck (>4 mm).
- Dome-to-width ratio of <2.
- Ruptured dissecting and blister aneurysms.
- Dysplastic, fusiform cerebral aneurysms that previously were only treatable by PVO, neurosurgical wrapping, or left untreated.

Antiplatelet therapy

- Current regimens include 75 mg of aspirin per day in the UK, typically continued indefinitely for most patients. For certain regions (e.g. proximal to the ICA bifurcation), some operators choose to discontinue the treatment after 1 year. Aspirin is usually commenced 5–7 days pretreatment. Alternatively, aspirin may be given intraprocedurally IV prior to stent placement.
- Added to aspirin are one of the following agents: clopidogrel, prasugrel, or ticagrelor (a comprehensive discussion of antiplatelets is given in Chapter 3, P2Y12 inhibitors, p. 103).
- Platelet function testing may be utilised to ensure that adequate inhibition is achieved.
- There are multiple case series of single-antiplatelet use in a range of FDSs (i.e. omitting aspirin). Currently, the COATING trial is assessing the use of a single antiplatelet (prasugrel or ticagrelor) with the Phenox p64 MW HPC flow diverter.

Patient preparation

- *As for coil embolization* (see 'Coil embolisation of intracranial aneurysms', p. 247).

Access

- There are two main options, depending on tortuosity and expected challenges with stability:
  - If access to the aneurysm is straightforward, a 6 Fr guide catheter, such as Benchmark, or 7 Fr, such as RIST, can be used with a delivery catheter. It is also possible to use a coiling catheter alongside the flow-diverter delivery microcatheter using such a system (e.g. inserting an Echelon-10 alongside a 0.027" microcatheter inside a Benchmark). Note that 6 Fr systems offer less support than 8 Fr, and can make accurate deployment of the FDS more difficult.
  - If access is likely to be difficult (e.g. tortuous anatomy) and multiple devices, and/or possibly coiling, are anticipated, it is recommended to use a triaxial system with an intermediate catheter, such as Navien 0.072". This requires 8 Fr vascular access.
- Transradial or transfemoral approaches can be utilised but in patients with smaller radial arteries (<2.5 mm) a 6 Fr system is less likely to cause problems with spasm.

- Systemic heparinisation is undertaken after the vascular access is achieved.

Aneurysm and vessel assessment

- Once the guide/intermediate catheter is placed, perform whole head baseline angiography in standard projections. Biplane equipment is essential.
- 3D-RA is recommended for flow diversion for assessment of aneurysm and parent vessel sizes.
- Review all previous imaging; assess for any change in anatomy. Note: if the aneurysm was partially thrombosed, this may reduce in volume while the patient is on pretreatment antiplatelets and alter the treatment plan.
- Software such as PreSize (Oxford Heartbeat) or Sim & Size (Sim & Cure) to assess the size of the required device and wall apposition may be useful.
- Considerations in choosing a device:
  - Access: some FDSs require larger delivery microcatheters, which may be more difficult to navigate and cause distortion of the arteries during deployment. The Silk Vista Baby (Balt) and Derivo2 (Acandis) can be deployed through low-profile 0.017" microcatheters.
  - Sizes of proximal and distal parent artery: most flow diverters have a wide range of sizes; however, at the extremes (very small or very large), certain companies offer more suitable sizes.
  - Personal experience with the device: each device behaves differently during deployment and may have certain 'quirks'. If you are unfamiliar with the device, bring an experienced colleague to oversee and a representative from the supplier who has technical expertise.
  - Tolerance to antiplatelet therapy: some FDSs, such as Pipeline Shield/Vantage, Derivo, P48,64 have coatings designed to reduce thrombogenicity. Hence, there is a theoretical benefit in utilising these, particularly in aSAH.

Adjunctive coil embolisation

- Coil embolisation in addition to flow diversion can be performed to increase the speed and chance of aneurysm occlusion and reduce the risk of early post-treatment haemorrhage. Strongly consider this if the aneurysm is >10 mm.
- Reasons not to coil include an increase in the complexity and potential risk of the procedure and a theoretical increase in the persisting mass effect post-treatment.
- Unlike standard stents, it is impossible to cross the struts of a deployed FDS to enter the aneurysm.
  - If the aneurysm is narrow necked, it may be coiled first with or without balloon assistance.
  - If the neck is wide, the microcatheter is usually 'jailed'. This involves first navigating the microcatheter inside the aneurysm. A partial coil loop is then deployed to secure the microcatheter in place. Next, the flow diverter is deployed, followed by the coiling of the aneurysm. The coil catheter can then be withdrawn from the aneurysm alongside the FDS without risk of dislodging it or pulling it back. Note that the microcatheter has a tendency to slip back or forward during

deployment of the flow diverter. This must be monitored for during deployment and the microcatheter adjusted if necessary.

- Flow diverters have limited capacity to withstand external pressure. Oversizing the coil diameter is not necessary and can cause parent artery compromise, as the flow diverter can be narrowed by a large stiff framing coil.
- Packing density is also less of an issue as the flow diverter will reduce luminal filling.

Deployment

(See Figure 8.17.)

- Study the 3D angiography on the console to obtain biplane projections suitable for measuring and deploying the device in the parent artery across the neck of the aneurysm (there must be good views of the proximal and distal landing zones in particular), and catheterising the aneurysm (if coiling is employed).
- There are two approaches to distal device placement:
  - Navigation of the delivery catheter some distance distal to landing zone, partial deployment then slow withdrawal of both to the desired position ('drag and drop').
  - Placement of the delivery catheter just distal to landing zone, navigating the stent to desired location within the catheter, and withdrawing the catheter to expose the flow diverter in this location without dragging it back.
- In the past, the former was recommended for certain flow diverters; nowadays, it is really a matter of personal preference.

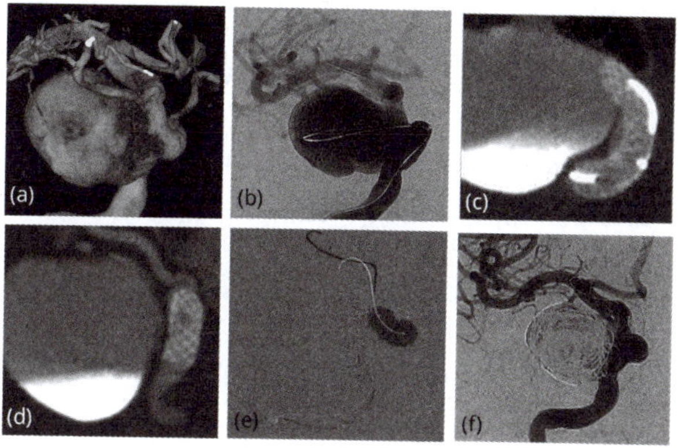

Figure 8.17 Flow diversion for a giant internal carotid artery aneurysm. (a) 3D rotational angiography of unruptured wide-necked giant internal carotid artery aneurysm. (b) Microcatheter and coil loop 'jailed' within the aneurysm during flow diverter deployment. (c, d) Post-deployment VasoCT demonstrates flow diverter deployed across the neck of the aneurysm. (e) Compliant balloon temporarily inflated within the flow diverter to improve vessel wall apposition. (f) Finally, the aneurysm is packed with coils.

- Once the distal end of the stent has emerged from the delivery catheter, the deployment must be gradual and controlled. Forward pressure is applied with the right hand while maintaining some tension on the delivery catheter with the left hand.
- Forward tension on the delivery catheter is important to reduce risk of slipping back and deploying the stent too proximally. It also promotes distal stent opening, 'anchoring' it in place. This is the key to easy flow diverter deployment.
- Most flow diverters have a central delivery wire for stability. This needs to move forward freely as the stent is deployed. There is the potential for vessel damage with uncontrolled movement. For this reason, these devices may be deployed into a more distal straight segment of vessel (e.g. M1) to allow free exit of the flow diverter and supporting wire. Both can then be withdrawn into position to continue deployment.
- While the tip of the delivery wire is designed to be soft, if it enters a perforator during deployment and force is applied, it may rupture the vessel (see Figure 8.19, p. 295). Therefore, carefully watch the wire (two operators are ideal for this purpose) to avoid this complication.
- The shape of the device, once exited from the delivery catheter, should be scrutinised. The ideal shape is a 'wine glass' with parallel sides against the vessel wall and proximal concavity. If the device has more of a 'martini glass' shape, with limited wall apposition and very shallow concavity, then there is too much forward tension. If the device looks like a 'champagne flute' with a long proximal taper and limited wall apposition, then there is not enough tension. In both situations, the device is likely to move and will not have enough wall apposition to be effective.
- The mid-deployment should be neutral with forward pressure on the delivery wire while allowing the delivery catheter to withdraw proximally.
- When deploying around tight bends, it is often necessary to pull back on the system (microcatheter and device together) to centre it in the middle of the vessel, as it tends to veer towards the outer curve.
- At the aneurysm neck, you may choose to deploy with more forward pressure to alter the orientation of the strands to become more densely packed with reduced porosity, which has a greater effect on diminishing aneurysm inflow.
- Similarly, if deploying across a bifurcation aneurysm (e.g. basilar tip from P1 to basilar main trunk), it is necessary to create some forward tension as the device crosses the neck of the aneurysm. If not, the device may simply follow the curve and not cover the neck at all. Devices are flexible and supple enough to almost mould into shape across the neck.
- Once proximal to the aneurysm neck, a more neutral deployment is required to balance deployment with withdrawal. Slow down as you approach the point of no return and ensure you are fully familiar with the markers of various devices. Most will have a marker (80–90% of deployed length) where the device cannot be resheathed and deployment is inevitable.
- The final deployment of the flow diverter should be performed without excessive forward tension. You will see the device open and the proximal end appose the vessel wall. It may retreat distally very slightly as it does so. 'Fish-mouthing' is a descriptive term for when the proximal stent does not fully open. Both of these can be avoided by ensuring there is

not too much forward force when deploying the final part of the device, so unsheathe the device, and do not push the device at its final extent.
- The delivery catheter and supporting delivery wire will now move independently of the device.

Assessment of deployment success

- At this stage, assess for device position and apposition. Most devices require at least 5 mm of anchorage distally and proximally.
- Cone beam CT with diluted (20%) contrast may be usefully employed either routinely or selectively. Review it on the biplane console in axial, sagittal, and coronal planes with the slice thickness set to the minimum level. It is particularly useful in complex anatomy and where more than one device has been deployed. It is less useful if the aneurysm has been coiled due to excessive metallic artefact.
- On 2D angiography:
  - Review both subtracted and non-subtracted images to assess position and shape of the device. Compare unsubtracted images without and mid-contrast opacification to assess for flow outside the lumen.
  - The stent should appose the vessel without stenosis or proximal/distal lips.
  - There should be no lines not explained by the stent structure (no twisting).
  - Look at the proximal and distal markers to ensure they align in the same plane and apposed to the vessel wall.

Post-deployment manipulation

Device mal-deployment

- The commonest issue is the device slipping proximally during deployment. This can occur with insufficient forward tension on the system in tortuous vessels. Too rapid deployment is also a factor.
- The device should be gently retrieved if not fully deployed. Re-advance the delivery catheter to the starting position with the device inside, if possible. Re-attempt deployment, more slowly and with greater forward force.
- Alternatively, if it is considered likely that the problem will recur, re-advance the catheter with the device more distally, partially deploy the device into the vessel, so the distal end opens, then slowly withdraw to deployment position ('drag and drop'). The partially deployed device may act as a 'brake', slowing the retreating delivery catheter due to friction with the vessel wall, and offer more control of the catheter movement.

Vessel apposition

- If the device is not properly apposed, there is a risk of endoleak leading to inadequate aneurysm occlusion, thrombosis forming between the stent and vessel wall, and stenosis of the vessel.
- Removal of any jailed microcatheters (once coiling has been completed) may resolve this.
- If not, there are some manoeuvres that may help:
  - Re-entry of the delivery microcatheter through the device over the deployment wire to encourage better apposition to the vessel wall. The risks include (i) foreshortening and 'fish-mouthing' of the proximal

end of the device during re-entry, and (ii) movement of the device such that there is insufficient coverage of the neck (if there is pre-existing device instability).

- Balloon inflation within a deployed device to improve wall apposition and the flow-diverter effect. The compliant balloon should be sized slightly larger than the vessel. To introduce the balloon inside the stent you can either (i) bring the delivery microcatheter through the stent over the delivery wire and then insert an exchange microcatheter, remove the microcatheter, and insert the balloon; or (ii) insert the balloon directly over a wire (a 'J' shape on the wire helps). Microwire exchange procedures risk vessel perforation and should be used carefully and selectively.
- Stent retrievers can also be used to improve wall apposition. These are unsheathed at the site of mal-apposition and then resheathed. The benefit is that the same microcatheter used for flow diverter deployment can be used for the stent retriever. The main disadvantage is cost.
- Deployment of another overlapping ('telescoped') stent or flow diverter either proximally or distally if it is the end that is affected and the above-listed manoeuvres have not resolved it.
- Retrieval of the flow diverter: this is an advanced last-resort manoeuvre that should only be performed by experienced practitioners. It may be achieved by snaring the device.

Tips

Crossing the aneurysm

- Occasionally, navigating a larger catheter (0.021" or 0.027"), typically required for flow diversion, into the distal vessel can be challenging. This is particularly true for large, very wide-necked ICA aneurysms.
- The microcatheter may become caught at the proximal or distal neck of the aneurysm due to the size difference between the microcatheter and the wire, known as the 'ledge' effect. This can be mitigated by inserting an additional 'buddy' wire into the microcatheter. In addition to a standard 0.014" microwire, a 0.027" microcatheter can accommodate a 0.010" wire, while a 0.021" microcatheter can accommodate a 0.007" wire.
- Sometimes, it is necessary to deflect the wire across the wall of the aneurysm to enable it to enter the distal vessel ('going around the world'; Figure 8.18). If the microcatheter can be safely advanced distally over the wire, its midsection may also remain prolapsed within the aneurysm, prohibiting the advancement of a flow diverter. Occasionally, gently tugging the microcatheter may straighten it, removing the prolapse, though this may also pull the distal end of the microcatheter back proximally. Alternatively, inserting and deploying a stent retriever into the distal vessel can anchor the microcatheter distally, allowing for midsection straightening. It may be necessary to use an exchange-length microwire with a smaller microcatheter initially, then exchange for the larger stent-delivery microcatheter when the wire is straightened (Traxcess wire with docking addition to rapidly convert standard wire to exchange length can be helpful).

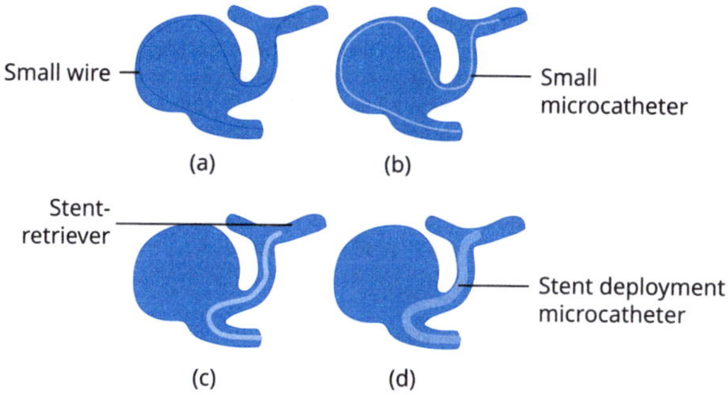

Figure 8.18 Technique to navigate the microcatheter distal to a giant wide-necked aneurysm. (a) A wire is passed around the aneurysm into the distal parent artery. (b) A small microcatheter is tracked over the wire. (c) A stent retriever is deployed to provide distal anchorage. The microcatheter is straightened and then removed. (d) The stent delivery microcatheter is inserted over the stent retriever, which is subsequently removed.

Multiple devices

- Multiple telescoped devices may be required for large aneurysms. These are usually laid distal to proximal. The second flow diverter diameter must be at least as large as the first (often greater).
- The choice of devices may be determined by the access and delivery catheter. Most operators would deploy the same manufacturer's device.
- An older technique was to place a scaffold (e.g. large braided stent) first, then line this with telescoped flow diverters.

Covering branch vessels

- Patent branch vessels are associated with continued aneurysm filling after flow diverter placement as runoff persists and maintains flow with an aneurysm. However, some remodelling is usual with the aneurysm diminishing over time.
- If it is not possible to occlude the vessel, then careful surveillance may be required.
- Coiling the aneurysm at the time of flow diverter placement may reduce this risk.
- Covering small branches (e.g. perforator branches, the anterior choroidal artery) does not *usually* cause any issues and there is no requirement to alter antiplatelet therapy. However, it should be avoided, where possible, to reduce the risk.
- Covering branches at bifurcation points (e.g. the MCA) can result in delayed branch closure. Depending on the collateral efficiency, this may or may not have neurological consequences.
- Covering the A1 origin may be necessary if there is not enough anchorage in the distal ICA for a more proximal aneurysm. In this case, the presence of a contralateral A1 and patent ACOM will likely determine the fate of the occluded A1. It may remain patent if required to supply A1/A2 vessels. Otherwise, it generally occludes. Occlusion is usually clinically silent.

- The ophthalmic artery will be covered in ophthalmic aneurysms treated using flow diverters. The rate of closure is around 8–10% (acute or delayed) and is usually without clinical consequence as collateral flow from the ECA will be sufficient. While some report a low incidence of ophthalmic ischaemic complications (1–3%), it is also reported that as many as 18% of patients experience permanent ophthalmic complications (mild to severe) and some are only detected with extensive ophthalmic investigation (Rouchaud et al., 2015). Optic perineuritis, responsive to steroids has also been reported.

Patient aftercare and discharge

- *As for stent deployment* (see 'Deployment', p. 284).

Imaging follow-up

- *As for stent deployment* (see 'Deployment', p. 284).

Complications

Delivery wire perforation

(See Figure 8.19.)

- When deploying the flow diverter, the delivery wire tip that the device is unsheathed from can enter perforators, and if too much force is applied, it can pass into the subarachnoid space. As attention is usually directed towards unsheathing of the flow diverter, this may be missed. Angiography, additionally, may not reveal haemorrhage at the time of perforation as the hole is sealed by the wire. Only when the wire is withdrawn back into the vessel, at the end of the procedure, is extravasation evident.
- Prevention involves paying attention to this wire, and avoiding it entering perforators. This task may be delegated to a second operator, if scrubbed. It is important to carefully scrutinise angiography at the end of the procedure for signs of extravasation, which may be subtle. Many operators perform on-table cone beam CT after deployment to look for haemorrhage.

Ischaemia

- Clinically significant ischaemia occurs in up to 10% of patients, usually intra- or periprocedural. However, >30% of events occur after 1 month.
- Intraprocedural thrombosis may relate to device malfunction, including twisting, mal-apposition/poor opening, or physical damage during placement.
- If thrombus is observed during a case, check the device and remove it if considered damaged and not fully deployed. If fully deployed and damaged, a second device can be placed, or the faulty device snared and removed.
- *Management is otherwise as for thrombosis during stent deployment.*

Stent migration

- This can often be predicted if the device is positioned just distal to the aneurysm neck with insufficient anchorage. There is a risk it will retreat further post-procedure in the parent artery or even into the aneurysm itself.

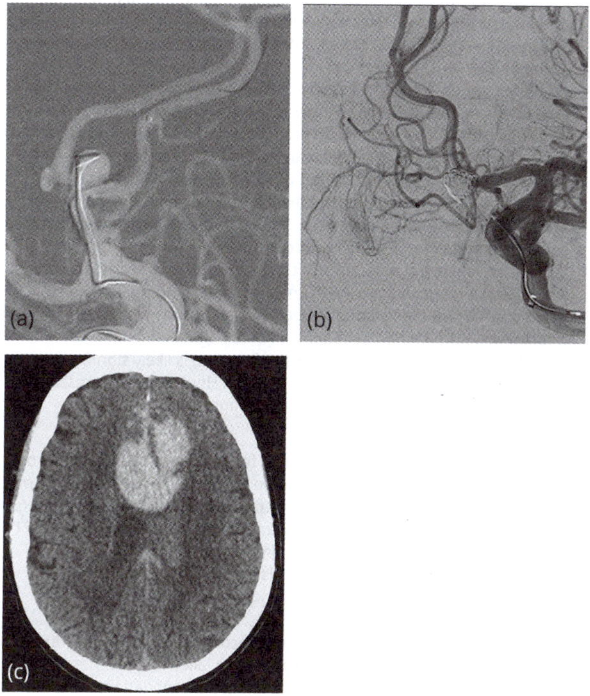

Figure 8.19 Delivery wire perforation. (a) Roadmap performed during the deployment of a flow diverter across the neck of an anterior communicating artery aneurysm, showing the delivery wire tip in a perforating vessel. (b) Digital subtraction angiography showing upon removal of the wire, extravasation is visible in the distal anterior cerebral artery, with bleeding stemmed by temporary balloon inflation. (c) A large parenchymal haemorrhage is observed on the post-procedure computed tomography scan.

- If there is migration during the case, or it is visible on follow-up imaging (with continuing aneurysm filling), the best option is usually to deploy a second device through the first to improve aneurysm coverage and anchoring of the distal end of the deployed device.
- Generally, no alteration to antiplatelet regimen is required.

Failure to occlude the aneurysm

- Aneurysm occlusion usually occurs hours, days, weeks, or months post device deployment. The usual reason for non-occlusion is suboptimal wall apposition by the device.

- This can result from poor sizing, discrepancy between proximal and distal vessel diameters, excessive tortuosity, device malfunction (twisting or damage), and device slippage proximal or distal to aneurysm neck (acute or delayed).
- A covered aneurysm with a vessel arising from the neck or lumen can maintain flow, reducing the efficacy of the flow-diversion effect.
- It may be possible on a follow-up procedure to gain access to the aneurysm via this branch vessel (e.g. via the PCOM) to catheterise and coil the persistent aneurysm. Alternatively, insertion of a second flow diverter inside the existing one at the neck of the aneurysm may help achieve thrombosis. The sizes usually need to match closely. Additional balloon inflation may also be required.
- If these options are too technically challenging, then a decision to accept a suboptimal result with ongoing imaging surveillance may be the best option. Stopping all antiplatelets (if suitable) may also encourage thrombosis.
- Even if the aneurysm persists, the risk of rupture is likely significantly lowered by the presence of the flow diverter. However, a progressively enlarging aneurysm has the potential for rupture.

Post-treatment rupture

- After flow diverters became established for aneurysm treatment, reports emerged of catastrophic delayed haemorrhage from treated aneurysms. The mechanism is still not fully understood but appears to occur in large intradural aneurysms after a delay of a few days to several weeks. DAPT meant that the haemorrhages were almost always fatal.
- The most widely accepted hypothesis is that inflammatory intra-aneurysmal thrombus itself is detrimental to the integrity of the aneurysm wall.
- To mitigate against this risk, it has been recommended that intradural aneurysms >10–14 mm should be coiled via a jailed microcatheter at the time of flow diverter placement. Since this recommendation, ruptures have diminished significantly.
- Rarely, too rapid thrombosis can lead to rupture of the aneurysm. This typically occurs in giant aneurysms that have been coiled tightly and flow-diverted.

Neointimal hyperplasia

- This is a reaction to endothelial damage and occurs in up to 20–30% of cases.
- Risk factors include diabetes, female sex, the presence of systemic inflammation, the presence of turbulent flow, poor device vessel wall apposition, and with certain flow diverters, e.g. Silk.
- It can be displayed angiographically as a line separating luminal contrast from the device.
- The reaction can be so severe as to lead to ischaemia due to embolic or haemodynamic stroke.
- There is a relationship between neointimal hyperplasia and aneurysm occlusion, and it may represent an exaggerated intimal response to the flow diverter.
- It does not necessarily require additional treatment but may need prolongation of DAPT. Balloon angioplasty can be attempted.

- The condition tends to subside from 6 months post-treatment.
- Drug-eluting balloons have been tried with some success, but clinical experience is limited.
- Simultaneous bilateral ICA or vertebral artery flow diversion risks ischaemia if neointimal hyperplasia develops in both stents. Staging the treatment may be less risky.

Intracranial haemorrhage

- Haemorrhages remote from site of deployment of device have been reported.
- There are multiple possible causes: coexisting pre-existing micro-haemorrhages or latent cerebral amyloid angiopathy, procedurally related subclinical microwire perforation, haemorrhagic transformation of occult embolic infarcts, or change in downstream pulse pressure and/or change in vessel compliance.
- Some clearly relate to antiplatelet over-responders.
- They do not need treatment specifically (unless very large requiring surgical evacuation), but will require a reassessment of DAPT and response.

Late ischaemic complications

- Delayed vessel occlusion.
- Causes include poor responder to antiplatelets, drug interactions, non-compliance with medication, and ignorance of the medical fraternity regarding their importance, e.g. discontinuation of antiplatelets for minor surgical procedures. Ensure that information on their importance is clearly documented and communicated to patients themselves and any medical practitioners.

Further reading

Caroff J, Iacobucci M, Rouchaud A, et al. The occurrence of neointimal hyperplasia after flow-diverter implantation is associated with cardiovascular risks factors and the stent design. J Neurointerv Surg. 2019;11(6):610–613.

Rouchaud A, Leclerc O, Benayoun Y, et al. Visual outcomes with flow-diverter stents covering the ophthalmic artery for treatment of internal carotid artery aneurysms. AJNR Am J Neuroradiol. 2015;36(2):330–336.

Intrasaccular devices

There has been much interest in devices which sit within the aneurysm and either provide flow disruption at the neck (WEB, Microvention, Contour, Stryker, and Artisse, Medtronic), or keep the coils within wide-necked aneurysms without the need for stents or flow diverters (Neqstent, Nautilus). These devices employ various designs to obtain a high fine-mesh density at the interface between the aneurysm neck and parent vessel. A full description of these devices is provided in Chapter 4, 'Intrasaccular devices', p. 134. Usage of the most widely used device, WEB, is described below. Subsequent nuances of other device usage are then presented.

Usage of the WEB

Indications

- Both ruptured and unruptured aneurysms.
- Bifurcation and side-wall aneurysms with wide necks.

Antiplatelets

- These are not routinely required, an advantage in ruptured aneurysms. However, loading with DAPT allows the use of adjunctive stents if necessary.
- Postprocedural antiplatelets are not mandated, but many continue aspirin for 6–12 weeks.

Access

- Accessing the aneurysm is the same as for coil embolisation. A 6 Fr guide catheter is generally required. A triaxial system can be used for extra support.

Device selection

- It is important to achieve significant compression of the device in the width dimension. For this reason, the WEB should be oversized in relation to the diameter of the aneurysm. *Correct sizing is crucial to achieve adequate aneurysm occlusion.*
- A sizing chart is provided with the device to aid selection of the correct device.
- In general, 1 mm (for small aneurysms) or 2 mm (for larger aneurysms) should be added to the average width of the aneurysm (obtained in orthogonal planes), and the height should be subtracted by a similar amount to account for the vertical growth of the device caused by horizontal compression.
- The SLS (Single Layer Sphere; Figure 8.20b) is spherical, designed to treat spherical or ovoid aneurysms that have necks that taper down (1.5:2 dome-to-neck ratios). The SL (Single Layer; Figure 8.20a) is cylindrical, designed to treat more barrel-shaped aneurysms with wider necks. The latter device is much more widely used.
- Irregularly shaped aneurysms with lobules can be treated if the device is fitted well to the neck. Lobules at the neck itself, however, can hinder this, resulting in an inadequate seal and incomplete occlusion.
- The smallest WEB is the 17 SL 3 mm (width) × 2 mm (height); therefore, the smallest treatable aneurysm is 2 mm wide and 3 mm height.

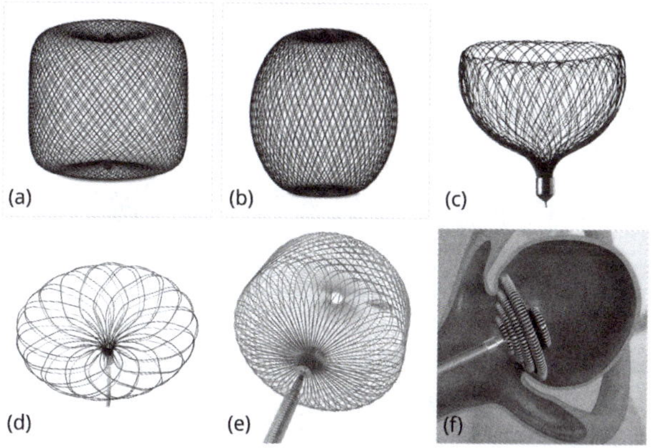

Figure 8.20 Intrasaccular devices for aneurysm treatment. (a) WEB SL. (b) WEB SLS. (c) Contour. (d) Neqstent. (e) Artisse. (f) Nautilus. Courtesy of Microvention, Stryker, Medtronic, and Endostream.

- The largest is the 11 SLS, which is 11×9.6 mm; therefore, the largest treatable aneurysm is 9–10 mm in width and 9.5–10.5 mm in height.
- The VIA microcatheter must be used, and the specific size depends on the size of the WEB device.

Deployment

(See Figure 8.21.)

- The aneurysm is catheterised with the microcatheter. Note: the VIA is stiffer than standard coiling catheters and care must be taken not to rupture the aneurysm. The distal 1 mm is not radiopaque.
- For sharply angulated aneurysms, 45° and 90° pre-shaped VIA catheters are available, or you may steam-shape them yourself.
- The WEB device is tested by inserting the wire end into the detachment device (without pressing the button). A green light will flash and there will be an audible notification. Some practitioners unsheathe the device under water to remove adherent bubbles, but this is not mandatory or recommended. Similar to stents, the WEB sheath must be flushed within the microcatheter hub.
- The device is pushed through the microcatheter under fluoroscopic visualisation of the microcatheter, as the microcatheter tip may move forwards or backwards in the aneurysm due to the stiffness of the device. There are distal and proximal markers for ease of visualisation.
- Unsheathe the device within the aneurysm slowly. Initially, the constrained WEB tip is sharp and so it must not be pushed against the aneurysm wall. When a sufficient amount of device emerges, it will 'blossom' and is much softer. It can then be more assertively repositioned in the aneurysm. The WEB will tend to self-centre as it expands within the aneurysm.

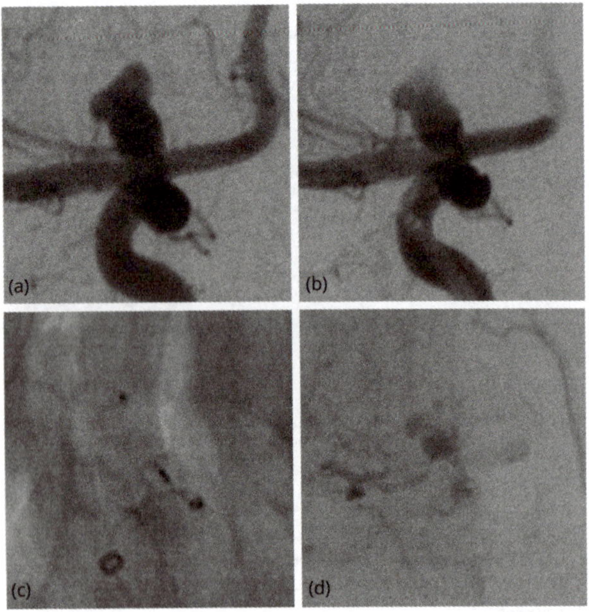

Figure 8.21 Treatment with the WEB device. (a) Wide-necked internal carotid artery termination aneurysm. (b) Subtracted and (c) unsubtracted angiography demonstrate the WEB SL device unsheathed and positioned in the aneurysm using a VIA 17 microcatheter. (d) After WEB detachment, stasis is observed within the aneurysm extending into the venous phase, indicating likely aneurysm occlusion.

- The inferior margin of the device should be positioned at the neck of the aneurysm. Once fully deployed, if correctly sized, it should be difficult to change the position or configuration of the device.
- The proximal marker often ends up in the parent artery and is not a significant thrombotic risk (as opposed to the mesh components of the WEB which are thrombogenic).
- Perform post-deployment angiography using standard biplane and flat panel cone beam CT with 20% diluted contrast if more detailed visualisation is required. Stasis should be seen in the aneurysm and there should not be impingement of the parent vessels. Contrast stasis predicts adequate occlusion at follow-up.
- If there is doubt regarding impingement on the parent artery, a period of a few minutes of observation before detachment might be prudent.
- Before detaching, ensure that the microcatheter and intermediate catheter do not have excessive load either forwards or backwards, to ensure that device displacement does not occur after detachment. The VIA microcatheter should be retracted 1–2 mm proximal to the detachment zone.

- Detachment is achieved using the handheld electrothermal detachment system. Screen the device while detaching. Successful detachment is indicated by minor movement of the proximal marker band relative to the microcatheter tip. Occasionally detachment does not work first time and multiple attempts must be made.

Complications

- Catheterisation and deployment: these become more difficult as the angle between the long axis of the aneurysm and the parent artery increases. Pre-shaped or steam-shaped VIA microcatheters are helpful.
- Non-symmetrical branches at the base of the aneurysm: this can risk vessel impingement or leaving 'dog-ear' remnants. Using a balloon catheter during deployment to reorient the device before the WEB is fully expanded might occasionally be necessary.
- Parent artery impingement: if this occurs prior to detachment the device can be recaptured and manipulated or exchanged for another size. If it occurs due to movement after deployment, a stent may be needed. If the stent is not able to remedy the impingement, the WEB can be often be retrieved using an Amplatz gooseneck microsnare (Microvena Corp, White Bear Lake, Minnesota, USA).
- Rupture during WEB deployment: this is very rare and occurs when the sharp tip of the constrained WEB exits the catheter and forward movement is applied against the aneurysm, puncturing the aneurysm dome. The usual protocol for rupture should be followed: reversing heparinisation and reducing the BP. The WEB should be deployed, as it creates a haemostatic seal. Temporarily inflating a balloon in the parent vessel can also promote haemostasis.
- The retreatment rate is around 10%. Adequate occlusion is dependent upon neck size, aneurysm height and width, intra-aneurysmal thrombus, irregular shape, and device compaction/compression >50%.
- Thromboembolic complications are reported in around 15%. Most are not clinically significant. Around 3% of patients experience permanent deficit.
- Rebleeding in ruptured aneurysms is reported in up to 2.5%.
- Device related morbidity is 0–4% and mortality 0–3%.

Follow-up

- DSA is the gold standard for follow-up, but IV DSA or MRA may be an acceptable alternative.
- The WEB Occlusion Scale has been developed for assessing follow-up imaging. Note that filling of the proximal marker recess is an expected finding in a completely occluded aneurysm, distinct from filling of the aneurysm neck.
- Compaction may occur, which is a decrease in the height of the device. It is not uncommon even with correctly sized devices and does not necessarily herald aneurysm recurrence. However, if the device is undersized, recurrence can occur.
- Device migration may rarely occur, when the WEB moves into the aneurysm with the aneurysm size remaining stable, and this is due to undersizing of the device in large or partially thrombosed aneurysms. WEB should not be used in known partially thrombosed aneurysms because of this.

- Recurrent aneurysms may be treated using conventional techniques such as coiling, stent coiling, flow diversion, or clipping.
- Satisfactory aneurysm occlusion is achieved in 85–90% of medium-sized wide-necked aneurysms.

Usage of the Artisse

(See Figure 8.20e.)

- The Artisse (Medtronic) is a comparable intrasaccular device consisting of a dual-layer, 72-wire mesh basket.
- Deployment is via a 0.021" microcatheter and the Rebar (Medtronic) is recommended. It includes an atraumatic, off-centre distal tip to prevent aneurysm dome damage during deployment. The tip of the device is much softer than the WEB when constrained, and so the initial unsheathing of the device can be done by pushing if necessary which makes unsheathing easier in shallow and angulated aneurysms.
- Choosing the device is aided by a supplied sizing chart. Just like the WEB, the device is oversized in comparison to the aneurysm.
- Similar to the WEB, the Artisse does not require long-term DAPT. Aspirin may be administered depending on the operator's preference.

Usage of the Contour

(See Figure 8.20c.)

- The Contour (Stryker) is an intrasaccular device manufactured from braided nitinol with platinum markers. Deployment is electrolytic. It adopts a cup-like configuration, conforming to the shape of the lower half of the aneurysm.
- The Contour device is therefore designed to sit at the aneurysm neck, and it is not necessary to reach the dome. For this reason, choosing the correct size (widest aneurysm diameter = equatorial plane) is relatively simple and a smaller inventory of devices is necessary (5 mm, 7 mm, 9 mm, 11 mm, and 14 mm).
- The device is deployed via 0.021" or 0.027" microcatheters depending on the size of the device.
- Like the Artisse, during the initial stages of unsheathing within the aneurysm the tip of the device is not sharp. During deployment the marker, at the base of the device, is positioned in the parent vessel and the Contour is kept as low as possible by giving it a gentle tug. This manoeuvre, in addition to oversizing the device in relation to the aneurysm, and achieving a good neck seal, are key to aneurysm occlusion.
- Detachment is electrolytic.
- Using the device alone, adequate occlusion is reported in 85–100% at 1 year. There are insufficient data in the setting of ruptured aneurysms to confirm suitability at present.
- In the authors' opinion, it is recommended to jail a microcatheter and deploy coils in larger aneurysms (such as those >8–9 mm) to maximise the occlusion effect. However, coils are not specifically indicated in the instructions for use for Contour.
- Loading with DAPT prior to the procedure is practised by many in case 'bail-out' stenting is required. Post-procedure, if no vessel encroachment

is observed, the patient is usually kept on DAPT for 4–6 weeks followed by aspirin for 12 weeks.

Usage of the Neqstent

(See Figure 8.20d.)

- The Neqstent (Stryker) is also designed to sit at the neck of wide-necked aneurysms; however, it provides minimal flow diversion compared to the Contour and so coiling of the aneurysm is required.
- Similar to the Contour it is also manufactured from braided nitinol with platinum radiopaque markers and is delivered via 0.021" and 0.027" microcatheters.
- Device sizes are 7 mm, 9 mm, 11 mm, and 14 mm to bridge aneurysm neck sizes of 3–10 mm.
- Once the device is deployed, a 0.017" microcatheter can be introduced via the struts of the device and used to fully coil embolise the aneurysm (this is not possible with the Contour, the microcatheter must be jailed).
- The device can be used in the acute setting. IV aspirin may be administered just prior to deployment but is not mandatory. Some operators leave the patient on aspirin for 6 weeks post-procedure.
- Thromboembolic events have been reported in two of a series of 20 patients, with permanent deficit in one (Islim et al., 2024).
- Immediate occlusion was reported in 90% with 94% adequate occlusion at 6 months.

Usage of the Nautilus

(See Figure 8.20f.)

- Nautilus (EndoStream Medical, Israel) is also a fully retrievable, nitinol-braided, detachable neck-bridging device with sizes ranging between 4 and 7 mm.
- The device has a spiral configuration when deployed with a 1 mm central hole to allow passage of a microcatheter.
- The device is deployed through a 0.0165–0.017" microcatheter in the midline of the aneurysm and then carefully retracted and adjusted to cover the neck. A second microcatheter is then navigated through the central hole for coil delivery (but can also be navigated through the struts).
- The Nautilus device is detached at the end of the procedure by breaking the pusher wire and pulling an inner strand (mechanical detachment).
- There is limited evidence for its usage, at present. A series of 41 patients is reported, all without antiplatelet medication. There was one minor asymptomatic ischaemic event, detected on brain imaging. Complete immediate aneurysm occlusion was achieved in 73%, neck remnant in 22%, and an aneurysmal remnant in 5%. At 3–6 month follow-up, complete occlusion was reported in 95% (Sirakov et al., 2023).

Further reading

Fiorella D, Arthur A, Byrne J, et al. Inter-observer variability in the assessment of aneurysm occlusion with the WEB aneurysm embolisation system. J Neurointerv Surg. 2015;7(8):591–595.

Goyal N, Hoit D, DiNitto J, et al. How to WEB: a practical review of methodology for the use of the Woven EndoBridge. J Neurointerv Surg. 2020;12(5):512–520.

Griessenauer CJ, Ghozy S, Biondi A, et al. Contour Neurovascular System for endovascular embolisation of cerebral aneurysms: a multicenter cohort study of 10 European neurovascular centers. J Neurointerv Surg. 2025;17(4):399–404.

Islim FI, Saleem N, Patankar T. Large single-center experience with short-term follow-up of Neqstent-assisted coiling. AJNR Am J Neuroradiol. 2024;45(5):605–611.

Sirakov A, Bhogal P, Sirakova K, et al. Endovascular treatment of wide-necked intracranial aneurysms using the Nautilus Intrasaccular System: initial case series of 41 patients at a single center. J Neurointerv Surg. 2023;15(10):989–994.

Complications of subarachnoid haemorrhage

aSAH can affect all organ systems. Even patients initially quite well can succumb to one or several complications. However, over the last 30 years, there has been an improvement in non-dependent survival. Overall, around 50–60% of patients presenting with aSAH will achieve a Modified Glasgow Outcome Score of 1–2. Outcome depends upon clinical status, age, and extent of aSAH.

Neurological

Cerebral ischaemia

- Ischaemia can result from aSAH, vasospasm, aneurysm treatment (coiling or clipping), and insertion of ventricular drainage catheters.
- Delayed cerebral ischaemia (DCI) is one of the commonest yet most difficult sequelae of aSAH to manage. It is an important topic with a dedicated section (see 'Vasospasm and delayed cerebral ischaemia', p. 310).

Hydrocephalus

- Symptomatic hydrocephalus occurs in up to 20% of all patients. It resolves within 24 h in one-third but can worsen.
- Risk factors include more extensive blood (high Fisher grade), poor neurological condition at admission, and aneurysm rupture during treatment.
- It usually presents as a decreased level of consciousness, without focal neurological deficit.
- There are two types:
  - Communicating: with generalised ventricular dilatation due to diffuse subarachnoid blood obstructing CSF absorption pathways.
  - Obstructive: where an intraventricular clot obstructs intraventricular CSF flow. For example, the lateral ventricles are expanded due to a third ventricular clot.
- For communicating hydrocephalus, treatment options include therapeutic LP or drainage. This is contraindicated in obstructive hydrocephalus.
- An EVD is necessary to manage obstructive hydrocephalus. Suboptimal drainage in the presence of a large ventricular clot may occur and occasionally more than one drainage catheter is necessary. After several days, the tube may be clamped to test the resolution of hydrocephalus; if well tolerated, the tube can be removed (reducing the 8% risk of infection).
- Some patients (around 7%) require ongoing CSF diversion involving a permanent ventriculoperitoneal or atrial shunt.

Rebleeding

- Re-haemorrhage from the culprit aneurysm before treatment is a feared complication with a mortality rate of >50%.
- Rebleeding occurs in at least 4–10% in the first 24 h, 8–23% in 72 h.
- For a ruptured dissecting aneurysm, it is as high as 50% in 24 h.
- Risk factors for higher rates of rebleeding are: systemic hypertension >160 mmHg, poor condition at admission, posterior circulation

aneurysms (higher morbidity and mortality from rebleeding), and larger aneurysms.

- In the ensuing 10–14 days, rebleeding occurs in 15–25%. Thereafter, rebleeding risk diminishes by 0.5% per day up to day 30.
- Securing the aneurysm early (within 24 h of diagnosis) prevents rebleeding in approximately 90% of cases and enables more effective management of other potential complications such as DCI.
- Tranexamic acid reduces the risk of rebleeding but does not improve clinical outcomes (ULTRA trial; Post et al., 2020).

Seizures/epilepsy

- Seizures at onset of haemorrhage are not uncommon and often are isolated events.
- There is an increased risk with subdural or intra-parenchymal haematomas, following aneurysm clipping, ventricular drainage, and cerebral infarction.
- Between 7% and 12% of aSAH survivors will develop epilepsy and there is an association between epilepsy and poor functional outcome following aSAH. The rate after clipping is significantly higher than after coiling.

Cranial nerve palsy

- Cranial nerve palsies occur in up to 10%.
- Oculomotor nerve palsy is the most common:
    - It may result in ptosis from levator palpebrae superioris paralysis, 'down and out' ocular deviation from unopposed lateral rectus and superior oblique muscles, pupillary dilation, and diplopia.
    - There are several causes: increased ICP (often causing bilateral signs), compression from PCOM aneurysms (causing unilateral signs), and damage after surgical clipping of PCOM or basilar termination aneurysms.
- Abducens nerve palsy may occur due to raised ICP. It can occasionally result from compression by a basilar, AICA, or PICA aneurysm.
- Aneurysms of the ophthalmic artery can compress the optic nerve and/or chiasm, leading to progressive visual loss or visual field defects.

Hormonal/electrolyte

Hyponatraemia

- Hyponatraemia (<130 mmol/L) is the most common electrolyte imbalance after SAH, occurring in up to 50% of patients.
- The most common cause probably is the syndrome of inappropriate antidiuretic hormone secretion (SIADH), but other causes include the use of diuretics, hypervolaemic therapy for DCI, and cerebral salt wasting.

SIADH

- This may be due to acute ACTH deficiency.
- Diagnosis is supported by normovolaemic hyponatraemia with high urine sodium concentration and low urine volume.

Cerebral salt wasting

- There is excessive secretion of natriuretic peptides provoking hyponatraemia and increased urine output and volume contraction making it difficult to maintain sufficient BP for the management of DCI.

- Poor grade aSAH and ruptured anterior communicating aneurysms predispose.
- Diagnosis is established by hypovolaemic hyponatraemia and high urine volumes.
- Infusion of hypertonic saline (to replace lost salt) and hydrocortisone or fludrocortisone are the treatments of choice and have been shown to reduce the incidence of DCI.
- It is usually self-limiting, resolving in 2–4 weeks, but occasionally progresses into a chronic condition.

Diabetes insipidus

- The onset is usually 1–3 days post aSAH. It occurs in up to 15% of aSAH.
- It is associated with the clipping of ACOM aneurysms and hypothalamic ischaemia.
- The condition is characterised by polyuria and polydipsia, although assessment may be challenging if the patient is obtunded or intubated.
- Diagnosis involves the presence of hypernatraemia (>145 mmol/L) and urinary hyponatraemia, alongside polyuria and low osmolality.
- While the condition is usually transient, it can occasionally last for months after onset.

Hyperglycaemia

- This is very common after aSAH.
- It is independently associated with increased rates of DCI and poorer outcomes.
- However, aggressive management strategies to maintain strict normoglycaemia have not been shown to improve clinical outcomes.

Pulmonary

Neurogenic pulmonary oedema and acute respiratory distress syndrome

- This is stimulated by several neurological insults, particularly those associated with a rapid increase in ICP. There is a risk associated with excessively high tidal volume ventilation.
- The cause of the oedema is not fully understood, but is believed to result from a catecholamine surge and can occur almost immediately after an insult or be delayed by up to 24 h.
- It is characterised by a clinically rapid onset of respiratory distress (dyspnoea, tachypnoea) with hypoxia. Pink frothy sputum and decreased air entry with crackles are observed, indicating the presence of oedema.
- Management is directed towards the underlying condition and reducing ICP. Diuretics reduce oedema if tolerated, but are contraindicated with DCI. Maintenance of positive end-expiratory pressure and prone ventilation can be beneficial.

Venous thromboembolism

- Patients with aSAH are hypercoagulable and at high risk from venous thromboembolism. Pulmonary embolism predicts poor inpatient and late clinical outcomes.
- Early securing of the aneurysm allows initiation of prophylactic therapy in accordance with the local hospital policy. Protocols vary, but many units commence venous thromboembolism prophylaxis as soon as or within 24 h of securing the aneurysm endovascularly.

- In case of a delay, mechanical compression devices, namely graduated compression stockings or intermittent pneumatic compression devices, may be used.

Aspiration and ventilator-associated pneumonia

- These are the most common nosocomial infections in aSAH patients.
- Acidic stomach contents are highly toxic, posing a risk of long-term damage.
- They are associated with prolonged time on a ventilator, which in itself is related to poor acute clinical condition.
- These infections can coexist with other pulmonary complications.

Cardiac

Takotsubo cardiomyopathy

- Takotsubo cardiomyopathy, also known as 'stress' cardiomyopathy, is a non-ischaemic cardiomyopathy resulting from a significant catecholamine surge producing global hypokinesia and lusitropy (reduced myocardial relaxation), poor cardiac output, and the development or exacerbation of pulmonary oedema. This is referred to as 'neurocardiac neurogenic pulmonary oedema'.
- The condition is typically transient but can significantly hinder the management of cerebral vasospasm, as inotropes to elevate BP can exacerbate cardiac dysfunction.

Arrhythmia

- These may also result from a catecholamine surge.
- Often temporary, the most common manifestation is atrial flutter and fibrillation, increasing the risk of thromboembolism. Sinus tachycardia and bradycardia often reflect ICP.
- ECG changes in aSAH are common, ranging from 25% to 90%. ST segment depression, T-wave inversion, and QT prolongation are also observed and are associated with poorer outcomes.
- ECG changes may also be secondary to electrolyte imbalance, and a significant proportion of patients may have pre-existing cardiac conditions.

Renal

- Acute kidney injury is common and can occur at various stages of admission for SAH. The incidence is as high as 30–40%.
- Minimising IV and intra-arterial contrast usage as much as is reasonable during interventions and diagnostic radiological investigations is necessary. Patients with hypertension are already vulnerable to acute kidney injury, and multiple overlapping factors contribute.

Cognitive

- Cognitive dysfunction is related to global cerebral damage and additional specific parenchymal loss.
- Short-term memory loss is the most common sequelae of SAH, affecting at least 50% of patients.
- Other consequences include dysfunction of spatial awareness and processing, concentration, personality, language, and executive functioning.

- Specific neuropsychological issues related to aneurysm location are contentious. Nevertheless, some studies have demonstrated higher levels of personality change and risk-taking behaviour after rupture of ACOM aneurysms related to damage to the orbitofrontal cortex.
- Specific neurological deficits such as hemianopia, hemiparesis, and synaesthesia all impact psychological recovery.

Psychological

- The incidence of depression following aSAH is around 30%.
- In a small proportion of patients this condition can be severe and difficult to treat and may rarely present a suicide risk.
- Anxiety disorders persist in >30%.
- Up to two-thirds of patients report fear of recurrent haemorrhage. The presence of partially secured aneurysms, fear of recurrence of endovascularly treated aneurysms, and presence of additional untreated lesions are understandable risk factors.

Further reading

Campos-Fernandez D, Rodrigo-Gisbert M, Abraira L, et al. Predictive model for estimating the risk of epilepsy after aneurysmal subarachnoid hemorrhage: the RISE score. Neurology. 2024;102(8):e209221.

Kassell NF, Torner JC. Aneurysmal rebleeding: a preliminary report from the Cooperative Aneurysm Study. Neurosurgery. 1983;13(5):479–481.

Kienzler J, Marbacher S, Remonda L, et al. Outcome after in-hospital rebleeding of rupture of intracranial aneurysms. J Neurol Surg A Cent Eur Neurosurg. 2016;77(3):207–221.

Ohkuma H, Tsurutani H, Suzuki S. Incidence and significance of early aneurysmal rebleeding before neurosurgical or neurological management. Stroke. 2001;32(5):1176–1180.

O'Kelly CJ, Kulkarni AV, Austin PC, Urbach D, Wallace MC. Shunt-dependent hydrocephalus after aneurysmal subarachnoid hemorrhage: incidence, predictors, and revision rates. Clinical article. J Neurosurg. 2009;111(5):1029–1035.

Post R, Germans MR, Tjerkstra MA, et al. Ultra-early tranexamic acid after subarachnoid haemorrhage (ULTRA): a randomised controlled trial. Lancet. 2021;397(10269):112–118.

Yamada M, Kitahara T, Kurata A, Fujii K, Miyasaka Y. Intracranial vertebral artery dissection with subarachnoid hemorrhage: clinical characteristics and outcomes in conservatively treated patients. J Neurosurg. 2004;101(1):25–30.

Vasospasm and delayed cerebral ischaemia

Definitions

Vasospasm/angiospasm

- Cerebral vasospasm refers to the narrowing of cerebral arteries and is more appropriately termed 'angiospasm'. It may be mild and transient or severe.
- It contributes, probably in a small way, to DCI. Angiospasm/vasospasm and DCI are *not* the same entity.
- Angiospasm usually occurs on days 4–12 then typically slowly resolves.
- Angiospasm occurs in up to 70% of all patients.
- The Fisher scale is an objective and prognostically significant measure of SAH blood load (see 'Subarachnoid haemorrhage grading', p. 240). The incidence and severity of both angiospasm and DCI are related to the amount of subarachnoid blood.

Delayed cerebral ischaemia

- DCI is the major cause of significant delayed morbidity and mortality.
- The condition is diagnosed based on symptoms and signs (clinical and imaging) of early brain injury appearing days after the initial bleed. DCI is defined as new focal neurological deficit or a 2 or more point drop in GCS score.
- Diagnosis and treatment may be compromised by delays to diagnosis in intubated patients and coexistence with other physiological and metabolic complications after SAH.
- It remains a formidable challenge, especially as management of DCI is currently directed mainly to alleviation of angiospasm which can compromise other physiological states, e.g. cardiac impairment. However, the impact may sometimes be improved by timely interventions. Therefore, developing and maintaining technical skills to manage angiospasm are considered an important part of the neurointerventional armamentarium. This may be rather simplistic for the reasons below.

Incidence and pathophysiology of delayed cerebral ischaemia

- DCI is an important complex multifactorial condition and warrants a brief description.
- Early brain injury and DCI are a continuum of the same pathophysiological process involving endothelial cell damage and blood–brain barrier (BBB) breakdown.
- Following aneurysmal rupture, for a short time, ICP equals systolic BP with intracranial circulatory flow arrest, followed by restoration of flow, albeit reduced. This results in an ischaemic insult to all cells of the BBB and neurovascular unit. Mitochondrial function is disturbed and reduction in ATP production affects the function of membrane ion pumps including the Na^+/K^+-ATPase with neuronal and astrocytic swelling resulting in cytotoxic oedema.
- The endothelial cells of the BBB become corrugated, the glycocalyx is disrupted, and the cells fail to secrete their endogenous anticoagulants and vasodilators, including nitric oxide, prostacyclin (PGI2), and tPA. Subendothelial vWF and collagen are exposed and tissue factor is

released. Pericytes constrict and thromboxane A2 released, resulting in microvasoconstriction and microthrombosis.

- The ischaemic insult stimulates the release of hypoxia-inducible factor and vascular endothelial growth factor. The latter further disrupts the endothelial cell with degradation of the BBB, risking vasogenic oedema.
- At the same time, subarachnoid blood penetrates the perivascular spaces. Red blood cells lyse and blood products are released into the perivascular spaces.
- Released oxyhaemoglobin decreases PGI2 (impairing vasodilatation) and increases endothelin-1 release (a potent vasoconstrictor) by the ischaemic endothelium. Oxyhaemoglobin degradation forms superoxide which combines with nitric oxide to form perioxynitrite which further damages mitochondria and the endothelium and impairs vasodilatation. Reactive oxygen species form and damage the endothelial cell tight junctions of the BBB. Reactive oxygen species inhibit endothelial nitric oxide synthase, cause lipid peroxidation, and activate caspases, leading to a succession of events ending in apoptosis.
- Blood products in the perivascular spaces pass into the brain via gaps in the astrocytic endfeet which are swollen and detached as a result of the initial ischaemic ictus. These blood products activate microglia and recruit monocytes into the brain. Activated microglia release tumour necrosis factor alpha, interleukins, and other inflammatory cytokines. This inflammatory response can activate various apoptotic pathways and further damage the BBB.
- Dysfunctional astrocytes of the BBB have reduced ability to clear and detoxify glutamate from the synaptic cleft with resultant excitotoxicity, NMDA and non-NMDA receptor stimulation, cytotoxic oedema, and apoptosis.
- Damage to the cells of the BBB impairs neurovascular coupling.
- The mechanisms described above create a perfect storm for cortical spreading depolarisation.
- Additional factors exist that may also contribute to or exacerbate poor cerebral circulation, including diffuse oedema, hydrocephalus, and haematoma. These increase ICP and reduce the cerebral perfusion pressure.

Diagnosis

(See Figure 8.22.)

Clinical presentation

- Initial clinical indicators are a change in focal or global neurological function not explained by initial haemorrhage or other causes.
- Onset of DCI can be heralded by additional systemic problems such as acute respiratory distress syndrome, metabolic disturbances, or a surge in BP (the 'self-driving' patient).
- As the clinical changes can occur at almost any time and be abrupt, continuous clinical and invasive physiological monitoring on specialist HDUs or ICUs is required.
- This level of care can be rationed to those with high risk of developing spasm based on clinical and Fisher grades (combined in VASOGRADE criteria).

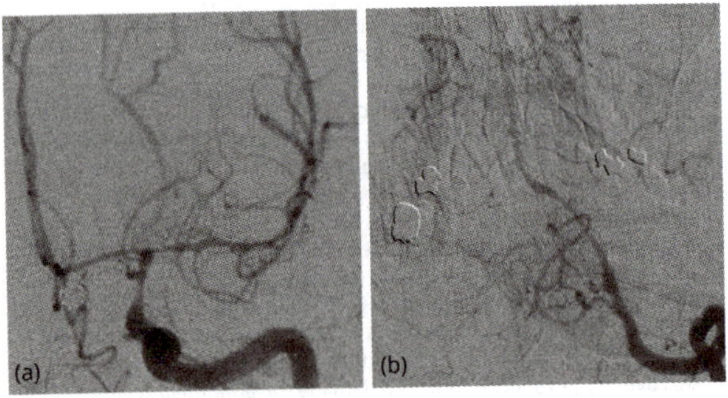

Figure 8.22 Angiographic vasospasm treatment. (a) Left internal carotid artery and (b) left vertebral digital subtraction angiography demonstrate diffuse intradural vasospasm.

Transcranial Doppler

- Utilised in many centres to detect angiospasm, this has the advantages of portability, repeatability, and lack of ionising radiation. It is particularly important when clinical assessment is not possible (e.g. on ITU), or complicated by neurological comorbidities or other metabolic complications of SAH.
- The pterion is insonated by a high-frequency probe to detect flow in intracranial vessels. Overall sensitivity approaches 80% for detecting spasm in large arteries.
- 2 MHz probes are required. Higher frequencies lack penetrative depth.
- It can be time-consuming to perform and approximately 10% of patients lack an adequate acoustic window. Additionally, it is suited to the anterior circulation vessels, particularly MCAs, although basilar artery insonation via the foramen magnum is possible.
- Multiple studies are required, including baseline at day 0/1 and at least once every 2 days to monitor the development/progress of angiospasm.
- Velocity in vessels is directly related to the presence of angiospasm. When spasm is present, the velocities are as follows: 110–120 cm/s in the ICA, 110 cm/s in the MCA, 120 cm/s in the ACA, and 80 cm/s in the basilar artery. In cases of severe spasm, the velocities increase to 130 cm/s in the ICA, >200 cm/s in the MCA, 180 cm/s in the ACA, and 115 cm/s in the basilar artery.
- The Lindegaard index is the ratio of peak velocity in affected vessel relative to cervical ICA and accounts for hyperaemic situation. A ratio >3 indicates spasm, >5 severe spasm.

CT angiography and perfusion

- CTA can be utilised in the absence of transcranial Doppler ultrasound availability. Caution is advised due to high radiation doses that will occur with repeated examinations, especially if performed in conjunction with CT perfusion (CTP).
- CTA has the advantage of availability of a comparison study performed at initial diagnosis. However, personal experience and some clinical

studies have shown it tends to overestimate the degree of vessel narrowing.

- Studies using CTP have reported variable correlation between areas of hypoperfusion and arterial territories affected, which is unsurprising given the more complex interaction between spasm and cellular injury/ DCI.
- Some objective criteria, however, have been established with mean transit times of ≥6 s correlating with development of DCI.

Catheter angiography

- While the gold standard investigation, angiography tends to be reserved for treatment rather than diagnosis.

Management

This is currently focused on enhancing cerebral blood flow (CBF). Many pharmacological studies addressing vascular biochemical abnormalities are ongoing. Currently, there is no reliable cure.

Removal of cerebral spinal fluid

- EVT has limited the scope for CSF washout as this would not be performed as a stand-alone therapy. Evidence for its efficacy is lacking, despite the pragmatic advantages.
- However, both drainage of obstructed CSF and blood (with or without intrathecal thrombolytics) via EVD, and cisternal CSF via lumbar drainage have shown some benefit in reducing the incidence of angiospasm and DCI.

Physiological

- Conventional management of DCI involves induced hypertension and normovolaemia to increase circulating volume and perfusion pressure. This is usually administered in ITU/HDU to monitor for complications, e.g. heart failure, and pulmonary oedema.
- Of all the components of 'triple H' therapy (induced hypertension, hypervolaemia, and haemodilution), only hypertension has been shown to be beneficial in the reducing risk of DCI.
- Due to the complexity of coexisting metabolic conditions, preventing hypovolaemia is the most likely achievable and safest therapeutic aim.
- Where this is difficult, or there are additional confounding conditions (e.g. cerebral oedema, pulmonary oedema, cardiac failure, or established cerebral infarction), additional direct endovascular measures may be required.
- Anaemia develops (haemoglobin <100 g/L) within 4 days in 50%. Transfusion may be necessary to enhance oxygen delivery to the brain.

Pharmacological

- The Co-operative Aneurysm Study first demonstrated the efficacy of nimodipine for prevention of cerebral vasospasm after aSAH. Since then, all patients admitted are administered nimodipine (60 mg, 4-hourly) and this will ordinarily continue for 3 weeks post haemorrhage. In patients with significant hypotension, it may be withheld. In those intubated, it is usually administered by nasogastric tube. IV nimodipine is not efficacious.

- The variable impact of nimodipine on large vessel calibre despite more consistent clinical benefit suggests a more diffuse benefit on peripheral small vessel spasm, and even on coagulation.

Chemical angioplasty

- Chemical angioplasty involves the intra-arterial infusion of calcium channel blockers directly into the cerebral circulation.
- It may be suitable for patients with clinically refractory angiospasm and/or in those who cannot tolerate physiological manipulation due to pre-existing cardiovascular disease, neurogenic pulmonary oedema, or Takotsubo cardiomyopathy.
- Contemporary CT head should reveal no established ischaemia in involved territory or territories.
- The treatment can be carried out under LA (by suitably experienced operators).
- Nimodipine given as a slow bolus of up to 2 mg per arterial territory titrated against invasively monitored systolic BP is the most common agent. Verapamil and milrinone can alternatively/adjunctively be used (see Chapter 3, 'Antispasmodics', p. 98).
- It can be used as the sole treatment if angiospasm is purely/predominantly peripheral.
- Ideally, angioplasty is performed soon after clinical deterioration to avoid irreversible ischaemia (preferably within 6 h and certainly 12 h). The therapy may need repeating several times.
- There is limited evidence for benefit at present. In practice, it is often requested too late and this may contribute to the mixed/disappointing results reported.

Balloon angioplasty

- This is reserved for proximal vessels and more severe spasm: ICA, basilar, and M1.
- Angioplasty of the A1 segments is more complex and comes with higher risk. A1 size shows significant variability and one must assess the size of the vessel on initial CTA to avoid potentially catastrophic overinflation. It is also more difficult to navigate into the A1 with a balloon.
- It can be combined with chemical angioplasty for combined proximal, intermediate, and microvascular therapy.
- There are two approaches: (i) using a small fixed-size coronary balloon to avoid overinflation or (ii) a soft, compliant intracranial balloon subtotally inflated to massage the vessels open.
- Newer microballoons allow for more peripheral angioplasty of M2/3, A2/3 vessels but beware of increased risks of fatal perforation and unproven efficacy.
- Heparinisation is desirable during the procedure.
- Spasm tends to involve long contiguous vessel segments and the balloon requires slow navigation to include the entirety of involved vessel.
- Biplane angiography is usually required to assess accurate balloon position in relation to spasm.
- The balloon is gently inflated using the right hand with the left hand needed to stabilise position. The balloon tends to behave like a 'melon

seed', slipping proximal or distal to the focal spasm, and so should be held in position during inflation.

- The inflation is staged: initially to 1–2 mm and then deflated. Progressively inflate to larger sizes before deflating: 2–3 mm, then possibly 3–4 mm, etc., depending on vessel size.
- Flow is related to the fourth power of the radius in accordance with Poiseuille's equation and so full dilatation of the vessel is *not* required.
- Distal to proximal, or vice versa, are both appropriate strategies, but it is preferable to stick to one as these tend to be uncommon procedures.
- After the first run of inflations, angiography is recommended to assess for the effect and exclude rupture or dissection (both are uncommon).
- It is often required to traverse the affected vessel several times to achieve the desired angioplasty result.
- Generally, angioplasty with compliant 4 mm balloons is sufficient for ICA and proximal MCA (but underinflated to 2–3 mm) and it is not commonly used in M2 vessels (increased perforation risk).
- The same technique may be applied to the contralateral ICA (often spasm is asymmetric in accordance with blood distribution) and the dominant vertebral and basilar artery if required.
- It is much less common for balloon angioplasty to need to be repeated compared to chemical angioplasty.

Stent-retriever angioplasty

- This is a newer technique that is gaining acceptance. The Tigertriever, in particular, allows controlled dilation.
- It is felt to be safer than balloon angioplasty.
- The stent retriever is deployed and left *in situ*, then either recaptured in the microcatheter or dragged proximally (as in MT).
- Some report inadequate radial force to open and dilate the vessel.
- The technique anecdotally works better without prior pharmacological vasodilatation. Presumably, the latter reduces the impact of stent retriever on the vessel wall. Some operators also utilise this approach for balloon angioplasty.
- There are reports of efficacy >70% in vessel dilatation and durability.
- This technique may be safer for distal vessels.

Further reading

Allen GS, Ahn HS, Preziosi TJ, et al. Cerebral arterial spasm—a controlled trial of nimodipine in patients with subarachnoid hemorrhage. N Engl J Med. 1983;308(11):619–624.

Peeyush Kumar T, McBride DW, Dash PK, Matsumura K, Rubi A, Blackburn SL. Endothelial cell dysfunction and injury in subarachnoid hemorrhage. Mol Neurobiol. 2019;56(3):1992–2006.

Chapter 9

Ischaemic stroke

Clinical presentation 318
Investigation 322
Intravenous thrombolysis 330
Patient selection for anterior circulation thrombectomy 334
Anaesthesia 339
Clot composition 343
Mechanical thrombectomy principles 344
Tandem carotid occlusion 355
Mechanical thrombectomy and intracranial atherosclerotic disease 365
Posterior circulation thrombectomy 368
Medium and distal vessel thrombectomy 378
Paediatric thrombectomy 381
Complications in mechanical thrombectomy 385
Postprocedural care 394
Organisation of care 397

Clinical presentation

History

- History can be obtained from multiple sources but must be rapid to confirm the clinical diagnosis of stroke and potentially exclude other entities.
- If utilising video assessment or telemedicine, this can begin in the prehospital setting. If not, history taking usually begins with the paramedic handover in hospital. Further history can be gathered by witnesses, friends/family, and the electronic patient record.
- Implementing pre-registration with the electronic patient record enables access to such records before the patient's arrival.
- A typical history is that of a persistent, sudden-onset, focal neurological deficit pertaining to a cerebrovascular arterial territory.
- Associated confusion or altered consciousness is rare for unilateral anterior circulation ischaemic stroke.
- Caveats include so-called chameleon presentations, which are suggestive of another condition but actually represent stroke. BAO can result in rapid progression to coma and, in basilar termination occlusion with bilateral thalamic ischaemia, fluctuating consciousness. This typically presents with focal neurological signs on detailed neurological examination, in contrast to presentations with more generalised alteration of consciousness seen in, e.g. drug intoxication and delirium.

Essential information to gather

- Symptom onset and course:
  - Exact time of symptom onset or when the patient was last known well.
  - Time the patient was found with symptoms.
  - Sudden versus gradual onset.
  - Fluctuation, progression, or improvement in symptoms.
- Nature of symptoms:
  - Weakness, numbness, speech difficulty, visual loss, dizziness, or imbalance.
  - Distribution and laterality.
  - Associated symptoms, e.g. headache, seizure, confusion, or altered consciousness.
- Eligibility for reperfusion:
  - Time since onset of symptoms.
  - Contraindications to treatments, e.g. recent surgery, bleeding disorders, or anticoagulant use.
- Risk factors and comorbidities:
  - Cardiovascular risk factors: atrial fibrillation, heart disease, hypercholesterolaemia, hypertension, or diabetes.
  - Lifestyle factors: smoking, alcohol, or recreational drug use.
  - Previous stroke or TIA.
  - Family history of stroke or cardiovascular disease.
- Medications and compliance:
  - Use of anticoagulants, antiplatelets, antihypertensives, or statins.
  - Recent changes to medication.
  - Adherence to prescribed treatments.

- Functional and social history:
  - Independence in daily activities before stroke (modified Rankin Scale (mRS)).
  - Mobility aids or support systems in place.

Modified Rankin Scale

- The mRS (Table 9.1) was developed as an outcome measure for functional status after stroke. It is commonly adapted for premorbid functional status to compare against guideline criteria backed by RCTs.
- Eligibility for MT usually involves functional independence, denoted by an mRS score of 0–2. People in this category are functionally independent in all activities of daily living, including shopping, managing one's own finances, cleaning, etc.
- If, on questioning, they cannot perform an activity, clarification must be sought on exactly why. A useful quick screening test is to ask the patient, or next of kin, could they be left alone for 1 month without any help from anyone at all?

Stroke mimics

- Seizures: seizure activity, particularly focal motor/sensory seizures with postictal phenomena, can mimic stroke presentations including hemiparesis or aphasia.
- Migraine with aura: transient visual disturbances, positive sensory changes, and motor deficits, or aphasia, can mimic focal neurological deficits seen in stroke.
- Hypoglycaemia: can result in neurological symptoms such as confusion and weakness, but also with focal deficits, mimicking stroke. Prompt bedside glucose testing will confirm.

Table 9.1 The Modified Rankin scale

0	No symptoms: no significant disability; the patient is able to carry out all usual activities without assistance
1	No significant disability: despite experiencing some symptoms, the patient is able to carry out all usual activities; symptoms do not interfere with lifestyle or work
2	Slight disability: not able to undertake all activities as previously but able to look after their own affairs without assistance
3	Moderate disability: the patient requires some help with activities of daily living but is able to walk unassisted
4	Moderately severe disability: the patient is unable to carry out most activities of daily living without assistance, including own bodily needs, and is unable to walk without assistance
5	Severe disability: the patient requires constant nursing care and attention; they are bedridden
6	Death

Reproduced from Van Swieten JC et al. (1988). Modified from the original Rankin Scale (J. Rankin, 1957). https://eprovide.mapi-trust.org/instruments/modified-rankin-scale

- Syncope: may present with transient loss of consciousness and bilateral motor weakness. Differentiating features include a prodromal symptom of lightheadedness and visual disturbance, typically with quick recovery.
- Functional disorders: can mimic stroke symptoms in the absence of organic pathology. Triggers can include psychological, physical, or a combination of these. The diagnosis relies on confirming an incompatibility between the symptoms/signs and a recognised neurological or medical condition and requires positive examination findings consistent with a functional disorder. Motor weakness is often variable and inconsistent with an upper motor neuron lesion. Well-known positive findings include a give-way/collapsing weakness, and Hoover's test. The latter assesses lower limb weakness by measuring involuntary movement in the 'normal' leg when the patient attempts to flex the contralateral leg (with hip flexion weakness) against resistance. When the normal leg's heel is felt pushing down, this suggests organic weakness, while a lack of movement indicates functional weakness, often associated with functional neurological disorder. Lip-pulling with tonic forced deviation of the lower lip towards the 'weak' side is a common finding in functional facial weakness.
- Meningitis/encephalitis: there may be physical signs of infection, and the neurological deficit is less likely to pertain to a vascular territory.
- Space-occupying lesions: can present with focal neurological deficits and seizures. The history is more often progressive rather than sudden onset.
- Drug use or intoxication.

Examination

- Initial assessment should start with assessment of airway, breathing, circulation, disability, and exposure (ABCDE).
- Early complications of stroke can lead to airway obstruction, either due to new neurological deficits or aspiration, respiratory compromise, or cardiovascular instability. Cardiac arrhythmias, including but not limited to atrial fibrillation with rapid ventricular response, are common.
- A focused and rapid neurological examination should be undertaken in addition to National Institutes of Health Stroke Scale (NIHSS) assessment. This quantifies the extent of neurological stroke deficit.
- The examination should include assessment of cranial nerves, the cerebellar system, and a motor sensory examination of the peripheral nervous system.
- In posterior circulation strokes, the NIHSS may underestimate functional disability. A scale to more accurately capture the deficits and prognosis associated with posterior circulation has been developed, the Posterior (POST)-NIHSS. This adds 3 points for gait/truncal ataxia, 4 points for dysphagia, and 5 points for abnormal cough.
- Current international guidelines for IVT and EVT eligibility are, however, aligned with the standard NIHSS. The benefit of thrombectomy for posterior circulation occlusions with lower NIHSS scores (<10) remains unproven.

Further reading

Alemseged F, Rocco A, Arba F, et al. Posterior National Institutes of Health Stroke Scale improves prognostic accuracy in posterior circulation stroke. Stroke. 2022;53(4):1247–1255.

Bruno A, Akinwuntan AE, Lin C, et al. Simplified modified Rankin scale questionnaire: reproducibility over the telephone and validation with quality of life. Stroke. 2011;42(8):2276–2279.

Intercollegiate Stroke Working Party. National Clinical Guideline for Stroke for the UK and Ireland [Internet]. 2023. http://www.strokeguideline.org

Nadarajan V, Perry RJ, Johnson J, et al. Transient ischaemic attacks: mimics and chameleons. Pract Neurol. 2014;14(1):23–31.

National Institute of Neurological Disorders and Stroke. NIH Stroke Scale [Internet]. https://www.ninds.nih.gov/health-information/stroke/assess-and-treat/nih-stroke-scale

Investigation

Protocols vary between centres, but the goal remains the same: to establish the correct diagnosis, and facilitate rapid management decisions regarding thrombolysis and EVT.

Computed tomography

- Often the standard for acute stroke due to speed, widespread availability, minimal contraindications, low cost, and ease of interpretation.
- A CT-based protocol should include a non-contrast CT head (NCCT; Figure 9.1a), CTA of brain and neck vessels, and, if available/indicated, CTP.
- Stroke windows: window level approximately 30–40 HU, width approximately 8–40 HU (i.e. narrow width and lower level than standard brain windows) optimise detection of early infarction.
- NCCT head excludes haemorrhage, assesses extent of infarction, and facilitates decision-making regarding IVT in eligible patients.
- Early infarction demonstrates loss of grey–white matter differentiation, low-attenuation change (Figure 9.1b,c), and local sulcal effacement. In carotid T and M1 segment occlusions, the earliest visible change is frequently within the basal ganglia and insula due to lack of collateralisation in lenticulostriate perforator territories.
- NCCT may help identify the site of arterial occlusion. Intra-arterial thrombus can be hyperdense on CT depending on composition, e.g. linear high density in a proximal artery such as the M1 (hyperdense artery sign; Figure 9.1a). Look more distally in the Sylvian fissure for a hyperdense 'dot' sign, indicative of an M2 occlusion. Other locations of hyperdense thrombus include the anterior interhemispheric fissure for an anterior cerebral occlusion, prepontine cistern for basilar thrombus, or ambient cistern for PCA occlusion. Review of 1 mm reconstructions is much more sensitive than 5 mm.
- Limitations: identification of very early infarcts, brainstem infarcts, and particularly with extensive small vessel disease and older infarcts.

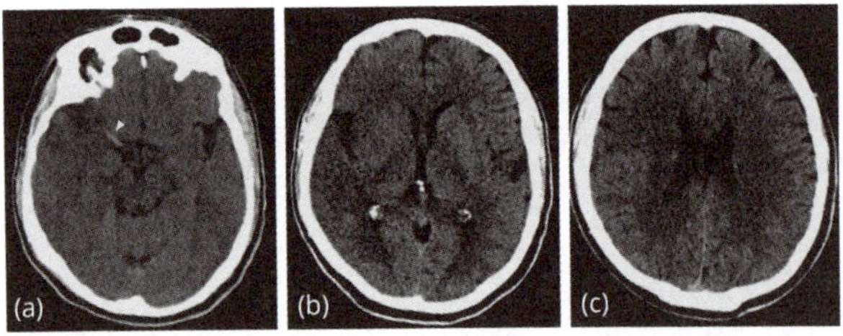

Figure 9.1 Computed tomography (CT) imaging findings. (a) Non-contrast CT head demonstrates hyperdense right M1 segment (arrowhead). (b) The same CT reveals hypodensity consistent with acute ischaemia involving the right insula and frontal/temporal operculum. (c) The hypodensity is also present more superiorly in the frontal lobe. Images courtesy of Dr Sarah Power.

Alberta Stroke Program Early CT Score (ASPECTS)

- This is a widely used scoring system developed to objectively analyse acute infarct extent in the MCA territory initially on NCCT.
- MCA territory is segmented into ten regions: caudate, lentiform, internal capsule, insula, and cortical zones M1–M6 (Figure 9.2). Zones M1–M3 lie at the basal ganglia level, extending from anterior to posterior. Zones M4–M6 are supra-ganglionic and also extend anteroposteriorly.
- 1 point is subtracted for an area of early ischaemic change, such as focal swelling, or parenchymal hypoattenuation, for each of the ten defined regions—where early ischaemic change is seen on at least two consecutive cuts.
- Many of the major RCTs providing evidence for the benefit of thrombectomy included ASPECTS as an imaging selection criterion. Higher ASPECTS scores are associated with better outcomes following stroke treatment.
- Limitations of ASPECTS include poor interobserver reliability and use limited to the MCA territory.
- The increasing use of artificial intelligence (AI) software platforms allows for automated ASPECTS analysis and can enhance inter-rater agreement and improve performance of non-expert readers.
- An ASPECTS scoring system has been developed for the posterior circulation, PC-ASPECTS. This is also a 10-point scoring system, with points lost for each region affected by early ischaemic change. In view of the high morbidity of brainstem infarction, the score is weighted, with pons and midbrain both assigned 2 points each. Other zones include bilateral thalami, occipital lobes, and cerebellar hemispheres (all of which have 1 point each). The lack of sensitivity for CT identification of early brainstem infarction is a limitation.

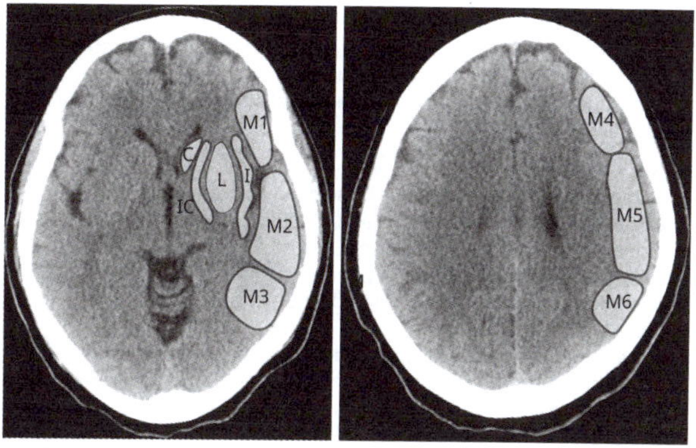

Figure 9.2 ASPECTS score. C, caudate nucleus; IC, internal capsule; L, lentiform nucleus; I, insula; M1–M6, cortical zones. The score is calculated by subtracting from 10 each involved region.

CTA

- This achieves rapid and highly accurate identification of proximal intracranial arterial occlusion.
- It should be performed from the aortic arch through to the vertex to evaluate extracranial carotid and vertebral arteries for occlusion, stenosis, dissection, or other pathology, which may impact patient outcome, treatment, and interventional technique.
- Thin slice imaging (≤1 mm), multiplanar reconstruction, and maximal intensity projection (MIP) images with a slice thickness of 6–10 mm aid in the detection of medium and distal arterial occlusions. Sagittal MIP is particularly useful for medium and distal M2 occlusion, ACA occlusion, and PCA P2–P3 occlusion (Figure 9.3). Coronal/sagittal MIPs help detect proximal M2, proximal ACA, and PCA occlusions.
- Many of the AI software platforms now include automated detection of anterior circulation LVO. However, AI LVO detection has been subject to a US Food and Drug Administration safety warning (April 2022) that they are a decision support tool and but should not be relied upon for definitive diagnosis of LVO.

Collateral scoring

- CTA allows evaluation of collateral arterial supply to an occluded territory, either antegradely via the circle of Willis or retrogradely through leptomeningeal collaterals.
- Good leptomeningeal collateral supply is associated with slower infarct growth ('slow progressors'), smaller final infarct volumes, and better functional outcome (Figure 9.3).
- Poor leptomeningeal collateral supply is associated with earlier signs of infarction (fast progressors), larger infarcts, and poorer outcomes.
- Many scoring/grading systems for collateral supply have been proposed without consensus on which to use. Most are confined to the MCA territory, and vary from binary (good vs bad) to 6-point scales. Evaluation usually compares extent of arterial contrast opacification in the occluded territory with the contralateral side, with the comparison expressed as a fraction or percentage. For example, <50% contrast opacification of arteries in occluded territory is considered poor, 50–75% moderate, >75% good, and 100% excellent. Use of thick axial MIP images facilitates rapid collateral evaluation.

Multiphase CTA and collateral grading

- Single-phase CTA lacks temporal resolution and can underestimate collateral supply, particularly if cardiac output is poor or there is a significant arrhythmia or proximal stenosis. Multiphase CTA can overcome these pitfalls. Typically, there are three phases: an arterial phase from arch to vertex, a delayed intracranial early venous phase, and a later venous phase.
- More comprehensive collateral grading systems have been developed for multiphase CTA that allow evaluation of delay across phases in addition to the extent of arterial contrast opacification in the occluded territory.
- Multiphase CTA evaluation of collaterals is a valuable tool in triage of patients for MT, and together with ASPECTS score on NCCT was utilised for patient selection in the ESCAPE/RESILIENT trials. It can enhance

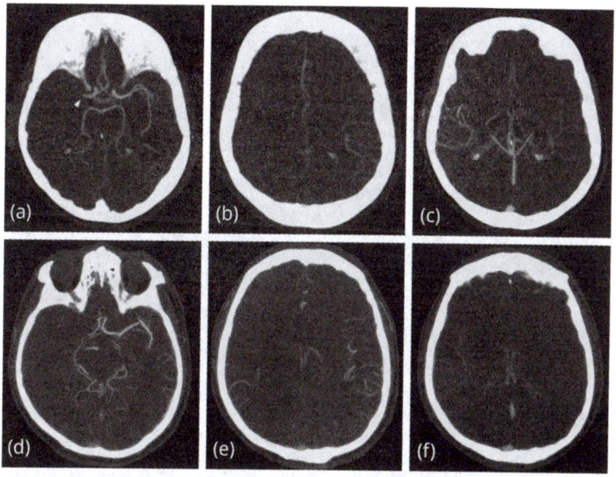

Figure 9.3 Collateral scoring on CTA. (a) A patient presented with sudden onset of left hemiplegia and dysphasia. CTA shows limited collateral flow into the right middle cerebral artery (MCA) territory. However, (b) the second and (c) third phase of the multiphase imaging demonstrate better collateral flow. (d) A second patient presented with severe left hemiparesis. Multiphase CTA revealed a tandem occlusion of the right internal carotid artery and the right carotid terminus. Arterial phase imaging shows poor collateral flow into the right MCA territory, which persists into the (e) second and (f) third phases. Images courtesy of Dr Sarah Power.

detection of medium and distal arterial occlusions by identifying delayed retrograde filling in the occluded territory over phases (Figure 9.3).

- Multiphase CTA helps to overcome pseudo-occlusion pitfalls caused by slow flow from severe proximal stenosis or distal occlusion, often seen in carotid-T occlusions. Single-phase studies may miss opacification of the proximal ICA, overestimating thrombus length and potentially deterring intervention. Accurate assessment of thrombus length is crucial for effective and safe MT.
- Many AI software platforms in stroke imaging now include analysis and scoring of collateral supply in MCA territory, with multiphase CTA analysis by some.

CTP

(See Figure 9.4.)

- Increasingly incorporated into imaging protocols, CTP evaluates the volume of infarcted tissue (core infarct) and volume of tissue at risk due to hypoperfusion but not irreversibly infarcted (penumbra). CTP facilitates the selection of extended-window patients for IVT, and late-window patients for MT. Another valuable usage is the identification of more distal occlusions, which can be challenging to detect.
- CTP is performed by sequentially imaging a defined section of brain tissue after administration of a high-flow IV bolus of iodinated contrast material. The raw imaging data require post-processing for

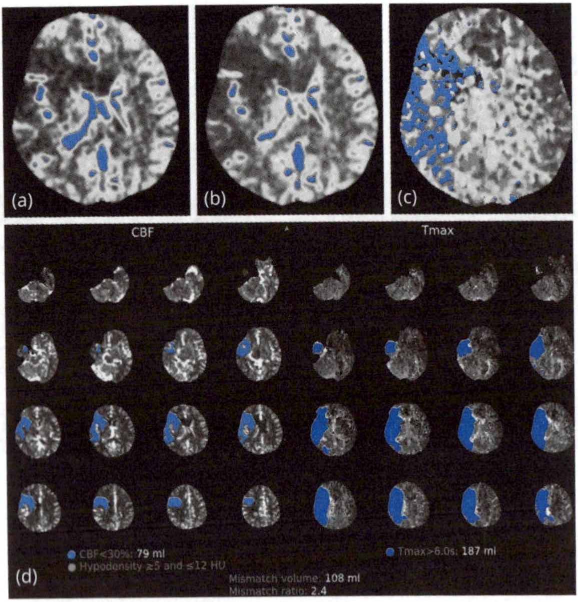

Figure 9.4 Computed tomography perfusion (CTP) imaging. Note that colours cannot be accurately reproduced in the figure due to limitations of this print. An elderly patient, last seen well 16 h earlier, was found with severe left hemiparesis. (a) Cerebral blood volume (b), cerebral blood flow (CBF), and (c) time to maximum contrast density maps are shown. (d) CTP imaging revealed a substantial 79 mL CBF <30% defect, affecting the right caudate nucleus, lentiform nucleus, insula, and M1, M2, and M4 cortical zones, with minimal involvement of the M5 zone. In comparison, the time to maximum (T_{max}) <6.0 s deficit measured 187 mL, resulting in a significant mismatch ratio of 2.4. It was noted that the at-risk territory (T_{max} >6.0 s) included the entire M5 and M6 cortical zones. The patient was selected for mechanical thrombectomy. Images courtesy of Dr Sarah Power.

interpretation and this is increasingly performed by fully automated software using deconvolution algorithms to create perfusion maps, including cerebral blood volume, cerebral blood flow (CBF), time to peak, mean transit time, and time to maximum (T_{max}).

- Many software platforms include automated post-processing of perfusion data. Reduced CBF <30% is the parameter most commonly used to reflect infarct core volume. T_{max} >6 s is most commonly used to reflect critically hypoperfused tissue at risk of infarction. Subtraction of core volume from volume of T_{max} >6 s gives penumbra volume. Most software platforms display a colour-coded summary map providing volume quantification of infarct core, T_{max} >6 s, mismatch, and calculated mismatch ratio. In addition, variable thresholds of T_{max} as well as CBF are frequently provided. Hypoperfusion intensity ratio can be calculated by dividing T_{max} >10 s volume by T_{max} >6 s volume and can be used to distinguish fast from slow progressors, with higher values (>0.5) in fast progressors. The hypoperfusion intensity ratio is a good surrogate of tissue collaterals. However, be aware that these perfusion parameters were largely developed using, and validated for, RAPID software, not other AI products.

- There are several potential pitfalls to CTP:
  - The CBF <30% threshold is not always an accurate reflection of ischaemic core in those presenting within 90 min from symptom onset/last seen well where infarct core can be overestimated. This is referred to as ghost core, and provision of additional CBF thresholds may help, with recommendation to use CBF <20% threshold in ultra-early presenters. Overestimation of core infarct can result in patients being erroneously deemed ineligible for MT.
  - There is variation in the calculated volume of key parameters between different software platforms. Although differences are not significant enough to impact decision-making, an exception arises with more distal occlusions. In these, the volumes of relative CBF <30% and T_{max} >6 s are inherently smaller, meaning minor differences in calculated volumes can have a greater impact on the mismatch ratio calculation.
  - Further pitfalls include delay in arrival of contrast bolus to intracranial vessels in patients with poor cardiac output resulting in resultant truncation of time–density attenuation curves. This can lead to inaccurate perfusion maps and calculations. Proximal carotid stenosis can overestimate the territory at risk, while chronic carotid occlusion/stenosis can cause a false-positive penumbra. Close correlation with CTA and additional T_{max} thresholds can aid interpretation in these situations. Additional pitfalls are motion artefact, poor contrast bolus with poor signal-to-noise ratio, and the inability of many CT scanners to perform whole brain coverage perfusion.
- The technical adequacy of a CTP study should be checked before interpretation and decision-making. Arterial input function and venous output function time–density curves should be inspected to ensure they are appropriately shaped, smooth, and have returned to baseline. The arterial input and venous output selections should be checked for accuracy.
- CTP in thrombectomy may become less relevant given recent late time window and large core infarct trial outcomes, with the ability to treat even large infarcts and/or out to 24 h based on NCCT ASPECTS or CTA collateral score.
- CTP remains valuable in detecting medium (MeVOs) and distal vessel occlusions (DiVOs), which can be difficult to identify and are easily missed on CTA. However, the benefit of MT in these groups remains unproven after neutral results in two recent trials (DISTAL and MeVO).

Magnetic resonance imaging

(See Figure 9.5.)

- DWI: diffusion restriction in acute infarcts is represented by high signal on B1000 images, with corresponding low signal on apparent diffusion coefficient maps. Diffusion restriction is visible within 20 min of stroke onset.

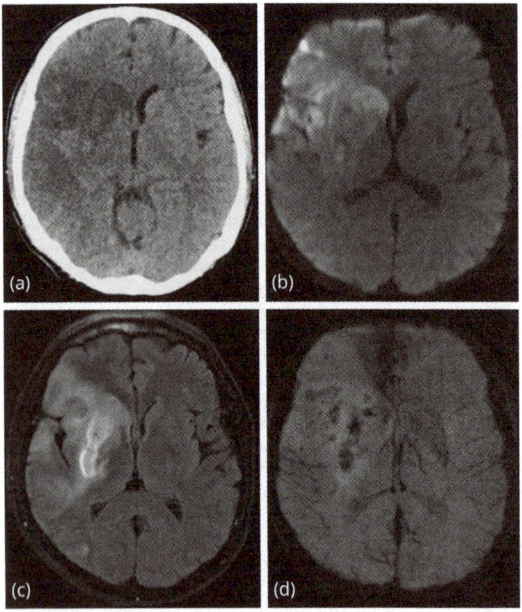

Figure 9.5 Magnetic resonance image of acute stroke. (a) Non-contrast CT brain for the same patient as in Figure 9.4, performed 24 h after a successful thrombectomy, reveals an unchanged infarct volume involving the right caudate nucleus, lentiform nucleus, insula, and M1, M2, M4, and anterior M5 cortical zones, with an ASPECTS score of 3. Notably, the posterior M5 and M6 zones, which were at risk, are spared. (b) Magnetic resonance diffusion-weighted imaging performed 8 days post-procedure confirms acute infarction in these areas. (c) Fluid-attenuated inversion recovery and (d) susceptibility-weighted imaging show petechial haemorrhagic transformation within the infarct. The patient remained hospitalised for 6 days and had a follow-up modified Rankin Scale score of 1 at 90 days. Images courtesy of Dr Sarah Power.

- FLAIR: hyperintensity is an indicator of irreversible acute infarction. It may take up to 6 h for FLAIR hyperintensity. Therefore, FLAIR:diffusion mismatch has been used as imaging selection criterion in RCTs, especially for IVT in wake-up strokes.
- MRA: for acute stroke it is advisable to include neck vessels. Techniques include time-of-flight or contrast-enhanced MRA.
- Gradient-recalled echo or susceptibility weighted imaging (SWI): iron (haem)-sensitive sequences. Evaluates for the presence of haemorrhage, acute or old. Depending on composition, thrombus in an artery may demonstrate blooming (red blood cell rich).
- T2 weighted: optional in hyperacute triaging stroke protocol. It does, however, allow preferential evaluation of the brainstem and cerebellum

over FLAIR. Used commonly in standard non-treatment triaging stroke protocol.
- MR perfusion: optional.

Re-imaging after transfer

- Patients may improve or deteriorate during interhospital transfer to a MT capable centre, potentially rendering them ineligible for treatment. There is currently no clear consensus or evidence-based guideline regarding re-imaging after transfer.
- Re-imaging, including at least a NCCT head, is reasonable if the last imaging was performed >2 h earlier. This time could be extended if the ASPECTS score at the referral site was high (≥7), with good collateral supply, and with no clinical deterioration/substantial improvement in NIHSS score during transfer. Biplane angiography suites allow on-table CT, although the detail is not as high as dedicated scanners.
- Additional imaging, or re-imaging, may be required.
- If a patient has significant clinical improvement on arrival, re-imaging, including CTA, is of value as the occlusion may have recanalised. Repeat CTA may demonstrate recanalisation of the initial occlusion, but the presence of a more distal occlusion, and with repeat neurological assessment and NIHSS scoring, facilitate decision-making as to whether thrombectomy is still appropriate.
- If a patient has clinically deteriorated, repeat imaging should be performed with NCCT to exclude haemorrhage within the infarct or complete infarction of the territory.
- In patients likely to be fast progressors, i.e. ASPECTS already lower on imaging, poor collateral supply on CTA, or high hypoperfusion intensity ratio on perfusion imaging, repeat NCCT prior to MT should also be considered. While there is evidence of benefit of MT even in large core infarcts, the greatest benefit is in patients with an ASPECTS score of 3 or above, with anterior circulation LVO, and excellent baseline function of mRS 0–1.
- In posterior circulation stroke, with basilar occlusion, and an obtunded patient, particularly if in coma at presentation, or requiring intubation, re-imaging should be considered on arrival and MRI is helpful to evaluate the extent of brainstem infarction.

Further reading

Ma H, Campbell BCV, Parsons MW, et al. Thrombolysis guided by perfusion imaging up to 9 hours after onset of stroke. N Engl J Med. 2019;380(19):1795–1803.

Maguida G, Shuaib A. Collateral circulation in ischaemic stroke: an updated review. J Stroke. 2023;25(2):179–198.

Menon BK, d'Esterre CD, Qazi EM, et al. Multiphase CT angiography: a new tool for the imaging triage of patients with acute ischaemic stroke. Radiology. 2015;275(2):510–520.

Sarraj A, Hassan AE, Abraham MG, et al. Trial of endovascular thrombectomy for large ischaemic strokes. N Engl J Med. 2023;388(14):1259–1271.

Vagal A, Wintermark M, Nael K, et al. Automated CT perfusion imaging for acute ischaemic stroke: pearls and pitfalls for real-world use. Neurology. 2019;93(20):888–898.

Yoo J, Choi JW, Lee SJ, et al. Ischaemic diffusion lesion reversal after endovascular treatment. Stroke. 2019;50(6):1504–1509.

Intravenous thrombolysis

Clinical pharmacology of thrombolytic agents

- Thrombus contains a mesh of cross-linked fibrin and platelets. Plasmin is a serine protease that dissolves fibrin. *In vivo*, endothelial cells produce tPA, an enzyme that cleaves plasminogen to the active form plasmin, leading to dissolution of thrombus.
- Alteplase is recombinant human tPA (rtPA). Alteplase is relatively inactive in the circulation, but is enzymatically active once bound to fibrin in thrombus.
- Alteplase is rapidly cleared, with a plasma half-life of 4–5 min. Despite the short half-life, the coagulopathy associated with alteplase treatment may last up to 24 h.
- Tenecteplase is a variant of native alteplase with amino acid substitutions that confer some biological advantage when compared to alteplase including a longer half-life allowing administration as a single bolus without subsequent infusion, enhanced fibrin specificity, and resistance to plasminogen activation inhibitor-1.

Evidence

- See Cochrane systematic review (Wardlaw et al., 2014) and an individual patient meta-analysis by the Stroke Thrombolysis Trialists' Collaboration (IST-3 Collaborative Group et al., 2012).
- Existing analyses emphasise the importance of rapid treatment (Emberson et al., 2014). Patients who are >80 y old with mild or severe stroke, and those with early signs of infarction on initial brain imaging, all benefit from treatment.

Considerations prior to administration

The summary of product characteristics for Actilyse outlines contraindications to treatment with rtPA in acute stroke, some of which can be considered absolute and some relative. The American Heart Association has published a comprehensive document outlining the scientific rationale for inclusion and exclusion criteria for rtPA in acute stroke that is a useful resource for the clinician. The non-exhaustive list below outlines some common considerations:

- **Acute blood in any compartment on cranial CT or symptoms consistent with SAH (even if acute blood is not immediately visible):** an absolute contraindication.
- **BPs >185/110 mmHg:** should be reduced to <185/110 mmHg prior to the administration of thrombolysis. If this cannot be achieved, the risk of rtPA-related ICH is considered to outweigh the benefit.
- **The administration of oral anticoagulants within the last 48 h:** this is usually considered a contraindication to thrombolysis, though expert consensus views in the European Stroke Organisation guidelines suggest that if urgent anti-factor Xa assay is available, administration of tPA can be considered if anti-factor Xa activity is <0.5 U/mL. For direct thrombin inhibitors, tPA can be considered if thrombin time is <60 s or if idarucizumab is readily available. Patients on oral vitamin K antagonists can receive thrombolysis once the INR is <1.7.

- **Prior treatment with antiplatelet agents:** does not appear to independently increase the risk of poorer functional outcome after IV tPA.
- **Prior ICH:** where the aetiology of previous ICH is non-recurring, e.g. a past history of a remote SAH with subsequent aneurysm coiling, this would likely not contraindicate treatment with rtPA.
- **Unruptured aneurysms:** a systematic review and meta-analysis of observational data by Goyal et al. (2015) showed that with rtPA treatment, the risk of sICH did not differ between patients with and without unruptured aneurysms.
- **Pregnant and paediatric patients:** these were excluded from the RCTs of tPA in acute ischaemic stroke. Data on this patient group are from case reports and registries. Expert consensus states that if pregnant patients otherwise meet criteria for thrombolysis of stroke, treatment with tPA should be considered on an individual basis. In practicality, urgent consultation should be made with obstetric colleagues to inform this individual risk:benefit analysis.

Complications

- Bleeding is the most feared complication, particularly ICH. The ECASS-II definition is a widely used radiological description that divides the appearance of haemorrhage into four categories: haemorrhagic infarction 1 (HI1), haemorrhagic infarction 2 (HI2), parenchymal haematoma 1 (PH1), and parenchymal haematoma 2 (PH2). PH2 describes blood in >30% of the infarct area with space-occupying effect and is the class of haemorrhage most consistently associated with poor outcome.
- The 2014 meta-analysis by Emberson et al. (2014) showed that the occurrence of PH2 in alteplase treatment for acute stroke was 5.2%.
- The management of ICH post thrombolysis is based on case reports and expert opinion. Reversal of tPA is considered reasonable up to 24 h post administration. This includes administration of cryoprecipitate or fibrinogen and tranexamic acid. In patients on warfarin, fresh frozen plasma, prothrombin complex concentrate, and vitamin K are also considered.
- Orolingual angio-oedema is a potentially life-threatening complication of IV tPA; however, the presentation is usually clinically mild. It is associated with use of angiotensin-converting enzyme inhibitors and insular infarction. Expert airway management may be required.

Late-window thrombolysis

- Recently, CTP and MRI perfusion/FLAIR/DWI imaging have explored extending the window in which thrombolysis can be administered.
- Thrombolysis for wake-up stroke/stroke of unknown time onset and thrombolysis for stroke with known onset 4.5–9 h ago can be considered two distinct clinical scenarios, even though in some trials both were evaluated together in one treatment group.

Thrombolysis for wake-up stroke/stroke of unknown time onset

- A patient-level meta-analysis published in 2020 included data from 843 individuals from four trials: WAKE-UP, EXTEND, THAWS, and

ECASS4-EXTEND. Patients were selected with a combination of CTP core–penumbra mismatch, MRI diffusion–perfusion mismatch, and MRI DWI–FLAIR mismatch. 60% of patients were from the WAKE-UP trial which used DWI–FLAIR mismatch, which is considered an imaging marker of stroke onset within 4.5 h. All four trials also stopped early, adding a risk of bias.

- European Stroke Organisation guidelines recommend that patients with wake-up stroke with either MRI DWI–FLAIR mismatch or CT/MRI core–penumbra mismatch within 9 h from the midpoint of sleep be treated with alteplase if MT is *not* planned.

Thrombolysis for stroke with witnessed onset 4.5–9 h

- Campbell at al. (2019) published a meta-analysis of three trials, EXTEND, ECASS4-EXTEND, and EPITHET, using CT or MRI core–penumbra mismatch to select patients for extended-window thrombolysis. This included patients with wake-up stroke (51%) as well as stroke with known onset at 4.5–9 h.
- rtPA is recommended for patients with known onset 4.5–9 h ago if perfusion imaging shows an appropriate core–perfusion mismatch and if thrombectomy is not indicated or planned.
- There is currently no evidence to guide the combination of extended-window alteplase in combination with MT.

Thrombolysis and mechanical thrombectomy

- Current European Stroke Organisation/European Society of Minimally Invasive Neurological Therapy recommendations (based on meta-analysis of six RCTs: DIRECT-MT, DEVT, SKIP, SWIFT-DIRECT, and DIRECT SAFE) are that patients with LVO who are eligible for rtPA and thrombectomy should receive both treatments prior to transfer to a thrombectomy capable centre.
- There is also RCT evidence that giving intra-arterial tenecteplase after successful MT (Thrombolysis in Cerebral Infarction (TICI) 2B or above) improves functional outcome at 90 days (ANGEL-TNK).

Post-thrombolysis care

- It is standard practice in most stroke units to intensively monitor patients for at least the first 24 h post thrombolysis. Neurological and BP assessment is recommended every 15 min for the first 2 h, every 30 min for the next 6 h, and hourly thereafter.
- Urgent cranial CT to assess for haemorrhage is recommended if there is a sudden increase in BP, any new headache, nausea, or vomiting, or a neurological deterioration. It is reasonable to proceed to repeat vessel imaging with neurological deterioration without haemorrhage.
- Routine cranial imaging is performed on all patients at 24 h post-thrombolysis before antiplatelet treatment is commenced, although there is some evidence that routine cranial CT does not alter treatment in clinically stable patients.

Further reading

Berge E, Whiteley W, Audebert H, et al. European Stroke Organisation (ESO) guidelines on intravenous thrombolysis for acute ischaemic stroke. Eur Stroke J. 2021;6(1), I–LXII.

Emberson J, Lees KR, Lyden P, et al. Effect of treatment delay, age, and stroke severity on the effects of intravenous thrombolysis with alteplase for acute ischaemic stroke: a meta-analysis of individual patient data from randomised trials. Lancet. 2014;384(9958):1929–1935.

Goyal N, Tsivgoulis G, Zand R, et al. Systemic thrombolysis in acute ischaemic stroke patients with unruptured intracranial aneurysms. Neurology. 2015;85(17):1452–1458.

IST-3 Collaborative Group; Sandercock P, Wardlaw JM, et al. The benefits and harms of intravenous thrombolysis with recombinant tissue plasminogen activator within 6 h of acute ischaemic stroke (the third International Stroke Trial [IST-3]): a randomised controlled trial. Lancet. 2012;379(9834):2352–2363.

Qiu Z, Li F, Sang H, et al. Intravenous tenecteplase before thrombectomy in stroke. N Engl J Med. 2025;393(2):139–150.

Turc G, Tsivgoulis G, Audebert HJ, et al. European Stroke Organisation–European Society for Minimally Invasive Neurological Therapy expedited recommendation on indication for intravenous thrombolysis before mechanical thrombectomy in patients with acute ischaemic stroke and anterior circulation large vessel occlusion. Eur Stroke J. 2022;7(1):I–XXVI.

Thomalla G, Boutitie F, Ma H, et al. Intravenous alteplase for stroke with unknown time of onset guided by advanced imaging: systematic review and meta-analysis of individual patient data. Lancet. 2020;396(10262):1574–1584.

Wardlaw JM, Murray V, Berge E, del Zoppo GJ. Thrombolysis for acute ischaemic stroke. Cochrane Database Syst Rev. 2014;2014(7):CD000213.

Patient selection for anterior circulation thrombectomy

<6 h: RCTs and HERMES

- Since 2015, nine RCTs have established MT in the treatment of anterior circulation stroke with LVO within 6 h of symptom onset.
- The HERMES meta-analysis (Goyal et al., 2016) demonstrated the superiority of MT, with or without bridging IVT, over IVT alone, with a number needed to treat of 2.6 to achieve a 1-point reduction in the mRS.
- These trials were relatively restrictive in their patient selection, incorporating only adults aged 18 years or older with acute ischaemic stroke involving the proximal anterior circulation, as demonstrated by CTA. Exclusions included posterior circulation strokes, strokes beyond 6 h, MeVOs or DiVOs, large infarct cores (e.g. ASPECTS <6), children, and patients with a baseline (pre stroke) mRS >2. Further trials have attempted to address these issues.

6–24 h

- This was addressed by two trials evaluating the late time windows: DAWN (n = 206) and DEFUSE-3 (n = 182) (Table 9.2) (Albers et al., 2017; Nogueira et al., 2018).
- DAWN recruited patients up to 24 h from stroke onset, with a clinical radiological mismatch, i.e. large clinical deficits, as defined by the NIHSS, which were used as a surrogate for ischaemic penumbra and compared with the smaller ischaemic cores seen on MRI. In contrast, the DEFUSE-3 trial used radiological perfusion markers for both ischaemic core and penumbra in patients within 6–16 h from last seen well.
- Both trials included a large subgroup of wake-up syndromes.
- Both trials concluded that with advanced imaging techniques, late-window acute stroke patients with a core–penumbra mismatch benefited from MT.
- The AURORA individual patient data meta-analysis combined individual-level patient data from six trials in late-window (i.e. >6 h) patients, including DAWN and DEFUSE-3 (Jovin et al., 2022). In this study, a range of prespecified subgroups retained a significant benefit for thrombectomy. In these late-window patients, the number needed to treat was 3. Furthermore, it confirmed that patients with witnessed syndromes in the late window benefited from MT.
- Evidence continues to evolve and a recent multinational cohort study of 1604 patients by Nguyen et al., comparing CT with perfusion scans for patient selection, showed that an increased number of thrombectomies guided by CT/CTA alone in the later time window did not lead to any significant difference in clinical outcomes (Nguyen et al., 2022).
- This was validated by the MRCLEAN-LATE RCT, using NCCT and collateral flow status in 500 patients to show that MT guided by these imaging modalities was still effective in the later time window. Patients in this study actually achieved a similar treatment effect to those in HERMES, indicating that late-window thrombectomies can achieve good clinical outcome without advanced imaging techniques (Olthuis et al., 2023).
- In summary, MT is reasonable in patients with LVO of the anterior circulation presenting between 6 to 24 hours from symptom onset, with NIHSS and ASPECTS $\geq$ 6.

Table 9.2 Inclusion criteria for DEFUSE 3, DAWN, and MR CLEAN-LATE trials

	DEFUSE 3	DAWN	MR CLEAN-LATE
Occlusion location	Extra- or intracranial ICA, proximal MCA, or both (tandem occlusion)	Intracranial ICA, proximal MCA, or both (tandem occlusion)	Intracranial ICA, proximal MCA, or both (tandem occlusion)
Mismatch	Initial infarct volume <70 mL NIHSS ≥6 Ratio of ischaemic tissue volume to infarct volume ≥1.8 Absolute penumbra volume ≥15 mL (T max >6 s on RAPID MRI)	Group A: ≥80 years old, NIHSS ≥10, infarct <21 mL Group B: <80 years old, NIHSS ≥10, infarct <31 mL Group C: <80 years old, NIHSS ≥20, infarct 31–50 mL	Perfusion imaging was not used
Age and functional status	Age 18–90 years, mRS 0–1 at baseline	At least 18 years old, mRS 0–1 at baseline	At least 18 years old, mRS 0–2 at baseline
Time since last seen well	6–16 h	6–24 h	6–24 h
Other imaging	ASPECTS ≥6	Hypodensity <⅓ of MCA territory	Collateral flow was graded: 1 (≤50% filling but >0%), 2 (>50% but <100% filling), or 3 (100% filling). Patients with 1 or above were included in the study On plain CT, hypodensity of <⅓ of the MCA territory
Alteplase	tPA given if within 4.5 h of onset	Presenting outside tPA window *or* received tPA but had persistent vessel occlusion at time of eligibility	Treatment with tPA was permitted

Large core

- In the early MT trials, including those in the HERMES collaboration, patients with large early ischaemic change with ASPECTS of <6, were largely excluded.
- RESCUE-Japan LIMIT was the first RCT to randomise 203 patients with an ASPECTS of 3–5 to MT (Yoshimura et al., 2022). MT in patients with large ischaemic cores were associated with better functional outcomes (mRS 0–3, 31% vs 12.7% RR 2.43 95% CI 1.35–4.37) compared with patients treated with best medical therapy.
- These results prompted early termination of the SELECT-2 and ANGEL-ASPECTS trials, but in both, their interim analyses showed that EVT in patients with large core stroke (ASPECTS 3–5) was significantly associated with a +1 point mRS shift at 90 days (Huo et al., 2023; Sarraj et al., 2023).

Secondary outcomes for both RCTs also showed improved rates of functional independence (mRS 0–2).

- There were some differences between the trials. RESCUE-Japan LIMIT utilised MRI-ASPECTS which tends to overestimate infarct volume whereas a significant proportion of patients in the ANGEL-ASPECTS and SELECT-2 trials underwent CTP imaging, with ischaemic core volumes ranging from 70 to 100 mL, and 50 mL or greater, respectively. Nonetheless, as a result of these three trials, large core MT in selected patients is now classed as indicated in the UK National Clinical Guidelines for Stroke, provided other clinical/mRS criteria are met.
- The LASTE trial evaluated patients (less than 80 years old) with ASPECTS 0 to 2, selecting patients with MRI-DWI within 6.5 hours, demonstrating 13.3% functional independence for the EVT group vs 7.5% for the medical group.
- In summary, MT is reasonable in patients witrh ASPECTS 3 to 5 younger than 80 years with anterior LVO presenting 6 to 24 hours with NIHSS ≥ 6 and mRS 0 to 1. In those with ASPECTS 0 to 2 it may be reasonable if the patient presents within 6 hours.

Medium vessel occlusion

- See 'Medium and distal vessel thrombectomy', p. 378.

Low NIHSS score

- Mild or minor stroke has many definitions but an NIHSS score of 6 or less is commonly accepted.
- These patients tend to have good leptomeningeal collaterals but are at risk if the collaterals become exhausted and up to one-third of all minor stroke patients become dependent (mRS 3–6) at 90 days.
- Currently there is no robust evidence to support MT in patients with minor stroke, even in the presence of an LVO, as most of the trials excluded these patients, including five out of seven studies in the HERMES analyses.
- Current evidence is therefore mostly from non-randomised cohort studies. A multicentre study comprised of 301 patients showed no significant difference in excellent functional outcomes at 90 days (mRS 0–1) between MT and medically treated patients (Dargazanli et al., 2017), although 24 patients (18%) in the medical group had rescue MT because of neurological worsening. Similarly, the Swiss Registry, comprising 312 patients, found no difference in functional outcomes but a trend towards higher mortality in the MT arm (9.3% vs 2.8%; P = 0.06) (Manno et al., 2019).
- Currently, two RCTs (MOSTE and ENDOLOW) are recruiting patients to provide definitive answers regarding thrombectomy in patients with minor stroke.

High pre-morbid mRS score

- Most trials excluded patients who were not functionally independent (mRS 3 and above). A meta-analysis of six retrospective cohort studies comprising 591 patients with a mRS score of 3 or higher before MT, showed a higher rate of poor functional outcomes and mortality as compared with patients who were functionally independent pre-MT (Adamou et al., 2022). Despite this, some of the patients treated with MT showed an ordinal shift in the functional outcomes or remained at baseline, suggestive of a benefit for MT in selected patients.

- In another meta-analysis with 1530 patients not functionally independent pre-stroke, MT had a higher likelihood of the patient returning to pre-stroke mRS score (Yang et al., 2022).
- More evidence is needed to determine which subset of patients with existing disability will benefit from MT as this is likely to be a very heterogeneous group. Currently, LVO patients with baseline mRS scores of 3 are considered on a case-by-case basis in some centres.

Carotid occlusion with patent circle of Willis

- Isolated acute ICA occlusions (without MCA or ACA occlusion) may respond poorly to IVT because of the large clot burden.
- There are, however, concerns about embolising clot into the MCA or ACA during MT. As there is often supply to the hemisphere from the ACOM or PCOM, there may be uncertainty regarding whether a clinical deficit is due to insufficient perfusion across collateral pathways, or distal emboli that do not show up on CTA.
- Small studies indicate improved functional outcomes for MT in moderate-to-large strokes (NIHSS score ≥6), but with relatively high distal embolisation risks (up to 20%) (Riegler et al., 2024). Some series suggest medical therapy may be equally effective in select cases.
- Perfusion imaging can guide MT eligibility in isolated ICA occlusions (Ter Schiphorst et al., 2021; Waters et al., 2022). A study found that treatment based on clinical–imaging mismatch or progressive neurological deterioration after 24 h led to successful recanalisation in 92% of cases, with good functional outcomes in 65% and significant NIHSS score improvement in nearly half. No increased sICH risk was observed. Another study linked core–perfusion mismatch volumes >40 mL to neurological decline on medical therapy.

Further reading

Adamou A, Gkana A, Mavrovounis G, Beltsios ET, Kastrup A, Papanagiotou P. Outcome of endovascular thrombectomy in pre-stroke dependent patients with acute ischaemic stroke: a systematic review and meta-analysis. Front Neurol. 2022;13:880046.

Albers GW, Lansberg MG, Kemp S, et al. A multicentre randomised controlled trial of endovascular therapy following imaging evaluation for ischaemic stroke (DEFUSE 3). Int J Stroke. 2017;12(8):896–905.

Costalat V, Jovin TG, et al. LASTE Trial Investigators. Trial of Thrombectomy for Stroke with a Large Infarct of Unrestricted Size. N Engl J Med. 2024; 9;390(18):1677–1689.

Dargazanli C, Arquizan C, Gory B, et al. Mechanical thrombectomy for minor and mild stroke patients harbouring large vessel occlusion in the anterior circulation: a multicentre cohort study. Stroke. 2017;48(12):3274–3281.

Goyal M, Menon BK, van Zwam WH, et al. Endovascular thrombectomy after large vessel ischaemic stroke: a meta-analysis of individual patient data from five randomised trials. Lancet. 2016;387(10029):1723–1731.

Goyal M, Ospel JM, Ganesh A, et al. Endovascular treatment of stroke due to medium-vessel occlusion. N Engl J Med. 2025;392(14):1385–1395.

Huo X, Ma G, Tong X, et al. Trial of endovascular therapy for acute ischaemic stroke with large infarct. N Engl J Med. 2023;388(14):1272–1283.

Intercollegiate Stroke Working Party. National Clinical Guideline for Stroke for the UK and Ireland [Internet]. 2023. http://www.strokeguideline.org

Jadhav A, Panczykowski D, Jumaa M, et al. Angioplasty and stenting for symptomatic extracranial non-tandem internal carotid artery occlusion. J Neurointerv Surg. 2018;10(12):1155–1160.

Jovin TG, Nogueira RG, Lansberg MG, et al. Thrombectomy for anterior circulation stroke beyond 6 h from time last known well (AURORA): a systematic review and individual patient data meta-analysis. Lancet. 2022;399(10319):249–258.

Manno C, Disanto G, Bianco G, et al. Outcome of endovascular therapy in stroke with large vessel occlusion and mild symptoms. Neurology. 2019;93(17):e1618–e1626.
Nguyen TN, Abdalkader M, Nagel S, et al. Non-contrast computed tomography vs computed tomography perfusion or magnetic resonance imaging selection in late presentation of stroke with large vessel occlusion. JAMA Neurol. 2022;79(1):22–31.
Nogueira RG, Jadhav AP, Haussen DC, et al. Thrombectomy 6 to 24 h after stroke with a mismatch between deficit and infarct. N Engl J Med 2018;378(1):11–21.
Olthuis SGH, Pirson FAV, Pinckaers FME, et al. Endovascular treatment versus no endovascular treatment after 24 h in patients with ischaemic stroke and collateral flow on CT angiography (MR CLEANLATE) in the Netherlands: a multicentre, open-label, blinded endpoint, randomised, controlled, phase 3 trial. Lancet. 2023;401(10385):1371–1380.
Prabhakaran S, Gonzalez NR, Zachrison KS et, al. Peer Review Committee. 2026 Guideline for the Early Management of Patients With Acute Ischemic Stroke: A Guideline From the American Heart Association/American Stroke Association. Stroke. 2026 Jan 26.
Psychogios M, Brehm A, Ribo M, et al. Endovascular treatment for stroke due to occlusion of medium or distal vessels. N Engl J Med. 2025;392(14):1374–1384.
Riegler C, von Rennenberg R, Bollweg K, et al. Endovascular therapy in patients with internal carotid artery occlusion and patent circle of Willis. J Neurointerv Surg. 2024;16(7):644–651.
Sarraj A, Hassan AE, Abraham MG, et al. Trial of endovascular thrombectomy for large ischaemic strokes. N Engl J Med. 2023;388(14):1259–1271.
Ter Schiphorst A, Gaillard N, Dargazanli C, et al. Symptomatic isolated internal carotid artery occlusion with initial medical management: a monocentric cohort. J Neurol. 2021;268(1):346–355.
Waters MJ, McMullan P, Mitchell PJ, et al. Endovascular therapy versus medical therapy for acute stroke attributable to isolated cervical internal carotid artery occlusion without intracranial large vessel occlusion. Stroke Vasc Interv Neurol. 2022;2(2):e000174.
Yang JC, Bao QJ, Guo Y, et al. Endovascular thrombectomy in acute ischaemic stroke patients with pre-stroke disability (mRS ≥2): a systematic review and meta-analysis. Front Neurol. 2022;13:971399.
Yoshimura S, Sakai N, Yamagami H, et al. Endovascular therapy for acute stroke with a large ischaemic region. N Engl J Med. 2022;386(14):1303–1313.

Anaesthesia

- MT is either performed under GA, with conscious sedation, or with LA.
- Anaesthetic practice currently varies significantly between centres, from almost all procedures performed under local LA/conscious sedation to almost all procedures performed under GA.
- The choice should be individualised and based on patient presentation including neurological status, comorbidity, and procedural considerations by the interventionalist.

Standards

- All patients undergoing MT should preferably be cared for by anaesthesia personnel who can provide airway management and emergent induction of GA if required.
- Pre-anaesthetic assessment should focus on neurological status and degree of cardiovascular comorbidity.
- Standard monitoring during the procedure includes ECG, pulse oximeter, non-invasive BP, and temperature.
- Capnography should be used for all patients who undergo MT in GA or conscious sedation, to avoid respiratory depression and hypercarbia.
- Patients should maintain a flat head position on the bed during induction of anaesthesia. The ZODIAC trial results demonstrated an overwhelming clinical benefit to maintaining a zero-degree flat head position in LVO patients awaiting thrombectomy, showing it significantly prevents early neurological deterioration compared to a 30-degree upright position.

Local anaesthesia

- LA should preferably be selected for patients who are awake and alert, can protect their own airway, and can fully cooperate with the procedure (typically patients with low NIHSS score and/or non-dominant acute ischaemic stroke).
- Advantages include the option of continuous neurological evaluation, stable haemodynamics, a potentially shorter delay to reperfusion, and reduced risk of postoperative respiratory complications.
- Disadvantages include uncontrolled patient movement which may prolong the procedure, increased risk of procedural complications, and an unprotected airway.
- Maintain oxygen saturation >94% using nasal cannulae with end-tidal CO_2 monitoring and temperature in the range of 36–37°C.
- A plan should be in place for patient deterioration, necessitating emergent conversion to GA.

Conscious sedation

- CS is similarly preferable in patients who are awake and alert, can protect their own airway, and can fully cooperate with the procedure (typically patients with low NIHSS score).
- Advantages include, depending on the depth of sedation, the option of continuous clinical neurological evaluation, stable haemodynamics, and a potentially shorter time delay to reperfusion.
- Disadvantages include uncontrolled patient movements (which may prolong the procedure and increase the risk of procedural complications) and an unprotected airway.

- Maintain oxygen saturation >94% using nasal cannulae with end-tidal CO_2 monitoring and temperature in the range of 35–37°C.
- A plan should be available if the patient deteriorates and airway management and/or emergent conversion to GA is necessary.

Technique

- Use rapid-onset short acting agents to facilitate titration of the level of sedation.
- Individualise and titrate the depth of sedation to the level where the patient can easily respond to verbal commands and without induction of respiratory depression.
- Higher doses of sedative drugs may facilitate uncontrolled movements, vomiting, respiratory depression, and, ultimately, conversion to GA.
- If airway obstruction occurs, reduce the level of sedation and consider jaw thrust and/or place oral or nasopharyngeal airway until the patient is responsive.
- Examples of conscious sedation protocols:
  - Fentanyl 0.5–1 mcg/kg bolus dose titrated to effect.
  - Propofol infusion 25–100 mcg/kg/min, with or without supplementary boluses of propofol 10–20 mg to facilitate onset.
  - Remifentanil may be added for pain control (0.05–0.2 mcg/kg/min).

General anaesthesia

- GA is preferable for patients with poor neurological presentation (high NIHSS score), who cannot cooperate, have involuntary movements, complex interventional cases (tandem, stenting, distal occlusions), or those who are at risk of airway compromise, aspiration, and likely conversion.
- The advantages are patient immobilisation, full airway protection, and a pain-free procedure.
- The disadvantages are a higher risk of haemodynamic instability, possibly procedure delay, and potential postoperative respiratory complications.
- Poor outcomes associated with GA in early retrospective studies is most likely related to confounding by indication (patients with poor neurological presentation receiving GA) and lack of meticulous attention to BP management.
- Dedicated RCTs have reported no difference in primary outcomes between GA and conscious sedation. Recent meta-analyses reported improved functional outcomes and revascularisation rates in patients subjected to GA. No substantial difference in time to revascularisation or complications has been reported.
- These findings suggest that the use of specialised anaesthesia personnel and meticulous BP and physiological management are more important determinants of outcome than choice of anaesthetic regimen.

Technique

- The optimal choice of anaesthetic drugs has not been established.
- Rapid sequence induction (using, e.g. alfentanil, propofol, and suxamethonium/rocuronium) is indicated due to uncertainty of last oral intake with increased risk of aspiration.
- Anaesthesia is maintained with IV anaesthetics (propofol, remifentanil/fentanyl) or volatile anaesthetics (supplemented by remifentanil or

fentanyl). The choice and doses of anaesthetics should be individualised and titrated according to age and comorbidity.

- Fraction of inspired oxygen (FiO_2) should be titrated to an oxygen saturation >92% and partial pressure of oxygen (PaO_2) >60 mmHg.
- Controlled ventilation is applied and titrated to maintain normocapnia ($PaCO_2$) between 35 and 45 mmHg.
- Neuromuscular blockade may be considered to facilitate the procedure and avoid procedural complications. Be aware of the increased risk of postoperative respiratory complications.
- Fluids should be administered to achieve and/or maintain normovolaemia, as hypovolaemia may be associated with reduced cerebral perfusion. Hypotonic fluids should be avoided due to the risk of cerebral oedema.
- Blood glucose should be monitored during the procedure to achieve or maintain normoglycaemia as both hypo- and hyperglycaemia may negatively influence outcome.
- Patient temperature should be monitored and maintained between 35°C and 37°C. If necessary, consider warming devices/blankets.
- Patients should be extubated as soon as possible after the MT procedure to avoid postoperative respiratory complications. The decision to extubate immediately after the MT procedure is based on individual patient and procedural considerations. In some cases, it may be preferable to delay extubation and admit the patient to the ICU for later and smooth extubation.

Blood pressure management

- The optimal procedure BP targets, and whether to aim for systolic or mean arterial BP targets, has not been determined.
- Retrospective and observational studies suggest poor functional outcomes in association with mean arterial pressures <70 mmHg and >90 mmHg.
- A systolic BP between 140 and 180 mmHg is recommended before revascularisation.
- Intra-arterial BP monitoring would ideally be used in all patients undergoing thrombectomy. However, usage is a compromise as it does add time to preparation and some units omit for this reason. Invasive BP monitoring should be preferred in patients undergoing thrombectomy in GA and patients with high cardiovascular comorbidity.
- After revascularisation, the systolic BP should be determined in collaboration with the neurointerventionist and stroke physician. A systolic BP between 120 and 140 mmHg may be considered to lower the risk of hyperperfusion and haemorrhagic transformation.
- BP can be maintained with infusion of vasopressor agents (phenylephrine or noradrenaline are the most commonly used agents). The choice of vasopressor should be considered in relation to cardiovascular comorbidity.
- Hypertension (systolic BP >180 mmHg) may be controlled using nicardipine or labetalol.

American Heart Association/American Stroke Association guideline

- The American Heart Association/American Stroke Association guideline currently recommends that the anaesthetic technique for MT should be selected on the basis of an individualised assessment of patient risk factors, technical performance of the procedure, and other clinical characteristics.

- The current American Heart Association/American Stroke Association recommendations suggest maintaining systolic BP <180/105 mmHg during and for 24 h after the thrombectomy procedure.

Further reading

Campbell D, Butler E, Campbell RB, et al. General anesthesia compared with non-GA in endovascular thrombectomy for ischaemic stroke: a systematic review and meta-analysis of randomised controlled trials. Neurology. 2023;100(16):e1655–e1663.

Rasmussen M, Schönenberger S, Hendèn PL, et al. Blood pressure thresholds and neurologic outcomes after endovascular therapy for acute ischaemic stroke: an analysis of individual patient data from 3 randomised clinical trials. JAMA Neurol. 2020;77(5):622–631.

Talke PO, Sharma D, Heyer EJ, Bergese SD, Blackham KA, Stevens RD. Republished: Society for Neuroscience in Anesthesiology and Critical Care expert consensus statement: anaesthetic management of endovascular treatment for acute ischaemic stroke. Stroke. 2014;45(8):e138–e150. [The current BP management practice in many centres originates from this publication.]

Clot composition

- Most clots in LVO stroke are embolic in origin, typically arising from the heart or the carotid bifurcation.
- However, clots can also form *in situ*, similar to those in acute myocardial infarction, due to intracranial atherosclerotic disease (ICAD). The latter is relatively rare in Caucasians, commoner in Black and Hispanic populations, and most prevalent in Asian populations.
- Embolic clots are primarily composed of red blood cells and dense fibrin, though the proportion of these components can vary significantly. They also contain smaller amounts of substances such as vWF and neutrophil extracellular traps. These additional elements may serve as potential targets for future advancements in pharmacological therapy.
- Clots rich in red blood cells are generally easier to remove. However, the primary challenge lies in minimising the loss of small clot fragments during the process. These fragments can lodge in the microvasculature, potentially contributing to the 'no-reflow' phenomenon, where the patient experiences poor or suboptimal outcomes despite a seemingly rapid and complete MT.
- At the other end of the spectrum are highly fibrin-rich, rubber-like clots. These can be resistant to removal despite repeated attempts.

Mechanical thrombectomy principles

Access

(See Chapter 6, 'Access', p. 175.)

- Arterial access should ideally be achieved with ultrasound guidance to reduce complications.

Femoral

- The femoral artery typically accommodates larger introducer sheaths due to its greater diameter. Femoral access is necessary for many (typically older) BGCs.
- Many find it to be quicker, important for reducing recanalisation time.

Wrist

- Wrist access (radial or ulna) has been shown in large cardiology series to have a lower complication rate with similar procedural efficiency, although this has not been proven in MT.
- It may have particular utility in catheterisation of the right vertebral artery (if puncturing the right radial artery) and left vertebral artery (for left radial punctures).
- It may also be easier to access the left CCA when arising from the innominate at an unfavourable angle for the femoral approach.
- There are limitations regarding the size of the guide catheters available through this route. 8 Fr catheters can be accommodated if used sheathless and the size of the vessel is at least 2.5 mm.

Brachial

- Brachial artery puncture is not recommended routinely due to its comparatively smaller size and, unlike the radial artery, a post-treatment occlusion can result in severe consequences, including devastating arm/hand ischaemia distal to the occlusion.
- If bleeding occurs from a brachial puncture site, it can be more difficult to control. A haematoma at the puncture site can spread in the medial brachial fascial compartment to cause neural compression and tissue compromise.

Carotid

- Ultrasound-guided direct carotid puncture (see Chapter 6, 'Carotid', p. 187) is a last resort in patients for whom access through the femoral or radial routes is impossible. So careful consideration of prognosis ± MT is required.
- GA is recommended for airway protection. Haemostasis is with common closure devices or closed directly with sutures by a vascular surgeon.
- Manual compression has been described, but there is a concern that the puncture site may bleed after completing the compression, particularly if the patient is being treated with thrombolysis, anticoagulation, or antiplatelets.
- Direct vertebral punctures have been described although this may be viewed as even more complex.

Balloon guide catheters

(See Chapter 4, 'Balloon devices', p. 125.)

- BGCs usefully achieve flow arrest in the ICA, reducing the chance of distal emboli into other territories during retrieval.

- Available BGCs include FlowGate and Merci (Stryker), Cello (Medtronic), Walrus (QÁpel Medical), EmboGuard (Cerenovus), and Bobby (MicroVention/Terumo). Note that the Flowgate doesn't accept larger intermediate/aspiration catheters (the largest compatible device is the Catalyst 7).
- RCT evidence so far on BGCs has not been positive, with no benefit demonstrated in one study (PROFATE), and harm observed in another (PROTECT-MT).

Techniques

Multiple techniques are described for MT (Figure 9.6). None is clearly superior.

Direct contact aspiration

(See Figure 9.7.)

- Direct contact aspiration is used to remove a clot without crossing it, thereby reducing the risk of distal emboli that can occur if a microcatheter or microwire passes between the clot and the vessel wall. This technique has fewer steps and uses less material, potentially leading to savings in time and consumable/device costs.

Technique

- Introduce an aspiration catheter through the guide catheter or BGC and navigate to the clot face, either alone ('snaking technique'), over a microwire, or with the aid of a microcatheter and microwire. These are removed when the catheter is in position.
- The catheter must face the clot end-on, not at an angle. Suction is then applied to the aspiration catheter using a 60 mL syringe (with forceps maintaining vacuum on the plunger), a dedicated VacLok (Merit Medical), or an aspiration pump. The clot is engaged by the aspiration catheter until completely ingested or lodged ('corked') at the catheter tip and removed as a whole.
- It is important to be in contact with the clot for effective aspiration. There should not be a significant distance between the clot and the aspiration catheter tip as the vessel segment between the two may collapse.
- Navigating the ophthalmic bend in more tortuous anatomy can be challenging and can be mitigated by using larger microcatheters, more robust microwires, or specially designed adjunctive devices that reduce the size discrepancy and ledge effect between the aspiration catheter and microcatheter. The Wedge microcatheter (Microvention/Terumo), Offset (Stryker), and SENDit (Penumbra) are examples of such devices. Similarly, steam-shaping the aspiration catheter tip can be a useful technique for better tracking (the RED catheter comes with a mandrel for this purpose). If impossible to advance the aspiration catheter over these devices, a stent retriever may need to be deployed, which provides distal anchorage.
- Pump versus hand aspiration: while both syringes and aspiration pumps have proven effective for MT, benchtop experiments have shown that syringe methods achieve the highest initial flow and suction force but this falls off as the syringe is filled. The suction force is also dependent on the catheter diameter and the catheter tip not collapsing under the pressure. Furthermore, cyclic or pulsatile aspiration force from the newer aspiration pumps has been suggested to be more effective at ingesting the clot with less distal emboli. Another anecdotal method to enhance aspiration thrombectomy force is to apply aspiration to the microcatheter as well, if it has not already been removed.

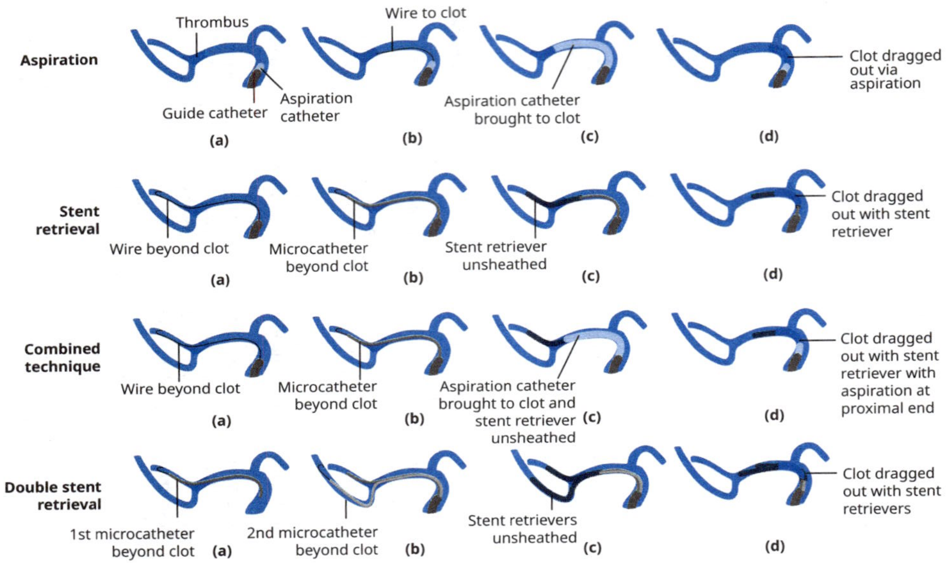

Figure 9.6 Techniques of mechanical thrombectomy.

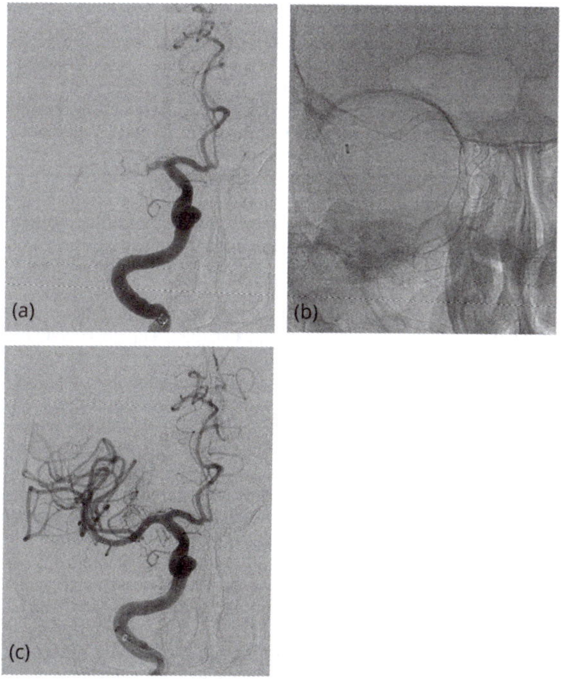

Figure 9.7 Direct contact aspiration. (a) Digital subtraction angiography shows right M1 middle cerebral artery proximal occlusion. (b) A 0.072" aspiration catheter was advanced over a 0.014" microwire to the face of the clot. Note that the catheter extends distal to the apparent occlusion site on the angiogram, likely indicating that the catheter has engulfed the proximal extent of the thrombus. (c) After aspiration is applied, the catheter is removed, and the artery is successfully recanalised.

- After a period of time, the aspiration catheter is withdrawn into the guide catheter and out of the body.
- The guide catheter RHV is removed prior to removing the aspiration catheter to avoid fragmenting clot.
- The guide is then aspirated thoroughly to remove any clot debris.
- DSA is performed to confirm that the artery has been successfully recanalised.
- Further thrombectomy passes are made, as necessary.

Stent retrieval

- Stent retrievers were developed prior to aspiration.
- If the aspiration catheter gets stuck proximally and cannot be brought to the clot face, a stent retriever must be used.
- Stents can be used alone or in combination with aspiration.

Devices

- The Solitaire (Medtronic) was the first stent retriever introduced to the market and continues to be one of the most widely used devices. Diameter ranges between 3 and 6 mm. When constrained within the microcatheter, the device is folded onto itself. Consequently, when an oversized Solitaire is used in a comparatively small vessel, it does not fully unfold and acts as a double-layer device.
- Another commonly used device is the Trevo (Stryker), designed with an optimised strut diameter and configuration. Also available in diameters ranging from 3 to 6 mm, it has been shown to benefit from being gently pushed while unsheathing, followed by a slight additional push ('fluffing') to maximise interaction with the clot. This device has a higher radial force than the Solitaire.
- Many other stent retrievers based on the same clot penetration principles are also available, including Catch (Balt), ERIC (MicroVention/Terumo), and Preset (Phenox) among others.
- The Tigertriever family, while still relying on clot penetration, features a unique design that allows the operator to manually adjust the device diameter using a slider on the handle. This adjustment ranges from 0.5 mm (Tigertriever 13 and 17) to 6 mm (Tigertriever), enabling customisation to match the vessel size and the presumed clot type.
- The Embotrap (Cerenovus) and Neva (Vesalio) stent retrievers are designed to 'trap' the clot through openings in the struts, rather than relying primarily on penetrating the clot with radial force. Additionally, these retrievers feature a meshed distal tip to prevent the loss of small clot fragments during retrieval. The proximal end of these devices should be deployed at the proximal end of the thrombus for maximum effectiveness (also essential for applying the pinching technique with the Nimbus device).
- The Nimbus (Cerenovus) is specifically designed to manage refractory, mostly fibrin-rich, thrombi that are difficult to remove. It has a proximal spiral section and distal barrel section. The proximal spiral section is designed to maximise device–clot interaction with wide opening angles to engage with clot and multiple pinch points. The device is deployed with its proximal marker at the proximal end of the clot, and fully unsheathed. No wait time is required. The technique for retrieval is to advance the microcatheter over the proximal end of the device, partially resheathing the device until resistance is felt. This indicates the clot is pinched between the spiral section of device and microcatheter. Forward pressure is maintained while retrieving the device with concomitant aspiration through distal aspiration catheter and/or BGC, depending on the access used. The clot is therefore pinched and removed from its proximal end. The distal barrel section is more like a regular stent retriever and is designed to maintain control of the clot during retrieval and to funnel the clot/device into the receiving aspiration/guide catheter.

Stent retrieval technique

- The classical stent retriever method typically involves positioning a guide catheter/BGC proximal to the occlusion site using a select catheter and a guidewire, ideally, in the petrosal segment of the ICA.
- The clot is approached and passed with a microcatheter with the aid of a microwire. While 0.027" microcatheters can be used, a smaller-bore microcatheter (0.021") is preferred. Some groups have found that

crossing the clot with the microcatheter alone without a leading wire has fewer complications.

- Microcatheter angiography can be performed to confirm that the clot has been crossed and to evaluate vessel size, anatomy, and runoff.
- Thereafter, the stent retriever is deployed across the clot, ideally with its proximal end a few millimetres prior to the proximal part of the thrombus.
- A period of 3–5 min is allowed for clot integration. During this time, a 50–60 mL syringe is attached to the guide catheter and a vacuum is created within by withdrawing the plunger and locking it either with forceps or by using a specialised 'VacLock' syringe while keeping the three-way valve locked (so that the vacuum is not yet applied to the catheter).
- After the waiting time is over, the BGC (if used) is inflated under fluoroscopy and the stent retriever and microcatheter are then slowly withdrawn together. The valve connecting the vacuum syringe to the guide catheter is released before pulling the stent/clot across the bifurcation to stagnate or reverse the flow in the ICA.
- The stent retriever and microcatheter are then pulled until they enter the guide catheter.
- Pulling the stent retriever through the RHV of the guide catheter can damage the stent and fragment the clot. To avoid this, it is important to unscrew and remove the guide catheter RHV first, allowing the stent to be withdrawn without passing through it.
- After removing the stent, the guide catheter is thoroughly aspirated to remove clot fragments.
- The BGC is then deflated.
- DSA is performed to determine whether the artery has been successfully recanalised.
- Further thrombectomy passes are made, as necessary.

Combined technique

(See Figure 9.8.)

- The stent retrieval technique can be modified by adding an intermediate/aspiration catheter which is brought in contact with the tail of the clot and negative aspiration force applied.
- A considerable number of variations have been described but all are essentially accomplishing the same thing, e.g. SAVE, partial SAVE, SOLUMBRA, modified SOLUMBRA, BADASS, Dual SAVE, etc.
- The stent retriever is typically deployed first, as its deployment provides distal anchoring, which facilitates the advancement of the aspiration catheter.
- Rather than pulling the stent into the aspiration catheter (which risks shearing off the clot), the entire construct is then pulled into the guide catheter or BGC. This 'pinching manoeuvre' involves the clot being trapped between the aspiration catheter and the stent retriever.
- Ensure that the stent retriever is not progressively drawn into the aspiration catheter during retrieval itself. To prevent this, release any tension in the intermediate or aspiration catheter before starting to pull the construct, and continue with a slow, steady withdrawal.
- An optional manoeuvre is to remove the microcatheter after deploying the stent retriever, leaving the stent in place. This increases the cross-sectional area available for suction.

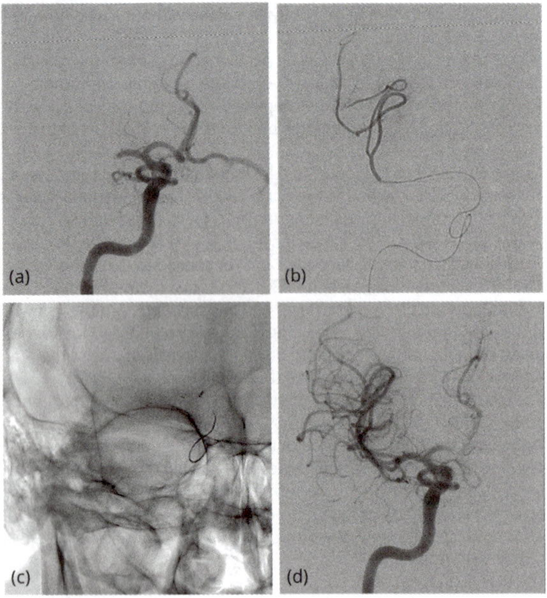

Figure 9.8 Combined technique for mechanical thrombectomy. (a) Digital subtraction angiography shows a right proximal M1 middle cerebral artery (MCA) thrombus. (b) An 0.021" microcatheter is advanced distal to the clot, and microangiography is performed. (c) An unsubtracted exposure reveals a 6 × 20 stent retriever deployed across the clot, with an 0.072" reperfusion catheter positioned as close as possible to the clot face. The microcatheter has been removed to maximise aspiration space within the reperfusion catheter. Aspiration is applied to both the reperfusion catheter and guide, and the reperfusion catheter is removed together with the stent, without retracting the stent within the reperfusion catheter. (d) The territory is fully recanalised. Note a common appearance of the right A1 flash filling. It is not occluded, both A1s are supplied contralaterally, and flow from the right internal carotid artery is now directed into the right MCA.

Double stent retriever technique

- A more recent development to address refractory clots is the double stent retriever technique. This involves deploying two stent retrievers in parallel, typically in two branches originating from a bifurcation, and withdrawing them simultaneously (Figure 9.9). Typically, a BGC is also used, but is not mandatory.
- First described in 2015, this method has since been proposed as a first-line technique, with promising outcomes reported in a case series of 39 patients with M1 or T-occlusions. It successfully recanalised all targeted vessels, achieving TICI 2C/3 in 69% of cases with a single pass (first-pass effect), without an increase in symptomatic intracerebral haemorrhages.
- This technique is particularly suited for MCA bifurcations or ICA terminus (T-) occlusions presenting as saddle thrombi and has outperformed other approaches in experimental flow-model comparisons.

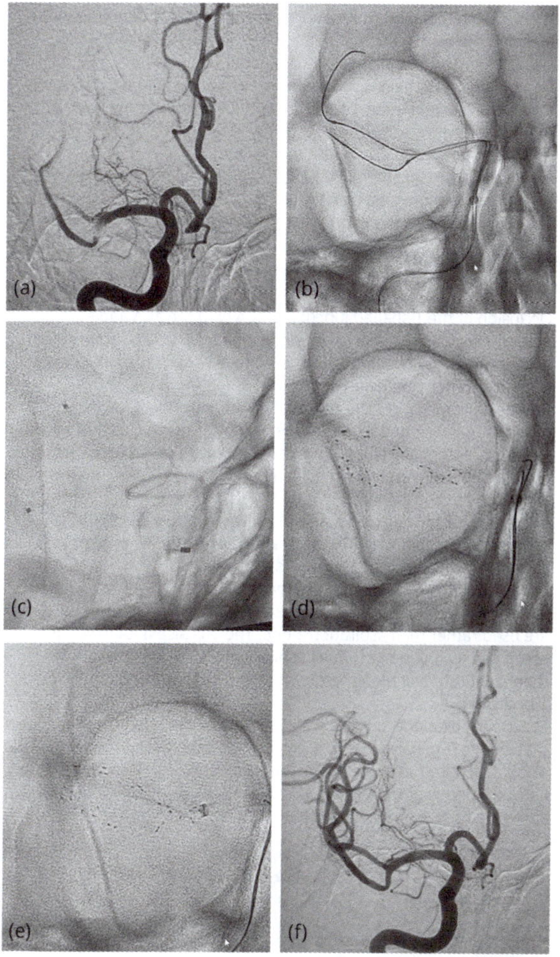

Figure 9.9 Double stent retriever technique. (a) Digital subtraction angiography showing thrombus at the right middle cerebral artery (MCA) bifurcation. (b) Unsubtracted imaging showing two 0.021" microcatheters positioned in both MCA divisions. (c) The microwires are removed. (d) Two 6 × 40 stent retrievers are deployed. (e) After removing both microcatheters, a 0.070" reperfusion catheter is advanced into the M1 to the clot face. (f) The entire construct is removed together, fully recanalising the vessel. Images courtesy of Dr Tommy Andersson.

- It is suggested to place both microcatheters in the different vessels (keeping the wire in the first before cannulating the second to aid visualisation) before unsheathing the stent retrievers.
- Depending on the vessel size, options include using two 6 mm stent retrievers, a combination of a 6 mm and a 4 mm stent retriever, or two 4 mm stent retrievers.
- An aspiration catheter can additionally be used.
- A pilot RCT from Spain (TWIN2WIN) has indicated promising results with a significantly higher first-pass effect for dual stent retriever technique (over single, 47 vs 24%) with no safety concerns.

Carotid T-occlusion

(See Figure 9.10.)

- Occlusion of the T-shaped junction of ICA with the ACA and MCA accounts for 20–30% of anterior circulation LVO. It is associated with poorer functional outcomes compared to M1 or other more distally located anterior circulation occlusions.
- Reasons include larger clot burden (longer and wider), lower successful reperfusion rates, and higher incidence of distal embolus during MT with clots potentially embolising into both the ACA and MCA territories. Additionally, collateral flow between the ACA and MCA is compromised with both territories involved.
- MT can be performed using stent retriever, aspiration only, or combination techniques. The most effective technique in removing large carotid terminus thrombus remains unclear.
- Some studies suggest higher first-pass effect and lower rate of embolism to new territory when stent retrievers and in particular longer devices are used rather than aspiration alone. There is also data to suggest combined technique of contact aspiration and stent retriever rather than stent retriever alone results in higher reperfusion grade in carotid T-occlusion.
- For aspiration alone, it is likely that superbore catheters, more closely matched to luminal size of ICA, have increased efficacy. A crossing double stent retriever technique has also been described for refractory carotid T occlusion.

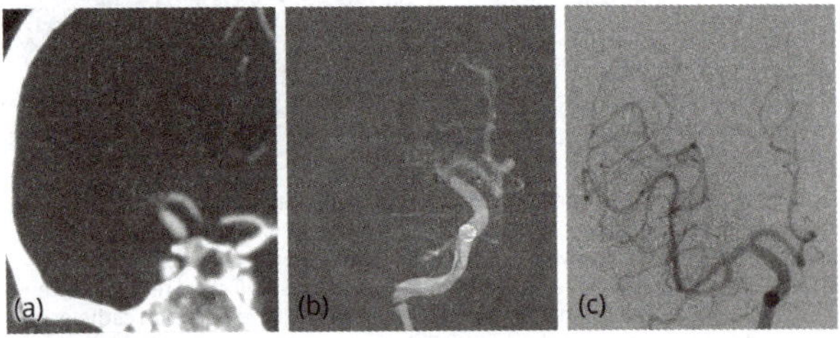

Figure 9.10 Carotid-T thrombectomy. (a) Computed tomography angiogram showing thrombus within the terminal right internal carotid artery extending into the middle cerebral artery and anterior cerebral artery. (b) A 0.072" reperfusion catheter is advanced to the clot face. (c) After a single pass, the catheter is removed, reperfusing the vessel.

Thrombolysis In Cerebral Infarction scores

- The main goal of MT, regardless of technique, is to achieve reperfusion of the ischaemic area, and this is graded by the TICI system, which was first described in 2003 (Table 9.3).
- This evolved into the modified system (mTICI), where reperfusion initially was considered successful if 50% or more of the affected territory was vascularised (defined as mTICI 2B–3).

Table 9.3 mTICI and eTICI scores

Score	mTICI	eTICI
0	No perfusion	No perfusion
1	Reduction in thrombus but limited, absent, or very slow filling of distal arterial branches	
2A	Partial perfusion of <50%	
2B	Partial filling of ≥50% territory	2B50: partial perfusion of 50–66%
		2B67: partial perfusion of 67–89%
2C	Near-complete perfusion except for some small distal vessels	Extensive perfusion of 90–99%
3	Complete perfusion	

- Subsequently, a 2C grade was added, defining a near-complete reperfusion except for a few distal vessels.
- More recently, the expanded treatment in cerebral ischaemia (eTICI) score has been used where the 2B grade has been divided into 50–66% (2B50) and 67–90% (2B67) of the affected area with clinically significant different functional outcomes. eTICI is probably more relevant in the research field than routine clinical practice.
- Achieving complete recanalisation on the first pass during thrombectomy, known as the 'first-pass effect', has been identified as an independent predictor of good clinical outcomes. This effect is likely a subset of what is termed 'sudden recanalisation', emphasising the importance of removing the entire clot in a single attempt rather than in a stepwise, piecemeal fashion.
- However, if the initial attempt fails, it is still beneficial to achieve mTICI 2C or 3 recanalisation in subsequent attempts.
- While the rate of revascularisation is a well-established independent predictor of good outcomes, it does not automatically lead to them. Tiny clot fragments can remain lodged in the microvasculature, contributing to incomplete reperfusion. Additionally, mechanisms such as neutrophil activity and neurovascular remodelling may also play critical roles.
- Looking ahead, the focus must shift from merely achieving clot removal to optimising techniques to ensure excellent outcomes for an even greater number of patients.
- The CHOICE study found that adding intra-arterial rtPA to a good MT significantly ($p = 0.05$) increased the primary outcome (rate of patients with excellent functional outcome, mRS 0–1), although the (usually more statistically powerful) shift analysis of mRS outcome was neutral.

However, CHOICE terminated early after only 121 were randomised and it enrolled just 16% of the LVO population meeting the trial angiographic criteria (TICI 2B or better after MT) and only 7% of the whole MT population.

Further reading

García-Tornel Á, Rubiera M, Requena M, et al. Sudden recanalisation: a game-changing factor in endovascular treatment of large vessel occlusion strokes. Stroke. 2020;51(4):1313–1316.

Liebeskind DS, Bracard S, Guillemin F, et al. eTICI reperfusion: defining success in endovascular stroke therapy. J Neurointerv Surg. 2019;11(5):433–438.

Renú A, Millán M, San Román L, et al. Effect of intra-arterial alteplase vs placebo following successful thrombectomy on functional outcomes in patients with large vessel occlusion acute ischaemic stroke: the CHOICE randomised clinical trial. JAMA. 2022;327(9):826–835.

Zaidat OO, Yoo AJ, Khatri P, et al. Recommendations on angiographic revascularisation grading standards for acute ischaemic stroke: a consensus statement. Stroke. 2013;44(9):2650–2663.

Tandem carotid occlusion

Tandem occlusion refers to the simultaneous occlusion of an extracranial vessel and a more distal artery within the intracranial circulation. It occurs in 10–20% of LVOs and is more common in patients with atherosclerotic disease. The most common site is the proximal ICA and MCA, which we focus upon in this chapter, but the same principles can be applied to the posterior circulation (see 'Posterior circulation thrombectomy', p. 368).

Types

- Preprocedural CTA reveals no opacification from the carotid bifurcation to the MCA, with distal MCA branches filling retrogradely by the collateral circulation. In patients with poor collateral circulation, these branches may be completely absent.
- The underlying pathology may not be clear before the procedure and could include any of the following:

    1. A long thrombus extending from the ICA to the MCA/ACA, potentially from emboli originating in the heart.
    2. Atherosclerotic stenosis proximally and embolus distally. Often, there is calcification in the proximal ICA with evidence of atherosclerotic disease elsewhere, and the patient typically has known risk factors.
    3. Dissection proximally and embolus distally, often seen in younger patients without risk factors or other signs of atherosclerotic disease.
    4. A carotid web ± thrombus proximally with an embolus distally.
    5. Chronic ICA occlusion with embolus via collateral route.
    6. Pseudo-occlusion, which occurs due to a distal carotid occlusion that slows flow in the proximal ICA, can mimic a tandem lesion on CTA but actually involves only one occlusion site.

Initial technique

- The guide catheter is positioned in the CCA and angiography is performed. The ICA may appear completely occluded, or there may be a small, slow-filling central channel. At this point, the pathology often remains unclear.
- First gain access to the ICA:
    - Aspiration at the site of proximal occlusion may remove enough clot to visualise a channel.
    - Stepwise progression using a 0.014" microwire and microcatheter is a safe method, followed by an aspiration catheter and guide catheter, if passage is possible. This can be challenging with tight stenosis or in the presence of dissection, where care must be taken to avoid entering the false lumen.
    - Alternatively, a 0.035" wire can be used to advance a 5 or 6 Fr selective catheter or the inner dilator of a long sheath/guide over the wire into the ICA. The guide catheter can then be advanced into the ICA over this construct. Even with severe stenosis at the occluded ICA origin, applying forward force often can be successful. If the inner select catheter or long sheath successfully crosses into the ICA but the guide catheter cannot follow, try replacing the wire with a stiffer one (e.g. Glidewire Advantage, Terumo).

- If only a microcatheter and wire, but not aspiration or guide catheter, can be advanced and stenosis is suspected, it must be addressed through angioplasty to facilitate the rest of the procedure. Confirm your position within the ICA lumen with a gentle microcatheter angiogram, remove the microcatheter over an exchange-length microwire, and use a 4 mm angioplasty balloon to dilate the stenosis. If this remains unsuccessful, the select catheter/inner dilator can be exchanged in to reduce the ledge effect and provide additional support to advance the guide catheter into the ICA. Occasionally, additional angioplasty with a larger 6 mm balloon may be required to gain access to the ICA with the guide catheter.
- Once successful, try to progressively advance the aspiration and guide catheter into the ICA over the balloon wire.
- Once the guide catheter reaches the ICA, the inner devices are removed, followed by aspiration to retrieve any thrombus from the ICA lumen—an essential step. Further clot can be removed by passing an aspiration catheter up as far as it goes and then dragging it back while aspiration is applied. Once accomplished, gentle angiography can be performed. If clot clearance is observed, continue the procedure progressively distally using aspiration and stent retrievers.
- Note, once access to the ICA is gained do *not* perform vigorous angiography injection as this may result in rupture of the ICA. This situation occurs when the system is closed, i.e. when the distal ICA is occluded by thrombus and the proximal end is obstructed by a combination of stenosis, thrombus, and guide catheter. There is no outlet for the injected contrast and the build-up in pressure can result in extravasation.

Tandem occlusion with atherosclerotic stenosis

- The cervical ICA occlusion can be managed conservatively with treatment focused solely on the intracranial occlusion, or it can be addressed with balloon angioplasty and stenting. This can be done either *before* addressing the intracranial occlusion (antegrade approach) or *afterwards* (retrograde approach). Currently, there is no consensus on which approach is best.
- If stenting is considered, on-table cone beam CT is recommended to first exclude haemorrhage, particularly if the case is prolonged with multiple passes, or if there is a large core of infarction.
- Whether stenting is performed before or after MT, it is important to repeat cerebral angiography afterwards to check for any additional emboli that may have been dislodged during the stenting.

Angioplasty and stent first (antegrade approach)

- Advantages include improved blood flow and collateralisation to the affected territory, and a reduced risk of re-occlusion from slow or stagnant flow during ICA treatment. Disadvantages include longer time to intracranial revascularisation, the need for at least one antiplatelet agent at the time of stenting, an increased risk of haemorrhagic conversion of an existing infarct (especially with a large core or unsuccessful revascularisation of large intracranial territories), and the risk of in-stent thrombus or occlusion.

- A distal protection device may be considered to reduce the risk of embolisation. The SpiderFX can be inserted over any 0.014" wire. Alternatively, if a BGC is used, the balloon can be inflated and aspiration applied in the CCA for proximal flow reversal.
- Angioplasty is typically performed with a 4 mm balloon, followed by placement of a carotid stent sized to match the CCA diameter and of sufficient length to cover the underlying stenosis. Subsequent in-stent angioplasty with a 6 mm balloon is often necessary to address any residual in-stent stenosis. The angioplasty and stenting technique is discussed in Chapter 10 'Carotid artery stenting', p. 400.
- Antiplatelet regimens are discussed in 'Antiplatelet regimen after stenting', p. 363.
- When using proximal flow control, aspiration through the BGC should be performed before proceeding further to remove any thrombus ahead of the guide catheter in the artery. The balloon should remain inflated until this step is complete.
- It is particularly important, when performing stent retriever thrombectomy, to advance the guide catheter beyond the carotid stent to avoid the stent retriever becoming entangled in the carotid stent struts during retrieval.
- The guide catheter can be advanced into the ICA over the angioplasty balloon, the distal protection device, a microcatheter and wire, or an aspiration catheter. To improve support and avoid the ledge effect while crossing the stent, it may be necessary to insert a 5 or 6 Fr select catheter through the guide to lead.
- Since thrombus is often present in the ICA beyond the stenosis, aspiration through the guide or aspiration catheter in the ICA should be performed to clear the artery. Once the guide catheter is positioned within the ICA, the intracranial occlusion can be addressed.
- An alternative antegrade approach is the Retriever Wire-Supported Carotid Artery Revascularisation (ReWiSed CARe) technique. Here, the ICA occlusion is crossed with a microcatheter and wire, and the stent retriever is deployed across the intracranial arterial occlusion. The microcatheter is then stripped from the stent retriever wire, and carotid angioplasty and stenting is performed using the 0.014" wire of the stent retriever.

Angioplasty and stent last (retrograde approach)

(See Figure 9.11.)

- Advantages of this approach include faster reperfusion of the intracranial circulation, avoiding commitment to antiplatelet therapy, and the ability to forgo stenting if there is a perceived high risk of intracranial bleeding. Disadvantages include the need to navigate the ICA blindly, which carries a risk of distal embolisation and damage, further embolisation during the procedure, and the potential loss of access to the ICA.
- Access to the ICA is first achieved (see above). If the guide catheter cannot pass into the ICA, angioplasty may be required to dilate the stenosis.
- After intracranial MT, management options for the ICA should be considered, as underlying stenosis at the ICA origin or carotid bulb is usually present. Wire access should be maintained in the ICA with a 0.014" wire, or alternatively, a distal protection device (e.g. Emboshield NAV6 Embolic

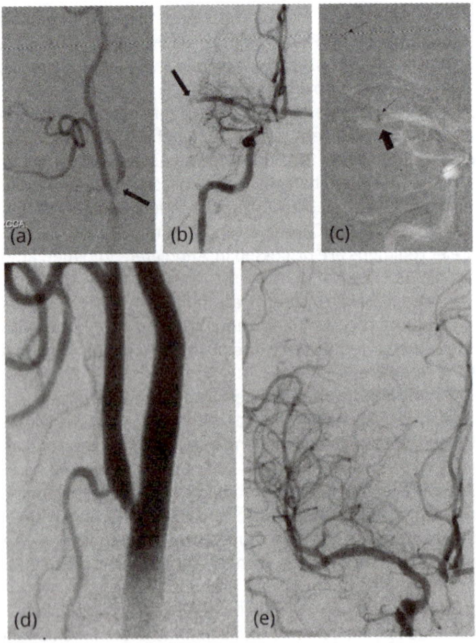

Figure 9.11 Tandem internal carotid artery (ICA) occlusion retrograde approach. (a) Digital subtraction angiography of the right common carotid artery shows a severe focal atherosclerotic stenosis (black arrow) at the carotid bifurcation with poor antegrade flow. (b) Frontal right ICA angiogram shows a complete occlusion of the left M1 segment (arrow). (c) Fluoroscopic image shows a stent retriever (small black arrows) with a reperfusion catheter (thick black arrow) at the site of thrombus. (d) After thrombectomy and stent placement in the ICA, the image shows a widely patent left ICA and (e) left middle carotid artery. Images courtesy of Dr Joseph Gemmete.

Protection System, Abbott). The device's wire can maintain access across the stenosis to facilitate angioplasty or stenting if required. The guide catheter should then be retracted into the CCA with aspiration applied to remove any remaining or re-accumulated thrombus. Angiography in the CCA allows assessment of residual stenosis and its severity.

- Management options include leaving the residual stenosis without acute intervention and delaying definitive ICA treatment (stenting or carotid endarterectomy (CEA)) provided the ICA remains patent. This approach may be preferred when the residual stenosis does not appear severe, there is already a large burden of cerebral infarction, or there are concerns about increased bleeding risk, thereby avoiding early antiplatelet therapy. A delayed on-table angiogram should be considered. If the stenosis worsens, thrombus develops, or the ICA begins to occlude, further intervention with angioplasty alone or stenting is usually necessary. In early-window cases with a small infarct burden and no thrombolysis, stenting with or without angioplasty may be the best option.

Tandem occlusion with dissection

(See Figure 9.12.)

- Dissection can lead to significant narrowing of the true lumen of the artery, occlusion, or the formation of thrombus with subsequent distal embolisation. Tandem occlusion caused by dissection can be very challenging to manage.
- The retrograde approach, where the intracranial occlusion is treated first, facilitates more rapid restoration of intracranial arterial flow, particularly if antegrade collateralisation through the circle of Willis is possible.
- Care must be taken to access the true ICA lumen. Erroneous entry into the false lumen can extend the dissection or expand the intramural haematoma, potentially worsening narrowing or causing complete occlusion or even rupture.

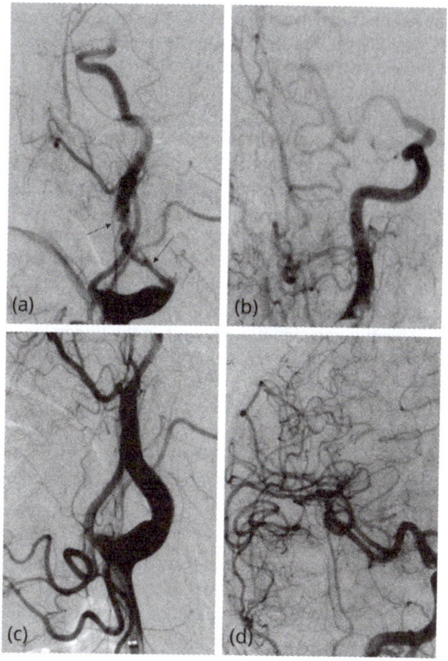

Figure 9.12 Internal carotid artery (ICA) tandem dissection. (a) Lateral right common carotid artery (CCA) angiogram shows a long segment of narrowing with filling defects (small black arrows) in the ICA, consistent with thrombus related to a dissection and poor antegrade flow. (b) Frontal right ICA angiogram shows sluggish filling of the intracranial circulation. (c) Lateral right CCA angiogram after suction thrombectomy and stent placement shows a widely patent right ICA with excellent antegrade flow. (d) Frontal right ICA angiogram after thrombectomy and stent placement shows improved filling of the intracranial circulation. Images courtesy of Dr Joseph Gemmete.

- If the true lumen in the cervical ICA is only narrowed but has a wide patent channel, it can usually be accessed with a select catheter under roadmap guidance. The guide catheter can then be advanced into the ICA distal to the dissection site. Aspiration through the guide catheter before proceeding is critical to clear any thrombus from the true lumen.
- If the true lumen appears extremely narrowed or completely occluded, access may require a 0.014" microwire and microcatheter. A good indicator that the true lumen has been accessed is if the wire moves freely without obstruction to the petrous or cavernous segment. If the wire enters the false lumen, it may fail to advance easily, display a corkscrew-like appearance, or meet an obstruction after initial easy movement. In such cases, the wire should be withdrawn to the CCA and access re-attempted.
- A microcatheter angiogram in the distal ICA can confirm placement within the true lumen. The guide catheter should not be advanced into the ICA until true luminal access is confirmed.
- An alternative approach involves using a large-bore aspiration catheter with a soft, flexible distal segment, such as the Sofia Plus 070. When advanced alone into the ICA, the catheter often locates the true lumen due to its size. If the catheter enters the false lumen, while there is a risk of extending the dissection, aspirating thrombus can help to collapse the false lumen and improve the calibre of the true lumen.
- Once access to the true lumen is achieved, an aspiration pass should be performed to clear any thrombus present. If thrombus is retrieved, repeated aspiration should be conducted until no further thrombus is recovered. A gentle angiogram can be performed to assess for a trapped segment, determine if the distal ICA is clear, and provide roadmap guidance to the intracranial occlusion.
- It is not recommended to pull a stent retriever across a dissected ICA segment, as this can significantly worsen the dissection. Ideally, the guide catheter should be positioned above the dissection site. Alternatively, the stent retriever can be pulled into the aspiration catheter before removal (although this does risk shearing off clot).
- After clearing the intracranial occlusion, if stenting is considered, it is essential to maintain wire access in the ICA to ensure positioning within the true lumen and facilitate decision-making regarding ICA management.

Conservative management of dissection

- Passage of guide or aspiration catheters within the ICA may be sufficient to restore the true lumen to a reasonable calibre. A delayed angiogram can be used to assess for worsening calibre, thrombus formation, or arterial occlusion, which may necessitate a change in management.
- If intracranial MT fails or achieves only limited recanalisation, avoiding stenting and the associated need for antiplatelet therapy would be beneficial, given the likelihood of extensive infarction. Literature supports conservative management in these cases for several reasons: recurrent embolisation from dissection is uncommon; the circle of Willis is often functional; carotid artery stenting (CAS) can be technically challenging due to the length of the involved section and the frequently tortuous underlying artery with a cervical loop; and the delayed carotid re-occlusion rate after emergency stenting is appreciable.

- With conservative management of dissection in tandem occlusion, immediate antiplatelet therapy is not mandatory but should be initiated as soon as deemed safe—usually at the 24 h mark, following a CT/CTA assessment.

Angioplasty

- Angioplasty may be performed to address significant residual stenosis of the true lumen, either as a standalone procedure or prior to stenting. However, there is a significant risk of causing thrombus trapped in the dissected segment to embolise distally.
- It may not be necessary if stenting is performed.
- Angioplasty should be performed more gently than in cases of atherosclerotic occlusion, as the artery is already compromised. The luminal narrowing is primarily due to mass effect from intramural haematoma rather than calcific atherosclerotic plaque. A compliant balloon may be all that is required.

Stenting

- Stenting can help prevent the ICA true lumen from narrowing or re-occluding. However, the decision to stent carries risks, including potential worsening of the dissection, perforation, or clot formation/ embolisation.
- Perforation of the carotid artery within the carotid sheath generally carries low morbidity and can often be managed conservatively, although an expanding haematoma in the neck can rarely lead to airway compromise. Perforation within the intradural ICA obviously can lead to life-threatening SAH.
- Acute stenting may be considered in cases of persistent brain hypoperfusion (e.g. isolated anterior circulation or incomplete circle of Willis), high-grade residual stenosis, early ICA re-occlusion after intracranial recanalisation, or the presence of thrombus at the level of dissection.
- Stenting is more straightforward if the dissection is limited to the cervical segment. Standard techniques can be applied. Ideally, the entire length of the dissection should be stented to minimise the risk of distal progression or recurrence.
- Stenting the mid and distal cervical ICA can be technically challenging in the presence of significant tortuosity or vascular loops. In such cases, the use of flexible and navigable carotid stents like Roadsaver (Terumo) may be beneficial. Alternatively, the ICA can be straightened using a stiff wire. An intermediate catheter can then be advanced, and a flexible guide catheter navigated over it into the distal ICA. The stent is inserted, the guide catheter is withdrawn with the stent in place, and the stent is deployed. This process can be repeated by progressively withdrawing the guide catheter down the ICA to place consecutive stents.
- Most ICA dissections originate at the level of the skull base, though they may extend proximally and, less commonly, distally over varying lengths. Stenting the cervical ICA to cross and secure the proximal end of the dissection, thereby tacking down the intimal flap, may suffice. A self-expanding carotid stent is typically used, followed by gentle angioplasty. However, in cases involving significant narrowing of the entire cervical ICA, distal cervical ICA, or intracranial ICA, a more extensive longitudinal stent construct with overlapping stents may be required. This is

generally performed from distal to proximal to fully cover the dissected segment.

- For dissections extending into the petrous or cavernous ICA, the transition from cervical to intracranial ICA can be challenging to stent due to vascular tortuosity and the smaller calibre of the parent artery. Rigid self-expanding carotid stents are often difficult to use in these situations and may exacerbate the situation. There are reports of flow diverters and braided stents being used effectively for the intracranial portion of dissections. Additionally, self-expanding laser-cut intracranial stents can be considered, provided they are of sufficient diameter.

Tandem occlusion with internal carotid artery web

(See Figure 9.13.)

- A 'web' is a shelf-like intimal flap originating from the posterior wall of the internal carotid bulb, projecting into the arterial lumen. Thrombus can form at this site and embolise distally. The pathogenesis of carotid web is not well understood and, due to its rarity, there are currently no evidence-based guidelines.
- If thrombus remains visible attached to the web at the beginning of the procedure, it can often be retrieved using an aspiration catheter, to avoid recurrent embolisation during the procedure.
- If the intracranial occlusion is treated but the carotid web remains untreated, there is a high risk of recurrent embolism. A systematic review in 2022 by Patel et al. reported that in patients with stroke attributable to

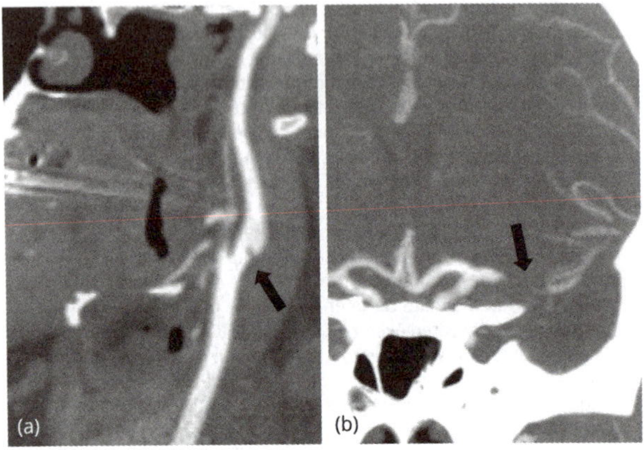

Figure 9.13 Tandem web dissection. (a) Lateral maximal intensity projection (MIP) computed tomography angiography (CTA) image of the left carotid artery shows a small linear filling defect in the proximal internal carotid artery (black arrow), consistent with a web. (b) Coronal MIP CTA image of the intracranial circulation shows thrombotic occlusion of the left M1, due to embolisation of thrombus from the web. The thrombus subsequently lysed after the administration of intravenous tissue plasminogen activator. Images courtesy of Dr Joseph Gemmete.

an ICA web, intervention (either stenting or CEA) was associated with no recurrent ischaemic events, compared to a recurrence rate of 26.8% in the untreated group.

- The decision to stent must be carefully weighed against the risk of haemorrhagic conversion of an existing infarct due to the necessity of initiating antiplatelet therapy. Other management options include treatment with antiplatelet therapy alone, anticoagulation, delayed stenting by a few days, or CEA.

Antiplatelet regimen after stenting

- Multiple antithrombotic regimens are available, but no clearly superior option has been identified. The choice should be based on factors such as infarct volume, time from symptom onset, and the potential risk of sICH:
  - Aspirin alone (300 mg loading dose) can be administered at the time of stenting (IV, nasogastric tube, or rectally) or shortly afterward when the patient is awake, followed by a loading dose of clopidogrel or ticagrelor at 24 h, provided a CT head excludes haemorrhage and a CTA confirms stent patency. The disadvantage is the risk of stent thrombosis within the first 24 h when using aspirin alone (this is not always symptomatic, however, depending on collaterals).
  - DAPT (aspirin plus clopidogrel or ticagrelor) loading doses can be given at the time of stenting or shortly after (administered orally, rectally, via nasogastric tube, or IV for aspirin). These are then continued at 24 h following a CT/CTA. This regimen provides higher stent patency rates compared to aspirin alone. However, the drawbacks include an increased risk of ICH and the lack of reversibility once the agents are administered.
  - GP IIb/IIIa or inhibitors (e.g. eptifibatide or tirofiban) can be given as an IV bolus dose at the time of stenting, followed by an infusion until dual antiplatelets are loaded at 24 h after the CT/CTA. An overlapping period of 2 h is recommended after administering oral antiplatelet medication. The advantage of this approach is the higher stent patency rates and the ability to discontinue the infusion if ICH develops. The disadvantage is a higher haemorrhage risk compared to aspirin alone. This can be given following thrombolysis: the SNIS Standards and Guidelines Committee states:

    > In patients undergoing CAS during emergent large vessel occlusion ischaemic stroke treatment, it may be reasonable to administer a loading dose of intravenous or oral glycoprotein IIb/IIIa or P2Y12 inhibitor followed by maintenance intravenous infusion or oral dosing to prevent stent thrombosis whether or not the patient has received thrombolytic therapy (Class IIb, C-LD).

- Cangrelor has been used with some success. This is an IV non-thienopyridine ATP analogue P2Y12 antagonist (see 'Glycoprotein IIb/IIIa receptor inhibitors', p. 103). It is non-competitive, reversible, and requires no metabolic activation. The agent has a rapid onset of action of 2–6 min. An advantage is that normal platelet function resumes 60–90 min after cessation, in cases of haemorrhage. It is given as an IV bolus dose followed by IV infusion, with conversion to ticagrelor agents at 24 h (the infusion is stopped following a 1 h overlap).

- Data from the TITAN registry, a collaborative effort to evaluate the best therapeutic approach for acute stroke due to tandem lesions, suggests that CAS with antithrombotic agents results in better recanalisation rates and functional outcomes. An ongoing RCT (also called TITAN) is currently addressing this question.
- The use of unfractionated heparin during acute stenting is discouraged due to higher risks of sICH.

Further reading

Behme D, Knauth M, Psychogios MN. Retriever wire supported carotid artery revascularisation (ReWiSed CARe) in acute ischaemic stroke with underlying tandem occlusion caused by an internal carotid artery dissection: technical note. Interv Neuroradiol. 2017;23(3):289–292.

Gory B, Piotin M, Haussen DC, et al. Thrombectomy in acute stroke with tandem occlusions from dissection versus atherosclerotic cause. Stroke. 2017;48(11):3145–3148.

Marnat G, Lapergue B, Sibon I, et al. Safety and outcome of carotid dissection stenting during the treatment of tandem occlusions: a pooled analysis of TITAN and ETIS. Stroke. 2020;51(12):3713–3718.

Min X, Du J, Bai X, et al. Antegrade or retrograde approach for the management of tandem occlusions in acute ischaemic stroke: a systematic review and meta-analysis. Front Neurol. 2022;12:757665.

Patel SD, Otite FO, Topiwala K, et al. Interventional compared with medical management of symptomatic carotid web: a systematic review. J Stroke Cerebrovasc Dis. 2022;31(10):106682.

Sgreccia A, Desilles JP, Costalat V, et al. Combined technique for internal carotid artery terminus or middle cerebral artery occlusions in the ASTER2 trial. Stroke. 2024;55(2):376–384.

Wilson MP, Murad MH, Krings T, et al. Management of tandem occlusions in acute ischaemic stroke intracranial versus extracranial first and extracranial stenting versus angioplasty alone: a systematic review and meta-analysis. J Neurointerv Surg. 2018;10(8):721–728.

Mechanical thrombectomy and intracranial atherosclerotic disease

ICAD accounts for 5–10% of strokes in the European population, but the prevalence is significantly higher in the Asian population, reaching 40–50%. Globally, it may represent the most common cause of stroke.

ICAD represents the most common reason for failed MT. Patients with failed reperfusion are known to have higher rates of severe disability and death. However, there is disagreement regarding the safety of angioplasty and stenting due to the need for antiplatelet therapy.

Recognition

ICAD may be seen directly as a visible stenosis, causing underperfusion of the territory despite the vessel still being patent. However, if severe stenosis or *in situ* thrombus formation leads to vessel occlusion, the underlying cause is usually not immediately apparent. A degree of suspicion is warranted in the presence of the following:

- Mural calcification in the occluded vessel.
- Absence of CT hyperdense sign or MRI susceptibility sign.
- Evidence of atherosclerotic disease in other vessels.
- Old watershed infarcts in the territory.
- The presence of well-developed collaterals (which form gradually as the stenosis progresses).
- Disproportionally low clinical deficit compared to occlusion location/ tissue at risk.
- Absence of atrial fibrillation.
- The location of occlusion in the mid-section of the vessel (truncal type occlusion) rather than at a branch point.
- A visible stenosis becoming evident after thrombectomy.
- Early re-occlusion of the vessel after thrombectomy. This occurs due to *in situ* thrombosis caused by activated plaque, which can be exacerbated by the microtrauma associated with MT.

Evidence

- Retrospective studies have shown promising reperfusion results after acute stenting in terms of mRS score, functional independence, and mortality.
- The ANGEL-REBOOT RCT looked at rescue therapies in MT. It involved 348 patients over 18 months at Chinese stroke centres, in patients with ICAD-related LVO. Most patients received only balloon angioplasty, with stents used in just 35.2% of cases. The study found no treatment effect for this strategy.
- At the time of writing, no RCTs have evaluated the effects of early bail-out stenting in thrombectomy ICAD-related or otherwise. The ICARUS RCT evaluating this question is ongoing.

Technique

(See Figure 9.14.)

- For MT in ICAD both stent retrievers and aspiration catheters can be used. However, be aware that the vessel may be more fragile due to the pre-existing disease.

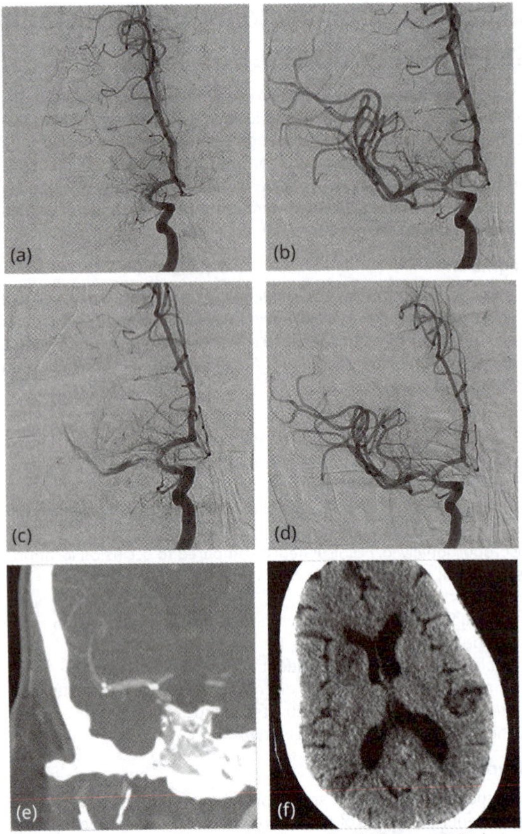

Figure 9.14 Acute stenting of intracranial atherosclerotic disease (ICAD) during mechanical thrombectomy. (a) Digital subtraction angiography shows proximal right M1 middle cerebral artery occlusion in a patient with dense left-sided weakness. (b) After the first aspiration thrombectomy pass, the artery recanalised with residual stenosis. (c) A second angiogram after 2 min shows thrombus reaccumulating and vessel shutdown. (d) After a second pass the same issue occurred, therefore a 4.5 × 21 Atlas stent was deployed across the stenosis using an SL-10 microcatheter, achieving persistent recanalisation. (e) Computed tomography angiography 1 day post-procedure shows the vessel open between stent markers. (f) Plain computed tomography reveals a small basal ganglia infarct, common after stent placement in ICAD due to occlusion of vessel perforators.

- After successful clot removal, stenosis will be visible. A brief observation period of a few minutes is recommended to monitor for re-occlusion. If improving on delayed angiograms, the appearance may represent spasm rather than a true stenosis and it may be observed further.

- A second thrombectomy pass is reasonable if there is continued doubt or suspicion that the cause is resistant thrombus.
- However, multiple attempts at thrombectomy in ICAD-associated LVO may dissect or even perforate the vessel. If stenting is considered, it is probably better to do earlier in the procedure rather than as a bail-out after multiple failed passes.
- In cases of significant residual stenosis or recurrent re-occlusion, balloon angioplasty or intracranial stenting may be indicated. Stenting will necessitate concurrent antiplatelet therapy, which might not be appropriate in the presence of large infarction cores or delayed presentations.
- Balloon angioplasty can be performed alone if there is valid reason to avoid DAPT. Evidence suggests this will provide a less durable result than angioplasty and stenting, however.
- Bolus IV antiplatelet agents also have been used successfully if stenting is not going to be performed.
- On-table cone beam CT first excludes haemorrhage particularly if the case is prolonged with multiple passes.
- The technique for angioplasty and stenting is described in 'Intracranial atherosclerotic disease stenting', p. 410. Both balloon-mounted and laser-cut stents can be used. For specifics relevant to the posterior circulation, see 'Posterior circulation thrombectomy', p. 368.
- Consider using an angioplasty balloon that allows stent deployment through it, eliminating the need for an intracranial microwire exchange, such as the NeuroSpeed PTA Balloon with the CREDO Stent (Acandis). If an exchange is necessary, shaping the microwire tip into a 'J' configuration can help prevent complications of perforation or dissection.
- Perform submaximal angioplasty up to maximum of 80% of the normal arterial diameter, selecting the balloon diameter accordingly and ensuring it covers the stenosis.
- Use an inflation device with a manometer and refer to the compliance chart included with the balloon packaging for nominal and burst pressure guidelines. Slow inflation and submaximal angioplasty help prevent snowploughing plaque into perforator origins and reduce the risk of arterial rupture or dissection. Angioplasty should be conducted before stenting and, if needed, again after stent deployment if there is significant residual stenosis.
- Many antiplatelet regimens are available (see 'Tandem occlusion', p. 355). The risk of in-stent thrombosis is significant, and the authors recommend a maximalist approach, starting with a bolus of GP IIb/IIIa inhibitors or cangrelor followed by a continuous infusion. This can be converted to oral DAPT after the procedure, stopping the infusion after a suitable overlap.

Postprocedural management

- Close neurological monitoring is necessary, preferably in an HDU or ICU.
- Clear instructions are essential for managing the antiplatelet regimen, as uncertainty regarding the use of antiplatelet infusions and tablets has led to cases of stent thrombosis.

Further reading

Mohammaden MH, Haussen DC, Al-Bayati AR, et al. Stenting and angioplasty in neurothrombectomy: matched analysis of rescue intracranial stenting versus failed thrombectomy. Stroke. 2022;53(9):2779–2788.

Posterior circulation thrombectomy

Approximately 10–20% of LVO stroke affects the vertebrobasilar system, with significant morbidity, dependence, and mortality.

Evidence

- Two initial RCTs, BASICS and BEST, did not show significant improvement in functional outcome mRS 0–3 at 90 days for MT-treated patients, but recruitment was slow with high crossover rates.
- Two subsequent recent RCTs in 2022 showed positive results for posterior circulation MT:
  - BAOCHE randomised basilar artery occlusion (BAO) patients presenting 6–24 h from onset, with NIHSS score >6, posterior circulation ASPECTS (PC-ASPECTS) score of ≥6, and pons midbrain index score of ≤2.
  - ATTENTION randomised patients with BAO presenting within 12 h of onset, with NIHSS score >10 and PC-ASPECTS ≥6.
- The proportion of favourable outcomes with MT was similar in all four RCTs, but the majority of the effect was due to the outcomes of clinically poor patients in the non-MT group in both ATTENTION and BAOCHE. In the subgroup of patients with a NIHSS score<10, a meta-analysis of the BASICS and BAOCHE showed no difference in outcomes between thrombectomy and best medical therapy. The number of patients with NIHSS score <10 was, however, low as they were excluded from the ATTENTION trial, and BAOCHE only included 17 such patients.
- However, as trials excluded those >80 years (BAOCHE) or 85 years (BASICS) and one required better imaging/mRS if >80 years (ATTENTION), and only one trial (BAOCHE) enrolled >12 h post symptom onset, these two subgroups are very under-represented in RCTs; therefore, caution is required regarding performing MT in these groups.
- Whether BAO patients with mild symptoms should be treated with MT, IVT with more inclusive criteria (as in the BASICS trial), or carefully monitored for clinical deterioration without immediate reperfusion therapy remains unclear.
- NIHSS score (anterior circulation) underestimates clinical severity in posterior circulation stroke. It is important to identify BAO patients presenting with low NIHSS scores with potentially disabling symptoms, who might benefit from MT.
- The posterior NIHSS score is a modified version of the anterior circulation NIHSS including additional points for gait/truncal ataxia and bulbar signs. Use of the posterior NIHSS is recommended.
  - Posterior NIHSS shows higher prognostic accuracy and may be useful to identify patients with anterior circulation NIHSS score <10 at higher risk of poor outcome.
  - This score consists of the standard NIHSS score + the following: gait/truncal ataxia (3 points), dysphagia (4 points), abnormal cough (5 points).
- Exclusions in BAOCHE and ATTENTION included cerebellar infarction with a significant space-occupying effect, complete bilateral thalamic or bilateral brainstem infarction, and simultaneous occlusions in both the anterior and posterior circulation.

- The percentage of patients treated with angioplasty and/or stenting was high in the three Chinese trials (BEST, ATTENTION, and BAOCHE), ranging from 30% to 55%, reflecting the high rate of ICAD seen in Asian populations.
- **In conclusion, the present data suggest optimum therapy if NIHSS score ≥10 is IVT + MT. Caution should be exercised regarding MT if extensive bilateral and/or brainstem ischaemic changes.**

Indications

Basilar occlusion

- MT in addition to best medical therapy is recommended in patients presenting with BAO up to 24 h from onset/last seen well with moderate to severe stroke symptoms, and without extensive ischaemic changes on baseline (PC-ASPECTS 7–10). Quality of evidence overall is low and only considers patients with NIHSS score ≥10. Treatment effect for MT is stronger for proximal and middle BAO.
- There is some evidence that patients with mild stroke symptoms and BAO may not benefit from MT due to a higher rate of sICH over best medical therapy, and lack of evidence demonstrating improved functional outcome with MT over best medical therapy alone. These patients should be very closely clinically monitored as neurological deterioration can occur, and MT may then be warranted.
- In BAO with infarction at baseline more extensive than included in RCTs (i.e. PC-ASPECTS 0–5), consider other prognostic variables such as pre-stroke handicap, age, and frailty before offering reperfusion therapy.
- In BAO, if there is very extensive bilateral established infarction, particularly bilateral extensive brainstem involvement, thrombectomy is unlikely to benefit the patient, with likely poor outcome, high level of disability and dependence, and possibly 'locked-in' syndrome.

Isolated V4 occlusion

- Evidence is lacking for best medical therapy of isolated V4 segment vertebral arterial occlusion. It is considered an LVO.
- Consider MT if stroke symptoms are moderate to severe and ensure ataxia and bulbar symptoms are not overlooked in decision-making.
- Indications for V4 segment MT include a contralateral occluded or hypoplastic V4 segment, risking the entire posterior circulation, particularly if the posterior communicating arteries are absent or small.
- Also consider V4 segment MT if thrombus is covering the PICA origin, there are significant stroke symptoms, and PICA territory is not already infarcted.

PCA thrombectomy

- Evidence for PCA vessel MT is also lacking. The P1 segment is a relatively large-calibre artery, and given the multiple perforating arteries that can arise from this segment, occlusion can be associated with significant stroke symptoms.
- For isolated P2 and more distal PCA occlusions, indication for MT remains individualised as MeVO trials have failed to demonstrate consistent benefit.

Imaging

- The goal of imaging is to exclude haemorrhage and identify acute infarction and site of arterial occlusion. CT or MRI can be used.
- The extent of acute infarction can be evaluated using the PC-ASPECTS score on NCCT or MRI DWI:
  - The PC-ASPECTS is a 10-point scoring system, with points lost for each region affected. In view of the high morbidity of brainstem infarction, the score is weighted with pons and midbrain both assigned 2 points each. Other zones include bilateral thalami, occipital lobes, and cerebellar hemispheres (all of which have 1 point each).
  - Lower PC-ASPECTS scores indicate more extensive infarction. PC-ASPECTS score was used as an imaging selection criterion for inclusion in trials including ATTENTION and BAOCHE and is incorporated into the guidelines for posterior circulation stroke.
  - Interpretation of PC-ASPECTS on CT can be difficult due to beam hardening artefact at the skull base, with poor evaluation of brainstem. DWI is more sensitive for detection of acute infarction.
- The pons–midbrain index is an 8-point scoring system which can also predict clinical outcome in BAO:
  - This evaluates extent of low attenuation in the pons and midbrain on CTA source images or on DWI.
  - A score of 0 implies no low attenuation in the brainstem and a score of 8 implies >50% low attenuation bilaterally in the pons and midbrain.
  - The pons–midbrain index was utilised together with PC-ASPECTS as an imaging section criterion in the BAOCHE RCT, with cut off score for inclusion at ≤2.
- The Basilar Artery on Computed Tomography Angiography (BATMAN) score is a 10-point scoring system that evaluates collateral circulation and thrombus burden, which can predict functional outcome after BAO. This scoring system has not been validated.
- There is no current recommendation for the use of advanced imaging using perfusion or MRI DWI–FLAIR mismatch for decision-making in posterior circulation stroke. Perfusion may be helpful in PCA occlusion evaluating established infarction and penumbra in the occluded territory which includes the thalami. MRI is more sensitive for brainstem infarction and is helpful in patients found with low GCS score, or who deteriorate prior to or during transfer from primary (PSCs) to comprehensive stroke centres (CSCs), requiring intubation with long transfer time. The likelihood of established brainstem infarction is higher these patients.

Technique

- Carefully evaluate available vascular imaging. Determine the site of occlusion and normal variant anatomy that can affect decision-making or contribute to complications if not identified, such as foetal-type PCA which can be misinterpreted as PCA occlusion on DSA. Assessment of the extracranial vertebral arteries is essential, evaluating for stenosis, occlusion, free-floating thrombus, and dissection.
- MT for BAO or other posterior circulation stroke can be performed using stent retriever, aspiration alone, or combined techniques. 4 mm stent retrievers are commonly used in the basilar artery and P1 PCA, with 3 mm devices for the more distal PCAs. 6 mm stent retrievers can be used in large-calibre basilar arteries.

- There is no RCT evidence to support the best first-line technique for posterior circulation stroke, but some evidence supports aspiration thrombectomy. A recent meta-analysis demonstrated that patients with posterior circulation stroke receiving aspiration thrombectomy achieved better recanalisation, first-pass effect, and shorter procedure time. Expert opinion in the latest European Stroke Organisation/European Society of Minimally Invasive Neurological Therapy guideline recommended direct aspiration as the first approach instead of stent retrievers.
- Many dominant vertebral arteries can accommodate 8 Fr guide catheters. If the calibre is smaller than average or very tortuous, a 6 Fr catheter might be needed.

Top of basilar strategy

(See Figure 9.15.)

- Occlusion of this location is most likely embolic, either artery-to-artery embolus or cardioembolic, and is atypical for underlying atherosclerotic disease.
- Aspiration is favoured as first-line technique. Consider the calibre of the basilar artery. The basilar can usually accommodate a large-bore 0.068–0.072" catheter. The aspiration catheter can be advanced alone to the occlusion from the guide catheter in the vertebral artery with the snaking technique, but tortuosity, particularly at the V3 segment, may require insertion of a microwire and microcatheter. If there is still significant tortuosity and difficulty navigating, consider insertion of a device reducing ledge effect, e.g. Wedge (MicroVention), AXS Offset Delivery Assist Catheter (Stryker), or SENDit (Penumbra). These also help the aspiration catheter navigate to the proximal end of the occlusion.
- Allow at least two passes with a first-line technique, before moving to second-line rescue therapy. If aspiration is used first, stent retrieval would be second line, and vice versa.

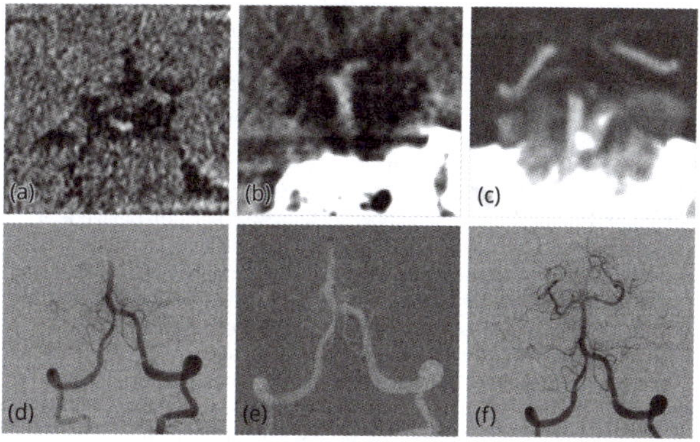

Figure 9.15 Basilar artery aspiration thrombectomy. (a) Axial computed tomography shows a hyperdensity in the distal basilar artery. (b, c) The hyperdense clot extends into the proximal posterior cerebral arteries. (d) Digital subtraction angiography via the left vertebral artery confirms distal basilar thrombus. (e) Fluoroscopy shows a 0.072" aspiration catheter in the distal basilar. (f) Post-procedure imaging confirms complete recanalisation of the vessel.

- For stent retrieval, navigation of wire and microcatheter should ideally be into one of the PCAs. If one PCA is occluded and other is patent, navigate into the occluded PCA, beyond the thrombus, and then deploy the stent retriever.
- Beware inadvertent navigation into a small SCA (thinking it is the PCA) because subsequent deployment of a stent retriever can result in haemorrhage.
- Combination technique with an aspiration catheter or retrieval into the aspiration catheter or guide catheter should be with concomitant aspiration.
- If it is not possible to navigate into the PCA, the stent retriever can be deployed from microcatheter position at the tip of the basilar, and while the thrombus is not fully covered, retrieval may still result in a successful recanalisation.
- If resistant clot is suspected, with failure to recanalise with second-line therapy, consider further change of technique, including use of NIMBUS geometric clot extractor (CERENOVUS), a device designed specifically to target tough clot, or dual stent retriever technique deployed from each PCA back into basilar providing there is no imaging evidence to indicate a hypoplastic P1 segment.

Proximal basilar strategy

- This may be of embolic aetiology, but be aware this is a common site for ICAD.
- Mild stroke symptoms despite proximal BAO or fluctuating symptoms can be associated with ICAD-related occlusion. Imaging frequently demonstrates atherosclerotic disease also involving V4 segments of the vertebral arteries with mural calcification and variable degrees of stenosis. Parenchymal imaging may suggest posterior watershed infarcts, or old brainstem lacunar infarcts as further clues for underlying ICAD.
- Aspiration can still be the first-line technique at the proximal end of the occlusion, particularly if the aetiology is unknown. Stent retrieval, or a combination technique, can also be used. If thrombus is retrieved and the artery recanalised, evaluate on angiography for any underlying arterial narrowing. If there is no narrowing, residual occlusion, or thrombus, further intervention is not necessary.
- If the artery is recanalised with underlying narrowing, this may reflect ICAD; alternatively, iatrogenic vasospasm or partially occlusive thrombus. If narrowing is not flow limiting, wait, perform delayed angiography, and re-evaluate. If improving on delayed angiograms, this is likely spasm. If stable, and not worsening, there may be underlying ICAD but acute intervention with angioplasty/stenting may not be required. The patient should, however, be very closely monitored for any neurological deterioration post-procedure as there is a risk of re-occlusion, and further MT may be required if clinically appropriate.
- If post-pass narrowing is worsening on delayed angiography or the artery re-occludes, consider ICAD or, less likely, propagation of partially occlusive thrombus. Perform at least one further pass, using a stent retriever. Deployment of a fully radiopaque stent retriever allows best evaluation for areas of poor stent opening/narrowing which can indicate underlying stenosis from ICAD (Figure 9.16). Antegrade flow during angiography with the stent *in situ* suggests stenting will be effective.

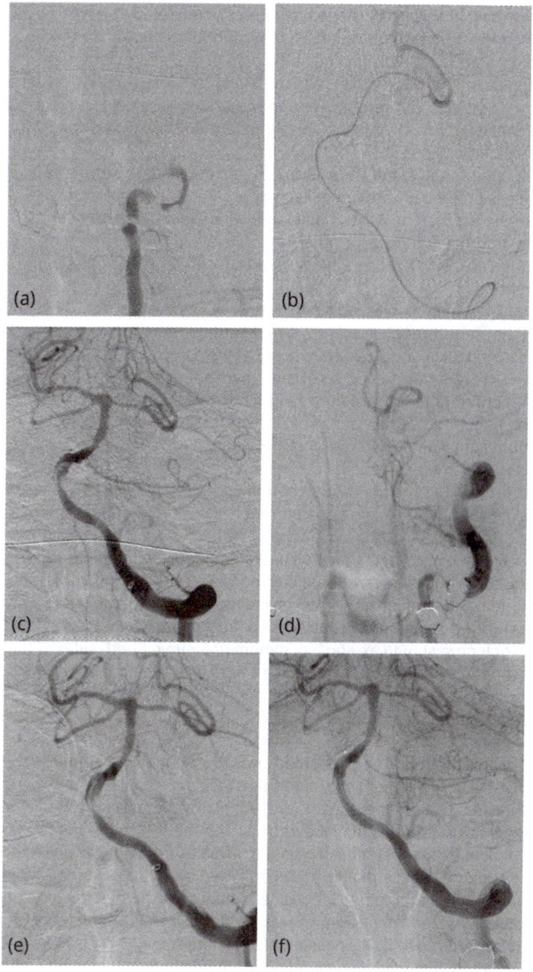

Figure 9.16 Acute intracranial atherosclerotic disease basilar stenting. (a) Digital subtraction angiography reveals occlusion in the left vertebral artery. (b) Four aspiration catheter passes failed to clear it. Switching to a Trevo 4 × 30 mm stent retriever successfully recanalised the V4 segment and basilar artery, with minor residual stenosis. Intravenous aspirin was given. (c) Angiography confirmed the artery was open, and the patient was woken up. (d) The patient, however, deteriorated 4 h later, with re-occlusion confirmed by angiogram. (e) Aspiration thrombectomy and EMBOTRAP stent retriever reopened the vessel. (f) A 3 × 23 mm balloon-expandable stent was deployed to improve blood flow. Post-procedure, 300 mg of clopidogrel was administered, leading to patient improvement. Images courtesy of Dr Sarah Power.

Post-pass, if the artery is open, and the clot retrieved, this may have been resistant thrombus, but as a precautionary measure, delayed angiography should again be performed. If the artery continues to have significant underlying stenosis, worsening stenosis, remains occluded, or re-occludes, further intervention with 0.014" wire navigation across stenosis/occlusion, and angioplasty ± stenting should be strongly considered.

- On-table cone beam CT first excludes haemorrhage, particularly if the case is prolonged with multiple passes.
- Angioplasty can be performed alone if there is concern for contrast staining/haemorrhage or other reason to avoid DAPT. Literature suggests this will provide a less durable result than angioplasty and stenting.
- Consider an angioplasty balloon that will allow subsequent deployment of the stent through it, thereby avoiding requirement for an intracranial microwire exchange manoeuvre, e.g. NeuroSpeed PTA Balloon and CREDO Stent (Acandis). If an exchange manoeuvre is necessary, forming a 'J' configuration to exchange length microwire tip can be protective, and help avoid complications of wire perforation or dissection.
- Submaximal angioplasty up to a *maximum* of 80% of the normal arterial diameter should be performed. Choose the balloon diameter accordingly. Purge the balloon before use, typically with 50:50 contrast saline solution. The same concentration is used for inflation, and an inflation device with a manometer should be used. Refer to the compliance chart in the balloon packaging detailing nominal and burst pressure—the diameter of the balloon varies with inflation pressure. Submaximal angioplasty protects against snowploughing plaque into perforator origins, and reduces risk of arterial rupture or dissection.
- Stent length should extend a minimum of 3 mm on both sides of the stenotic lesion. The stent should be a little oversized to the maximal normal diameter of the artery. The degree of oversizing varies by stent type, with recommended vessel size usually provided on stent packaging.
- Angioplasty should be performed prior to stenting and, if required, also post-stent deployment with significant residual stenosis.
- Once the decision is made to stent, antiplatelet medication should be administered. GP IIb/IIIa inhibitors are commonly used as the primary antiplatelet agent at time of stenting, given as a weight-calculated bolus (consider 50% of cardiology dose), followed by an infusion for 12–24 h prior to transition to DAPT. Consider additional aspirin at the time of stenting, which can be administered IV if available. Continue DAPT for 6 months, followed by a single antiplatelet agent.

V4 strategy

- Indications are outlined above. Aspiration thrombectomy can be considered first line; however, stent retrieval and combination techniques can be used. A V4 segment occlusion can reflect underlying ICAD, and management is similar to that outlined above for BAO.

PCA strategy

- The P1 segment is of relatively large calibre and will often accommodate a large-bore aspiration catheter, which can be navigated into the artery over a microcatheter or device to reduce ledge effect if needed. As catheter size is closely matched to the artery, aspiration is very effective. Stent retrieval and combined techniques can also be used.

- Smaller aspiration catheters, e.g. 3–5 Fr, can be used for more distal P2 and P3 segment occlusions. Stent retrievers, e.g. 3 mm diameter, are appropriate in P2 and P3 segments and as the PCA is relatively straight, there is less shear effect and vessel straightening than in M3 MCA occlusion. Addition of an aspiration catheter into the PCA P2 segment to allow co-aspiration/combination technique is protective for the basilar artery.
- P2 or P3 thrombectomy is probably most frequently currently performed in chasing distal emboli from a more proximal pass.
- For isolated P2 and more distal PCA occlusions, indications for thrombectomy remain individualised.

Tandem occlusion in posterior circulation

- The procedural and technical approach for tandem occlusion in the posterior circulation is similar to that of the anterior circulation (see 'Tandem occlusion', p. 355).
- Options also include antegrade versus retrograde approaches, similar strategies for guide catheter access into the vertebral artery as for the ICA, aspiration of vertebral artery thrombus, access to intracranial arterial occlusion, and consideration of definitive management of underlying vertebral artery stenosis with stenting. The retrograde approach is preferred with BAO as it allows for more rapid recanalisation of the intracranial occlusion.
- If the tandem involves a single vertebral artery, with patency of the contralateral vertebral artery, with minimal or no disease, of reasonable calibre, without a hypoplastic V4 segment, then access through the 'clean' vertebral artery is preferred because of more rapid access to and recanalisation of the intracranial occlusion, and avoidance of risk of distal emboli from accessing the diseased vertebral. The diseased occluded vertebral is likely asymptomatic given a patent contralateral good-calibre vertebral and can be managed conservatively.
- If variant anatomy with a hypoplastic contralateral vertebral artery and/or V4 segment, then access to the intracranial occlusion will be through the diseased/occluded/stenosed dominant vertebral.
- Following recanalisation of the intracranial occlusion, definitive management of the diseased dominant vertebral artery should be considered if there is residual significant stenosis, to secure inflow to the posterior circulation (Figure 9.17). Consider stenting acutely or angioplasty and deferred stenting if there is concern regarding high bleeding risk with early antiplatelet administration.
- If both vertebral arteries are diseased and occluded or significantly stenosed, or bilaterally dissected, if co-dominant, consider access through the least diseased artery, otherwise access the dominant vertebral artery and secure recanalisation of the dominant artery following intracranial MT.
- For stenting across the vertebral artery origin, the proximal end of the stent should project into the subclavian. Smaller-calibre carotid or balloon-mounted stents, e.g. 5 mm diameter, are usually appropriate. Ensure 0.014" wire access is maintained across the stenosis/dissection and origin of the vertebral following MT.

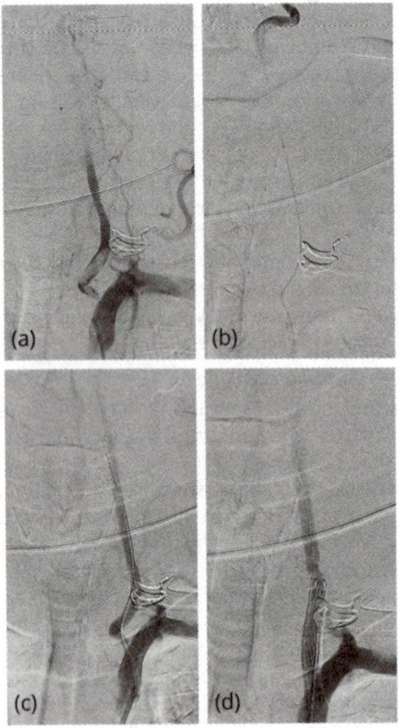

Figure 9.17 Tandem occlusion in the posterior circulation. (a) Angiography via the left subclavian artery identifies severe left vertebral stenosis and distal thrombus. (b) An 8 Fr guide catheter is placed in the subclavian artery, and the stenosis is crossed with a 0.014" microwire and microcatheter (0.035" wire attempts failed). Microcatheter angiography confirmed intraluminal position. (c) Angioplasty with a 4 × 30 mm non-compliant balloon and thrombus aspiration was performed. (d) Due to a contralateral hypoplastic vertebral artery, stenting was necessary. Repeat angioplasty with a 6 × 30 mm balloon was followed by placement of a 6 mm carotid stent. Images courtesy of Dr Sarah Power.

- While a distal protection device can be used, the orientation of the stent in the subclavian post-deployment, particularly on the right, and poor proximal support given guide catheter position in the subclavian, can make it difficult to re-enter the stent with recapture of the sheath of the distal protection device. For the same reasons, it can be difficult to navigate an angioplasty balloon into the proximal end of the stent, particularly on the right after deployment. Avoiding use of a distal protection device and performing angioplasty with a 4 mm and subsequently a 6 mm balloon at the site of stenosis prior to stent deployment can avoid these issues.

Further reading

Alemseged F, Rocco A, Arba F, et al. Posterior National Institutes of Health Stroke Scale improves prognostic accuracy in posterior circulation stroke. Stroke. 2022;53(4):1247–1255.

Huo X, Xiong Y, Huang X, et al. Aspiration versus stent retriever for posterior circulation stroke: a meta-analysis. CNS Neurosci Ther. 2023;29(2):525–537.

Intercollegiate Stroke Working Party. National Clinical Guideline for Stroke for the UK and Ireland [Internet]. 2023. http://www.strokeguideline.org

Jovin TG, Li C, Wu L, et al. Trial of thrombectomy 6 to 24 hours after stroke due to basilar-artery occlusion. N Engl J Med. 2022;387(15):1373–1384.

Langezaal LCM, van der Hoeven EJRJ, Mont'Alverne FJA, et al. Endovascular therapy for stroke due to basilar-artery occlusion. N Engl J Med. 2021;384(20):1910–1920.

Liu X, Dai Q, Ye R, et al. Endovascular treatment versus standard medical treatment for vertebrobasilar artery occlusion (BEST): an open-label, randomised controlled trial. Lancet Neurol. 2020;19(2):115–122.

Strbian D, Tsivgoulis G, Ospel J, et al. European Stroke Organisation (ESO) and European Society for Minimally Invasive Neurological Therapy (ESMINT) guideline on acute management of basilar artery occlusion. J Neurointerv Surg. 2024;16(9):e7.

Tao C, Nogueira RG, Zhu Y, et al. Trial of endovascular treatment of acute basilar-artery occlusion. N Engl J Med. 2022;387(15):1361–1372.

Xu J, Chen X, Chen S, et al. Endovascular treatment for basilar artery occlusion: a meta-analysis. Stroke Vasc Neurol. 2023;8:e001740.

Medium and distal vessel thrombectomy

- MeVO accounts for 25–40% of ischaemic stroke (largely depending on M2 classification).
- Disability outcomes for MeVOs are lower than those for LVOs. However, 50% of patients do not achieve an excellent clinical outcome and 9% die within 90 days despite optimal medical management, including IVT.
- Recanalisation is closely linked to better functional outcomes, but is achieved in just 20% of patients who do not receive IVT and in fewer than 50% of those who do.
- MT may enable higher rates of recanalisation; however, there are concerns about increased complication rates in smaller, more distal arteries.

Evidence

- Post hoc analysis of seven RCTs in HERMES identified significant benefit for proximal M2 MCA thrombectomy but there were insufficient data to analyse the distal M2 occlusion subgroup.
- While non-randomised data suggested benefit for MeVO MT, two RCTs (ESCAPE-MeVO and DISTAL) found no difference in 90-day mRS, with sICH higher in the EVT group for both studies and mortality also higher in one trial.
- Two recent trials have produced conflicting findings. ORIENTAL MeVO reported improved functional outcomes with EVT in distal or medium vessel occlusion and moderate to severe deficits, with a risk ratio of 1.24 (95% CI 1.07 to 1.44; $P = .004$). The benefit was confined to patients with baseline NIHSS ≥ 8, with no effect in those scoring < 8. DISTALS, using the low profile Tigertriever 13, achieved a composite endpoint of successful reperfusion at 24 hours without sICH in 86.3% of the thrombectomy group compared with 27.7% of controls.
- Current treatment decisions therefore are made on an individual basis.
- For more distal occlusions (DiVOs) there is no robust evidence and procedures are generally only undertaken for very eloquent, easily accessible areas, typically where MT of more proximal occlusion has been performed.

Definitions

Location

- There are varying definitions for the anatomical location of MeVOs due to the inconsistent nomenclature in the existing literature. There is not even a consistent definition for the commencement of the M2 segment (see Chapter 2, 'Middle cerebral artery', p. 44).
- This remains true for ongoing RCTs, with definitions varying as follows:
  - MCA: *proximal*—any part of the M2, non-dominant/co-dominant M2, distal M2; *distal*—M3, M4.
  - ACA: *proximal*—A1; *distal*—A2, A3.
  - PCA: *proximal*—P1, P2; *distal*—P3.

Primary versus secondary

- Primary MeVO results from the same mechanisms that cause LVO, including cardioembolism, arterioembolism, and ICAD.
- Secondary MeVO is due to the dissolution of an LVO, either spontaneously or iatrogenically (during thrombolysis or after MT). This

latter constitutes 20–40%, and is associated with worse outcomes than primary MeVOs.

Imaging

- More distal occlusions are challenging to diagnose on conventional CTA but newer technologies allow for increased detection:
  - Multiphase CTA enhances the conspicuity of DiVO as vessel segments distal to the point of occlusion achieve peak enhancement later than corresponding non-occluded vessels. This enables a thorough examination of the proximal feeding vessels for potential occlusion sites.
  - CTP is useful, allowing the easy identification of perfusion defects. The proximal vessels supplying this territory are then carefully scrutinised for occlusions.
- Additional training and awareness of the significance of diagnosing distal occlusions, the utilisation of more specialist neuroradiologists, together with double reporting, can also reduce the rate of misses.

Indications

- **Due to the conflicting evidence of benefit in RCTs, the exact indications for performing MT in MeVO patients are unknown yet to be determined at time of writing.**
- **Many centres continue to perform MT on proximal M2 MCA vessels in the dominant hemisphere in those presenting less than 6 h with NIHSS and ASPECTS ≥ 6.**

Technical considerations

- Given the distal occlusion site and small vessel size, even slight movements by the patient can lead to complications of vessel rupture or dissection. In addition, navigation is challenging with movement. GA is recommended to minimise patient movement, particularly in those likely to have poor compliance. As always, meticulous BP control is mandatory.
- Identifying the occluded vessel can be more challenging than with LVO. Inspect the pre-procedure imaging to know what to look for. Scrutinisation of the capillary or venous phase on DSA may reveal slow contrast flow proximally into a vessel stump. If the occluded vessel is at a bifurcation point, it may be extremally difficult to visualise angiographically. In this situation, the occlusion may be located by studying areas of reduced perfusion and working backwards to the likely vessel origin. Attempts are then made to probe the expected location of the branch point with a wire or microcatheter.
- The use of longer devices may be necessary to prevent exhausting catheter length.
- It is probable that aspiration catheters are less traumatic than stent retrievers in the distal circulation. Catheters such as the 3MAX, RED 43, ZOOM 35/45/55, Q3/Q4 (MIVI neuro), and Sofia 5 Fr may be utilised.
- Smaller stent retrievers are now available, such as the Solitaire or Trevo 3 mm, pRESET LITE, CatchView mini, and the Tigertriever 13. Smaller, longer, microcatheters are used with these stents. The CatchView mini can be used with the 0.013" Headway Duo 167 and the Tigertriever 13 can be used with Headway Duo 167 or Marathon.

- Distal arteries tend to be more tortuous and can straighten with the withdrawal of a stent retriever producing shear stress at the origin of perforator vessels, resulting in SAH. This can partly be mitigated by utilising an intermediate catheter, which acts as an extra joint, reducing stress on the vessel wall and changing the vector of force during stent withdrawal.
- Given the lack of evidence, adopting the approach that minimises risk may be the appropriate one. This might involve not proceeding, proceeding more slowly and carefully, and bailing out if initial attempts prove unfruitful.

Further reading

Duloquin G, Graber M, Garnier L, et al. Incidence of acute ischaemic stroke with visible arterial occlusion: a population-based study (Dijon Stroke Registry). Stroke. 2020;51(7):2122–2130.

Goyal M, Ospel JM, Ganesh A, et al. Endovascular treatment of stroke due to medium-vessel occlusion. N Engl J Med. 2025;392(14):1385–1395.

Menon BK, Hill MD, Davalos A, et al. Efficacy of endovascular thrombectomy in patients with M2 segment middle cerebral artery occlusions: meta-analysis of data from the HERMES Collaboration. J Neurointerv Surg. 2019;11(11):1065–1069.

Ospel JM, Menon BK, Demchuk AM, et al. Clinical course of acute ischaemic stroke due to medium vessel occlusion with and without intravenous alteplase treatment. Stroke. 2020;51(11):3232–3240.

Psychogios M, Brehm A, Ribo M, et al. Endovascular treatment for stroke due to occlusion of medium or distal vessels. N Engl J Med. 2025;392(14):1374–1384.

Paediatric thrombectomy

Paediatric arterial ischaemic stroke is rare, constituting 1–2% of all strokes (1.6 per 100,000 per year in the UK), yet it may result in significant morbidity in children. Stroke-specific mortality rate is reportedly around 3–6%. Among survivors, around one-third suffer moderate to severe long-term disability. In those with LVO treated conservatively, nearly three-quarters experience moderate to severe disability or death at 3 months.

Advances in neuroimaging and interventional techniques have increased the feasibility of MT. However, the limited incidence of paediatric stroke and its more varied aetiology pose major challenges for diagnosis and treatment trailing.

Clinical presentation

Symptoms may be non-specific and stroke recognition in children is often delayed. Clinical manifestations vary by age:

- Infants often present with seizures, irritability, or evolving hemiparesis.
- Older children typically exhibit focal neurological deficits.

Aetiology

About half of childhood stroke is due to arteriopathies such as focal cerebral arteriopathy (FCA), dissection, and moyamoya. After age 8, cerebral haemodynamics become similar to those of adults, with comparable mechanisms and implications for stroke.

- FCA: the most common cause of anterior circulation stroke in the non-cardiac paediatric patient. It is characterised by unifocal and unilateral stenosis or irregularity of the large arteries of the anterior circulation. The FCA-i (inflammatory) subtype is due to an inflammatory or infectious process. Post-varicella arteriopathy (occurring within a year of varicella zoster virus infection) accounts for up to one-half of cases. FCA-i often demonstrates unilateral arterial irregularity, stenosis, or occlusion usually involving the M1, A1, or terminal ICA. Banding in the M1 MCA is pathognomonic.
- Dissection: classified as subtype FCA-d (dissection), it is more common in the posterior circulation. Trauma is the most common cause.
- Moyamoya (Japanese, 'puff of smoke'): a chronic non-inflammatory steno-occlusive arteriopathy.
  - Moyamoya *disease* is stenosis of the supraclinoid ICA with the development of an extensive collateral network, giving rise to the name of the condition.
  - Moyamoya *syndrome* is secondary to other medical disorders, e.g. Down syndrome, sickle cell disease, or neurofibromatosis.
- Cardiac disease: including congenital heart disease, structural heart defects, cardiac procedures, and cardiomyopathy. Cardioembolic stroke should be suspected with a history of cardiac disease. Multiple vascular territories involved suggests embolism.
- Haematological disorders: include genetic prothrombotic disorders and sickle cell disease.
- Infections: meningitis and viral infections including varicella zoster virus (see above).

- Cancer: due to a variety of mechanisms including radiotherapy-induced cerebrovascular changes, mass effect from tumours, and cancer-related coagulopathy.
- Metabolic stroke: disorders such as mitochondrial diseases (e.g. MELAS (mitochondrial encephalomyopathy, lactic acidosis, and stroke)), amino acid metabolism disorders, or hypoglycaemia lead to brain energy failure rather than vascular occlusion. Prior to 8 years old, paediatric brains are more metabolically active, making them more vulnerable to energy failure. They often do not follow vascular territories. Diagnosis involves biochemical tests and genetic screening, while management focuses on treating the metabolic disorder, supportive care, and preventing triggers.
- Perinatal stroke: usually due to placental embolism through the foramen ovale, venous infarction, or cervical traction injury.
- Stroke mimics: stroke mimics are more prevalent in children. Migraine, postictal paralysis, Bell's palsy, metabolic disturbances, inflammatory disease, and infections can closely resemble stroke.

Imaging

As with adult stroke, imaging should be performed promptly:

- MRI is preferred because it differentiates stroke from mimics. Sequences should include MRA, DWI, FLAIR, gradient-recalled echo or SWI, and T1 and T2.
- CT/CTA should be performed if MRI will incur delay.

Intravenous thrombolysis in children

- The international multicentre phase I TIPS study was terminated early due to poor recruitment, largely caused by delays in stroke diagnosis, and there remains no consensus on IVT in children.
- IVT is currently not approved in those <16 years but can be given in selected cases by paediatric neurologists.
- Higher doses may be required in children due to lower levels of endogenous TPA and its faster hepatic clearance.

Indications for mechanical thrombectomy

A MDT, incorporating paediatric neurointervention and neuroimaging, stroke neurology, paediatrics, neurosurgery, and haematology, should ideally be involved in decision-making. Evidence stems from retrospective single-arm studies.

- Location: anterior and posterior circulation LVO. MT has been performed in M2 and M3 branches, but caution is advised and benefit is uncertain.
- Neurological deficit: there are no specific paediatric guidelines. Based on adult studies, MT is considered when NIHSS score is >6. The median PedNIHSS score in SaveChildS on admission was 14.0 (interquartile range 9.2–20.0).
- Infarct volume: younger children exhibit greater neural plasticity than adults and this may enable more effective recovery from even large existing infarct volumes.
- Timing: paediatric stroke is often diagnosed late. Children may still benefit >6 h from onset (in SaveChildS, MT achieved good outcomes up until 16.2 h with good outcomes). A clinical–radiological mismatch, and DWI–FLAIR mismatch, predicts benefit.

Contraindications

- Non-embolic aetiologies, e.g. vasculopathies.
- Caution is advised in children <5 years, due to smaller vessel diameters and increased procedural risk. In those <2 years the balance of risk may not favour MT. An exception might be a cardiac paediatric patient with a known source of embolism.

Procedural considerations in children

- Refer to Chapter 7, 'Paediatric angiography', p. 216, for general advice regarding paediatric angiography, and Chapter 6, 'Paediatric', p. 190, for access advice.
- GA is mandatory.
- Outside of specialist paediatric units, great caution should be observed in performing MT on paediatric stroke patients <2 years old. The arteries are very small, and more prone to vasospasm and potential rupture.
- In children 2–5 years old, 4 Fr groin sheath and systems are suitable.
- For children >5 years, the size of the brain arteries approaches 95% that of adult patients. The groin arteries are still relatively small, but a 5 Fr sheath should be tolerated. Intermediate catheters are useful adjuncts in paediatric age groups.
- Device selection:
  - Smaller stent retrievers and aspiration catheters are favoured due to their compatibility with smaller vessels. In Save ChildS, the most common device was a 4 × 20 stent retriever. Aspiration catheters were used less frequently.
  - Combined techniques using aspiration with stent retrievers have shown efficacy.
- If the lesion is resistant to standard MT techniques, vasculopathy or dissection should be suspected. Avoid stenting vasculopathy.
- Given the lack of RCT evidence and the fragility of developing vessels, an angiographically imperfect result may be acceptable.

Complications

- The safety profile of MT in children appears comparable to adults (see 'Complications in mechanical thrombectomy', p. 385).
- In Save ChildS, there were no periprocedural complications other than transient vasospasm, resolving with nimodipine. There was one patient with post-interventional intracerebral haemorrhage, and a second with malignant infarction.

Postprocedural care

- Multidisciplinary input is required after MT.
- The child should be managed in the HDU or ITU.

Outcomes

- The retrospective Save ChildS study reported favourable outcomes in 80% at discharge and 86% at 6 months—significantly better than the adult series. Similar to adults, favourable outcome relates to severity of NIHSS score at presentation and successful reperfusion.

- Lack of RCTs limits the evidence for MT in paediatrics, necessitating extrapolation from adult data and observational studies. Ethical and logistical barriers to conducting trials in this population remain significant.

Further reading

Bernard TJ, Manco-Johnson MJ, Lo W, et al. Towards a consensus-based classification of childhood arterial ischaemic stroke. Stroke. 2012;43(2):371–377.

Rennie A. UKNG Guidance Document for Paediatric Mechanical Thrombectomy. Great Ormond Street Hospital; 2021. https://ukng.org.uk/about/standards_guidelines.aspx

Sporns PB, Sträter R, Minnerup J, et al. Feasibility, safety, and outcome of endovascular recanalization in childhood stroke: the Save ChildS study. JAMA Neurol. 2020;77(1):25–34.

Sun LR, Lynch JK. Advances in the diagnosis and treatment of pediatric arterial ischaemic stroke. Neurotherapeutics. 2023;20(3):633–654.

Complications in mechanical thrombectomy

- Complications in MT are inevitable. The Hermes collaboration documented a rate of serious intracranial complications at 5–10%.
- Prompt recognition and management of these complications are crucial but they should also be regarded as learning opportunities to refine technical skills, improve patient selection, optimise procedural planning, and enhance team preparedness.

General advice

- Key principles:
  - Early recognition of when things are starting to go wrong is critical.
  - Decision-making is often time-sensitive: set clear time limits for each approach and know when to change strategy.
  - Team preparation and communication is vital: clear protocols improve outcomes.
  - Backup strategies should be in place.
- Prevention remains the best strategy:
  - Careful patient selection.
  - Meticulous technique.
  - Equipment familiarity.
- Participation in quality improvement processes is important:
  - Regular team training.
  - Team debriefing after complications.
  - Regular case reviews and morbidity and mortality meetings.
  - Participation in audits and national databases.
  - Protocol updates based on experience.

Difficult arch navigation

- Vascular access:
  - Time is critical, so choose your fastest and most reliable access approach.
  - If the iliac arteries are excessively tortuous, consider exchanging the short femoral sheath for a longer one that can straighten and reduce friction on the catheters.
- Evaluate anatomy on pre-procedure CTA:
  - Consider the aortic arch type, including any variant anatomy, and note vessel tortuosity. Excessive tortuosity and unfavourable angulation of the carotid arteries make catheterisation difficult and increase the risk of guide catheter herniation. Vascular loops in the ICAs increase the risk of dissection.
  - In excessively tortuous anatomy, consider the use of a long sheath such as the 8 Fr Arrow-Flex. This can be placed in the proximal ICA and conventional 8 Fr guide or balloon catheters can then be inserted within.
  - Simmons select catheters might be considered first line for the MT typical demographic. Berenstein catheters can be considered in younger age groups. If needed, stiffer diagnostic catheters can be used, e.g. a 6 Fr Weinberg.

- Set clear time limits for each approach:
  - Avoid tunnel vision when dealing with challenging anatomy. Keep an eye on the clock and set a maximum time for the initial access attempt, typically <20 min.
  - Always have a backup strategy ready before starting and switch approaches promptly if difficulties arise.
- Technical pearls for difficult anatomy:
  - For support, use a variable stiffness 0.35" guidewire, e.g. the Advantage Guidewire.
  - If you are unable to track the guide catheter over the select catheter, consider catheterisation with a soft conventional diagnostic catheter and using an exchange-length wire to exchange for the guide catheter. Alternatively, you might catheterise the origin of the vessel and progressively track a microcatheter and aspiration catheter more distally to provide support.
  - BGCs can be challenging to navigate in difficult anatomy. One technique is temporary inflation of the balloon in the CCA, which straightens the catheter shaft proximally. This provides an anchor or support for the distal catheter tip and facilitates the advancement of a stiff wire in the ICA, a technique known as the 'grappling technique'.

Alternative access approaches

- Transradial access:
  - Primary consideration should often be given when a type III arch is present, femoral attempts have failed, or in basilar occlusions, particularly depending on the angle of the take-off of the vertebral artery.
  - Use purpose-designed radial access systems and employ ultrasound guidance to reduce spasm and complications. A meticulous technique can help avoid spasm.
- Direct carotid puncture:
  - Reserve this approach as a last resort where other methods fail. Although feasible, it is risky and has decreased in popularity as radial approaches have become more common. It is probably safer in younger patients.
  - Ultrasound guidance is mandatory, and additional roadmap guidance should be used if available. Select the puncture site below the carotid bifurcation and plan the closure strategy before puncture.

Multiple passes and strategy change

- The first-pass effect is strongly associated with good outcomes. Success rates decrease with each pass, while the risk of complications increases.
- After 2–3 unsuccessful attempts, consider changing your strategy. It is important to balance the benefits of continued attempts against the risks. For instance, achieving TICI 2B might be reasonable in a large core infarct rather than making several more passes with diminishing returns.

Optimising for success

- Adequate guide catheter support is essential, particularly given the typically tortuous vessels encountered during MT procedures. If the guide catheter is not sufficiently positioned distally in the ICA (distal cervical or petrous segments), it may buckle and prolapse into the aortic

arch during MT attempts. This can slow down the procedure or make it impossible to carry out.
- Have a range of devices readily available in your inventory and become familiar with the nuances of their use. Careful device selection is important to optimise for first-pass success. It is important to confirm complete clot coverage and carefully consider the optimal retrieval technique.
- Be mindful of your progress, and recognise early signs of futility.
- Injury to a vessel can decrease the chances of success due to complications, which include rupture or endothelial damage (which may lead to thrombosis or dissection). To minimise trauma, gently manipulate the catheter, avoid aggressive retraction, and avoid excessive straightening of the vessel.

Changing strategies

- Indications for strategy change:
  - No clot engagement despite a good position.
  - Repeated loss of clot during retrieval.
  - Evidence of clot fragmentation.
  - Suspicion of underlying pathology such as dissection or atheroma/ ICAD.
- Strategy modification:
  - Consider switching from aspiration to a stent retriever, or vice versa.
  - Change the device size or switch to another device. Larger-bore aspiration catheters may be tried if they will fit into the vessel, or conversely, smaller-bore ones may be necessary to achieve contact with the thrombus. Larger stent retrievers can be used if thought they will not excessively traumatise the vessel.
  - Consider alternative stent retriever designs. The Embotrap is quite different in design from the Solitaire, for example.
  - Consider using a balloon guide if it is not already in use.
  - Consider using combined techniques like SAVE, Solumbra, or BADASS.
  - Consider the double stent retriever technique for large clot burden, resistant clots, and branch occlusions. Note that this carries a higher risk of vessel injury and haemorrhage.
  - Use devices specifically designed for tough/resistant clots, such as the Nimbus device if suspected. Calcified clots are especially resistant to retrieval.

When to stop

- Decision factors: consider the total procedure time, radiation dose, number of passes, development of complications, changes in clinical status, and baseline patient prognosis.
- Hard stops:
  - New significant haemorrhage (either on angiography or on-table CT).
  - Vessel injury/perforation.
  - Significant clinical deterioration.
  - Clear futility after multiple approaches.
- Relative stops:
  - 90–120 min without progress.
  - 3–4 different strategies tried.
  - Progressive vessel trauma.
  - Diminishing returns with each attempt.

Artery reocclusion

Recognition and initial assessment

- Assess for underlying aetiology:
  - ICAD: risk factors include focal stenosis, vessel irregularity, calcification on initial CT, and Asian ethnicity.
  - Dissection: more common in younger patients and in the posterior circulation.
  - Residual thrombus.
  - Embolisation from proximal source.
- Immediate steps:
  - Rule out guide catheter-induced flow limitation.
  - Obtain multiple projections if unsure.
  - Consider concurrent vasospasm (and treatment of such).

Management strategy

- If ICAD suspected:
  - Allow 5–10 min observation period if the vessel is still open.
  - Consider intra-arterial vasodilators.
  - Maintain systolic BP >140 mmHg.
  - Prepare for possible angioplasty/stenting.
- If residual thrombus likely:
  - Consider additional passes.
  - Switch retrieval strategy.
  - Assess for a proximal source.
- Pharmacological options:
  - Intra-arterial nimodipine/verapamil for spasm.
  - GP IIb/IIIa inhibitors if platelet-rich thrombus.
  - Consider direct intra-arterial microcatheter thrombolysis in selected cases for very distal thrombi that are not otherwise accessible.
- Mechanical options:
  - Angioplasty: use submaximal dilation to minimise the risk of vessel rupture, and apply slow inflation speeds for added safety.
  - Rescue stenting and antiplatelet therapy.

Rescue angioplasty and stenting

- Indications:
  - Failed multiple retrieval attempts.
  - Underlying stenosis identified or suspected clinically or from imaging, e.g. diabetic patients with multiple vascular risk factors, low NIHSS relative to clot location, excellent collaterals, presence of large T_{Max} on CTP.
  - Vessel re-occlusion after a successful pass. This may happen immediately, or gradually over a few minutes (a period of observation and repeat angiography is recommended if suspected).
  - Evidence of ICAD.
- Technical considerations:
  - Obtain new runs to assess true vessel size.
  - Choose appropriate stent sizing.
  - Consider using a stent which will deploy through a balloon (e.g. Neurospeed and Credo).
  - Consider need for pre/post dilation.

- Submaximal angioplasty (80% of vessel) decreases the risk of vessel damage.
- Plan post-procedure antiplatelets in collaboration with the stroke neurology team. Patients who already have large infarct cores may not be suitable for antiplatelets (and hence stenting).

Embolism to other vascular territories

- A major concern here is that other territories might be providing collateral supply to the originally occluded area. This essential supply is lost when embolism occurs.
- High-risk scenarios:
  - Heavy clot burden.
  - Long segment clot.
  - Tortuous anatomy.
  - Procedures requiring multiple passes.
- Technical considerations:
  - Use of BGC when feasible.
  - Maintain continuous aspiration during retrieval.
  - Ensure optimal guide catheter position distal in the ICA.
  - Consider switching to larger-bore aspiration catheters.
  - Ensure careful device sizing and minimise the number of passes if possible.
- Procedural modifications:
  - Slow, steady, retrieval in tortuous anatomy.
  - Consider combined techniques for large clots.
- Management options:
  - Additional MT can be performed.
  - Consider intra-arterial thrombolysis for distal emboli.

Intraprocedural subarachnoid haemorrhage

Causes

- After stent retrieval (Figure 9.18), typically in small vessels or those with an underlying susceptibility, such as dissection.
- Microcatheter injection into an occluded or small vessel.
- Wire perforation.

Temporary solutions

- Immediate actions:
  - Reverse heparin if given with protamine.
  - Alert the anaesthesia team and lower the BP.
  - If a BGC is used, this can be inflated to stop proximal inflow of blood.
- Compliant balloons or temporary coils can be used to try to stop the bleeding:
  - Balloon inflation: prepare and inflate a compliant balloon at the site of extravasation. Gently inflate, just sufficient to stop the contrast leak. Perform angiography to confirm that the balloon has stopped the haemorrhage. Keep the balloon inflated 5–10 min at a time and repeat the inflation if necessary.
  - Temporary coiling: place a large, long coil at the site of extravasation but do not detach. The thrombogenic coil helps the formation of a platelet plug to restore haemostasis.

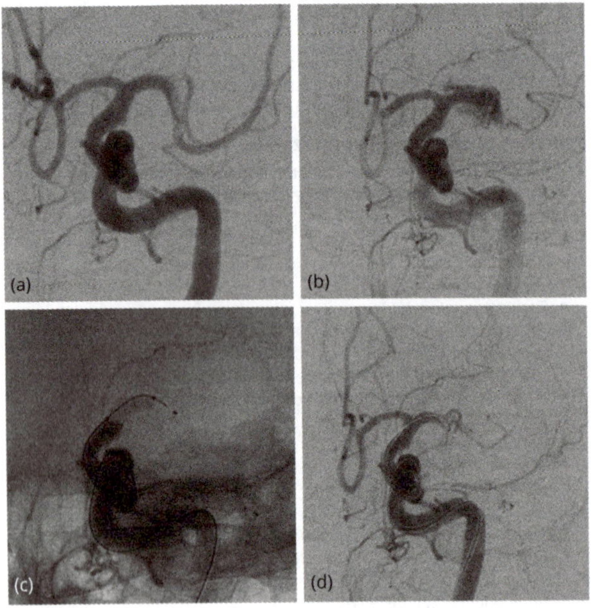

Figure 9.18 Vessel rupture during thrombectomy. (a) Digital subtraction angiography shows thrombus located within the left middle cerebral artery (MCA) divisions. (b) After a single stent retrieval pass, repeat angiography reveals contrast extravasation. (c) Unsubtracted angiography shows a Scepter XC balloon inflated in the distal internal carotid artery and extending into the MCA. Stasis is confirmed, as no contrast flows past the balloon upon gentle injection. (d) The balloon was deflated after 3 min, achieving haemostasis. No further thrombectomy attempts were made due to the risk of re-rupture.

Permanent solutions

- Indications for permanent solutions:
  - Continued extravasation despite repeated balloon inflation or temporary coil usage.
  - Massive haemorrhage.
  - Balloon or temporary coiling does not slow the bleeding.
  - Haemodynamic instability.
- Either parent vessel occlusion with coils or the use of covered stents can be employed.
  - Vessel occlusion with coils: assess collateral supply before occlusion to assess the consequences of occlusion. Insert a coiling catheter to the site of the extravasation and deploy coils to form a dense pack. The initial coil should be sized larger than the vessel.
  - Covered stent: difficult to handle in cerebral vessels and should only be used by experienced operators. Control bleeding first (e.g. with a

compliant balloon). The aspiration catheter may need removal due to length constraints. Precise placement is essential. DAPT is usually needed post-placement.

Once the bleeding is controlled

- Perform an on-table CT head to review the volume of blood and assess for hydrocephalus.
- Obtain a neurosurgical consultation.
- Consider EVD placement.
- Serial neurological monitoring is required in the ICU setting.
- MDT meeting with relatives should be arranged in a suitable environment as soon as possible to explain and break the news regarding the likely grim prognosis.

Iatrogenic arterial dissection

Recognition

- Angiographic signs: double lumen appearance; irregular vessel calibre; delayed contrast clearance; intimal flap visualisation.
- Risk factors:
    - Excessive wire manipulation.
    - Guide catheter trauma (especially common with BGCs).
    - Forceful contrast injection against the wall of the vessel.
    - Resistant clot retrieval.
    - Underlying vessel disease.
- Immediate actions:
    - Assess flow limitation and collateral supply.
    - Consider anticoagulation if flow compromised.
- Treatment strategy:
    - If non-flow-limiting, aspirin can be given.
    - Consider stenting if flow limitation, clinical deterioration, poor collaterals, or continued embolisation.
- Plan follow-up imaging at 3–6 months.

Stent detachment/retention

- The unintended detachment of stent retrievers during MT is an extremely rare complication and linked to poor clinical outcomes. It is less common with newer-generation devices. The usual site of detachment is the connection of the stent retriever to the pusher wire.
- Risk factors: excessive rotation of delivery wire; atherosclerosis; tortuous anatomy; calcified vessels; long clots requiring multiple passes; previous stenting; excessive size of stent retriever compared to vessel.
- Elongation and tension of the stent retriever are possible signs of potential detachment.

Interventions

- Initial response:
    - Stop manipulation immediately.
    - Assess distal flow and collaterals.
- Retrieval options:
    - Micro-snares can be utilised to capture and retrieve the device. Multiple attempts may be needed.
    - The Tigertriever and other stent retrievers have also been used for this purpose.

- Bail-out options:
  - Deploy fully if retrieval fails.
  - Consider emergency stenting.
  - Institute post-procedure DAPT if the vessel remains open. If the vessel has thrombosed, this is unnecessary.
  - Early follow-up imaging.

Postprocedural subarachnoid haemorrhage

- Common mechanisms: use of stent retrievers (common to have small-volume SAH); subarachnoid extension of haemorrhagic infarct; unrecognised wire perforation; multiple microcatheter injections into 'wedged' occluded system; vessel friability post-thrombectomy; underlying vascular abnormality.
- Risk minimisation:
  - Gentle wire/catheter manipulation.
  - Careful review of final angiogram runs.
  - Multiple projections before procedure end.
  - Careful use of microcatheter injections and control of force used.
  - Lower threshold for on-table CT in high-risk cases: multiple passes, vessel tortuosity, distal access required, prolonged procedure time.

Management strategies

- Immediate actions:
  - Full clinical evaluation including airway, breathing, and circulation assessment.
  - Stop/reverse anticoagulation.
  - BP control (target systolic BP <140 mmHg).
  - Early neurosurgical consultation.
- Ongoing care:
  - Small-volume post-thrombectomy SAH is common especially after stent-retrieval usage and is usually a self-limiting phenomenon.
  - Consider CTA ± emergent DSA if focal/extensive.
  - Early EVD if hydrocephalus present.
  - ICU admission.
  - Frequent neurological monitoring.
  - Delayed vessel imaging to rule out underlying lesion.

Haemorrhagic conversion of infarct

Risk factors and identification

- Clinical risk factors: LVO; prior anticoagulation; delayed presentation; high NIHSS score; hyperglycaemia; poor collaterals.
- Imaging risk factors: large core infarct on initial imaging; early ischaemic changes (ASPECTS ≤7); poor collateral status; extensive clot burden; BBB disruption on CTP; malignant perfusion profile on CTP (T_{max} >8 s is >85 mL volume or potentially any tissue with T_{max} >14s).
- Procedural risk factors: multiple passes; prolonged procedure time; combined IV-tPA and MT; complete reperfusion of large core.

Intervention options

- Initial management:
  - Full clinical evaluation including airway, breathing, and circulation assessment.

    - Immediate CT head if suspected.
    - ICU admission and endotracheal intubation may be required.
- BP control:
    - Immediate systolic BP reduction to <140 mmHg.
    - Consider more aggressive targets if expanding.
    - Regular BP monitoring.
- Anticoagulation management:
    - Stop heparin if running and reverse with protamine if recently given.
    - Fresh frozen plasma or vitamin K can be given if on warfarin.
    - Consider prothrombin complex concentrate for direct oral anticoagulants.
    - Consider stopping GP IIb/IIIa infusions.
    - Consider platelet transfusions.
- Supportive care:
    - Early neurosurgical assessment.
    - Consider ICP monitoring.
    - Seizure prophylaxis if large.
    - Serial neurological monitoring.

Postprocedural care

Functional outcomes following thrombectomy remain suboptimal with 40–50% of patients not achieving functional independence despite good recanalisation rates of >80%. Mortality remains high at 10–20%. Reasons include late or incomplete reperfusion (most cases), reperfusion injury, BBB breakdown, and procedural complications.

Close neurological monitoring is necessary, usually in a hyperacute stroke unit or neurointensive care unit. Emergent brain and vessel imaging is required if there is significant neurological deterioration.

Although it is well recognised that post-thrombectomy care is critical for optimising clinical outcomes, there is a lack of high-quality evidence to guide peri- and postprocedural management.

Blood pressure

- Both low and high baseline BP are associated with poor outcome post-thrombectomy.
- Low BP risks hypoperfusion via poor collateral flow and high BP may increase risk of haemorrhage or reperfusion injury.

Induced hypertension

- Although it is reasonable to treat symptomatic hypotension, there are no data to support routine use of induced hypertension.

Intensive lowering of BP

- Several RCTs have addressed BP lowering after MT (OPTIMAL-BP, BEST-II, BP-TARGET, ENCHANTED2/MT). Despite differences between trials, collectively they failed to establish a clinical benefit of intensive BP lowering after thrombectomy and did not show any reduction in haemorrhagic transformation. Two of the trials reported worse clinical outcomes with intensive BP reduction.
- European guidelines recommend maintaining BP at <180/105 mmHg during MT and for 24 h afterwards, albeit with a very low quality of evidence and only a weak recommendation. No specific BP-lowering drug is preferred.
- Expert consensus agreed that the degree of reperfusion should be considered in the choice of BP target after MT. A lower BP target of 160/90 mmHg may be preferred with complete reperfusion.

Neurological agents

- There is renewed interest in intra-arterial thrombolysis as an adjunct to MT. The single-centre CHOICE RCT has shown benefit of intra-arterial alteplase in patients with successful reperfusion (eTICI 2B/3), perhaps due to improved microcirculatory reperfusion. However, the trial was terminated early and effect size may have been overestimated.
- CHOICE 2 is a multicentre RCT that will assess efficacy of intra-arterial alteplase in patients with successful reperfusion (eTICI 2B/3).
- The ongoing TECNO RCT will assess intra-arterial tenecteplase in MT patients with incomplete reperfusion.
- The successful reperfusion provided by MT has also renewed interest in neuroprotection or adjuvant therapies. Several agents/strategies have been investigated including uric acid, activated protein C,

nerinetide, otaplimastat, imatinib, verapamil, butylphthalide, edaravone, nelonemdaz, ApTOLL, regional hypothermia, remote ischaemic conditioning, normobaric oxygen, and nuclear factor erythroid 2-related factor 2. Although theoretically promising, there is yet to be robust favourable evidence from a large phase III RCT (trials neutral to date).

Blood sugar

- Hyperglycaemia is associated with worse outcome in ischaemic stroke.
- However, the efficacy of intensive treatment of hyperglycaemia has not been proven in RCTs. International guidelines recommend maintaining normal glucose levels.

Temperature control

- Elevated temperature post-stroke is associated with worse clinical outcome.
- European guidelines acknowledge that data are limited and, therefore, strength of recommendations is weak. Prophylactic administration of antipyretics to prevent hyperthermia is not recommended.
- Antipyretics should be initiated to treat any high temperature, and the underlying source of infection identified and treated.
- The potential benefit of routine induction of hypothermia has not been proven safe/effective and is not recommended.

Antithrombotics for secondary stroke prevention

- Standard management post-thrombectomy involves repeat brain imaging at around 24 h followed by standard antiplatelet therapy once significant haemorrhage is excluded. This has been inferred from the standard management used in positive IVT RCTs.
- In acute stroke and atrial fibrillation, several recent RCTs have demonstrated the safety of early initiation of anticoagulation with DOACs (e.g. the OPTIMAS trial).

Reperfusion injury

- Reperfusion injury is a consequence of restoring blood flow to ischaemic tissue. Preclinical studies suggest that abrupt reperfusion induces secondary brain damage responsible for up to 70% of the final ischaemic lesion size.
- Cerebral reperfusion syndrome, or cerebral hyperperfusion syndrome, is a rare but serious complication following rapid revascularisation of a partially or completely occluded artery with successful thrombolytic therapy, successful thrombectomy, CEA, or stenting. Clinical presentations include new headache, new or worsening contralateral focal neurological deficit, and seizure. Outcomes vary with early identification and treatment reducing sICH and improving prognosis. It is important to recognise and treat any precipitating factors, especially uncontrolled hypertension.

Contrast-induced encephalopathy

- Contrast-induced encephalopathy is another rare and often under-recognised complication after MT. The incidence is reported to be 1.7% in a case series of >400 consecutive patients.

- Consider with significant clinical worsening after MT. Intravascular contrast additionally disrupts the BBB with leakage of fluid and contrast.
- Urgent repeat brain imaging shows prominent contrast staining and oedematous change; more commonly in patients with renal dysfunction, hypertension, or prior history of stroke.
- Management is usually supportive with resolution over several days.

Re-occlusion

- Vessel re-occlusion after successful recanalisation may be the cause of early neurological deterioration.
- If confirmed, repeat MT can be considered. Early initiation of anticoagulation or antiplatelet therapy (either single or dual) can also be considered if haemorrhage or large infarct is excluded.

Further reading

Caroff J, Aubert L, Lavenu-Bombled C, et al. Antithrombotic therapies for neurointerventional surgery: a 2021 French comprehensive national survey. J Neurointerv Surg. 2023;15(4):402–407.

Chu YT, Lee KP, Chen CH, et al. Contrast-induced encephalopathy after endovascular thrombectomy for acute ischaemic stroke. Stroke. 2020;51(12):3756–3759.

Gao P, Wang D, Zhao Z, et al. Multicentre prospective trial of stent placement in patients with symptomatic high-grade intracranial stenosis. AJNR Am J Neuroradiol. 2016;37(7):1275–1280.

Jadhav A, Molyneaux BJ, Hill MD, Jovin TG. Care of the post-thrombectomy patient. Stroke. 2018;49(11):2801–2807.

Leslie-Mazwi T, Chen M, Yi J, et al. Post-thrombectomy management of the ELVO patient: guidelines from the Society of NeuroInterventional Surgery. J NeuroIntervent Surg 2017;9(12):1258–1266.

Ntaios G, Dziedzic T, Michel P, et al. European Stroke Organisation (ESO) guidelines for the management of temperature in patients with acute ischaemic stroke. Int J Stroke. 2015;10(6):941–949.

Schirmer CM, Bulsara KR, Al-Mufti F, et al. Antiplatelets and antithrombotics in neurointerventional procedures: guideline update. J NeuroInterv Surg 2023;15(11):1155–1162.

Turc G, Bhogal P, Fischer U, et al. European Stroke Organisation (ESO)–European Society for Minimally Invasive Neurological Therapy (ESMINT) guidelines on mechanical thrombectomy in acute ischaemic stroke. J NeuroInterv Surg 2023;15(8):e8.

Organisation of care

Clinical networks

- Formal MT networks consist of hub and spoke sites, where hubs are comprehensive stroke centres (CSCs) equipped to perform advanced interventions, including thrombectomy/decompressive craniectomy, and the spoke sites are smaller hospitals or stroke units called Primary Stroke Centres (PSCs) (or acute stroke centres) that provide the initial diagnosis, care, stabilisation, and transfer of patients to the hub for advanced treatment.
- Networks can work within, or in collaboration with, other local organisations (such as the Integrated Stroke Delivery Networks in England). The primary goal of these networks is to expedite patient transfer and reduce the time from stroke onset to reperfusion.
- The aim is to establish seamless patient care pathways across multiple organisations, involving a range of stakeholders including ambulance services, clinical stroke teams, radiologists, anaesthesiologists, intensive care physicians, and neurointerventional specialists from both referring PSCs and CSCs.

Spoke sites

- The majority (e.g. approximately 75% in England) of thrombectomy patients undergo their first assessment at a PSC prior to transfer. The PSC is instrumental in confirming the acute ischaemic stroke LVO diagnosis and delivery of initial treatment. Furthermore, the PSC can improve patient flow across a regional network by facilitating timely transfers for MT and efficient repatriation.
- Door-in to door-out (DIDO) times should be minimised for patients transferred for MT. Prolonged DIDO times negatively impact outcomes and may be the most significant modifiable factor to reduce time of onset to recanalisation. DIDO times can vary considerably among different PSC.
- It is the responsibility of the CSC to respond with a prompt decision. PSCs should target a median DIDO time of 45 min. Accurate data entry for national audit databases (SSNAP in UK) to record and share DIDO times across a network is valuable.
- The utilisation of shared regional rotas and telemedicine can facilitate the evaluation of stroke patients in the PSC by a specialist, particularly out of hours. AI platforms can assist with supporting decision-making around interpretation of clinical imaging, especially in hospitals without access to neuroimaging specialists. These tools identify regions of core infarction (including ASPECTS estimation and volume estimation), detect LVO, estimate collateral flow, and process perfusion imaging to delineate core infarct region and penumbra with volumetric evaluation.
- The administration of IVT should not be delayed. Local protocols should be established for the delivery of IVT before transfer. While the use of thrombolytics during secondary transfer by trained paramedics has been shown to be feasible, there is currently a lack of evidence supporting its effectiveness in reducing DIDO times. However, similar protocols have been successfully implemented in cardiology without any reported transfer-associated complications. Stroke nurses may supervise the delivery of thrombolysis during transfer, but this poses a significant

resource challenge for the PSC. Routine use of tenecteplase instead of alteplase will render this issue redundant.

- Networks that rely on paramedic transfer have reported minimal secondary transfer-related complications.
- If no complications arise in the PSC, it is acceptable to transfer the patient without a stroke nurse escort following IVT administration.
- Patients with a GCS score of ≤8 require rapid endotracheal intubation and transfer with an anaesthetic escort. Guidelines from the Neurocritical Care Society outlining safe transfer practices have been published, emphasising the importance of an ICU-to-ICU handover in such cases.

Hub sites

- Evidence from clinical trials supporting the positive clinical outcomes of patients treated with MT has predominantly come from higher-volume CSCs with fellowship-trained neurointerventionalists where patients have access to CSC-level acute stroke care.
- These findings indicate that optimisation in patient selection, technical execution of MT, and post-procedure care support the current practice of concentrating MT procedures at specialised (regional) thrombectomy centres with a hyperacute stroke unit integrated into a high-quality comprehensive stroke service. This setup should have access to neurosurgical, neurocritical care, and specialised in-patient and out-patient stroke services, as well as advanced brain imaging facilities and appropriate neurointerventional expertise.
- Endovascular stroke therapy should exclusively be administered by CSCs with the necessary expertise in performing such procedures. According to the international multisociety consensus guidelines document, 'Standards of practice in acute ischaemic stroke intervention' (Pierot et al., 2019), each institution providing MT should conduct 120 MT procedures annually, and each operator should carry out a minimum of 50 neuroendovascular procedures, including coiling/aneurysm treatment procedures, per year. This aligns with the published UK guidance recommending a minimum operator volume of 40 cerebral interventional neuroendovascular procedures per year.

Prehospital care

- Emergency medical services play a vital role in hyperacute stroke care and local protocols and algorithms should be in place for dispatch, assessment, prenotification, and transport strategies. All suspected stroke patients potentially eligible for IVT should be transferred immediately to the closest centre with hyperacute stroke services (PSC or CSC) with early notification of the specialist stroke team.
- Patients with suspected stroke and contraindications to IVT should be equally prioritised. In hospitals receiving acute stroke patients, pre-alert protocols may be extended to include patients presenting beyond 4.5 h and include wake-up strokes or strokes without an immediately apparent onset time. Time extension should be agreed locally by networks.

Further reading

Pierot L, Jarayaman M, Szikora I, et al. Standards of practice in acute ischaemic stroke intervention international recommendations. Can J Neurol Sci. 2019;46(3):269–274.

Chapter 10

Atherosclerotic disease

Carotid artery stenting *400*
Vertebral artery stenting *406*
Intracranial atherosclerotic disease stenting *409*

Carotid artery stenting

Around 20% of acute strokes are due to atherosclerotic plaque rupture or thrombosis from carotid stenosis.

CAS is increasingly used for extracranial carotid artery disease and appears to have a broadly similar perioperative risk to CEA. The recently released results of CREST-2 have resurged interest in the technique by demonstrating that carotid stenting plus intensive medical management significantly reduced stroke risk compared to medical therapy alone in asymptomatic patients, whereas carotid surgery failed to show a statistically significant benefit over modern medical management.

Indications

- Restenosis after endarterectomy or previous stenting.
- Stenosis secondary to radiotherapy.
- Difficult surgical access to carotid artery (e.g. postoperative neck scars, distal ICA stenosis, or other anatomy unfavourable for surgery).
- CCA stenosis.
- Patients unfit or unwilling to have surgery.
- To open up a stenotic ICA during acute MT.

UK National Clinical Guidelines for Stroke 2023

- The degree of carotid artery stenosis should be reported using the North American Symptomatic Carotid Endarterectomy Trial (NASCET) method.
- People with non-disabling carotid artery territory stroke or TIA should be considered for carotid revascularisation, and if they agree with intervention:
  - They should have carotid imaging (duplex ultrasound, MR or CT angiography) performed urgently to assess the degree of stenosis
  - If initial test identifies a relevant severe stenosis (≥50%), a second or repeat non-invasive imaging investigation should be performed to confirm the degree of stenosis. This confirmatory test should be carried out urgently to avoid delaying intervention.
- People with non-disabling carotid artery territory stroke or TIA should be considered for carotid revascularisation if the symptomatic internal carotid artery has a stenosis ≥50%. The decision to offer carotid revascularisation should be:
  - Based on individualised risk estimates taking account of factors such as the time from the event, gender, age and the type of qualifying event;
  - Supported by risk tables or web-based risk calculators.
- People with non-disabling carotid artery territory stroke or TIA and a carotid stenosis <50% should not be offered revascularisation of the carotid artery.
- Carotid endarterectomy for people with symptomatic carotid stenosis should be:
  - The treatment of choice, particularly for people who are 70 years of age and over or for whom the intervention is planned within seven days of stroke or TIA.
  - Performed on individuals who are neurologically stable and fit for surgery, using either local or general anaesthetic according to the person's preference.
  - Conducted as soon as possible, and within 1 week of the first presentation.
  - Deferred for 72 hours in patients treated for intravenous thrombosis.

- Only undertaken by a specialist surgeon in a vascular centre where the outcomes of carotid surgery are routinely audited.
- Carotid angioplasty and stenting should be considered for individuals with symptomatic carotid stenosis who are unsuitable for open surgery (e.g. high carotid bifurcation, symptomatic re-stenosis).

Pros and cons

- In favour of stenting:
  - Can be performed under LA (although there is evidence from the GALA trial that CEA can be performed equally safely).
  - Avoids neck incision and risk of lower cranial nerve palsy.
  - Short hospital stay.
- Against stenting:
  - Risks of embolisation.
  - Restenosis.
  - Implanted metal requiring antiplatelet therapy.

Evidence

- Endarterectomy became the treatment of choice for patients with recently symptomatic, severe (>70%) carotid artery stenosis following RCTs (NASCET and ECST) that demonstrated a significant reduction in the risk of recurrent stroke or TIA compared to best medical treatment alone. A smaller benefit was also observed in patients with 50–69% stenosis. For optimal outcomes, patients should be operated on soon after a TIA or stroke—preferably within 2 weeks, and within 48 h for very high-risk cases.
- A number of RCTs have compared CAS and CEA: SPACE, EVA-3S, ICSS (CAVATAS 2), and CREST. On the whole, the trials indicated that in symptomatic patients CAS generally has a higher risk of stroke or periprocedural death compared to CEA, with statistically significant differences observed in CREST and ICSS, but not in SPACE. Significant restenosis was more common after CAS and leads to a small excess of recurrent TIA and stroke.
- CEA therefore remains the treatment of choice for recently symptomatic carotid stenosis.
- The recently released CREST-2 results signal a paradigm shift in managing asymptomatic ≥70% carotid stenosis: while Carotid Artery Stenting (CAS) plus intensive medical management (IMM) significantly halved the 4-year stroke risk compared to IMM alone (2.8% vs 6.0%), Carotid Endarterectomy (CEA) failed to show a statistically significant benefit, suggesting modern pharmacotherapy has effectively neutralized the historical advantage of surgery in this population.

Technique

(See Figure 10.1.)

- Nuances of acute stenting during MT is discussed in Chapter 9 (see 'Tandem carotid occlusion', p. 355).
- DAPT is required. Clopidogrel, in addition to aspirin, is usually the agent of choice as many patients will have had recent strokes. Platelet function testing is recommended. Typically, patients are loaded for 7 days beforehand.
- LA, conscious sedation, or GA can be utilised. An anaesthetist should be present in any case. For elective CAS, conscious sedation is the standard of care in the UK.

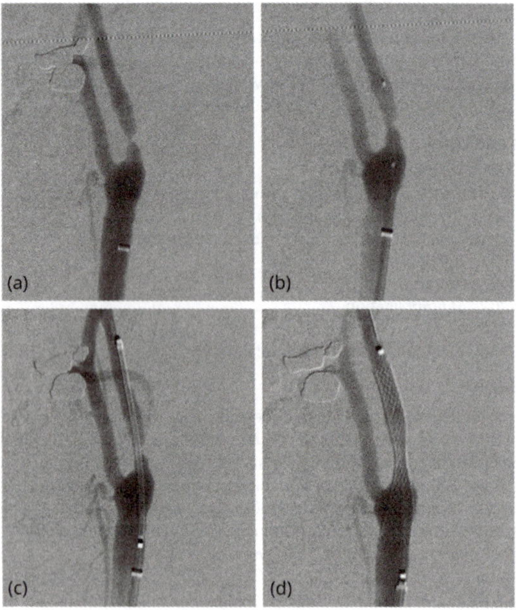

Figure 10.1 Carotid stenting technique. (a) Digital subtraction angiography shows symptomatic proximal internal carotid artery stenosis. (b) Post balloon angioplasty, with deflated balloon across the stenosis. (c) Stent within sheath placed across stenosis. (d) Post stent deployment. While there was some residual stenosis, this was deemed acceptable. The patient did not experience any further strokes at 6-month follow-up.

- An 8 Fr vascular sheath is inserted into the common femoral artery. Transradial access is also suitable.
- Systemic heparinisation is achieved with subsequent ACT monitoring.
- An 8 Fr guide catheter is positioned within the CCA and connected to a rotating haemostatic valve and heparin–saline flush. A select catheter can be used to aid catheterisation of the ICA.
- Cerebral protection devices, e.g. SpyderFx (Medtronic), can be deployed in the distal cervical ICA if desired. The usage of these devices is controversial. In ICSS, a higher proportion of stroke and fatal or disabling stroke was reported in the cerebral protection device group. In CASWEP, no benefit in terms of periprocedural TIA, stroke, death, or new ischaemic brain lesions on postprocedural diffusion-weighted MRI was found. However in CREST-2 usage was mandated and low rates of procedural stroke were observed.
- Angiography is performed to assess cerebral circulation and the cervical ICA. The detectors are positioned to optimise visualisation of the stenosis and arterial segments proximal and distal.

- Typically, a 0.014–0.018" microwire, such as the V-14 (Boston Scientific) or Synchro support (Stryker), is used. A slight curve is applied to the tip (do not over-shape the tip as it will be harder to cross the stenosis). The stenosis can often be crossed directly with the microwire alone. If necessary, a microcatheter can be used to facilitate crossing the stenosis, but an exchange-length microwire is required to exchange for the angioplasty balloon or stent.

Angioplasty

- If the stenosis is very narrow, it may be necessary to predilate with an angioplasty balloon. Non-compliant rapid exchange coronary dilatation balloons (e.g. Trek (Abbott), NC Emerge (Boston Scientific), or Sterling (Boston Scientific)) are suitable. Typically, 3 mm diameters are used for the carotid artery (slightly undersize the balloon with respect to the vessel).
- The balloon is prepared by purging the dead space with 50% contrast:saline mixture. This is performed by filling a 20 mL syringe and aspirating from the device's inflation port three times, for approximately 20 s each time, while gently tapping the port to displace air and allow the fluid to occupy the space. The port is then connected to an inflation device via a three-way stopcock.
- The wire is flushed and threaded retrogradely into the end of the balloon catheter.
- The balloon is then passed through the guide catheter and centred across the stenosis using the microwire under roadmap guidance.
- Atropine can be administered prior to balloon inflation to prevent severe bradycardia—typically 0.5 mg.
- Slowly inflate the balloon by rotating the handle on the inflation device under fluoroscopic guidance, until the nominal balloon pressure is reached (as specified on the pressure card provided with the device). The balloon sometimes slips forwards during inflation and may need to be tugged back gently.
- Wait a few seconds and then deflate the balloon by pulling back on the plunger of the inflation device and perform an angiogram to see the results. Additional angioplasty attempts can be performed if needed.
- Keeping the wire in place across the stenosis, remove the angioplasty balloon. It is necessary to fix the wire to the table, and screen the wire tip intermittently, in order to ensure the wire does not slip forwards or backwards.

Stenting

- Thread the stent onto the back end of the microwire and position it centred across the stenosis.
- The carotid stent diameter must be wider than the widest segment of artery to be stented. Tapered stents are available to manage proximal to distal vessel size discrepancies.
- Unsheathe the device in place.
- Repeat angiography to assess the stenosis.
- If required, should the stenosis remain >50%, additional angioplasty can be performed to further expand the stent and vessel, but this risks distal emboli.
- Cerebral angiography should be performed at the end of the procedure to confirm that no emboli have been dislodged into the cerebral circulation.

Post-procedure

- A baseline ultrasound or CTA can be performed immediately after stenting for later comparison.
- The patient is monitored overnight, ideally in an HDU.
- Different protocols exist for antiplatelets. Dual antiplatelets are given for 6 weeks to 6 months, with one agent (either aspirin or clopidogrel, depending on local protocols) continued for life.

Follow-up imaging

- Serial ultrasound or CTA can be used for follow-up.
- In symptomatic patients, formal catheter angiography is warranted.

Tips

- Most carotid stents will prove effective in the great majority of stenotic lesions. Particular stents may be advantageous in certain situations.

Vessel tortuosity

- Open-cell stents are flexible and therefore useful if the vessel is very tortuous. The disadvantage is reduced longitudinal strength, unequal cell size due to compression, elongation during delivery, and the potential for kinking.
- Some open-cell stents have smaller open-cell areas and more bridges between the rings, e.g. Acculink (Abbott). These trade flexibility for more longitudinal support.
- Roadsaver (Terumo) is a particularly flexible and navigable closed-cell stent.
- Carotid Wallstent and closed-cell stents such as NextStent (Boston Scientific) are the most rigid design. These are not optimal for tortuous vessels, however.

Vessel diameter mismatch

- Proximal ICA stenosis is very common, and the stent must bridge the distal CCA and the proximal ICA. As the CCA is generally larger than the ICA, there is a size discrepancy. This is often greatest when stenting across vessels that have previously undergone endarterectomy.
- The stent should be selected based on the size of the largest diameter, usually the CCA.
- The Carotid Wallstent is a good option in this situation as the woven mesh structure constrains well.
- Alternatively, a tapered stent may be used. The Protégé (Medtronic) has a punctuated decrease in stent calibre, and the XACT and Acculink (Abbott) have a more graduated decrease.

Calcified plaque

- Calcified lesions require high radial force in addition to moderate outward expansive force.
- Nitinol stents have a high outward radial force and are a good choice for calcified stenosis. Closed-cell stents, such as X-Act (Abbott), have the highest radial force.
- The Carotid Wallstent has a relatively low radial force which may not be great enough to prevent vessel recoil in calcified stenosis.

Complications

- **Bradycardia and hypotension:** may occur during angioplasty of the carotid bulb: Ensure that BP and heart rate monitoring is in place. If this occurs, immediately deflate the balloon. The condition is usually self-limiting but if not, atropine can be administered. Many operators administer atropine prophylactically.
- **Embolic stroke:** occurs in about 5%. Care must be taken during the procedure not to dislodge plaque with wires, catheters, or devices. If LVO occurs, MT can be performed. Note: do not pull a stent retriever through the carotid stent as it may become trapped in the struts. Instead, deploy the guide through the stent or pull the stent retriever into an aspiration catheter before crossing the stent. Results on use of carotid filters to catch distal emboli are mixed but two large trials (including ICSS) found no benefit.
- **Acute stent thrombosis:** occurs more commonly during acute stroke treatment. Risk factors include antiplatelet medication, non-compliance or resistance, overlapping stents, intrinsic prothrombotic disorders, stent edge dissection, atheroma disruption, and ICA kinking post-stent placement. Confirm first with CT/CTA. It might be necessary to take the patient back to the angiography suite and aspirate the thrombus or perform further angioplasty/stenting. Anticoagulant and thrombolytic agents may also be administered.
- **Hyperperfusion syndrome:** occurs in 3.1–6.8% of cases, resulting in haemorrhage in <1%. Symptoms tend to start within hours of the procedure and include severe headache, eye pain, and facial pain, often with elevated BP. Focal neurological deficits, seizures, and loss of consciousness occur less commonly. CT or MRI reveals patchy or diffuse white matter oedema, primarily affecting the posterior parieto-occipital lobe, along with focal infarction, petechial haemorrhage, or large haemorrhages in severe cases.
- **Late restenosis:** in asymptomatic cases, conservative management with continued antiplatelet therapy is recommended. For symptomatic cases, angioplasty (potentially using a cutting balloon) may be considered, or surgical intervention may be required.

Further reading

Barnett HJ, Taylor DW, Eliasziw M, et al. Benefit of carotid endarterectomy in patients with symptomatic moderate or severe stenosis. North American Symptomatic Carotid Endarterectomy Trial Collaborators. N Engl J Med. 1998;339(20):1415–1425.

Brott TG, Hobson RW 2nd, Howard G, et al. Stenting versus endarterectomy for treatment of carotid-artery stenosis. N Engl J Med. 2010;363(1):11–23.

Eckstein HH, Ringleb P, Allenberg JR, et al. Results of the Stent-Protected Angioplasty versus Carotid Endarterectomy (SPACE) study to treat symptomatic stenoses at 2 years: a multinational, prospective, randomised trial. Lancet Neurol. 2008;7(10):893–902.

Gorgulu S, Sahin M, Norgaz NT, et al. Carotid artery stenting without embolic protection: a randomized multicenter trial (the CASWEP trial). Interv Neuroradiol. 2023;29(4):419–425.

International Carotid Stenting Study investigators, Ederle J, Dobson J, et al. Carotid artery stenting compared with endarterectomy in patients with symptomatic carotid stenosis (International Carotid Stenting Study): an interim analysis of a randomised controlled trial. Lancet. 2010;375(9719):985–997.

Lin YH, Liu HM. Update on cerebral hyperperfusion syndrome. J Neurointerv Surg. 2020;12(8):788–793.

Mas JL, Trinquart L, Leys D, et al. Endarterectomy Versus Angioplasty in Patients with Symptomatic Severe Carotid Stenosis (EVA-3S) trial: results up to 4 years from a randomised, multicentre trial. Lancet Neurol. 2008;7(10):885–892.

Vertebral artery stenting

Around 20–25% of strokes involve the posterior circulation. Greater than 50% vertebrobasilar stenosis risks early recurrent stroke. Atherosclerotic stenosis of the vertebral artery, typically at its origin with distal embolisation, is a significant cause of posterior circulation strokes, accounting for roughly 20% of cases. The other main sites for posterior circulation stenosis are the distal intracranial vertebral and proximal basilar arteries. The optimal management of these patients is unclear, but in recent years angioplasty and stenting have been advocated as there are no acceptable surgical alternatives. Stenting of vertebral stenosis is technically possible but randomised trials are required to determine efficacy.

Evidence

- There is no randomised trial data (other than 16 cases in CAVATAS) but it is widely accepted that surgery on vertebral artery stenosis is high risk.
- Complication rates for EVT of extracranial vertebral (origin) disease are significantly lower than the risks associated with treatment for intracranial vertebrobasilar artery disease. The rate of any stroke or death within 14 months for proximal stenting is 2.3%, compared with 10.8% for distal stenting.
- In the UK, vertebral artery stenting is not routinely performed following the Vertebral Artery Ischaemia Stenting Trial (VIST) RCT, which ended prematurely due to poor recruitment (182 participants). The trial showed no periprocedural complications with extracranial stenting and two with intracranial stenting. While stenting showed some benefit, it was not statistically significant except in a small subgroup treated within 2 weeks of their last TIA or stroke.
- Markus et al. (2017) pooled data from the VIST, Vertebral Artery Stenting Trial (VAST), and Stenting and Aggressive Medical Management for Preventing Recurrent Stroke in Symptomatic Stenosis (SAMMPRIS) trials on stenting for symptomatic vertebral stenosis, analysing 354 patients. They found a higher early risk with stenting, mainly due to intracranial cases, with a 30-day periprocedural risk of 0.8% for extracranial stenting and 15.6% for intracranial stenting. Their analysis showed no overall statistical benefit in preventing recurrent strokes, especially for intracranial stenosis.
- **In summary, intracranial vertebral artery stenting carries additional risks, including brainstem perforator infarction and SAH, which is reflected in the higher morbidity observed in clinical trials. Extracranial stenting is safer and shows a trend towards improved outcomes, but larger trials are needed to confirm these findings.**

UK National Clinical Guidelines for Stroke 2023

People with ischaemic stroke or TIA and symptomatic vertebral artery stenosis should receive optimal secondary prevention including antithrombotic therapy, blood pressure treatment, lipid-lowering therapy and lifestyle modification. Angioplasty and stenting of the vertebral artery should only be offered in the context of a clinical trial.

Technique

(See Figure 10.2.)

- Antiplatelets: it is recommended to administer 75 mg of aspirin daily for at least 7 days prior to the procedure, or to give a 600 mg loading dose the day before the procedure, followed by 75 mg on the day itself. Additionally, clopidogrel should be given at a dose of 75 mg daily for at least 7 days before the procedure, or alternatively, a 600 mg loading dose the day prior, followed by 75 mg on the day of the procedure. Platelet function testing is recommended. If clopidogrel fails to provide adequate suppression, prasugrel or another alternative may be used.
- Most stenoses occur at the origin. Stenting within the foramina is generally not recommended, as neck movement can lead to stent fracture and occlusion.
- Stenting at the origin can be performed under LA with or without sedation.
- A 5 or 6 Fr common femoral artery puncture is required. Alternatively, transradial access is a viable option, with the right radial artery used for the right vertebral artery and the left radial artery for the left vertebral artery.
- Systemic heparinisation is achieved with ACT monitoring.
- Angiography of both subclavian arteries will assess the origins of the vertebral arteries, collateral flow, and provide views of the intracranial circulation. The guide catheter is placed in the relevant subclavian artery and attached to an RHV with a heparin–saline flush.
- A symptomatic stenosis should be ≥50% to warrant treatment.
- Sometimes the lesion requires pre-dilatation using a compliant balloon (e.g. Mini-Trek (Abbott)). Balloon diameter should be 0.5 mm less than that of the non-stenosed artery.
- Usually balloon-mounted stents are deployed under roadmapping. Rapid exchange (monorail) stents are preferred, and various types are available, including coronary and renal. The lesion is crossed with either

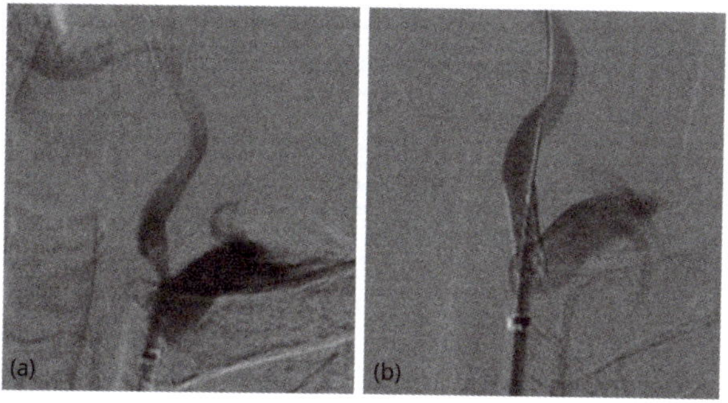

Figure 10.2 Vertebral ostium stenting. (a) Digital subtraction angiography shows symptomatic vertebral origin stenosis. (b) Post deployment of balloon-mounted stent. Note the proximal stent protruding into the subclavian artery.

a 0.014" or 0.018" wire, depending on the stent used, and a balloon-mounted stent is deployed across the stenosis, leaving a few millimetres of stent in the subclavian artery if necessary.

- Alternatively, self-expanding carotid stents have been tried with some success deployed from the vertebral ostium to the subclavian artery ('jailing' the distal subclavian artery).
- Following deployment, perform check angiography of the stented artery and cerebral circulation, and if the results are satisfactory, remove the delivery system.

Postprocedural care

- Extracranial patients should ideally be managed in an HDU overnight. Heparinisation is not necessary for extracranial stents.
- For intracranial stenting, it is essential that the patient is managed on an HDU or even an ITU overnight for close monitoring of BP and neurological parameters. Heparinisation is continued for 24 h.
- DAPT should be continued at 75 mg for at least 6 weeks, with one agent, usually aspirin, maintained at 75 mg daily for life.
- All patients have atheromatous disease and should be managed by a neurologist or stroke physician, with control of vascular risk factors.

Tips

- Accessing the right vertebral artery can be challenging. Sometimes, using a 7 Fr sheath with a wire guided into the subclavian artery can stabilise the system and facilitate access.

Imaging follow-up

- Non-invasive imaging such as ultrasound, particularly to look at flow through an origin stenosis, or CTA or MRA, is indicated.
- Angiography is reserved for those who become symptomatic or as follow up as part of a trial.

Further reading

Compter A, van der Worp HB, Schonewille WJ, et al. Stenting versus medical treatment in patients with symptomatic vertebral artery stenosis: a randomised open-label phase 2 trial. Lancet Neurol. 2015;14(6):606–614.

Derdeyn CP, Chimowitz MI, Lynn MJ, et al. Aggressive medical treatment with or without stenting in high-risk patients with intracranial artery stenosis (SAMMPRIS): the final results of a randomised trial. Lancet. 2014;383(9914):333–341.

Markus HS, Larsson SC, Kuker W, et al. Stenting for symptomatic vertebral artery stenosis: the Vertebral Artery Ischaemia Stenting Trial. Neurology. 2017;89(12):1229–1236.

Markus HS, Harshfield EL, Compter A, et al. Stenting for symptomatic vertebral artery stenosis: a preplanned pooled individual patient data analysis. Lancet Neurol. 2019;18(7):666–673.

Intracranial atherosclerotic disease stenting

Stenosis of the intracranial arteries occurs in approximately 40% of patients with ischaemic stroke and is likely to be a causative factor in around 7% of cases.

It is more frequent in Asian and Afro-Caribbean patients with some evidence that the risk is concentrated in women and those with stenosis >70%.

Stroke frequently occurs even with medical treatment. Recurrent stroke rates of up to 20% in 2 years were observed in the WASID trial (most within 12 months).

Stenting for symptomatic ICAD can be performed electively or as part of MT. However, there is very limited evidence to support its clinical benefit.

This section focuses on stenting for the anterior circulation. Posterior circulation stenting is commented on earlier in this chapter (see 'Vertebral artery stenting', p. 406).

Evidence

SAMMPRIS

In the SAMMPRIS trial, subjects were randomised to receive either the best medical treatment or stenting combined with best medical treatment. The trial was stopped prematurely after 451 out of the planned 764 subjects enrolled due to the demonstrated superiority of best medical therapy over stenting. The stroke/death rate in the stenting arm within 30 days was 14%, compared to 6% with medical therapy alone.

VISSIT

The Vitesse Intracranial Stent Study for Ischemic Stroke Therapy (VISSIT) trial compared the efficacy and safety of balloon-expandable stents combined with medical therapy against medical therapy alone in patients with symptomatic intracranial stenosis exceeding 70%. The stenting group exhibited a 24.1% rate of stroke or death within 30 days, compared to 9.4% in the medical group, corroborating the results of the SAMMPRIS trial.

WEAVE

The more recent Wingspan Stent System Post Market Surveillance (WEAVE) trial, published in 2019, revealed a much lower 2.6% rate of periprocedural stroke and death, suggesting the importance of careful patient selection, particularly excluding those with basilar and perforator strokes. Factors identified in the trial believed to contribute to improved outcomes include stenting >7 days after the qualifying event, experienced operators, and utilising optimal periprocedural management and protocols.

CASSISS

The China Angioplasty & Stenting for Symptomatic Intracranial Severe Stenosis (CASSISS) RCT published in 2022 enrolled 380 patients with a history of TIA or non-disabling ischaemic stroke linked to severe intracranial stenosis (70–99%), and who were beyond 3 weeks from their last ischaemic event. The results showed no statistically significant difference between medical treatment or medical therapy combined with intracranial stenting in terms of the incidence of stroke or death within the initial 30 days, and stroke in the qualifying artery territory at 1 year. Secondary endpoints also demonstrated no significant difference between the groups.

Reviews and guidelines

- A Cochrane review (2023) concluded that there was:

> moderate-certainty evidence that EVT plus conventional medical treatment (CMT) compared with CMT alone increases the risk of short-term stroke and death in people with recent symptomatic severe ICAS [intracranial atherosclerotic stenosis]. This effect was still apparent at long-term follow-up but appeared to be due to the early risks of EVT; therefore, there may be no clear difference between the interventions in terms of their effects on long-term stroke and death.

- NICE concluded there is insufficient evidence on the outcome of stenting and more research is needed.
- UK National Clinical Guidelines for Stroke 2023:

> People with ischaemic stroke or TIA due to severe symptomatic intracranial stenosis should be offered dual antiplatelet therapy with aspirin and clopidogrel for the first three months in addition to optimal secondary prevention including blood pressure treatment, lipid-lowering therapy and lifestyle modification. Endovascular or surgical intervention should only be offered in the context of a clinical trial.

Technique

(See Figure 10.3.)

- Acute intracranial stenting during MT is discussed in Chapter 9 (see 'Tandem carotid occlusion', p. 355).
- Patient selection should involve an MDT experienced in the management of stroke. The results of the WEAVE trial suggest that stenting should be performed at least 7 days after the ischaemic event.
- Antiplatelets: it is recommended to administer aspirin 75 mg daily for at least 7 days prior to the procedure, or alternatively a loading dose of 600 mg the day before, followed by 75 mg on the day of the procedure. Clopidogrel should be given at a dosage of 75 mg daily for at least 7 days before the procedure, or a 600 mg loading dose the day before, followed by 75 mg on the procedure day. Platelet function testing is recommended.
- GA is desirable due to the risks involved and procedural complexity.
- An 8 Fr vascular sheath is inserted into the common femoral artery. Transradial access is also suitable for the procedure.
- Systemic heparinisation is achieved with ACT monitoring.
- An 8 Fr guide catheter is positioned within the ICA and connected to a RHV and heparin–saline flush.
- An intermediate catheter, such as Navien, can be used for extra support.
- Angiography is performed to assess the cerebral circulation and site of stenosis. Cone beam CT is occasionally useful to optimise projections for navigation and stenting.
- A 0.014" microwire, e.g. Synchro (Stryker), is used. A gentle curve is applied to the tip (do not over-shape the tip as it will be harder to cross the stenosis).

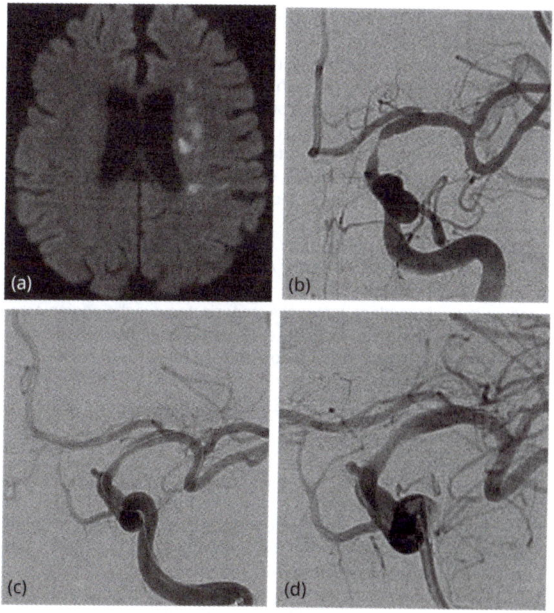

Figure 10.3 Intracranial atherosclerotic disease stenting. (a) Fluid-attenuated inversion recovery sequence demonstrating watershed ischaemic lesions. (b) Digital subtraction angiography shows distal internal cerebral artery stenosis. (c) After balloon angioplasty (deflated balloon across lesion). (d) After deployment of laser-cut stent (distal end markers seen in proximal middle cerebral artery), the vessel lumen is wider.

- The stenosis can often be crossed directly with the microwire. However, if needed, a microcatheter can be used to aid in crossing the stenosis with an exchange-length microwire. The microcatheter is then exchanged for the angioplasty balloon or stent. The risk of this manoeuvre is wire-tip perforation and SAH.

Angioplasty

- If the stenosis is very narrow, it may be necessary to predilate with an angioplasty balloon. Non-compliant balloons suitable for intracranial use include Neurospeed (Acandis), pITA (Phenox), and Mini-Trek (Abbott).
- Undersizing the angioplasty balloon in perforator-rich regions, including the M1 segment of the MCA or the pontine segment of the basilar trunk, has been shown to reduce the incidence of perforator strokes.
- The balloon is prepared by purging the dead space with 50% contrast:saline mixture. This is performed by filling a 20 mL syringe and aspirating from the device's inflation port three times, for approximately 20 s each time, while gently tapping the port to displace air and allow

the fluid to occupy the space. The port is then connected to an inflation device via a three-way stopcock.

- The wire is threaded retrogradely into the end of the balloon catheter.
- The balloon is then passed through the guide catheter and centred across the stenosis using the microwire and roadmap guidance. Angiography can be performed to confirm correct placement.
- Carefully (under)inflate the balloon by rotating the handle on the inflation device under fluoroscopic guidance, until the nominal balloon pressure is reached as specified on the pressure instructions accompanying the device.
- Deflate the balloon by pulling back on the plunger of the inflation device. Angiography will assess the result. Additional angioplasty attempts can be performed if needed.
- Keeping the wire in place across the stenosis, remove the angioplasty balloon. It is necessary to fix the wire to the table, and screen the wire tip intermittently to ensure the wire does not slip forwards or backwards.

Stenting

- The stent must be sized to the vessel segment proximal and distal to the stenosis. Oversizing can be employed to increase radial force.
- Various stents are suitable:
  - Atlas or other laser-cut stents: microcatheters such as the SL-10 can be used to deploy these.
  - The Neurospeed balloon (Acandis) can be used to deploy the Credo or Acclino HRF (Acandis) stents. This avoids the necessity of performing microwire exchange with its associated risks.
  - The Wingspan stent system (Stryker) is delivered through a supplied delivery microcatheter. Pre-dilatation of the lesion using the Gateway PTA balloon is necessary to approximately 75% of the diameter of the normal vessel before deployment of the stent.
  - Balloon-mounted coronary stents can also be used. Resolute Onyx (Medtronic) is a balloon-mounted coronary stent, available in both rapid exchange and over-the-wire versions, and has been used off-label for intracranial atherosclerotic disease, featuring a drug/polymer coating composed of zotarolimus within a BioLinx polymer.
- Prepare the stent. Laser-cut stents need simply to be flushed. Balloon-mounted stents must be prepared similarly to angioplasty balloons.
- If angioplasty is first performed, and it is desired not to recross the stenosis with a wire, microwire exchange must be performed to insert a deployment catheter unless the Neurospeed balloon is used (as this balloon microcatheter itself can be used to deploy the stent).
- Use a roadmap to centre the stent across the stenosis. Perform angiography to confirm correct device position.
- Unsheathe the device in place.
- Repeat angiography to determine residual stenosis.
- If necessary, balloon angioplasty can be performed to expand the stent and vessel further.
- Cerebral angiography should be performed at the end of the procedure to confirm absence of distal emboli.

Postprocedural care

- It is essential for the patient to have access to an HDU or potentially an ITU bed overnight for close monitoring of BP and other neurological parameters. Heparinisation may be continued for 24 h following the procedure.
- DAPT should be continued for 6 months. One agent, either aspirin or clopidogrel, should thereafter be continued for life.

Further reading

Alexander MJ, Zauner A, Chaloupka JC, et al. WEAVE trial: final results in 152 on-label patients. Stroke. 2019;50(4):889–894.

Chimowitz MI, Kokkinos J, Strong J, et al. The Warfarin-Aspirin Symptomatic Intracranial Disease study. Neurology. 1995;45(8):1488–1493.

Gao P, Wang T, Wang D, et al. Effect of stenting plus medical therapy vs medical therapy alone on risk of stroke and death in patients with symptomatic intracranial stenosis: the CASSISS randomized clinical trial. JAMA. 2022;328(6):534–542.

Luo J, Wang T, Yang K, et al. Endovascular therapy versus medical treatment for symptomatic intracranial artery stenosis. Cochrane Database Syst Rev. 2023;2(2):CD013267.

Zaidat OO, Fitzsimmons BF, Woodward BK, et al. Effect of a balloon-expandable intracranial stent vs medical therapy on risk of stroke in patients with symptomatic intracranial stenosis: the VISSIT randomized clinical trial. JAMA. 2015;313(12):1240–1248.

Cranial dural arteriovenous fistulas

Introduction 416
Imaging of dural arteriovenous fistulas (DAVFs) 419
Classification of DAVFs 421
Indications for treatment 423
Complications of treatment 425
Principles of endovascular treatment 426
Transverse-sigmoid sinus DAVF 430
Superior sagittal sinus DAVF 432
Tentorial DAVF 433
Lateral foramen magnum DAVF 436
Anterior cranial fossa DAVF 439
Indirect cavernous sinus DAVF 441
Direct carotid–cavernous DAVF 444

Introduction

Aetiology

- DAVFs are abnormal arteriovenous shunts within the walls of the dural venous sinuses or meningeal or cortical veins.
- They are most commonly supplied by meningeal arteries, although they can also be fed by pial arteries via their dural branches (10–15%) and drain into the dural venous sinuses (directly or indirectly), or into meningeal or cortical veins.
- They are considered acquired lesions, and two main hypotheses, which may coexist, account for their formation:
  - Physiological microshunts, present in the walls of sinuses, enlarge in the presence of increased sinus pressure caused by sinus thrombosis.
  - Venous hypertension caused by venous outflow obstruction (including, but not exclusively, sinus thrombosis) results in hypoxia, which stimulates the production of endothelial growth factors and triggers angiogenesis.
- DAVFs are seen with increased frequency with all causes of CVST including hypercoagulable states such as protein S deficiency, pregnancy, and oral contraceptive usage. They are also associated with otitis or sinusitis, phlebitis of the lower limbs, trauma, and surgery. AVMs predispose to the development of DAVF, possibly due to either venous hypertension or cerebral hypoxaemia in brain parenchyma surrounding an AVM.
- CVST may also occur secondary to a DAVF. Turbulent flow on the sinus induces intimal injury and thrombosis.
- Direct arteriovenous fistulas can arise from rupture of arteries adjacent to veins creating direct fistulous tracts, after trauma or surgery. These are separate entities from DAVFs but are included in this chapter as the treatment is similar.

Epidemiology and demographics

- The incidence of DAVF in the Scottish Intracranial Vascular Malformation Study (SIVMS) was 0.16 per 100,000 per annum. In the same study, AVMs were seven times more common (with an incidence of 1.12 per 100,000 per annum).
- They occur in adults most commonly between the ages of 40–60 years; however, they may also be seen in paediatric patients.
- The commonest sites are the transverse–sigmoid junction and cavernous sinus. Other frequently encountered locations include the tentorium cerebelli, superior sagittal sinus, and anterior cranial fossa.

Clinical presentation

- Symptoms may arise gradually after the onset of dural venous sinus thrombosis (which may have been clinically silent or undiagnosed).
- DAVFs may be diagnosed incidentally on cross-sectional or angiographic imaging performed for other purposes.
- Symptoms are related to arterialisation of the draining sinus or veins:
  - Pulsatile tinnitus: this is common due to the frequency of DAVFs involving the transverse and sigmoid sinuses and their closeness to

the inner ear. It reflects the turbulent vascular flow through the skull base. The onset is usually sudden and patients often recall the time of symptom onset. The sound is synchronous with the heartbeat and may be audible during auscultation. Symptoms may be alleviated by carotid or occipital artery compression.

- Spontaneous ICH: parenchymal, subdural, and subarachnoid haemorrhage are all possible. 20–30% present with ICH, with a poor prognosis in 30%. The risk is increased for DAVF with cortical venous reflux (CVR) and for those who have suffered a previous haemorrhage. The risk is also increased in symptomatic venous hypertension secondary to the CVR (18.2% vs 5.9% without symptoms). The risk of rebleeding is very high, 35% within 2 weeks.
- Venous infarction: secondary to venous congestion and can lead to haemorrhage. This is usually adjacent to the sinus and reflecting the frequency of transverse–sigmoid sinus DAVF, often in the temporal lobe.
- Retroauricular pain can coexist.
- Ophthalmic symptoms: raised intraocular pressure may result in potentially irreversible visual loss. Other symptoms include exophthalmos, diplopia, chemosis, pain, and bruit.
- Seizures: due to CVR.
- Dementia, Parkinsonism, hypersomnolence and focal deficits: due to venous congestion or raised ICP, typically for DAVF at the falcotentorial junction with reflux into the deep venous system.
- Intracranial hypertension: causes headache, papilloedema, and upward gaze palsy. If severe, this may result in a decreased level of consciousness.
- Cranial nerve palsies, commonly oculomotor and abducens, due to elevated ICP or venous compression. The hypoglossal nerve can be affected by fistulas of the anterior condylar canal (hypoglossal canal).
- Cervical myelopathy: with spinal venous drainage, patients may exhibit limb weakness, bulbar and autonomic dysfunction (e.g. postural hypotension, spontaneous bradycardia, and systemic hypertension).

Natural history

- Fistulas may evolve over time. They may rarely resolve spontaneously, show a change in symptomatology, or progress to a higher grade (0.8% per year). Venous stenoses and/or thromboses may complicate secondary to a high-flow venopathy. Consequently, any alteration in symptomatology, be it the emergence of new symptoms or their resolution, necessitates angiographic re-evaluation. For benign fistulas conservatively managed, annual follow-up is routinely recommended—MRI/MRA will often suffice rather than DSA.
- In a series of patients with CVR who declined treatment or had persistence of the fistula after treatment, the annual mortality was 10.4%, the annual haemorrhagic risk was 8.1%, and non-haemorrhagic neurological deficit was 6.9% (van Dijk et. al., 2002).

Further reading

Al-Shahi R, Bhattacharya JJ, Currie DG, et al. Prospective, population-based detection of intracranial vascular malformations in adults the Scottish Intracranial Vascular Malformation Study (SIVMS). Stroke. 2003;34(5):1163–1169.

Sachs E. Diagnosis and Treatment of Brain Tumours and Care of Neurosurgical Patient. Mosby; 1946.

Soderman M, Pavic L, Edner G, Holmin S, Andersson T. Natural history of dural arteriovenous shunts. Stroke. 2008;39(6):1735–1739.

van Dijk JM, terBrugge KG, Willinsky RA, Wallace MC. Clinical course of cranial dural arteriovenous fistulas with long-term persistent cortical venous reflux. Stroke. 2002;33(5):1233–1236.

Imaging of dural arteriovenous fistulas (DAVFs)

Cross-sectional imaging

- Non-contrast CT:
  - Often normal in benign fistulas.
  - May reveal parenchymal oedema, ICH, or enlarged vessels.
  - There may be prominent transcalvarial channels due to enlarged transosseous feeding arteries, especially in osteodural DAVFs.
  - Curvilinear calcification in the subcortical white matter reflects venous ischaemia/hypertension.
  - Carotid–cavernous fistulas typically result in enlarged superior ophthalmic veins and proptosis.
- CT angiography and venography: may reveal enlarged dural arteries, ectatic arterialised veins, and thrombosed sinuses.
- MRI:
  - Is more sensitive and may demonstrate oedema, haemorrhage (including chronic haemosiderin staining), and enlarged meningeal arteries and veins.
  - Arterialised veins may be detected as high signal on SWI sequences.
  - Dural venous sinus thrombosis may be observed surrounded by flow voids, representing feeding arteries.
  - Enlarged transmedullary veins may be seen, representing alternate venous drainage pathways.
  - Changes in cervical spinal or brainstem signal representing myelopathy may be the only feature of Cognard type 5 DAVF.

Digital subtraction angiography

- DSA is the gold standard for diagnosis and characterisation.
- Fast frame rates (≥5 frames/s) are useful as these are often high-flow lesions.
- A six-vessel cerebral angiogram is usually required to identify all feeding arteries and draining veins. Document normal cranial venous drainage pathways.
- It is especially important to identify CVR as this impacts prognosis and management. Tortuous engorged veins in the venous phase of angiography (not in the venous phase of the DAVF) reflect the effects of severe chronic venous hypertension. Venous aneurysms are an aggressive feature.
- 3D rotational cone beam angiography (Vaso or DynaCT) is helpful to characterise complex architecture.

Follow-up imaging

- 'Recurrences' probably represent angiographically occult but still anatomically present fistulas, rather than true recanalisation of a completely occluded fistula. In the Consortium for Dural Arteriovenous Fistula Outcomes Research (CONDOR) study, endovascularly 'cured' DAVF recurred in about 7% of cases. This number may be an overestimation, as a large number of cases were lost to follow-up. Most of these cases were clinically silent but have a statistically higher incidence of haemorrhage and neurological deficit. Therefore, it is important to follow up and treat if identified. Conversely, the persistence of symptoms was found to be common after cure and does not necessarily indicate that the fistula is still present.

- DSA is the gold standard and is typically performed 3–12 months after treatment. MRI/MRA may also be valuable as a less invasive alternative, or if the fistula or its sequelae (such as venous congestion) could be identified on the initial study. MRI can miss 'recurrences,' however.

Further reading

Abecassis IJ, Meyer RM, Levitt MR, et al. Recurrence after cure in cranial dural arteriovenous fistulas: a collaborative effort by the Consortium for Dural Arteriovenous Fistula Outcomes Research (CONDOR). J Neurosurg. 2021;136(4):981–989.

Classification of DAVFs

DAVFs may remain dormant and without clinical consequence or may result in devastating ICH. Several classification schemes have been developed to predict the natural history (Tables 11.1–11.3). The presence of CVR is the single most important architectural feature in classifying fistulas as high or low grade.

Table 11.1 Cognard classification of dural arteriovenous fistulas

Type 1	Drainage into sinus with antegrade flow	'Low' grade
Type 2a	Drainage into sinus with retrograde reflux into sinus	
Type 2b	Drainage into sinus with retrograde reflux into cortical veins	'High' grade
Type 2a + 2b	Drainage into sinus with retrograde reflux into sinus and cortical veins	
Type 3	Drainage directly into cortical veins	
Type 4	Drainage directly into cortical veins with venous ectasia	
Type 5	Drainage into spinal perimedullary veins	

Table 11.2 Borden classification of dural arteriovenous fistulas

Type 1	Drainage directly into dural venous sinuses or meningeal veins with antegrade drainage. In the spine, this includes drainage into Batson's epidural venous plexus
Type 2	Drainage into dural sinuses or meningeal veins with retrograde drainage into subarachnoid veins. In the spine, drainage is into both the epidural venous plexus and perimedullary veins (which are subarachnoid)
Type 3	Drainage into directly into subarachnoid veins. In the spine, most commonly these are supplied by meningeal branches of a radicular artery and drain intrathecally through a subarachnoid vein into the coronal venous plexus

Table 11.3 Barrow classification of carotid–cavernous fistulas

Type A	Direct ICA to cavernous sinus high-flow shunt	Direct fistula
Type B	Dural ICA branches to cavernous sinus	Indirect fistula
Type C	Dural ECA branches to cavernous sinus	
Type D	Both ICA and ECA dural branches to cavernous sinus	

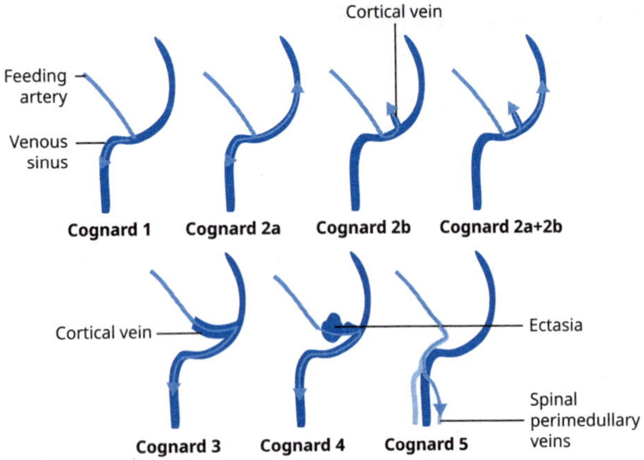

Figure 11.1 Cognard classification of dural arteriovenous fistula.

Cognard classification

(See Figure 11.1.)

Borden classification

The Borden classification is simpler and can also be used to grade spinal DAVF. Type 1 Borden roughly corresponds to type 1–2a Cognard, type 2 Borden to 2b Cognard and type 2a + 2b Cognard, and type 3 Borden to type 3–5 Cognard.

Barrow classification

The Barrow classification is of cavernous fistulas. Type A indicates a direct carotid–cavernous fistula, whereas types B–D indicate an indirect fistula.

Further reading

Barrow DL, Spector RH, Braun IF, Landman JA, Tindall SC, Tindall GT. Classification and treatment of spontaneous carotid–cavernous sinus fistulas. J Neurosurg. 1985;62(2):248–256.

Borden JA, Wu JK, Shucart WA. A proposed classification for spinal and cranial dural arteriovenous fistulous malformations and implications for treatment. J Neurosurg. 1995;82(2):166–179.

Cognard C, Gobin YP, Pierot L, et al. Cerebral dural arteriovenous fistulas: clinical and angiographic correlation with a revised classification of venous drainage. Radiology. 1995;194(3):671–680.

Indications for treatment

Cognard type 1

- These are considered benign, with very little risk of haemorrhage or neurological consequence. In the CONDOR study, there was no benefit in terms of neurological or functional outcomes for treating low-grade (Borden 1) fistulae. A conservative approach is therefore preferred.
- There is a small risk of progression to CVR due to spontaneous progressive thrombosis of venous outlets. Therefore, patients should be followed, or at least asked to re-present if symptoms change.
- Indications for treatment include severe life-impacting tinnitus, local pain due to irritation of the dura mater, or other symptoms impacting quality of life. Any treatment must carry the lowest risk. The patient must be aware that obliteration of the fistula may not necessarily cure the symptoms.

Intermittent manual compression

- There is limited evidence that intermittent compression over a period of time is effective in curing the fistula. The exact mechanism is unclear (possibly a reduction in arterial flow and/or venous drainage inducing thrombosis).
- The technique involves pressing on the ipsilateral carotid with the contralateral hand (which will fall away with induced ischaemia!) until the pulsatile tinnitus disappears (if present) 25–100 times a day for 10–30 s.
- It is contraindicated in those with carotid atherosclerosis, or if symptoms such as faintness or motor symptoms develop.

Cognard type 2a

- The risk of ICH remains very low; however, indications for treatment may additionally include intracranial hypertension and dementia.

Treatment of Cognard types 2b–5

- There is a strong indication for treatment because of the high risk of ICH and venous infarction due to arterialisation of the cortical veins.
- Annual risks include 10.4% mortality, 8.1% haemorrhage, and 6.9% non-haemorrhagic neurological deficit. The overall annual event rate is 15%.

Symptomatic or ruptured dural fistulas

- There is a high risk of rebleeding (35% within 2 weeks after the first haemorrhage) in DAVFs presenting with haemorrhage, often with grave consequences.
- These fistulas must therefore be treated within the acute phase, ideally within 24–48 h, similar to ruptured aneurysms.
- Patients with non-ruptured high-grade fistulas presenting with seizures and venous congestion are likely also at high risk for haemorrhage and should be treated promptly.

Further reading

Chen CJ, Buell TJ, Ding D, et al. Observation versus intervention for low-grade intracranial dural arteriovenous fistulas. Neurosurgery. 2021;88(6):1111–1120.

Duffau H, Lopes M, Janosevic V, et al. Early rebleeding from intracranial dural arteriovenous fistulas: report of 20 cases and review of the literature. J Neurosurg. 1999;90(1):78–84.

Satomi J, van Dijk JM, Terbrugge KG, et al. Benign cranial dural arteriovenous fistulas: outcome of conservative management based on the natural history of the lesion. J Neurosurg. 2002;97(4):767–770.
Schumacher M, Szczeponik N. Successful treatment of dural AV fistulas by manual compression: a matter of perseverance. Neuroradiology. 2007;49(6):495–498.
van Dijk JM, terBrugge KG, Willinsky RA, Wallace MC. Clinical course of cranial dural arteriovenous fistulas with long-term persistent cortical venous reflux. Stroke. 2002;33(5):1233–1236.

Complications of treatment

- Post procedural pain: due to dural ischaemia.
- Death: 1%.
- Ischaemia: 2.3%.
- Vessel perforation: 0.9%.
- Vessel rupture: 0.3%.
- Venous occlusion with non-haemorrhagic deficit: 0.6%.
- Venous occlusion with haemorrhage: 0.5%.
- Failure to occlude fistula: rate dependent on location and type of fistula (and operator experience).
- Recurrence: 7%.
- Pulmonary emboli: rare.
- Cardiac migration of embolic agent: can be the source of arrhythmias and may require anticoagulation and, rarely, cardiac surgery.
- Trigeminocardiac reflex:
  - Involves bradycardia and hypotension with potential progression to cardiac arrest upon injection of DMSO or LE material. It usually settles spontaneously without treatment, on stopping the injection. Slow injection of the LE can resume after.
  - May be treated with atropine and avoided by intra-arterial injection of 5–20 mg of lidocaine (e.g. 1 mL 2% lidocaine). There is no need to premedicate.
  - It is advisable to inform the anaesthetist before injecting these agents so that the haemodynamic status can be monitored closely.
  - The putative mechanism is stimulation of the trigeminal sensory nucleus via the Gasserian ganglion. This pathway connects with the reticular formation and motor nucleus of the vagus.
- Venous thrombosis: can occur with stagnation of blood flow. Heparinisation for 24–48 h is advisable if significant stagnation is identified.
- Additional shared risks of angiographic procedures: puncture site haemorrhage or ischaemia, radiation, contrast allergy, and those associated with GA.

Further reading

Abecassis IJ, Meyer RM, Levitt MR, et al. Recurrence after cure in cranial dural arteriovenous fistulas: a collaborative effort by the Consortium for Dural Arteriovenous Fistula Outcomes Research (CONDOR). J Neurosurg. 2021;136(4):981–989.

Hiramatsu M, Sugiu K, Hishikawa T, et al. Results of 1940 embolisations for dural arteriovenous fistulas: Japanese Registry of Neuroendovascular Therapy (JR-NET3). J Neurosurg. 2019;133(1):166–173.

Kobayashi A, Al-Shahi SR. Prognosis and treatment of intracranial dural arteriovenous fistulae: a systematic review and meta-analysis. Int J Stroke. 2014;9(6):670–677.

Sun Z, Wang R, Dong H, et al. Prophylactic intra-arterial injection of lidocaine: a novel strategy to prevent endovascular embolization-induced trigeminocardiac reflex. J Neurointerv Surg. 2023;15(5):473–477.

Principles of endovascular treatment

- DAVF is primarily a venous disease. The target for occlusion is therefore the proximal portion ('foot') of the vein, at the site of the fistula, whether treated via a transarterial, transvenous, or a combined approach.
- Proximal arterial occlusion alone will inevitably result in recanalisation of the fistula due to recruitment of collateral flow. Partial embolisation is acceptable only to alleviate (considerable) symptoms in benign fistulas.
- Shunts are most commonly in the wall of a sinus or involve a localised shunted venous pouch ('parasinus').
- EVT is considered first line for most DAVFs and the principles are relatively well established, in contrast to the strategy of treatment of AVMs, where there is still a lot of debate.
- While probably the majority of fistulas can be obliterated at one attempt, staging the treatment may be prudent in complex fistulas to reduce the risk of complications.
- If the fistula has multiple arteries supplying it, e.g. the ECA and vertebral artery, placing a diagnostic catheter in the second site is useful to ensure embolisation is not terminated early,
- A description of general principles is provided here. Tips for certain fistula locations are presented later.

Materials

- Refer to Chapter 4, 'Guidewires', p. 117; 'Sheaths and Catheters', p. 119; 'Copolymer liquid embolics', p. 140, and 'Cyanoacrylate glue', p. 137.

Characterisation

- A five- or six-vessel cerebral angiogram is recommended to define the architecture prior to treatment. Knowledge of arterial feeders and variants, extracranial to intracranial anastomoses, cranial nerve supply, venous drainage pathways, CVR, and arterialisation and thrombosis of sinuses and venous drainage pathways of the brain, is particularly important.
- High-resolution cone beam CT using transarterially injected 15% contrast can be useful in defining the anatomy in complex fistulas, e.g. when in close proximity to arterial feeders of the cranial nerves.
- Microcatheter angiography is indicated prior to every injection of embolic material.
- Understanding the site and shape of the fistula is necessary. 'Security margins' should be defined—these are lines beyond which it is dangerous for the LE to traverse. You can draw these on the monitor during injection of embolic agents for increased clarity.

General strategy

Cognard types 1–2a

- Transarterial embolisation with LEs with sinus preservation is usually the strategy.
- Occlusion of an involved sinus is contraindicated as the cortical veins are not arterialised and are necessary to drain the brain parenchyma.
- The sinus may be protected by placement of a large compliant balloon, however there still remains the risk that LE can enter the sinus and

travel along its wall into cortical veins. This may be difficult to detect. Therefore, the balloon should be inflated sufficiently to completely occluding the sinus.

Cognard type 2b

- Transarterial injection of LEs to occlude the fistula is a good strategy if possible.
- If the sinus and inserting cortical veins are arterialised, then occluding the whole sinus may be an option (this must be confirmed with ICA and vertebral injections). This can be achieved with transarterial injection of LE or transvenous placement of multiple large coils ± transvenous LE. It is best to target only the region of sinus involving the fistula.

Cognard types 3–5

- The usual approach is transarterial injection of LE to close the direct connections between dural arteries and cortical veins. This is often more straightforward than type 1–2b fistulas.
- A transvenous approach can also be employed. While it is probably safer to navigate through arteries compared to veins as they have thicker walls, this must be balanced against the risks of transarterial LE injection, which may be significant in certain locations.

Transarterial technique

- The technique involves injecting LEs into the fistula utilising blank roadmaps. Prolonged injections with LE can occlude multiple feeders through the fistula itself.
- Proximal arterial occlusion does not cure the disease even if the fistula no longer opacifies. While there may be temporary resolution of symptoms, these will likely recur with recruitment of more dural vessels over time, secondary to angiogenic growth factors.
- Injections are often limited by reflux proximal to the injecting position. A plug may be built up by injecting and then stopping when reflux is seen.
- It is important to position the microcatheter as close as possible to the fistulous point to aid penetration to the foot of the vein before the reflux limit is reached.
- When a distal position cannot be reached, balloon catheters such as the Scepter Mini used in combination with a low-viscosity agent such as Squid-12 can prevent reflux, allowing more distal penetration. Inflation may need to be increased, with care, as the procedure progresses.
- An alternative approach is the 'pressure cooker' technique, which involves positioning an additional microcatheter more proximally and using it to create a plug using glue and/or coils to prevent reflux.
- If multiple vessels are involved (for example ICA and VA) it can be useful to deploy a second angiographic catheter in the alternate parent vessel because: (i) angiography can be performed while the injecting catheter is still in place, helping to ensure that treatment is not ceased prematurely; and (ii) other arterial pedicles can be readily accessed during the same treatment if necessary.
- The fistula is occluded considered treated when it no longer fills from all potential arterial feeders and the proximal part of the vein is occluded.
- Avoid reflux into the cortical veins when injecting LEs by injecting slowly and progressively. It may take quite some time if a large volume needs filling.

- The best arterial pedicles for injection are those that: (i) do not supply cranial nerves or have anastomoses with pial branches, (ii) have straight courses that can be easily navigated, and (iii) are wide enough to be navigated with the catheter. Branches of the MMA are the most frequently used vessels because they often satisfy these criteria.
- The pedicle does not necessarily need to be very large. A smaller-diameter vessel is sometimes preferable as 'wedging' the microcatheter prevents reflux and encourages forward flow.
- The occipital artery can be treacherous even when it appears invitingly wide, as the course is often very tortuous and the catheter must traverse the skull to reach the fistula. Injecting through a balloon catheter (e.g. Scepter Mini) can be very helpful if a distal position cannot be reached. Note that the proximal occipital artery has links with the vertebral artery.
- The proximal ascending pharyngeal artery is risky to embolise due to its cranial nerve supply and dangerous anastomoses. Embolisation via the dural branches of the ICA (e.g. the ILT/MHT branches) are also hazardous due to the risk of reflux into the ICA and ischaemia of cranial nerves. If these branches are utilised, reaching a distal position with the injecting catheter combined with balloon protection of the ICA is recommended.
- The petrosal and lacrimal branches of the MMA should be protected to avoid, respectively, facial nerve palsy and retinal artery infiltration.
- A full discussion of dangerous anastomoses is covered in Chapter 2 (see 'Dangerous cranial anastomoses', p. 58).

Transvenous technique

- Occlusion of the entire venous drainage pathway with coils and/or LEs can cure the fistula but this *cannot be undertaken* if the venous channel is still used to drain the brain as it risks venous ischaemia (i.e. functional sinus).
- If the cortical veins are arterialised, the sinus is unlikely to significantly contribute to parenchymal venous drainage and can be safely occluded, preferably as close to the fistulous point as possible.
- Inflation of an arterially positioned balloon may help to prevent reflux across the fistula into dangerous anastomoses.
- It is helpful to define the exact point of fistulisation, potentially via 3D angiography, as this may be small and easily occluded (Figure 11.2).

Post-procedure

- Venous stagnation may occur after treating fistulas and, if marked, the patient may benefit from continued post-procedure heparinisation to reduce the risk of thrombus propagation. LMWH is probably best, and a suggested protocol is 1 week of full treatment dose and a further week of the lower preventative dose. In some centres this protocol is given routinely for every case.
- Corticosteroids may be given postprocedurally to reduce tissue swelling but there is limited evidence for their efficacy. A suggested regimen is dexamethasone 4 mg three times a day for 1 day, 4 mg twice a day for 1 day, and a single 4 mg dose on the third day. In cases of more extensive DAVF, a tapering dose over 5 or 7 days is sometimes prescribed.

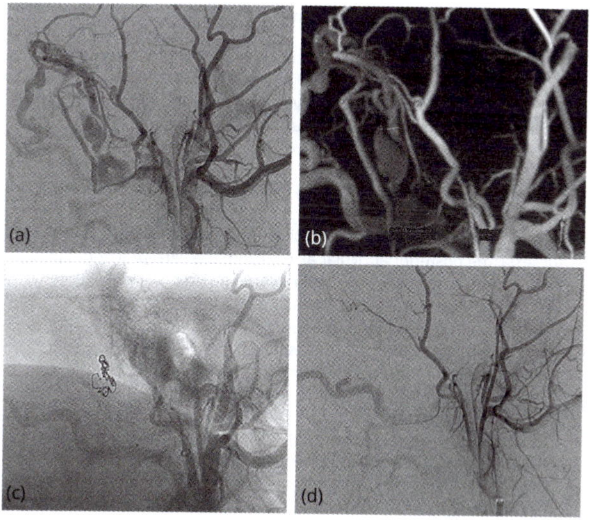

Figure 11.2 Transvenous treatment of Cognard type 3 dural arteriovenous fistula (DAVF). (a) DAVF with drainage via an ectatic intradural venous pouch into the transverse sinus. (b) The exact point of fistulation into the vein is clearly demonstrated on 3D rotational angiography. (c) This was occluded with detachable coils. (d) Obliteration of the fistula is confirmed.

Further reading

Bhatia KD, Lee H, Kortman H, et al. Endovascular management of intracranial dural arteriovenous fistulas: transarterial approach. AJNR Am J Neuroradiol. 2022;43(3):324–331.

Buell TJ, Raper DM, Ding D, et al. Development of an intracranial dural arteriovenous fistula after venous sinus stenting for idiopathic intracranial hypertension. J Neurointerv Surg. 2018;10(7):e15.

Lin YH, Lee CW, Liu HM. Clinical outcomes of adjunct sinus stenting in dural arteriovenous fistulas: role of flow restoration in steno-occlusion and cortical venous reflux. Clin Neuroradiol. 2022;32(2):455–464.

Transverse–sigmoid sinus DAVF

Together with the cavernous sinus, this is one of the two commonest locations of DAVF. Symptoms include pulsatile tinnitus, focal neurological deficits, cognitive decline, seizure, visual problems (occipital lobe), and haemorrhage, dependent upon venous drainage.

Anatomy

- Arterial: the MMA typically supplies this fistula and is the preferred pedicle for arterial injection. Other common feeders include the transmastoid branches of the occipital (more tortuous and less chance of success), the posterior auricular artery (from the vertebral or occipital), the marginal tentorial artery, the jugular/sigmoid branches of the neuromeningeal trunk of the ascending pharyngeal artery, and dural branches from the vertebral artery.
- Venous: the sigmoid or transverse sinus may be patent throughout, stenosed, or thrombosed distally or proximally, or both ('isolated sinus').

Treatment strategy

- Cognard types 1–2a: transarterial LE embolisation with preservation of the sinus. A compliant balloon placed in the venous sinus (usually the Balt Copernic) may provide protection from unintended migration of LEs into the sinus.
- Cognard type 2b (Figure 11.3): transarterial liquid embolisation is usually feasible. The sinus can also often be occluded via a transvenous approach if there is CVR. Coils are the safest and most straightforward method, although many large ones may be necessary. Injecting some LE or n-BCA at the end may be useful to complete the occlusion.
- Cognard types 3–5: usually transarterial with LEs ± balloon protection of the sinus.

Tips

- The simplest method for treating fistulas of isolated sinuses is often transarterial embolisation with LEs. If there is no suitable vessel for injection, however, it is often possible to reopen the blocked tract of an isolated sinus in order to occlude the fistula. This can be achieved with a microcatheter and wire, or by rotating a 0.035" guidewire using an angiographic catheter for support. There is a small risk of venous perforation and subdural haematoma during this manoeuvre. If this proves impossible, surgical access to the sinus through a burr hole can be obtained.
- When performing coil embolisation of a sinus, large, wide-diameter coils, such as the POD400/PAC400 coils (Penumbra), are preferred (these require the the PXSlim 0.020" microcatheter for delivery).

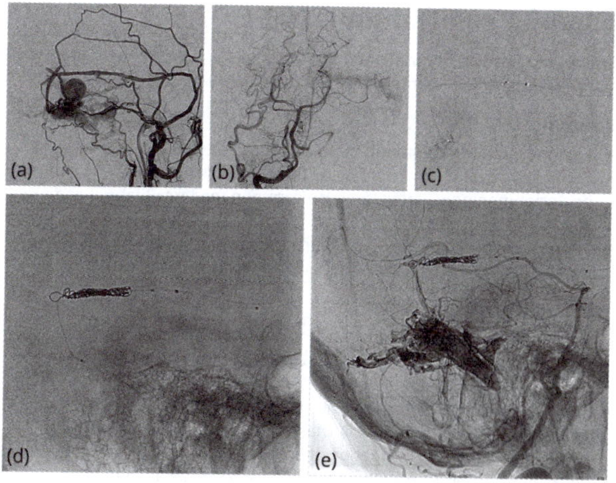

Figure 11.3 Treatment of a transverse sinus dural arteriovenous fistula (DAVF). (a) Digital subtraction angiography reveals a DAVF involving the transverse sinus with cortical venous reflux (CVR). A hypertrophied petrosquamosal middle meningeal artery (MMA) feeder is evident. (b) Feeders are also evident via dural branches of the SCA. (c) A detachable tip 0.013" microcatheter is inserted via the MMA feeder into the point of fistulisation and microcatheter angiography is performed. (d) Via a second, more proximal, microcatheter, detachable coils are released into the branch to reduce reflux of liquid embolics. (e) Final liquid embolic cast after occlusion of fistula.

Further reading

Gross BA, Albuquerque FC, Moon K, McDougall CG. Evolution of treatment and a detailed analysis of occlusion, recurrence, and clinical outcomes in an endovascular library of 260 dural arteriovenous fistulas. J Neurosurg. 2017;126(6):1884–1893.

Hendriks EJ, Lynch J, Swaminathan SK, et al. Embolization strategies for intracranial dural arteriovenous fistulas with an isolated sinus: a single-center experience in 20 patients. J Neurointerv Surg. 2022;14(6):605–610.

Superior sagittal sinus DAVF

These are usually high grade and not infrequently present with aggressive symptoms including haemorrhage, venous infarction, and seizures.

Anatomy

- Arterial: the MMA commonly supplies these fistulas. The superficial temporal, occipital, anterior falcine from the ophthalmic artery, and posterior meningeal artery are also common feeders. Bilateral and pial supply is not uncommon.
- Venous: shunting may be into the true superior sagittal sinus or into a parasinus.

Treatment strategy

- Transarterial embolisation with LEs via the MMA is usually a viable option (Figure 11.4). Balloon protection of the sinus is recommended if the brain depends on it for drainage.
- Transvenous occlusion of the sinus with coils ± LEs is an option if the sinus is arterialised with CVR. A triaxial setup is advisable, to provide more support during navigation. If access to the sinus is thrombosed, recanalisation with a microcatheter or rotational advancement of a 0.035" guidewire is often possible. There is a small risk of vessel perforation or subdural haematoma with this approach.

Tips

- As with other transarterial treatments, injecting from a balloon microcatheter may increase the chance of success due to reduced reflux during injection of LEs.

Complication avoidance

- Pial supply increases the risk of ischaemic complications.

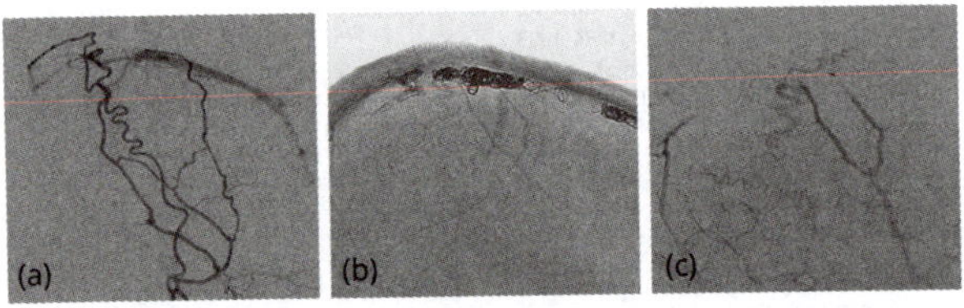

Figure 11.4 Superior sagittal sinus dural arteriovenous fistula (DAVF). (a) Digital subtraction angiography reveals a DAVF involving middle meningeal artery and superficial temporal artery feeders into the superior sagittal sinus. The anterior part of the sinus was arterialised. (b) The sinus is occluded with coils and liquid embolic. (c) The fistula no longer fills.

Further reading

Kurabe S, Kumagai T, Abe H. A comprehensive analysis of dural arteriovenous fistula involving the superior sagittal sinus: a systematic review. J Neuroendovasc Ther. 2021;15(1):1–7.

Tentorial DAVF

Tentorial DAVFs occur in the reflected double layer of dura of the tentorium and its attachments, which can extend from the clinoid process attachment and petrous ridges anteriorly to the torcula posteriorly. These are often complex, high-grade fistulas, with a poor natural history. CVR is common. They often present with haemorrhage or focal neurological deficits. Symptoms otherwise may include thalamic venous hypertension and dementia, coma, headache, exophthalmos, dysphagia, dysphonia, and ataxia.

Classification (Lawton)

- Galenic (anterior falcotentorial).
- Straight sinus (middle falcotentorial).
- Torcular (posterior falcotentorial).
- Tentorial sinus (paramedian tentorium).
- Superior petrosal (petrotentorial junction).
- Incisural (tentorial incisura).

Anatomy

- Arterial: different sites have predilections for certain arteries:
  - Galenic DAVF: PCA (artery of Davidoff and Schechter), SCA (Wollschlaeger and Wollschlaeger), posterior meningeal artery, MHT, anterior meningeal artery, pericallosal artery, MMA, occipital, superficial temporal. Posterior medial choroidal arteries supply 'mixed'-type fistulas.
  - Straight sinus DAVF: posterior meningeal artery, occipital artery, tentorial artery.
  - Torcular DAVF: posterior meningeal artery, occipital artery.
  - Tentorial sinus: MMA, scalp arteries.
  - Superior petrosal: tentorial artery.
  - Incisural: MMA, STA, tentorial arteries.
- Venous:
  - Galenic: drainage is commonly supra- and infratentorial. The straight sinus is often occluded, with venous drainage redirected retrogradely via the vein of Galen or its tributaries (BVR, precentral cerebellar vein). There may be drainage via cerebral and cerebellar cortical veins, and the lateral mesencephalic vein.
  - Straight sinus DAVF: infratentorially to vermian or superior cerebellar veins.
  - Torcular DAVF: medial and inferior occipital veins along the sagittal and transverse sinuses.
  - Tentorial DAVF: infra-occipital veins.
  - Superior petrosal sinus: infratentorially to the petrosal vein.
  - Incisural DAVF: medial and inferior temporal veins, lateral mesencephalic veins in the ambient cistern, or Rosenthal.
  - Cognard type 3 DAVF drain directly into cortical veins by definition.

Treatment strategy

- Transarterial is usually first line (Figure 11.5). The choice of vessel, as always, depends on tortuosity, risk of occlusion, and how close you can

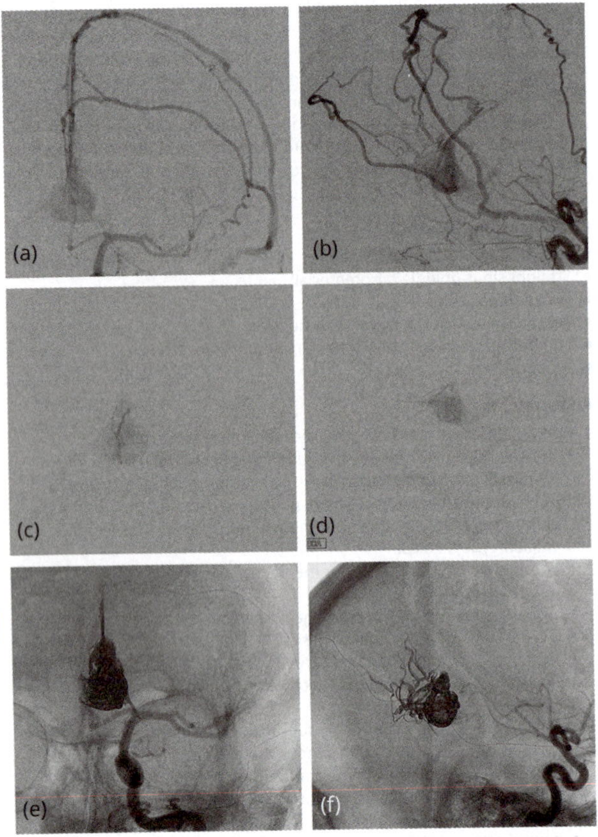

Figure 11.5 Galenic dural arteriovenous fistula. (a) Anteroposterior and (b) lateral digital subtraction angiography demonstrating fistulation into the vein of Galen via bilateral middle meningeal artery feeders. The internal cerebral veins were not draining via this channel (not shown). (c, d) Microcatheter angiography. (e, f) Final Onyx cast once occlusion of fistula had been achieved. Courtesy of Dr Parthiban Balasundaram.

get to the fistulous point. The MMA is a preferred vessel even if not the main feeder. The vein of Galen and straight sinus should not be occluded if at all possible.

- Transvenous: employed if transarterial therapy is impossible. Treatment with coils is safest.
- Complete obliteration is reported in 86.1% with clinical improvement in 88.8%.

Tips

- As these are often high-flow fistulas with large feeders, flow control with a large catheter (such as the Echelon-10), or balloon microcatheter, may be very helpful.

Complication avoidance

- These are high risk both in terms of natural history and treatment-related complications.
- For Galenic and straight sinus DAVF, it is important to first ascertain whether the internal cerebral veins are still draining conventionally via the vein of Galen and/or Rosenthal, or whether drainage is transmedullary via collaterals:
  - Occluding the vein of Galen or straight sinus when the internal cerebral veins depend on it for drainage may result in catastrophic venous ischaemia and potential haemorrhage. Collateral drainage is suggested if the vein of Galen is not visible on angiography when injecting vessels not supplying the fistula (i.e. Galen is arterialised or thrombosed).
  - Even if the vein is not seen, however, opacification and stagnation of the internal cerebral veins and a lack of collateral venous drainage of the ependymal veins is suggestive that the vein *is still* being used. Therefore, the deep venous system, or at the very least the junction between the BVR and internal cerebral vein, should be preserved.
- Pial feeders are a risk factor during transarterial treatment as reflux may occur into cortical arteries. It may be beneficial to occlude these first with coils.
- It may not always be possible to completely obliterate complex fistulas. Reduction of blood flow may suffice to temporarily reduce the risk of haemorrhage with the intention of bringing the patient back when the arterial feeders hypertrophy, allowing additional attempts.

Further reading

Byrne JV, Garcia M. Tentorial dural fistulas: endovascular management and description of the medial dural-tentorial branch of the superior cerebellar artery. AJNR Am J Neuroradiol. 2013;34(9):1798–1804.

Islak C, Bagcilar O, Nacar Dogan S, et al. Endovascular management of anterior falcotentorial dural arteriovenous fistulas: importance of functionality of deep venous system and existence of accompanying choroidal arteriovenous malformation. J Neurointerv Surg. 2022;14(6):599–604.

Lawton MT, Sanchez-Mejia RO, Pham D, et al. Tentorial dural arteriovenous fistulae: operative strategies and microsurgical results for six types. Neurosurgery. 2008;62(3 Suppl 1):110–124.

Lateral foramen magnum DAVF

These comprise a group of interconnected venous structures. Fistulous points may be single or multiple.

Locations

- Anterior condylar confluence and vein (otherwise known as hypoglossal canal).
- Posterior condylar canal.
- Marginal sinus.
- Jugular foramen.

Clinical

- Symptoms and signs are varied and include pulsatile tinnitus (very common), headache, and orbital symptoms such as chemosis and extra-orbital muscle palsies. Other symptoms include SAH, hypoglossal and trigeminal nerve palsy, and myelopathy.
- Imaging may reveal serpiginous vessels at the skull base and around the spinal cord, and spinal cord oedema. Venous thrombosis or large pouches might be seen.
- The presence of CVR and exclusive cortical venous drainage, similar to other DAVFs, correlates with haemorrhage and myelopathy.

Anatomy

- Arterial: ascending pharyngeal (hypoglossal and jugular branches), dural branches of the vertebral (anterior and posterior meningeal), occipital (mastoid and hypoglossal branches), MMA, and posterior auricular arteries and the meningohypophyseal and ILTs of the ICA. Bilateral supply is common.
- Venous:
  - Anterior condylar confluence/vein DAVF: involve the anterior condylar confluence located at the extracranial aperture of the hypoglossal canal and the anterior condylar vein located within the canal itself. McDougal divided drainage into: (i) type 1: antegrade into the IJV and/or vertebral venous plexus via the lateral condylar vein and posterior condylar vein, (ii) type 2: retrogradely into the cavernous sinus and/or orbital veins via the inferior petrosal sinus (IPS) and inferior petro-occipital vein, or (iii) type 3: directly into pial or perimedullary veins via the anterior condylar vein and marginal sinus.
  - Posterior condylar canal DAVF: involve the posterior condylar vein located within the posterior condylar canal. The posterior condylar vein drains into the IJV or suboccipital cavernous sinus.
  - Marginal sinus DAVF: this sinus is an inconstant intradural sinus ring lining the rim of the foramen magnum. Venous drainage is antegrade into the jugular bulb, retrogradely through the IPS and into the cavernous sinus, or retrogradely into cortical venous drainage.
  - Jugular foramen DAVF: these drain directly into the IJV or lateral medullary veins.

Treatment strategy

- It is important to comprehend the often-complex anatomy of the fistula before treatment. Superselective arteriography, venography, and cone beam CT can all be beneficial.
- The choice of transarterial or transvenous treatment depends on DAVF architecture.
- A transvenous approach is preferable, if feasible, as it is possible to access the fistula and safe to occlude the vein, as they usually do not drain cerebral parenchyma. The precise fistulous point needs to be occluded, and this can be accessed via its drainage pathway, often via the IPS or IJV. Coil embolisation is safest, but LEs and n-BCA may also be used.
- Transarterial treatment with LEs or glue has a higher risk of cranial nerve palsy, migration of agent to the vertebrobasilar circulation via anastomoses, and it can be difficult to achieve penetration into the vein (Figure 11.6). The approach may be necessary if the venous pouch cannot be reached due to stenosis or tortuosity or if drainage is directly into the IJV, risking major jugular occlusion with transvenous treatment.

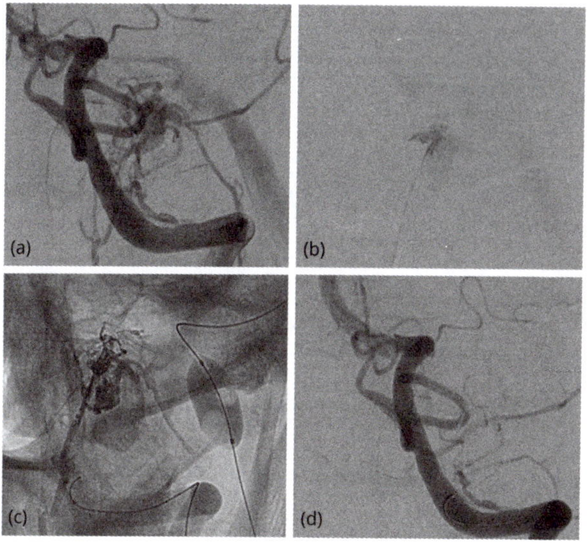

Figure 11.6 Foramen magnum dural arteriovenous fistula. (a) Digital subtraction angiography reveals an anterior condylar confluence fistula. (b) Microcatheter angiography via a dural feeder arising from the vertebral artery. It was not possible to achieve a stable position in the venous drainage channel and hence transarterial embolisation was performed. A balloon has been placed in the internal jugular vein to protect it. (c) Liquid embolic cast after embolisation via the same feeder. (d) Occlusion of fistula.

It is more successful in those with a single arterial feeder (uncommon). Transarterial access is more usefully employed as an adjunct after venous treatment to complete fistula occlusion.

Complication avoidance

- Avoid over-packing of the draining veins in this region to minimise the risk of postoperative cranial nerve palsy. Soft coils are preferable if placing within the hypoglossal canal to avoid palsy.

Further reading

Caton MT, Narsinh KH, Baker A, et al. Dural arteriovenous fistulas of the foramen magnum region: clinical features and angioarchitectural phenotypes. AJNR Am J Neuroradiol. 2021;42(8):1486–1491.

Li C, Yu J, Li K, Hou K, Yu J. Dural arteriovenous fistula of the lateral foramen magnum region: a review. Interv Neuroradiol. 2018;24(4):425–434.

Spittau B, Millán DS, El-Sherifi S, et al. Dural arteriovenous fistulas of the hypoglossal canal: systematic review on imaging anatomy, clinical findings, and endovascular management. J Neurosurg. 2015;22(4):883–903.

Anterior cranial fossa DAVF

Also known as ethmoidal or cribriform plate DAVFs, these usually drain directly into frontal cortical veins (making them Cognard type 3) and hence they often present with ICH.

Anatomy

- Arterial: anterior/posterior ethmoidal arteries and anterior falcine branches of the ophthalmic artery; facial artery; sphenopalatine artery; MMA; pial branches of the anterior cerebral artery; and superficial temporal artery.
- Venous: frontal basal cortical veins draining into the superior sagittal sinus; olfactory veins draining into the cavernous sinus; inferior and superior ophthalmic veins; and superficial and deep cerebral veins.

Treatment strategy

- Clip ligation of the draining vein has historically been considered the first-line treatment; however, newer endovascular techniques are able to achieve 80–90% occlusion rates comparable to other fistula sites.
- Transarterial (Figure 11.7): the ophthalmic artery beyond the origin of the central retinal artery (and hence choroidal blush, see Chapter 2,

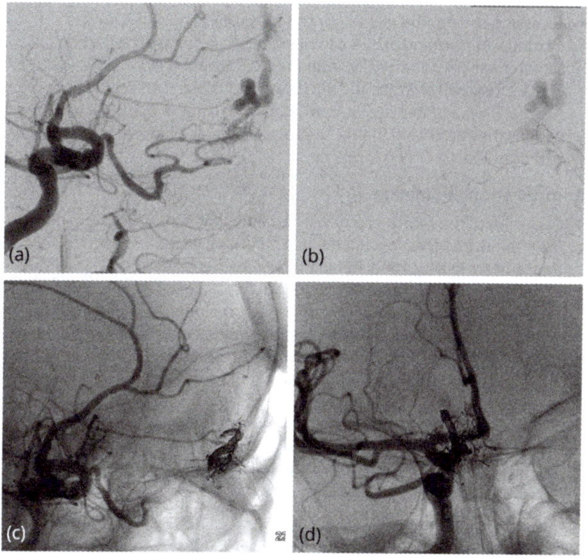

Figure 11.7 Anterior cranial fossa dural arteriovenous fistula. (a) Internal carotid artery digital subtraction angiography demonstrates the fistula with shunting into a frontal cortical vein. (b) Microcatheter angiography via distal ophthalmic artery at point of fistulisation. Note absence of choroidal blush (and hence distal to retinal artery). (c, d) Liquid embolic cast after embolisation. There was no significant reflux proximal into the ophthalmic artery.

'Internal carotid artery', p. 35) is the most common access site. The MMA and sphenopalatine artery may also be good choices if supplying, and reduce the risk of retinal ischaemia. As reflux is the limiting factor, a balloon catheter like the Scepter Mini may prove useful.

- Transvenous: from a distal access catheter placed in the anterior aspect of the superior sagittal sinus, a microcatheter can be navigated through the draining cortical vein until the site of the fistula is reached. Embolisation with LE agents ± coils can then be undertaken. This technique has the advantage of avoiding ophthalmic artery catheterisation and hence has a reduced risk of retinal ischaemia. In some series transvenous access has a higher rate of fistula occlusion.

Tips

- Venous drainage (and arterial supply) may be bilateral. Placing a second diagnostic catheter in the contralateral ICA for intermittent diagnostic runs can confirm occlusion of all feeding vessels as the fistula is embolised.
- Even if the MMA does not appear to supply the fistula on initial angiography, it may be a viable arterial pedicle. Microcatheter angiography often reveals a small contribution, which suffices for injection of LEs.
- Accessing the ophthalmic artery can be challenging if its origin is tortuous. Performing 3D-RA can help identify a suitable projection for catheterisation. Additionally, inflating a compliant balloon adjacent to the artery can stabilise the microcatheter during catheterisation. Alternatively, an intermediate catheter lodged at the ophthalmic origin, such as the Fargo Mini (Balt) can provide a stable platform for the distal microcatheter.

Complication avoidance

- Occlusion of the retinal artery will result in blindness. This can happen from reflux into this vessel, and also ophthalmic artery spasm from the catheter itself. A detachable tip microcatheter may be helpful in preventing damage or stretching of the ophthalmic artery during retrieval. Nimodipine infusion into the ophthalmic at the outset of treatment may reduce the risk of ophthalmic artery spasm.
- Cortical veins are more fragile than arteries and there is a higher risk of perforation and therefore navigation should be performed very carefully. A J-tip to the wire helps avoid this.

Further reading

Agid R, Terbrugge K, Rodesch G, Andersson T, Söderman M. Management strategies for anterior cranial fossa (ethmoidal) dural arteriovenous fistulas with an emphasis on endovascular treatment. J Neurosurg. 2009;110(1):79–84.

Dabus G, Kan P, Diaz C, et al. Endovascular treatment of anterior cranial fossa dural arteriovenous fistula: a multicentre series. Neuroradiology. 2021;63(2):259–266.

Su X, Gao Z, Ma Y, et al. Transarterial embolization for anterior cranial fossa dural arteriovenous fistulas: a retrospective single-center study. J Neurointerv Surg. 2024;16(7):684–690.

Indirect cavernous sinus DAVF

These are classified as Cognard type 1 or 2b depending on the presence of CVR. In the absence of reflux, treatment may be indicated due to deteriorating vision.

Clinical

- Signs/symptoms include chemosis, proptosis, ophthalmoplegia, visual disturbance, raised intraocular pressure, headache, and local pain.
- Imaging may reveal orbital venous congestion with a dilated superior ophthalmic vein, disc swelling (i.e. papilloedema), and dilatation/arterialisation of the cavernous sinus.

Anatomy

- Arterial: ILT and MHT ICA branches, artery of the foramen rotundum, middle/accessory/recurrent meningeal arteries, and ascending pharyngeal artery branches (clival and recurrent artery of the foramen lacerum). Note many arteries in the cavernous region supply, or have anastomoses to arteries that supply, cranial nerves.
- Venous: any tributary of the cavernous sinus such as the ophthalmic veins, inferior/superior petrosal sinuses, sphenoparietal sinus/middle cerebral veins, and frontal cortical veins.

Treatment strategy

- Involve the ophthalmic team. Intraocular pressures and visual fields should be documented.
- Conservative: spontaneous closure of indirect fistulas occurs in about 50% of cases. If sight is deteriorating, or this approach fails, then EVT is first line. Conservative management is not recommended with CVR.
- On-table cone beam CT with injection via the ECA can often show the exact point of fistulisation if studied closely.
- A transvenous approach is strongly favoured and usually successful, most commonly via the IPS (Figure 11.8). The origin of the IPS in relation to the jugular bulb is variable but mostly it arises from the medial aspect of the superior bulb of the IJV, at the level of the hypoglossal canal or slightly lower. Sometimes the IPS is a plexus. It is absent in around 17% of cases.
- If the IPS cannot be visualised angiographically, it may be thrombosed. Even when thrombosed, access is successful in about 50%. Perform a venous run from the IJV and a stump may be visible, which is your target. Try first with a microcatheter and wire. If this fails, using an angiographic catheter for support and rotating a 0.035" lubricious guidewire through the thrombosed IPS can be attempted, and is usually successful, albeit with a small risk of subdural haemorrhage. If you can reach the sinus with the 0.035" wire, do a roadmap with the wire in place. Removing the wire will yield a negative mask (a white line) of the wire, which you can then attempt to navigate through with the microcatheter and wire.
- Once the cavernous sinus has been accessed, a microcatheter angiogram should be performed to confirm you are in a part of the sinus that is involved in the fistula (the cavernous sinus is often compartmentalised in anterior, intercavernous, and posterior segments).

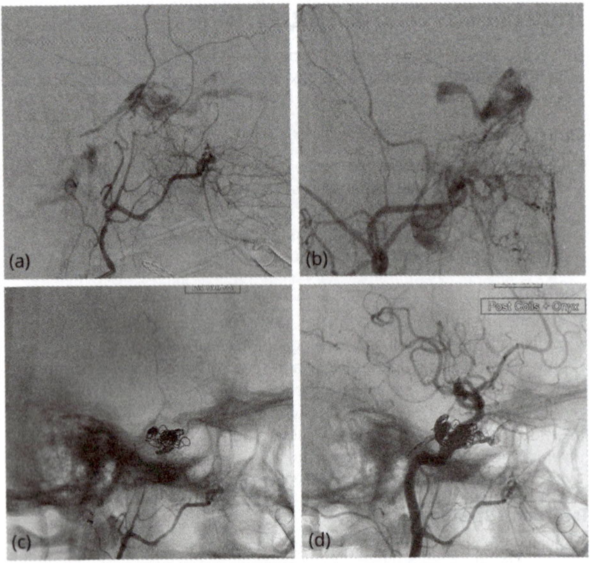

Figure 11.8 Indirect carotid–cavernous fistula. (a) Lateral projection external carotid artery digital subtraction angiography. The cavernous sinus is opacified, with drainage into the superior ophthalmic vein and inferior petrosal sinus (IPS). (b) Anteroposterior projection. (c) A microcatheter was inserted into the cavernous via the IPS and several coils placed. (d) A small amount of liquid embolic was injected to completely occlude the fistula.

If possible, a second microcatheter should be inserted into the sinus and positioned within the SOV, which can help if access is lost with the first.

- The principal target for treatment initially is any cortical venous drainage, as this carries the risk of haemorrhage. These routes should be coiled off first. It may also be sensible to coil off the intercavernous routes if there is drainage to the contralateral cavernous sinus.
- Coiling should then be performed at the fistula site, if this can be recognised.
- Transarterial injection of LEs in this region is generally avoided due to the high risk of cranial nerve deficit (other than as a limited adjunct to coiling; see Figure 11.8). In addition, these feeders are also often small, can be difficult to navigate, and LE reflux can occur into the carotid artery.

Tips

- If the IPS is occluded, other access pathways include a contralateral approach via the intercavernous sinus, the superior petrosal sinus, and the ophthalmic vein via the facial vein or superior temporal vein/ trochlear vein. To find the origin of the facial vein as it branches off the cervical IJV or external jugular vein, it may be necessary to create a roadmap by injecting through the ECA. Alternatively, the venous phase of the angiogram may reveal it.

- If conventional transvenous approaches (including direct transjugular approach) are impossible, direct puncture into the superior ophthalmic vein medial to the orbit (perhaps utilising cone beam CT) or directly into the cavernous sinus can be performed. This is often successful but the risk of this manoeuvre is retro-orbital haemorrhage and so it is advisable to have an ophthalmic surgeon on standby (alternatively, it may be a good idea to learn how to perform a lateral canthotomy to decompress the orbit in case of ocular compartment syndrome).

Complication avoidance and management

- Procedure-specific complications include ophthalmoplegia due to cranial nerve damage and delayed recurrence. There may be temporary worsening of eye symptoms after the procedure.
- Occasionally, cortical veins drain into the IPS and can be inadvertently cannulated (and even ruptured) during attempted cannulation of the cavernous sinus.
- Perforation of the IPS can also result in subdural haemorrhage. Usually this is well tolerated provided it is recognised early.

Further reading

Alexandre AM, Sturiale CL, Bartolo A, et al. Endovascular treatment of cavernous sinus dural arteriovenous fistulas. Institutional series, systematic review and meta-analysis. Clin Neuroradiol. 2022;32(3):761–771.

Guest W, Krings T. Transvenous approaches to embolization of dural arteriovenous fistulae of the cavernous sinus. J Neurovasc Ther. 2022;16(2):63–73.

Lekkhong E, Pongpech S, Ter Brugge K, et al. Transvenous embolisation of intracranial dural arteriovenous shunts through occluded venous segments: experience in 51 patients. AJNR Am J Neuroradiol. 2011;32(9):1738–1744.

Min XF, Yuan G, Si GY, Xu YN. Direct puncture the superior ophthalmic vein guiding by Dyna-CT to obliterating a traumatic carotid-cavernous sinus fistula: a case report and literature review. Medicine (Baltimore). 2022;101(43):e31560.

Direct carotid–cavernous DAVF

These are not DAVFs and therefore, strictly speaking, do not belong in this chapter, but as the treatment is similar, they are included.

Direct fistulas are usually caused by trauma (80%). They are rare nowadays in developed countries probably due to increased safety standards in cars and motorcycles. They can also arise iatrogenically from surgery or endovascular procedures. Spontaneous carotid–cavernous fistulas are most commonly due to rupture of cavernous aneurysms into the adjacent sinus. There is an association with Ehlers–Danlos syndrome, pseudoxanthoma elasticum, and fibromuscular dysplasia.

Clinical

- Signs/symptoms are due to ophthalmic vein congestion and include visual loss, bruit, chemosis, exophthalmos, orbital pain, diplopia, headache, and pain in the V1 nerve territory. Symptoms may be bilateral, but there is usually a preponderance on the side of the fistula. 5% may suffer ICH from CVR.
- Imaging may reveal similar features to indirect fistulas. Skull fractures may additionally be seen.
- Prompt treatment is necessary because of the risk of blindness and ICH. There is minimal chance of spontaneous resolution.

Anatomy

- The fistula is usually a single hole measuring 1–10 mm, or a small number of holes, directly connecting the carotid artery and cavernous sinus. Rarely, there may be involvement of the dural arteries of the ICA (perhaps due to recruitment or tearing in deceleration injuries). Venous drainage can be bilateral, usually across the intercavernous sinus, and only 1% of cases involve bilateral fistulas.
- The difficulty may be in identifying the size and location of the hole/s between the carotid artery and cavernous sinus. Cone beam CT or contralateral ICA or vertebral artery injections under flow arrest of the affected ICA may be helpful.

Treatment strategy

- Previously, detachable balloons were inflated within the cavernous sinus to occlude the fistula. While very effective, these are now unavailable, but controlled detachment coils can be used for the same purpose (Figure 11.9).
- It is helpful to inflate a compliant balloon in the cavernous ICA (e.g. Scepter C) while coiling the sinus. The coiling catheter can either be advanced via the arterial side into the sinus through the fistula, or directly into the cavernous sinus via the IPS. The latter approach may be easier, as coiling can be commenced at the site of the fistula working backwards into the sinus. Occasionally, stent or flow diverter-assisted coiling may be indicated, in case of a larger sized hole in the cavernous ICA.
- If the above strategy is impossible, then ICA occlusion can be performed if there is adequate cross-hemispheric circulation.

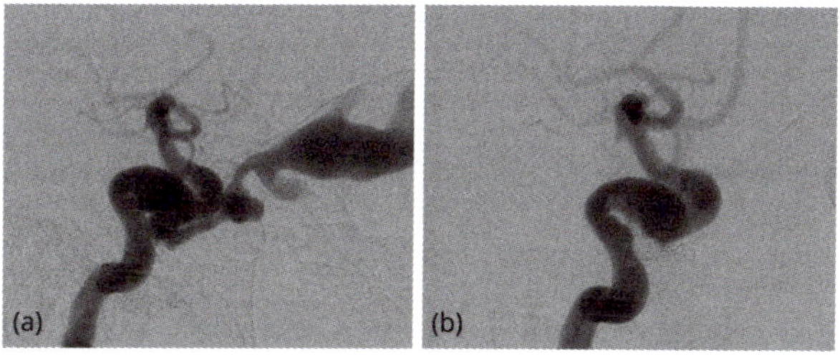

Figure 11.9 Direct carotid–cavernous fistula. (a) Internal carotid artery (ICA) digital subtraction angiography demonstrates fistula of inferior cavernous ICA segment into cavernous sinus with ectasia of the superior ophthalmic vein. (b) A coiling catheter was inserted from the ICA through the fistula into the vein and multiple coils placed, occluding the hole.

- Flow diversion has been used alone or in conjunction with coil embolisation, but the treatment requires antiplatelets, which may pose an increased risk in the context of trauma. Overlapping flow diverters are usually required. Efficacy in comparison to more established treatments has not been ascertained and flow diversion is not advocated as first-line treatment.

Tips

- LEs have been used as an alternative to balloons or coils to primarily occlude the cavernous sinus; however, there is high risk of migration of the agent, including into the ICA.

Complication avoidance and management

- ICA balloon test occlusion might be considered if vessel occlusion proves necessary.
- Coiling of the cavernous sinus carries the same risks as for indirect fistulas. There may also be temporary worsening of (cranial nerve or orbital) symptoms after treatment.

Further reading

Lindgren A, Ahmed SU, Bodani V, et al. Embolization techniques of spontaneous direct carotid-cavernous fistulae: a single-center experience. Neuroradiology. 2024;66(9):1625–1633.

Sumdani H, Aguilar-Salinas P, Avila MJ, et al. Carotid cavernous fistula treatment via flow diversion: a systematic review of the literature. World Neurosurg. 2021;149:e369–e377.

Brain arteriovenous malformations

Introduction 448
Imaging of brain arteriovenous malformations (bAVMs) 450
Classification of bAVMs 451
Indications for treatment 453
Complications of endovascular treatment of bAVMs 454
Materials 455
Treatment strategies for ruptured pial AVMs 458
Transvenous embolisation of AVMs 465
Pre-radiosurgical embolisation of unruptured pial AVMs 467
Vein of Galen malformations 468
Stereotactic radiosurgery 472

Introduction

Brain arteriovenous malformations (bAVMs) are one of the most difficult and complex neurovascular diseases to manage. They are heterogeneous entities with variable natural history and symptomatology.

Many who are affected are young and otherwise healthy, with few, if any, symptoms.

Management and treatment strategies are not universally agreed upon. Any treatment may radically, and not infrequently, detrimentally affect lives, and therefore a multidisciplinary approach is obligatory.

Presentation

- most present in their 20–40s. The estimated prevalence is 10–18/100,000 (more common than DAVFs). Detection is around 1–1.5/100,000 person years.
- Autopsy studies suggest that ≤12% become symptomatic during life.
- ICH is the commonest presentation, accounting for about 50%. Bleeding may be from the nidus or draining veins (commonly as a consequence of venous outflow obstruction).
- AVMs account for 4% of ICH overall but one-third of ICH in young adults. 9% present with SAH. 75% of haemorrhagic presentations occur before the age of 50 years.
- Seizures are reported in 18–40%. 30% are generalised and 10% focal. Seizures are more common with frontal and temporal AVMs, in younger people, size >3 cm, superficial cortical location, and with superficial venous drainage. They respond well to antiepileptic drugs.
- Headaches may be no more frequent than in the general population. There are no distinctive features, and they are unrelated to AVM site or size.
- Around 5–15% suffer progressive focal neurological deficits unrelated to ICH, likely due to venous hypertension/dilatation and mass effect rather than arterial steal.

Natural history

- AVMs are dynamic lesions that can change in size, and so haemorrhagic risk may vary over time. Over 50% grow over a mean of 8 years and 9% will decrease in size.
- The estimated annual risk of ICH from the Columbia database is 2.5% with deep venous drainage, 3.1% with deep location, and 4.5% with previous ICH. With all three risk factors, it is 34.4%, and with none, 0.9%.
- The annual risk of ICH in the MARS population-based meta-analysis was 1.3% for previously unruptured and 4.8% for previously ruptured AVMs.
- AVM ICH case fatality rate is 12% at 1 year. Rebleeding is likely to be the highest in the first few months after the initial bleed (18%) and decreases with time but probably never reaches baseline. The Columbia database reports that 47% sustain no deficit post ICH, 37% are mRS 1, 19% mRS 2–3. Therefore, 84% remain independent, 13% are moderately disabled, and 3% severely disabled. They report no significantly increased morbidity following the second bleed and mortality rate from rebleed events is low (3%).

- Mortality rates are 0.7–3.9% per annum.
- The 5-year survival rate is approximately 95% even for symptomatic AVMs.

Further reading

Ajiboye N, Chalouhi N, Starke RM, Zanaty M, Bell R. Cerebral arteriovenous malformations: evaluation and management. ScientificWorldJournal. 2014;2014:649036.

Kim H, Al-Shahi Salman R, McCulloch CE, Stapf C, Young WL; MARS Co-investigators. Untreated brain arteriovenous malformation: patient-level meta-analysis of haemorrhage predictors. Neurology. 2014;83(7):590–597.

Mohr JP, Parides MK, Stapf C, et al. Medical management with or without interventional therapy for unruptured brain arteriovenous malformations (ARUBA): a multicentre, non-blinded, randomised trial. Lancet. 2014;383(9917):614–621.

Imaging of brain arteriovenous malformations (bAVMs)

- It is necessary to define the size, location, feeders, draining veins, and flow dynamics.

Cross-sectional imaging

- MRI is essential to show the AVM location and precise relationship to eloquent cortex, especially when planning the surgical approach. Consider:
  - Is it in an eloquent area?
  - Is it deep or superficial?
  - Is it located in a sulcus or a gyrus?
  - How much dissection into the deep white matter is present?
  - Is it associated with a ventricle?
  - What are the interconnections between feeders and draining veins?
- In a ruptured AVM, haemorrhage (subarachnoid or intracerebral) can be clearly defined by NCCT, but CTA is helpful in demonstrating the presence of a pseudoaneurysm (if present, the likely rupture point), and relationship with the haematoma and nidus.

Digital subtraction imaging

- The gold standard is DSA, providing information about the flow dynamics (i.e. the velocity of the flow), the relative importance of the different feeders, the participation of the different arterial axis (right and left anterior, posterior circulation), type of nidus (diffuse vs compact), architecture of the venous drainage, presence of high-flow fistulas, existence of pseudoaneurysms, presence of minor feeders (perforators), and of minor venous drainage and stenosis.
- DSA must be a six-vessel study, including the ECAs because there may be dural recruitment into the AVM, more so in superficial and large AVMs.
- When needed, the study may be completed with superselective catheterisation of the different feeders, usually under GA.
- Modern angiographic machines offer useful diagnostic tools: 3D and 4D reconstructions, injected cone beam CT, colour maps, etc., which may provide superior anatomical definition and understanding.

Follow-up

- Any residual component of an AVM implies ongoing risk of haemorrhage and requires DSA. CTA and MRA will not suffice.
- To demonstrate signs of an early draining vein, many projections, magnification, and reconstructions are often needed.
- Delayed DSA at 1 year is superior to earlier follow-up because a minimal residuum may become more obvious with time.

Classification of bAVMs

Spetzler–Martin classification

- See Table 12.1.

- Spetzler–Martin is a *surgical* classification and not designed to apply to stereotactic radiosurgery (STRS) or EVT (although they commonly are, regardless).
- Summing the points gives five different grades ranging from I (the easiest to treat with the best outcomes) to V (the worst outcomes).
- It has been subsequently modified and simplified by Spetzler into three grades: grade A, the lowest (grades I and II of the previous classification); grade B, the middle (grade III); and grade C (grades IV and V), the most difficult to treat.

Lawton–Young supplementary classification

- Table 12.2.
- Used together with the Spetzler–Martin classification for a more detailed classification.

Table 12.1 The Spetzler–Martin classification of brain AVMs

Size	<3 cm	1
	3–6 cm	2
	>6 cm	3
Location	Non-eloquent location	0
	Sensory, motor, language, or visual cortex; hypothalamus or thalamus; internal capsule; brainstem; cerebellar peduncles; deep cerebellar nuclei	1
Venous drainage	Superficial drainage	0
	Any deep venous drainage	1

Table 12.2 The Lawton–Young supplementary classification

Age	<20 years	1
	20–40 years	2
	>40 years	3
Haemorrhage	Presentation with haemorrhage	0
	Non-haemorrhagic presentation	1
Nidus type	Compact	0
	Diffuse	1

Pollock–Flickinger radiosurgical classification

- This grading scale was devised using regression analysis to predict the outcome of bAVMs treated with radiosurgery considering the AVM volume, location, and the patient's age, and was later simplified as follows:
  - AVM score = (0.1)(volume in mL) + (0.02) (age in years) + (0.3) (hemispheric/corpus callosum/cerebellar location = 0; basal ganglia/ thalamus/brainstem = 1).
  - The volume of the AVM for this formula in mL can be approximated from *x*, *y*, and *z*-axis measurements (in cm) of the nidus using this formula: $V = (3\pi xyz)/4$.
- 'Excellent' outcomes range from almost 90% with a score ≤1 to 37% with a score of >2.0.

Indications for treatment

There is no consensus regarding the indications for treating bAVMs, particularly if asymptomatic and/or unruptured.

The consequences of treatment (neurological complications in young and otherwise healthy people) and conversely, of non-treatment (risk of brain haemorrhage in the same population) can be life-changing.

All bAVMs are unique. A variation of a few millimetres in size or location, a small difference in flow velocity in arteries or veins, their calibre, or the venous drainage may change an 'easy' AVM into a 'high-risk' one.

Ruptured AVMs

- Haemorrhage is the main indication, but even with a ruptured AVM, the risks of treatment with the intention to cure must be seriously considered, especially with very large and/or complex AVMs.
- An alternative approach may be to target architectural weak (bleed risk) points such as nidal aneurysms.

Unruptured AVMs

- The ARUBA trial was an RCT of ruptured (58%) and unruptured (42%) bAVMs. It showed that bAVM treatment with any modality significantly harms patients in the short/medium term more than conservative observation.
- Many have criticised the trial for multiple reasons, particularly the relatively short follow-up period, but one conclusion is clear: AVM embolisation carried a higher-than-expected risk of immediate complications (almost all the AVMs in the treatment arm were embolised).
- Patients are generally young with a long life expectancy. Living with a bAVM can be challenging, as it may bring with it problems such as epilepsy, drug consumption, uncertainty, and anxiety.
- Modern neurosurgical techniques have improved considerably in recent decades due to innovations such as routine microscope use, on-table angio facility (e.g. indocyanine green angiography), intraoperative monitoring (ultrasonography or electroencephalography) and 'brain lab' planning kit.
- STRS has also been shown to be efficacious in certain circumstances, generally for AVMs with a nidus <3 cm, and may be preferable if the AVM is located in eloquent cortex or deep in the brain.
- Taking into account the findings of the ARUBA study, it is concluded that there are enough indications to consider treatment of unruptured Spetzler–Martin grade 1–2 AVMs. There may be indications for treating patients with higher grades on an individual basis after consideration by an experienced MDT, with a treatment strategy with cure as the goal.
- The MDT may offer any treatment (surgery, STRS, embolisation, alone or combined) when the total estimated risk is <5–6%.

Further reading

Cenzato M, Boccardi E, Beghi E, et al. European consensus conference on unruptured brain AVMs treatment (supported by EANS, ESMINT, EGKS, and SINCH). Acta Neurochir (Wien). 2017;159(6):1059–1064.

Complications of endovascular treatment of bAVMs

- Haemorrhagic and ischaemic complications are the most common.
- Periprocedural haemorrhage occurs in up to 20% of cases, with the most common cause being venous occlusion. Veins become occluded when they fill with embolic material (whether intended or unintended). However, there are instances where veins may thrombose due to a sudden, significant drop in blood flow resulting from the occlusion of a critical sector of the AVM. Bleeding typically occurs during the procedure, but, on occasion, may also occur in the hours or days that follow. Unfortunately, the clinical consequences of a venous haemorrhagic infarct are often grim, even when haematomas are promptly surgically evacuated.
- Bleeding can also occur during vessel navigation, secondary to traumatic rupture of arteries or veins (veins are more fragile and difficult to navigate). Elevation in pressure due to the injection of contrast may also cause rupture, especially when intranidal. Other causes include traction on the bAVM when retrieving the microcatheter and excessive bAVM volume reduction in one session.
- Ischaemic adverse events relate to the usual problems with intracranial navigation of catheters and wires (dissections, emboli, thrombus formation), but also with inadvertent or inevitable LE occlusion of arteries supplying normal brain.
- The rate of adverse events increases progressively with progressive occlusion of the AVM and if embocure is the goal of the treatment, it is in the range of 8–20%, with the serious complication rate being probably not less than 5–10%. These are generally higher-than-accepted values for surgery (in Spetzler–Martin grade 1–2 lesions) or STRS.
- The other serious disadvantage of EVT is lack of efficacy. The probability of completely curing an AVM is low. The literature is unhelpful because of its extreme heterogeneity. Series are not easily comparable due to multiple differences in management, course, techniques, analysis of results and of follow-ups, and the inevitable publication bias (bad results are usually unpublished). A recent review would suggest that average cure rate by embolisation alone is around 20–25%.

Further reading

Baharvahdat H, Blanc R, Termechi R, et al. Hemorrhagic complications after endovascular treatment of cerebral arteriovenous malformations. AJNR Am J Neuroradiol. 2014;35(5):978–983.

Lv X, Zhang Y, Wang J. Systematic review of transcatheter arterial embolization of AVM: indications, bleeding complications, cure rate, and long-term bleeding risk. Neurol India. 2020;68(6):1285–1292.

Materials

Microcatheters

To enable catheterisation of small and tortuous feeding vessels, microcatheters and wires need to be soft and atraumatic.

Non-detachable tip microcatheters

- The Magic catheter (Balt) is the most supple. Its shaft becomes progressively thinner and softer with the tip being as small as 1.2 or 1.5 Fr.
- It is the only catheter which is really 'flow directed', meaning it easily advances only by blood flow without the need of a wire in most cases.
- A small curve on the tip makes it less traumatic and enables selection of the desired feeder. The curve is obtained by warming it with steam or with a heat-gun between the fingers.
- The catheter will occasionally take a wrong turn. The soft tip of the catheter may be directed by the injection of contrast or saline. The higher the pressure of injection, the more it will jump back (perhaps selecting a different vessel). Try using different concentrations of contrast, from pure contrast to pure saline. Pure contrast will not produce a jump but just a vibration of the distal part of the Magic, which allows progression in the same direction even when the many curves or the limited speed of flow are not enough to push it forward.
- Low-concentration contrast injected with a 2–3 mL syringe (but never a 1 mL syringe because of the excessive pressure that results) will cause the tip to jump back and possibly select a different branch. The more dilute the contrast, and the higher the pressure of injection, the more the catheter will jump.
- Using a Magic catheter needs some training but once mastered it is extremely useful and gratifying. Note: Magic cannot be used with DMSO-based LEs.
- Two other microcatheters are widely used/available: the Marathon (Medtronic) is also very small and supple but less so than the Magic, and consequently it does not usually advance without a wire. Similarly, the Duo microcatheter (Microvention), with one marker and a longer tip (167 cm) also requires a wire. Both are DMSO compatible.

Detachable tip microcatheters

- Microcatheters with detachable tips may reduce risks of AVM embolisation. Non-adhesive LEs do not 'glue' the catheters in place but the microcatheters can still be retained within the embolic material by friction.
- Detachable microcatheters have tips that detach and are left in place at the end of the procedure. The length of the detachable part varies and can be as long as 5–7 cm. Detachment is obtained by pulling.
- The Apollo (Medtronic) provides an internal tube that slips off from the external one.
- The Sonic (Balt) has a more detachable point when pulled, especially if it has been in contact with DMSO.
- A disadvantage is premature tip detachment during tortuous or prolonged navigation.

Embolic materials

LE materials range from adhesive agents (cyanoacrylates) to non-adhesive LE agents (EVOH or hydroxyethyl methacrylate (HEMA) dissolved in DMSO).

Cyanoacrylate glue

- Cyanoacrylates are adhesive, risk 'gluing' the catheter, and are not as efficacious in occluding large-volume bAVMs (see Chapter 4, 'Cyanoacrylate glue', p. 137).
- The first cyanoacrylate was iso-butyl-cyanoacrylate which later was modified to the current *N*-butyl-cyanoacrylate (Histoacryl by Braun or Glubran by GEM). They are rendered radiopaque by adding Lipiodol (Guerbet), an oil-based radiopaque contrast agent. Lipiodol can also modulate the speed of polymerisation—the more Lipiodol, the slower the solidification of the cyanoacrylate.
- Typically, one part cyanoacrylate is mixed with two or three parts of Lipiodol, but if needed, may be made more dilute for longer injections in slow-flow arteriovenous shunts or stronger for high-flow fistulas. The two elements must be carefully mixed, like oil and vinegar in a vinaigrette, to obtain a homogeneous emulsion and ionic solutions avoided. The microcatheter *must always* be first flushed with 5% glucose.
- Radiopacity of cyanoacrylate can also be achieved by the addition of micronised tantalum powder if it is disadvantageous to slow the rate of polymerisation (typically in very high-flow fistulas, such as vein of Galen malformations (VOGMs)).
- After glue injection, the microcatheter is rapidly removed to avoid tip retention.

Copolymer liquid embolics

- EVOH dissolved in DMSO is a non-adhesive material that can be injected for long periods of time, achieving more abundant diffusion and nidal penetration (see Chapter 4, 'Copolymer liquid embolics', p. 140).
- Onyx has been widely used since 2005. Squid (Balt) is similar in composition and behaviour to Onyx. A less concentrated form (Squid 12) is available which may allow deeper penetration but risks embolisation of too many vessels both proximal and distal to the nidus.
- On leaving the tip of the catheter, LEs will laminate on the vessel wall. Successive injections add further layers. Progressive stratification from the outside towards the centre will gradually occlude the vessel. Resistance to further filling increases until the material will find a different vessel (at random). The operator must decide whether the new vessel is appropriate to occlude (continue to push) or if not, stop, wait, and restart.
- Once precipitated, Onyx becomes a black rubber-like, cohesive solid material. It may be pulled out of the vessel in one block if needed, using a stent retriever, e.g. described with Tigertriever 13.
- PHIL (Microvention) is HEMA dissolved in DMSO. PHIL behaves differently to Onyx/Squid. It tends to precipitate in the centre of the vessel, in a cauliflower-like blob. It occludes faster than Onyx and has less reflux so that the injection time is reduced. On entering the veins, it will occlude them much faster, potentially risking haemorrhage. This behaviour might be desirable in the treatment of DAVFs, where occlusion of the foot of the vein is key. PHIL is rendered opaque with iodine and is less radiopaque than Onyx or Squid.

- The choice of which LE agent is a matter of training, experience, and personal preference. Some use cyanoacrylates in most cases, for occlusion of pseudoaneurysms in ruptured AVMs, and also presurgical occlusion of selected feeders.
- Onyx or Squid are often used transarterially and for the venous approach.
- PHIL may be used when the purpose of the treatment is to fill a significant portion of the nidus, avoiding any passage into the veins.

Particles

- Particulate materials are no longer used for bAVMs. They are not very visible and a high proportion end up in the lungs. They are inefficient at occluding the nidus.

Further reading

Chapot R, Stracke P, Velasco A, et al. The pressure cooker technique for the treatment of brain AVMs. J Neuroradiol. 2014;41(1):87–91.

Treatment strategies for ruptured pial AVMs

- Strategy and technique will vary depending upon the goal: (i) to occlude deep surgically inaccessible feeders, (ii) to occlude a high-flow arteriovenous fistula, (iii) to occlude perinidal/nidal aneurysms or pseudoaneurysms, or (iv) to penetrate the nidus as much as possible.
- GA is always necessary. Biplane angiography is mandatory—the injection of the embolising liquid must be controlled very carefully and requires two different planes. Severe complications can result due to the occlusion of vessels 'hidden' in the single projection.

Presurgical targeted embolisation

- With improvements in the surgical approach and technique, most AVMs (especially Spetzler–Martin 1–2) may be surgically excised without any endovascular contribution.
- The aim of presurgical embolisation requires detailed discussion with the neurovascular surgeon before the procedure. The risks of the two approaches are additive.
- Choose the endovascular technique that obtains the desired result with the minimal risk possible. Two approaches are described:

Occlusion of deep surgically inaccessible feeders

(See Figure 12.1.)

- Generally, feeders that are most helpful to embolise pre-surgery are the perforating arteries, pericallosal arteries, mesial branches of the posterior cerebral arteries, early branches of the cerebellar arteries, choroidal arteries, etc.
- Catheterisation of perforating arteries may be difficult, especially lenticulostriates originating from the M1 segment of the middle cerebral artery (MCA).
- It may be preferable to use a very soft, thin, flow-guided catheter (Magic 1.2 Fr) and cyanoacrylate as an embolic material in these circumstances (the Magic is not DMSO compatible). A very thin (0.007") guidewire may be necessary to fix and stabilise the catheter at the origin of the target vessel and to allow it to proceed towards the final destination. Lenticulostriate artery origin from the M1 is often very acutely recurrent: a small balloon in the M1 just beyond the origin, supporting perforator catheterisation may be helpful. Perforating arteries of the distal segments of the MCA and more rarely, feeders originating from A1, from P1 or even from the posterior communicating artery may also require embolisation (by experienced operators).
- The goal is to occlude the very terminal part of the perforating feeder, as close to the nidus as possible, avoiding occlusion of long segments which might cause ischaemic injury to the deep white matter. A small amount of cyanoacrylate (0.1–0.2 mL) is usually more than enough to obtain the desired result.

Deep/distal feeders:

- This strategy aims to occlude feeders supplying an AVM located deep in the surgical field and therefore difficult to manage surgically (e.g. a long distance from the surface, behind (to the surgeon) the nidus, behind the draining veins, etc.). The typical arterial site to occlude is the distal

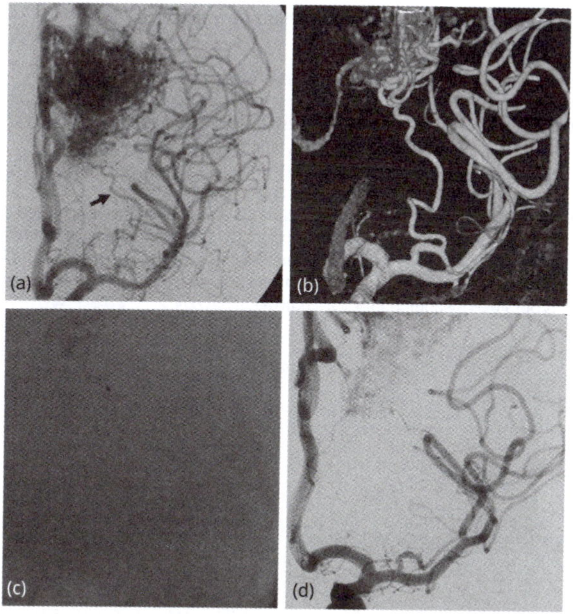

Figure 12.1 Treatment of a large frontal arteriovenous malformation (AVM) feeder. (a) Digital subtraction angiography anteroposterior view of the AVM. A deep lenticulostriate feeder is surgically inaccessible (arrow). (b) This is shown clearly on 3D rotational angiography. (c) Microcatheter angiogram via the feeder with a Magic microcatheter. (d) After glue injection the feeder is no longer present. Images courtesy of Dr Mariangela Piano and Dr Dodi Boccardi.

segment of the posterior cerebral artery in AVMs in the occipitotemporal lobe or branches of the pericallosal artery in AVMs of the mesial surface of the hemispheres.

- These can be tackled by 'endovascular clipping' where the feeding artery is occluded using a very small quantity of cyanoacrylate in a very precise segment—just like a surgical clip. This technique can be relatively low risk and extremely useful.
- In these cases, it is not required to inject the LE inside the nidus, a focal limited occlusion of the arterial feeder is sufficient. Avoiding nidal penetration considerably lowers the endovascular risks, X-Ray exposure, and procedural time, and allows endovascular and surgical operations to be undertaken sequentially under one anaesthetic.
- Timing relative to surgery is controversial—some say within 24 h, some say within days to avoid ICH and some advocate after 3 weeks to allow haemodynamic stabilisation and progressive thrombosis. Leaving it longer risks development of anastomoses to supply the AVM, which can complicate surgery.

Targeted occlusion of intranidal high-flow fistulas

(See Figure 12.2.)

- It may be helpful to occlude high-flow fistulas pre-surgery or as an adjunct to STRS.
- Occlude the arterial side of the fistula, avoiding the passage of embolic material into the venous side (occluding the veins of an AVM before having occluded the whole nidus is a bad idea). Either cyanoacrylates or LEs may be used, depending on operator preference.
- A controlled injection is required. With cyanoacrylates, this is achieved with a high concentration of the mixture (two parts of glue and one part of Lipiodol) and a very slow injection, but some operators may prefer a fast injection of pure glue. In this latter case, the radiopacity of the glue is obtained by adding tantalum powder.

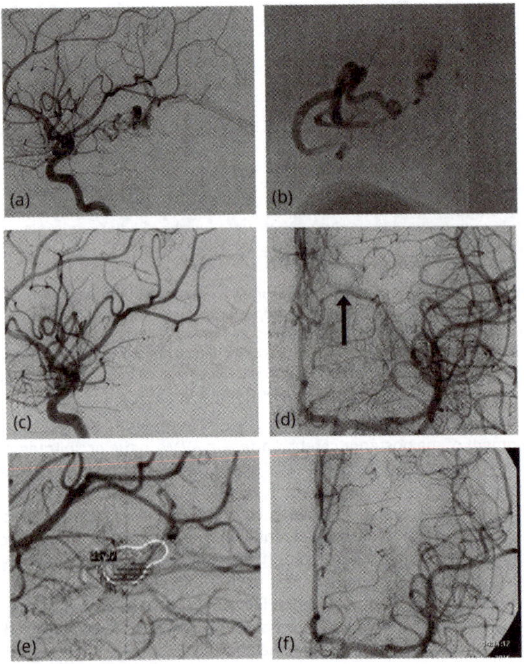

Figure 12.2 Treatment of a ruptured arteriovenous malformation (AVM) with glue followed by radiosurgery. (a) Left internal carotid artery injection in the lateral projection shows a choroidal AVM and associated aneurysm. (b) The artery was selectively accessed with a Magic 1.2 microcatheter and glue was injected (glue cast shown). (c) On the lateral view, the AVM appears obliterated. (d) The anteroposterior view, however, demonstrates a residual early filling deep vein (arrow). (e) Gamma Knife radiosurgery was performed 3 months after embolisation. (f) Follow-up digital subtraction angiography 4 years later confirms complete cure of the AVM. Images courtesy of Dr Mariangela Piano and Dr Dodi Boccardi.

- A small balloon may be used to temporarily stop/diminish the flow. New double-lumen balloons may be used to inject Onyx directly (not cyanoacrylate) without the need of a second catheter. Sceptre/Mini-Scepter (Microvention), Hyperform (Medtronic), Hyperglide (Medtronic), and Eclipse (Balt) balloon microcatheters are all DMSO compatible but beware that cyanoacrylate may rupture these balloons.

Targeted occlusion of perinidal/nidal aneurysms or pseudoaneurysms

(See Figure 12.3.)

- This may be indicated acutely in ruptured AVMs or prior to STRS or surgery. These are very small feeders (not uncommonly branches of the

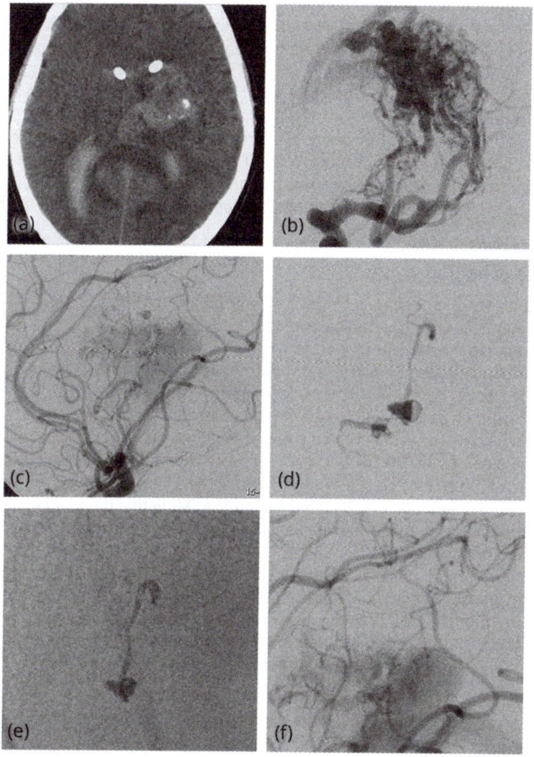

Figure 12.3 Treatment of a ruptured arteriovenous malformation (AVM)-associated pseudoaneurysm. (a) Intraventricular haemorrhage. (b) A deep left hemisphere AVM was detected on the left internal carotid artery (ICA) angiography. (c) Right ICA injection revealed a culprit pseudoaneurysm located on the superior surface of the lateral ventricle. (d) Superselective catheterisation of the small feeder was performed using a Magic 1.2 microcatheter. (e) Glue cast from injection. (f) Post-treatment images show the occlusion of the aneurysm.

choroidal arteries), not contained in the parenchyma, but rather in the subarachnoid space and therefore prone to rupture.

- Pre-STRS embolisation of nidal and perinidal aneurysms is advocated by some to reduce the risk post-STRS haemorrhage as AVM haemodynamics change following STRS.
- Ruptured pial AVMs historically were managed with less urgency compared to ruptured aneurysms because a second rupture immediately following the first is much less frequent. This is statistically true for all ruptured AVMs, but where a pseudoaneurysm (evidence of the point where a vessel has ruptured) is present, there is a place for an emergency procedure in the first 24–48 h.
- The goal is to occlude the vessel as close as possible to the pseudoaneurysm, preferably placing some embolic material within pseudoaneurysm if safe to attempt. It is often a small perforating and/or subependymal vessel (hence the frequent intraventricular haemorrhage in ruptured AVMs) and the technique is similar to that described above for perforating arteries. A ratio of 1:1 glue to lipiodol to glue is typically used.
- If and when the rupture point is secured, a ruptured AVM may be treated or followed as an 'unruptured AVM'. STRS may be considered. When the point of rupture is not found in a ruptured AVM, urgent surgical or EVT or even conservative treatment may be appropriate.

Embocure

(See Figure 12.4.)

- The goal of embocure may not be favoured by many due to the potentially unfavourable outcomes.
- Embocure is more likely with small and medium-sized superficial non-eloquent AVMs <3 cm in size with a compact nidus that is at least twice the size of the normal arteries, few superficial arterial feeders (<3), without en passant, choroidal, or lenticulostriate supply, and easily delineated and unobstructed views of the draining vein. Each arterial feeder should allow for 2–3 cm of reflux. If these criteria are satisfied, an AVM cure may be achieved in the majority. These, however, are also surgically appropriate (Spetzler–Martin 1) AVMs with a high success rate and low(er) complication rate and in many centres surgery would be the treatment of choice.
- In larger AVMs, where embocure is rare, often only partial occlusion of the nidus is obtained, multiple embolisation sessions are often needed with multiplication of procedural risks, X-ray exposure, costs, etc. The patient may then require surgery (or STRS) where the presence of the embolisation material may cause more problems than advantages.

Technique

- Periprocedural-induced hypotension (as with transvenous embolisation) may decrease the risk of periprocedural haemorrhage. Some give steroids periprocedurally. Bolus doses of heparin are generally not given because of the risks of periprocedural haemorrhage.
- The non-adhesive LE polymers (EVOH or HEMA, dissolved in DMSO) have been developed exactly for this purpose—to allow a long, slow injection from a single arterial feeder, in the proximity of the nidus (not necessarily inside), filling most of the small intranidal vessels. It is usually

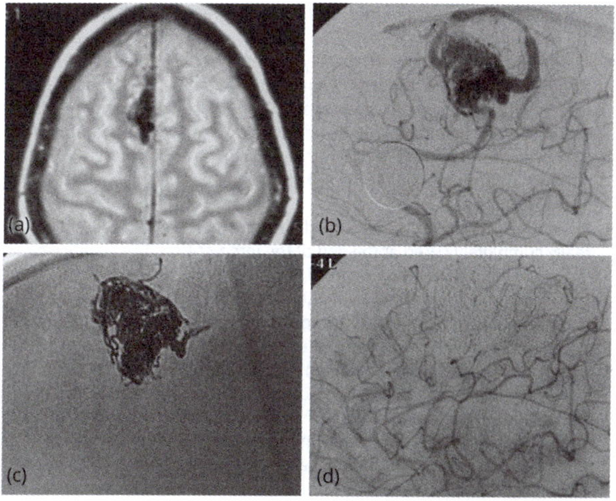

Figure 12.4 Curative embolisation of frontal arteriovenous malformation (AVM). (A) Magnetic resonance imaging and (B) digital subtraction angiography showing medial frontal AVM supplied by the pericallosal arteries, with drainage into the superior sagittal sinus. (C) Onyx cast after injection. (D) 1-year follow-up showing complete cure. Image courtesy of Dr Mariangela Piano and Dr Dodi Boccardi.

better to lodge the microcatheter in an artery of smaller calibre to avoid excessive reflux of the material.

- Initially the LE, after a short advancement into the nidus, will start to reflux (back-flow over the microcatheter). When this happens, stop injecting, restart after about 20–30 s, and stop again if it refluxes. Continue until you have formed a good plug around the tip of the catheter that will allow only forward injection. Sometimes this takes only a few minutes, but occasionally 20–45 min are required to achieve a good forward injection.
- Creating a good plug to allow the forward passage of material into the nidus may be facilitated by the 'pressure cooker' technique. An artificial plug is rapidly constructed using a few small coils and a small amount of cyanoacrylate. A detachable tip catheter through which the material will be injected is placed where desired while a second catheter is placed more proximal to allow the coils to be detached immediately proximal to the tip of the first. A few coils and a drop of glue will seal the vessel creating a plug. One can inject the material more rapidly because it will only flow forward.
- The 'pressure cooker' technique is also utilised in the venous approach to increase the amount and the speed of the intranidal filling and to limit the dissemination of the material in the venous system. The technique is complex and challenging, must be well mastered and correctly applied, and is only for experienced operators.
- Fill as much of the nidus as possible avoiding the veins. The vein should be the last structure to be filled and occluded only when the whole

nidus is completely eradicated. Occluding the vein is necessary to cure the AVM.

- Premature venous occlusion usually causes the most dreadful complications, i.e. intra/postprocedural haematomas, and is the main reason why many avoid transarterial EVT of AVMs. It is also the reason why most AVMs are *not* cured by embolisation since most operators stop prematurely, afraid of occluding the vein, having achieved nothing as far as managing the AVM (or even possibly increasing the haemorrhagic risk).
- It is not always straightforward to determine if an embolised AVM is really completely cured at the end of the intervention. The absence of a draining vein is not complete proof, especially with the ongoing unstable changes in the heart of the AVM and the presence of very radiopaque material obscuring any detail. Microcatheter angiography is superior to injections in the ICA/VA to determine residual filling.
- Microcatheter retrieval at the end of the injection may also cause haemorrhage. LE agents are non-adhesive, but catheters may remain stuck especially after long injections, when 2–3cm of the tip in a tortuous segment of a vessel is completely immersed in the embolic material. This can mostly be avoided with 'detachable tip' microcatheters.
- A control DSA angiogram at 8–12 months is necessary, but even then the stabilised result may not be so clear.

Palliative treatment

- This can be considered when the AVM causes severe and progressive neurological problems, often secondary to the excessive blood flow and venous hypertension.
- Embolising the main compartments of the AVM, the high-flow shunts, the direct arteriovenous fistulas, while diminishing the overall cerebral engorgement may result in a significant and sometimes stable neurological improvement. It must be considered a last-chance compassionate treatment.

Transvenous embolisation of AVMs

Primary transvenous approaches to AVM embolisation have been developed in response to the challenges of complete occlusion of an AVM transarterially. The rationale is that a complete cure may only be achieved by occluding the draining vein.

Indications

- When a treatment is definitely needed: ruptured AVM, when surgery or STRS are not options.
- When the nidus is small <3 cm and deep: most reports are for small ruptured AVMs with deep-seated choroidal supply although very experienced operators are treating larger, more complex AVMs.
- When the vein (preferably only one) is small and accessible.

Technique

(See Figure 12.5.)

- A triaxial system and a jugular approach is suggested for the venous access. This allows for better support when navigating via the veins, and reduced catheter length retention if impossible to retrieve.
- If occlusion of the vein is obtained at the same time as occlusion of the nidus, the risk of bleeding might be avoided. Onyx injected in the vein close to the nidus layers progressively and raises the resistance in the direction of the drainage and starts to back-flow towards the nidus. An experienced operator must obtain simultaneous occlusion of the nidus, the draining vein, and the arterial feeders, injecting retrogradely through the nidus—not easy, especially if the nidus is large, high flow, if the vein is big, and/or if there is more than one vein.
- It is more feasible if the nidus and the vein are small. Induced hypotension (systolic BP 20% below normal or mean BP 100 mmHg) may aid the retrograde reflux of embolic agent into the nidus. Consider also inflating a balloon on the arterial side.
- Onyx (or Squid) is preferred to PHIL because of the progression of the occlusion of the vein. Onyx will add successive layers inside the vein lumen, shrinking it gradually, and in so doing will favour the injection in the direction of the nidus. PHIL would achieve a more rapid venous occlusion, risking a rupture. Cyanoacrylates risk immediate venous occlusion. Obtura (IHT Medical) is a newer agent that also has shown promising utility for this purpose.
- Some suggest it might be safer to routinely cut off the microcatheter in the jugular vein to avoid traction on the AVM when removing the microcatheter at the end of the procedure to minimise AVM rupture.
- Cure is usually mandatory in one session because of venous occlusion.

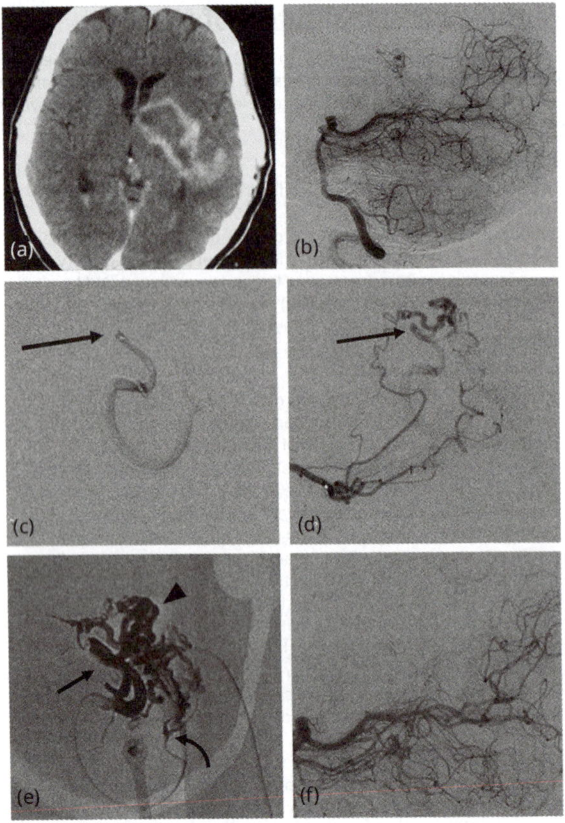

Figure 12.5 Transvenous embolisation of residual arteriovenous malformation (AVM) feeder post-surgery. (a) Computed tomography scan demonstrating haemorrhagic cavity in left basal ganglia. (b) Residual AVM post-surgery fed by the posterior choroidal artery. (c) Arterial access was not possible due to vessel tortuosity. A solitary draining vein is evident (arrow). (d) Microcatheter tip in the origin of the vein. (e) Onyx cast via venous injection. Arrow shows the vein. Arrowhead shows the filled nidus, curved arrow shows Onyx passed through the nidus to reach the arterial feeders. (f) Complete cure of the AVM. Images courtesy of Dr Mariangela Piano and Dr Dodi Boccardi.

Further reading

Koyanagi M, Mosimann PJ, Nordmeyer H, et al. The transvenous retrograde pressure cooker technique for the curative embolisation of high-grade brain arteriovenous malformations. J Neurointerv Surg. 2021;13(7):637–641.

Pre-radiosurgical embolisation of unruptured pial AVMs

- Whether EVT should be performed prior to STRS is currently contentious. STRS is more effective with a smaller target (nidus). Historically, it was considered that partial embolisation of an AVM could improve results with radiosurgery reducing both flow and nidal size.
- Current evidence, however, has yet to show benefit and it remains controversial. Usually embolisation does not achieve homogeneous occlusion of the part embolised, leaving areas of incomplete occlusion. The final target for STRS may therefore be unchanged. Embolisation may even reduce the efficacy of STRS. Embolic material results in artefacts and less reliable recognition of the target volume in the residual AVM. Embolisation induces ischaemia/hypoxia which upregulates angiogenesis. Embolisation may compartmentalise the AVM making STRS planning more difficult. If embolisation is too proximal, there may be recanalisation.
- Attenuation of STRS dose by LE material has also been suggested as a (probably theoretical) risk.
- It is important to closely liaise with the STRS team first to determine the best strategy if embolisation is considered.
- Pre-STRS embolisation of nidal and perinidal aneurysms is an indication to reduce the risk of post STRS haemorrhage as AVM haemodynamics change following STRS and the presence of aneurysms increases the risk of bleeding in the years following radiosurgery.
- Adverse effects of embolisation must be taken into account: symptomatic and non-symptomatic complications and the summation of the radiation effects on the brain.
- Radiation-induced long-term brain adverse events are more frequent in patients who have undergone at least two embolisation sessions before STRS.
- Complications of embolisation are not rare and if their rate, around 10% of symptomatic complications, is combined with the adverse events caused by STRS and related to overall success of the combined treatment, the results may not be favourable.
- If pre-radiosurgical embolisation is considered, the best strategy may be to only target direct fistulas within the nidus, as these are more resistant to treatment by STRS.
- A different (and, in the UK, increasingly common) approach may be to start with STRS and reserve embolisation to complete the treatment if and when needed. AVMs treated by STRS are smaller, the nidus is simplified, and there are fewer feeders and fewer veins. Potential residual direct fistulas are then usually readily occluded by embolisation.

Further reading

Russell D, Peck T, Ding D, et al. Stereotactic radiosurgery alone or combined with embolisation for brain arteriovenous malformations: a systematic review and meta-analysis. J Neurosurg. 2018;128(5):1338–1348.

Vein of Galen malformations

VOGMs refer to a rare paediatric subtype of high-flow AVM that involves the embryonic precursor of the vein of Galen, the median prosencephalic vein (MPV).

Aetiology

- The VOGM developmental defect occurs in first trimester of foetal development around 6–11 weeks. The exact mechanism remains unclear; however, an interplay between genetic and local environmental factors is likely, resulting in a small arteriovenous shunt that enlarges over time.
- Several associated germline gene defects have been identified, such as capillary malformation–AVM syndrome genes *RASA1* and *EPHB4*, often alongside other vascular malformations. High flow dilates and prevents the maturation of the MPV, which often persists, draining through a persistent primitive falcine sinus.

Clinical presentation

- Diagnosis is often made antenatally during the late second or third trimester via ultrasound. In regions where antenatal screening is less common, perinatal presentation may occur with high-output cardiac failure, or there may be a delayed presentation in infancy or childhood characterised by macrocephaly, hydrocephalus, and signs of venous hypertension such as seizures, facial venous congestion, developmental regression, and coma. Clinical presentation is primarily determined by the angioarchitecture of the VOGM.
- Classically, VOGM has two architectural subtypes:
  - Choroidal type: this is characterised by multiple fistulous points often interposed by a nidus from the choroidal and thalamoperforating arteries. Choroidal malformations tend to exhibit higher flow and exhibit a more aggressive course.
  - Mural type: this has fewer (1–3) direct fistulas typically entering the inferior aspect of the MPV.
- However, there is, in reality, a spectrum of the disease, with other factors, including the degree of constriction on the outflow from the MPV, being equally important as the above classification.
- Up to one-third of patients remain undetected in the perinatal period and present later with hydrovenous syndrome. Clinical features include headache, irritability, lethargy, developmental delay or regression, seizures, macrocephaly, and dilated facial veins.

Anatomy

- The shunt is located at the back of the third ventricle and is primarily supplied by the anterior and posterior choroidal arteries.
- Typically, persistence of the limbic arch connects the anterior cerebral pericallosal branches to this choroidal network and the shunt. Additionally, small thalamoperforating arteries arising from the P1 segments, along with dural branches from various sources, are involved. Secondary remote DAVFs have also been described, postulated to be induced by high flow.

Imaging

Antenatal

- Ultrasound: ultrasound conducted around 20 weeks may occasionally reveal a midline high-flow structure, although more commonly, the lesion remains undetectable during screening. By approximately 30 weeks, the dilated MPV is usually well seen as an anechoic midline structure. In severe cases, oligohydramnios and signs of antenatal high-output cardiac failure may be present.
- Foetal MRI: the brain is evaluated for indications of encephalomalacia, hydrocephalus, the degree of hypertrophy of the pial feeding arteries, and the diameter of the MPV outflow (a surrogate marker for flow rate). These aid prognostication.

Neonatal

- Echocardiogram: can guide the urgency of treatment. Indicative of a more severe course are diastolic flow reversal in the descending aorta, severe cardiac dysmotility, suprasystemic pulmonary hypertension, and coexisting cardiac defects. In many cases, with effective early intensivist care and careful medical management of cardiac failure, definitive interventional treatment can be delayed for 3–6 months.
- Neonatal/childhood brain MRI/MRA: critical for evaluating the presence and extent of brain parenchymal injury, which may influence treatment decisions. The assessment should include DWI and SWI sequences, as well as sagittal T2-weighted imaging. MRA is also useful for a gross assessment of the angioarchitecture and venous outflows, particularly the jugular outflows at the skull base.

Principles of endovascular management

- The timing of EVT is critical, as procedural complications are more likely in the first week. Early intervention is reserved for those with refractory cardiac failure to preserve life.
- The objective of treatment is to close the fistulous points to reduce high-output cardiac failure, lower pulmonary and venous pressures, and improve organ perfusion. Treatments are generally staged to allow for progressive reduction and vascular adaptation, thereby minimising complications such as venous thrombosis and reperfusion cerebral haemorrhage.
- Umbilical arterial access may provide a route for early embolisation and should be preserved when possible. Femoral arterial access must be protected at all costs, and groins should remain free of vascular access lines unless absolutely critical.
- The usual considerations for fluid and contrast doses in very small infants are heightened in cases of VOGM with associated organ failure.
- Techniques used to close the atrioventricular junction include the injection of highly concentrated n-BCA in free flow (Figure 12.6) or the use of detachable platinum coils delivered via transarterial or transvenous approaches supplemented with further injections of n-BCA or EVOH-based embolic agents. The use of intra- and postprocedural IV heparin varies between centres.

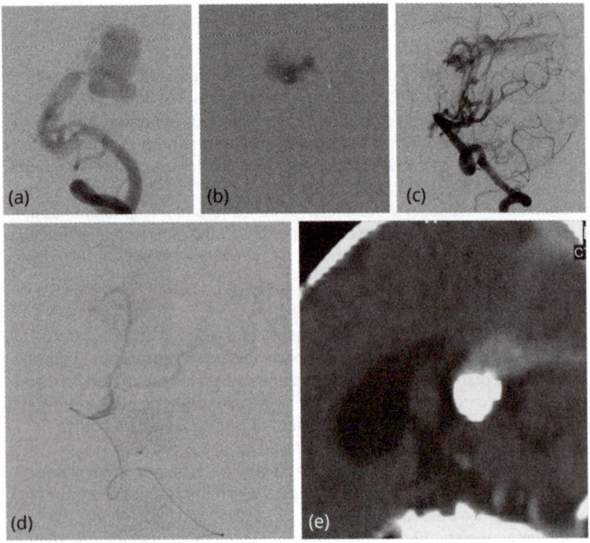

Figure 12.6 Endovascular treatment of a vein of Galen malformation. Cardiac failure had been well managed in the first 2 months medically and an echocardiogram revealed pulmonary arterial hypertension. (a) Diagnostic digital subtraction angiography showed a mixed-type vein of Galen aneurysmal malformation. (b) Glue injection. (c) Post-embolisation angiogram showed significant reduction in flow with residual choroidal-type fistulae. (d) Subsequent microcatheter hagiography in a branch during a further attempt to embolise the residual showed complete obliteration of the malformation, which had completely thrombosed at this point. (e) Post-embolisation computed tomography scan, showing hyperdense glue in the venous pouch. The baby made an excellent clinical recovery, catching up in weight and achieving normal milestones. Images courtesy of Dr Leve Joseph Sebastian.

- Antenatal treatment remains experimental at this stage. The technical feasibility of transuterine transtorcular access to the MPV for coil deployment has been demonstrated in a small number of cases, showing encouraging early results. This offers promise for those with very poor predictive imaging and clinical features in the third trimester.
- Management is complex, and care should be transferred to a designated VOGM centre with specialist antenatal, paediatric neurointerventional, cardiac, neurosurgical, and intensivist support at the earliest opportunity.
- Coordinated teamwork within experienced teams achieves the best outcomes. In the UK (population 67 million and 28 neuroscience centres), VOGM management is concentrated in just two centres, London and Liverpool.

Further reading

Berenstein A, Fifi JT, Niimi Y, et al. Vein of Galen malformations in neonates: new management paradigms for improving outcomes. Neurosurgery. 2012;70(5):1207–1213.

Raybaud CA, Strother CM, Hald JK. Aneurysms of the vein of Galen: embryonic considerations and anatomical features relating to the pathogenesis of the malformation. Neuroradiology. 1989;31(2):109–128.

Zhao S, Mekbib KY, van der Ent MA, et al. Mutation of key signalling regulators of cerebrovascular development in vein of Galen malformations. Nat Commun. 2023;14(1):7452.

Stereotactic radiosurgery

- STRS was pioneered in 1951 and, to date, several million patients have received treatment with STRS.
- The current gamma unit utilises an array of 192 separate cobalt sources focused at a fixed centre. Collimators focusing the radiation can produce a treatment volume as low as 5 mm^3.
- Linear accelerators predominantly utilised for body oncology irradiation have also been utilised for AVM treatment; however, they are somewhat limited by collateral dose and precision.
- A further evolution of the linear accelerator involves mounting it directly on a robotic arm for CT-guided, frameless robotic surgery—CyberKnife. Data on this modality remain relatively limited.
- AVMs represent a heterogeneous disorder in terms of angioarchitecture and neuroanatomy. Cases should be reviewed in a multidisciplinary setting, incorporating neurosurgical, neuroradiological, medical physics, and radiographer input.

Mechanism

- High-dose ionising radiation in radiosurgery causes endothelial damage within the AVM, leading to smooth muscle cell proliferation and extracellular collagen production in the nidus.
- This results in gradual stenosis and eventual obliteration of the AVM. Change in arterial versus venous flow may account for radiation-induced changes either by inducing venous stasis and vasogenic or cytotoxic oedema.

Indications

- AVMs with a history of haemorrhage carry an elevated risk of re-haemorrhage (mainly for the first few months), making prior haemorrhage a strong indicator for early treatment by surgery or EVT.
- Unruptured AVMs require a more nuanced approach, with careful consideration of the neuroanatomical eloquence of the location and the patient's age.
- Compact lesions in non-eloquent locations make ideal radiosurgery targets. Larger lesions in eloquent areas can be treated in a staged manner with a reasonable safety profile and obliteration rate.
- Small residual lesions following surgical resection are usually effectively treatable. However, lesions treated with LE agents can be challenging to target, with unpredictable effects on radiation scatter.
- Key factors to consider include proximity to cranial nerves and the orbits, especially when retreating lesions. Brainstem lesions are also approached with great caution, as even a mild radiosurgical response could be significantly symptomatic due to radiation-induced changes.
- A previous craniotomy is also a consideration, as it may interfere with the fixation of the Gamma Knife frame to the skull.

Radiosurgical treatment planning.

- Most patients are treated with LA alone. Those unable to tolerate frame fixation to the skull or requiring cerebral angiography may need GA. This is predominantly in paediatric patients and patients with movement disorders.
- Gamma Knife radiosurgery is a day-case procedure. A metal frame is affixed to the skull at four points, and a transparent cuboid box is fitted around most of the head. The box contains fiducial markers to enable co-registration of the 3D volume with MRI, CT, and angiographic images.
- A technique might involve performing T2- and proton density-weighted MRI, co-registered with DSA to localise the AVM. Gadolinium-enhanced MRI provides additional benefits for complex AVMs previously treated with surgery, embolisation, or radiosurgery. CTA is occasionally used when MRI is contraindicated.
- Transradial cerebral angiography is of particular benefit fòr this cohort of AVM patients who may undergo multiple angiograms.
- The entire process—from fitting the frame, imaging, and treatment to frame removal—can take between 3 and 8 h. Consequently, even well-informed and compliant patients may find the pathway challenging.
- Larger, staged lesions (around 10 mL) can be treated over weeks to months. For the second and third stages, only cross-sectional imaging is needed, which can be co-registered with the initial angiogram.

Outcomes and complications

(See Figure 12.7.)

- Nidus obliteration is achieved in about 65–85% of patients after a 3–5-year latency period (China, 2022).
- Radiation-induced changes are influenced by AVM volume, location, and treatment dose. Approximately 8% develop neurological symptoms and 3% will experience permanent neurological deterioration (including new seizure activity).
- Further delayed adverse effects, namely radiation necrosis and benign tumour and cyst formation, have been reported.

Clinical and radiological follow-up

- Patients are followed up clinically within weeks after radiosurgery. If no new symptoms arise, an MRI/MRA performed 3–4 years post-treatment is generally sufficient to assess the treatment response.
- If MR appearances suggest obliteration, angiography at 4 years from treatment should be performed, allowing time for the full effect of radiosurgery.
- If an obvious residuum persists on cross-sectional imaging, repeat radiosurgery may be indicated.

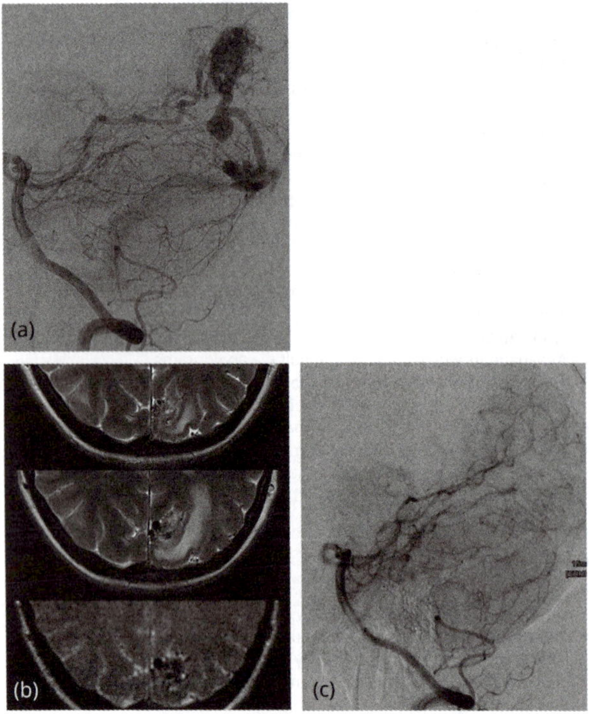

Figure 12.7 Stereotactic radiosurgical cure of an arteriovenous malformation (AVM). (a) Left occipital AVM fed by the posterior cerebral artery. (b) Pre-treatment magnetic resonance image demonstrating AVM (top), post-stereotactic radiosurgery revealing increased perilesional oedema (middle), and final result at 4 years (bottom). (c) 4-year digital subtraction angiography confirms exclusion of the AVM. Images courtesy of Dr George Tse.

Further reading

China M, Vastani A, Hill CS, Tancu C, Grover PJ. Gamma Knife radiosurgery for cerebral arteriovenous malformations: a systematic review and meta-analysis. Neurosurg Rev. 2022;45(3):1987–2004.

Venous procedures

Inferior petrosal sinus sampling *476*
Dural venous sinus pressure monitoring and stenting *479*
Cerebrospinal fluid–venous fistula embolisation *483*
Venous thrombectomy *488*

Inferior petrosal sinus sampling

Inferior petrosal sinus sampling (IPSS) is a diagnostic procedure to determine whether excess adrenocorticotropic hormone (ACTH) originates from the pituitary gland (typically a pituitary adenoma causing Cushing's disease) or from an external source (such as an adrenal tumour causing ectopic ACTH syndrome).

It is considered the gold standard for diagnosing Cushing's disease in patients with consistent ACTH-dependent Cushing's syndrome without a clear lesion on pituitary MRI.

The test involves comparing ACTH levels in blood samples from the IPSs (the draining veins of the pituitary gland) and peripheral blood, before and after the administration of corticotrophin-releasing hormone (CRH).

Indications

- ACTH-dependent hypercortisolaemia.
- No definite cause identified on gadolinium-enhanced pituitary MRI (lesions are usually <6 mm) and biochemical testing is discordant.
- Patients with biochemical Cushing's disease who have undergone previous subtotal hypophysectomy without clinical improvement or effect on ACTH secretion.

Contraindications

- The test is unsuitable for differentiating Cushing's disease from pseudo-Cushing's disease (where patients exhibit signs, symptoms, and abnormal cortisol levels associated with Cushing's syndrome, but the pathology is not caused by a problem with the hypothalamic–pituitary–adrenal axis).
- General contraindications to angiography: bleeding tendency, very impaired renal function (without dialysis), or contrast allergy.

Risks

- Venous puncture site complications (see Chapter 6).
- Venous thrombosis: at the puncture site or IPS.

Technique

(See Figure 13.1.)

- The procedure is performed awake or under conscious sedation.
- An IV cannula is required.
- A 4 or 5 Fr sheath is placed within one common femoral vein (CFV) and 6 Fr sheath in contralateral CFV. The 6 Fr sheath allows for simultaneous aspiration of peripheral venous blood during the procedure. Transarterial access is generally not required.
- Each IPS is catheterised with a 4 Fr angled catheter (30–45°) over a 0.035" hydrophilic wire. Venography can then be performed.
- Once satisfied with catheter position, sample collection can begin. A set of baseline samples (3 mL from each site) are from the right IPS catheter, left IPS catheter, and the peripheral sheath. A CRH bolus is then injected through a peripheral IV line (typically 100 mcg or 1 mcg/kg). Samples are taken from the three sites simultaneously at 1 min, 3 min, 8 min, and 15 min following CRH injection.

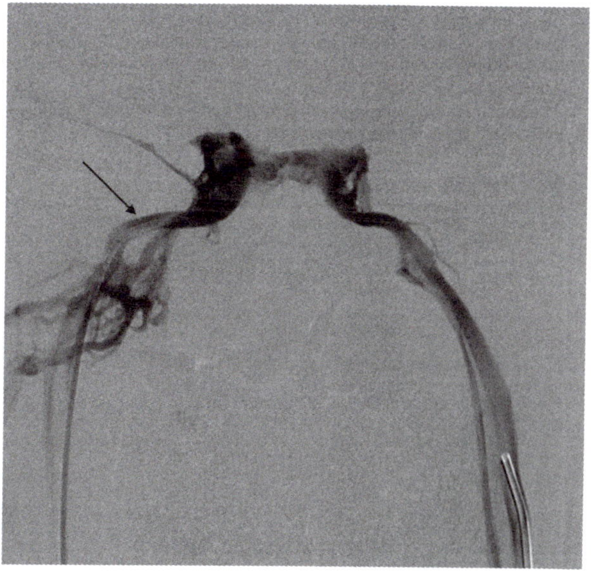

Figure 13.1 Venogram via right inferior petrosal sinus (arrow). Image courtesy of Dr Ayman Qureshi.

- The samples are transferred to chilled EDTA tubes before immediate transportation to the laboratory. A heparinised flush prevents catheter clot formation. Therefore, 5 mL of blood should be aspirated and discarded before each sample is taken.
- After sheath removal, 5 min of compression achieves haemostasis for each groin.

Post-procedure

- The procedure is tolerated as a day case. Patients can be discharged following 2 h of bed rest.

Interpretation

- An IPS/peripheral ACTH ratio of >2 at baseline or >3 following CRH stimulation suggests a central cause for elevated ACTH.
- IPS/IPS ratio of >1.4 indicates the side of the lesion.

Tips

- A second scrubbed pair of hands can help with the simultaneous sampling of three sites and bifemoral haemostasis.
- Study any cranial cross-sectional imaging to assess venous anatomy. If the IPS cannot be catheterised, sampling can be performed in the IJV, but this reduces test accuracy.

- The IPS runs in the petroclival synchondrosis, seen on the AP fluoroscopic view, usually arising from the anteromedial IJV. Therefore, the catheter tip should point medially on AP, and anteriorly on the lateral view. Once the first sinus is catheterised, venography can be performed to demonstrate the contralateral IPS, which can then be catheterised under roadmap guidance (biplane equipment facilitates this).

Further reading

Zampetti B, Grossrubatscher E, Dalino Ciaramella P, Boccardi E, Loli P. Bilateral inferior petrosal sinus sampling. Endocr Connect. 2016;5(4):R12–R25.

Dural venous sinus pressure monitoring and stenting

- Idiopathic intracranial hypertension (IIH) (or pseudotumour cerebri) is a disorder of raised ICP without apparent cause. It occurs primarily in overweight women of child-bearing age.
- The condition is uncommon, with an annual incidence in 2020 of approximately 5 per 100,000. It is significantly more prevalent in young, obese women, with incidence rates reaching 15–19 per 100,000.
- Medical management involves weight loss and reducing ICP with acetazolamide and topiramate.
- Venous sinus stenosis is found in ≥80% and is an addressable cause of venous outflow obstruction that can result in elevated ICP. There is probably a feedback loop whereby stenosis is caused by, and then exacerbates, the raised ICP.
- First performed in 2002, venous stenting is gaining acceptability as a treatment modality. Published data report 89% improvement in papilloedema, 88% alleviation of diplopia or visual disturbance, 79% reduction in headaches, and 95% improvement in pulsatile tinnitus.
- Alternative treatments are optic nerve sheath fenestration and CSF diversion. The latter is associated with a significant complication rate and revision rates of up to 42%. An ongoing RCT is currently comparing venous stenting and CSF diversion in *de novo* fulminant IIH patients (the IIH Intervention Trial).

Clinical presentation

Symptoms and signs

- Incapacitating headaches, nausea, and vomiting.
- Visual deterioration: ranging from transient obscuration of vision and visual defects, to blindness if untreated.
- Pulsatile tinnitus.
- Papilloedema: typically bilateral but may be unilateral. May be asymptomatic.

Modified Dandy criteria for diagnosis (all criteria required)

- Signs and symptoms of raised ICP.
- No localising neurological signs except abducens nerve palsy.
- Raised CSF pressure (>25 cmH_2O), without cytological or chemical abnormities.
- Normal CT/MRI findings without evidence of venous sinus thrombosis.

Imaging

- Orbital: optic nerve sheath distension and tortuosity, posterior globe flattening, papilloedema.
- Arachnoid cave outpouching: empty sella, Meckel's cave enlargement, prominent perivascular spaces.
- Sinuses: transverse sinus stenosis, which may be unilateral or bilateral. Other sinuses may also be affected.
- Cerebellar tonsillar ectopia.

Indications for stenting

- Risk of permanent visual loss.
- Failure or intolerance to medical management.
- More controversially, severe tinnitus or headaches. If performed for these reasons, it should significantly impact the patient's quality of life.

Risks

- ICH: <2%.
- Temporary headaches are common (in up to 50%), thought to be caused by dural stretching.
- Postprocedural thrombosis or stenosis, or stent-adjacent stenosis requiring retreatment: 9%.
- Permanent neurological morbidity: <2%.
- Mortality: <1%.
- *Other general complications associated with cerebral angiography, such as puncture site complications and contrast allergy.*

Technique

Pressure measurement

(See Figure 13.2a, b.)

- The most accurate measurement of pressures is obtained under LA as GA tends to markedly reduce pressures and gradients. GA can be administered bearing this limitation in mind.
- A 5 Fr sheath is inserted in the CFV. A 4 or 5 Fr sheath is inserted in the common femoral artery.
- A diagnostic catheter is positioned in the ICA ipsilateral to the stenosis. It is attached to an RHV and a continuous heparin–saline infusion. The catheter is utilised to conduct angiography in the venous phase to look for venous stenosis and to generate roadmaps for venous navigation.
- A 5 Fr guide catheter is positioned in the left IJV. It can be helpful to slightly oblique the lateral detector to throw off the contralateral transverse sinus.
- Utilising a venous roadmap, a 0.021" microcatheter connected to a continuous heparin–saline flush is navigated into the cerebral venous sinuses over a microwire (preferably J-tip). For pressure measurements, the RHV is removed and the microcatheter hub is connected to tubing flushed with saline, subsequently connected to a manometer (this is typically the same device used for gauging arterial line pressures on the anaesthetic machine).
- The transducer should be zeroed to atmospheric pressure when placed at the level of the external meatus (the approximate level of the foramen of Monro).
- Pressure measurements typically start at the superior sagittal sinus, and the microcatheter is pulled back to the confluence of sinuses, right and left transverse sinus proximal and distal to the stenosis (if present), the sigmoid sinuses, and the IJVs. Pressure recordings should be made over 30 s and patients should be instructed not to talk or hold their breath. Flush the catheter first if you suspect it is obstructed.
- The key factor is the pressure gradient across the stenosis. There is no clear agreement regarding the necessary gradient for stenting, with cited values varying from 4 to 8 mmH_2O, while others suggest that lower figures are acceptable.
- After measurements are complete, venous haemostasis at the groin is typically achieved with 5 min of manual pressure. Either manual pressure or closure devices are utilised for the arterial puncture site.

Venous stenting

(See Figure 13.2c–f.)

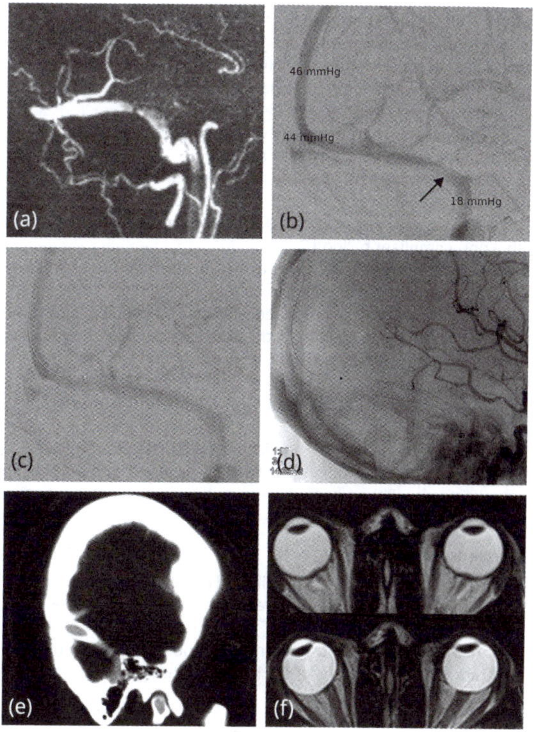

Figure 13.2 Transverse sinus stenosis stenting. (a) Magnetic resonance venography demonstrating transverse sinus stenosis. (b) Venous phase angiogram does not show the stenosis so clearly, but a large pressure gradient (26 mmHg) is measured at the arrow. (c) Subtracted and (d) unsubtracted angiography demonstrate the 7 × 40 Wallstent deployed across the stenosis. (e) Computed tomography venogram 1 month later demonstrates stent patency. (f) T2-weighted magnetic resonance imaging demonstrates papilloedema pre-treatment (top) with resolution post-treatment (bottom).

- Load patients with dual antiplatelets (DAPT) (no particular regime has been demonstrated to be superior).
- Stenting is performed under GA.
- An 8 Fr sheath is placed in the CFV (or the IJV, if more support is required). A 4 or 5 Fr sheath is inserted into the common femoral artery.
- Systemic heparinisation is initiated.
- A diagnostic catheter is positioned in the ICA ipsilateral to the stenosis. It is attached to an RHV and continuous heparin–saline infusion. This is utilised to conduct angiography and to generate roadmaps for venous navigation and to check for complications.
- An 8 Fr guide catheter is placed in the sigmoid sinus, if possible, or IJV, if not. Newer guide catheters with soft tips and supportive shafts such

as the Cerebase (Cerenovus) are recommended. A Berenstein tip select catheter and Terumo wire may aid guide catheter advancement. The guide catheter is attached to an RHV with a heparinised–saline flush.

- An intermediate catheter, e.g. Navien 0.072", may be utilised for extra support.
- Angiography is performed and the venous phase is inspected for stenosis, typically in the transverse sinus.
- If not already performed, pressure measurements are undertaken, most importantly pre- and post-stenosis. Decide whether or not to proceed.
- If the stenosis is very tight, it may be necessary to perform angioplasty with a non-compliant balloon.
- The diameters of the venous sinus before and after stenosis are measured, along with the length of the sinus to be stented. Typically, 7 mm, 8 mm, or 9 mm diameter stents are required. They must be self-expanding with sufficient radial force to counteract the external stenosis arising from the raised ICP. They should extend >10 mm proximal and distal to the stenosis. Long stents are typically necessary.
- The stent is deployed across the stenosis, and pressure measurements again performed.
- Final angiography is obtained and inspected for complications.
- Venous haemostasis at the groin is typically achieved with 5–10 min of manual pressure. Either manual pressure or closure devices are utilised for the arterial puncture site.

Postprocedural care

- DAPT is continued for 6 months, followed thereafter by aspirin.
- Usually the patient is monitored overnight, and discharged the following day.
- Post-intervention imaging usually involves one CT venogram or MR venogram within 12 months of the intervention.

Tips

- In addition to GA, therapeutic lumbar CSF drainage, acetazolamide, topiramate, and caffeine can potentially cause misleading ICP measurements.
- To provide extra support, the venous short sheath can be exchanged for a long sheath such as the 8 Fr Arrow-Flex (Terumo).
- Numerous stents are suitable for IIH stenting, such as Zilver 518 (Cook Medical), SMART (Cordis), Protégé Everflex (Covidien), Precise (Cordis), and Wallstent (Boston Scientific). A stent designed specifically for venous sinus stenosis, the BossStent (Sonorous), has recently been developed.

Complication avoidance and management

- Observe carefully for the wire snagging on cortical veins, as they are very delicate and can rupture, leading to ICH.
- Stent and sinus thrombosis may rarely occur.

Further reading

Azzam AY, Mortezaei A, Morsy MM, et al. Venous sinus stenting for idiopathic intracranial hypertension: an updated meta-analysis. J Neurol Sci. 2024;459:122948.

Cagnazzo F, Villain M, van Dokkum LE, et al. Concordance between venous sinus pressure and intracranial pressure in patients investigated for idiopathic intracranial hypertension. J Headache Pain. 2024;25(1):153.

Kalyvas A, Neromyliotis E, Koutsarnakis C, et al. A systematic review of surgical treatments of idiopathic intracranial hypertension (IIH). Neurosurg Rev. 2021;44(2):773–792.

Cerebrospinal fluid–venous fistula embolisation

CSF–venous fistulas are increasingly identified as a cause of spontaneous intracranial hypotension. They consist of a pathological connection between the spinal subarachnoid space and adjacent intervertebral/foraminal veins. Symptoms range from mild to debilitating and typically manifest as severe postural headaches, neck stiffness, photophobia, nausea, and occasionally hyperacusis. Imaging techniques, such as digital subtraction myelography (see Chapter 5, 'Dynamic fluoroscopic myelography', p. 153) and dynamic CT myelography, have enhanced their detection. Embolisation has proven to be effective and extremely safe.

Alternative treatment options

- Targeted blood patching, targeted fibrin glue embolisation, and surgical ligation are potential alternative options. These must be discussed in a multidisciplinary setting.

Anatomy

- Venous blood from the posterior aspect of the axial skeleton of the trunk, including the spine, primarily drains through the azygos system. This consists of the azygos, hemiazygos, and accessory hemiazygos veins.
- The venous drainage of the spinal cord and vertebral column can be categorised into three compartments: intradural, extradural, and paraspinal (Figure 13.3). The extradural and paraspinal compartments are of primary interest in CSF–venous embolisation:
  - The epidural (extradural) compartment is located within the spinal canal and encompasses the spinal epidural venous plexus (or internal vertebral venous plexus). This plexus has no valves, making it easily navigable with a microcatheter. While it surrounds the entire dura, there are four longitudinal channels where the plexus is more prominent: two anteriorly and two posteriorly. Venous rings at the mid-level of each vertebral body facilitate communication between the anterior and posterior plexuses and are seen clearly on angiography.

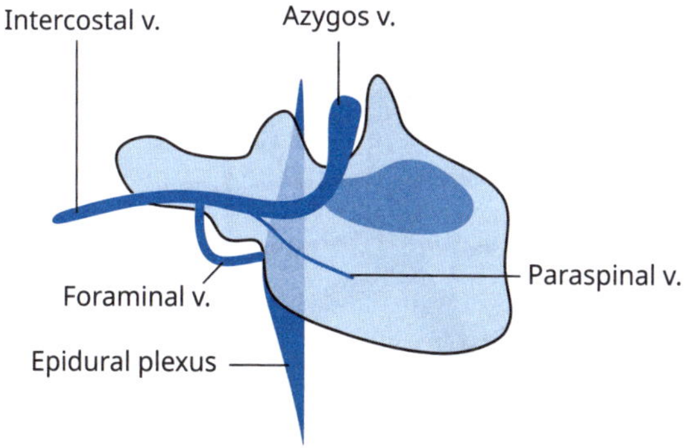

Figure 13.3 Intersection of the epidural space with azygos system.

    - The paraspinal compartment (or external vertebral, paravertebral, or paraspinal venous plexus) is located outside the canal. It also consists of two anterior and two posterior columns. The anterior external plexuses are located adjacent to the vertebral bodies and drain the basivertebral and foraminal veins. The posterior external plexuses run outside the lamina and drain the deep paraspinal muscles. They also communicate with the posterior internal plexuses and, in the cervical region, anastomose with the vertebral, occipital, and deep cervical veins.
- The epidural and paraspinal compartments are connected through each intervertebral foramen via the intervertebral foraminal veins, which form a plexus surrounding each nerve root. In the thoracolumbar spine, the veins drain directly into the adjacent segmental vein (an intercostal vein) at each level. The intervertebral foraminal veins are usually the site of the CSF–venous fistula.
- The above systems can be accessed via the azygos vein, entered via the superior vena cava (Figure 13.4).

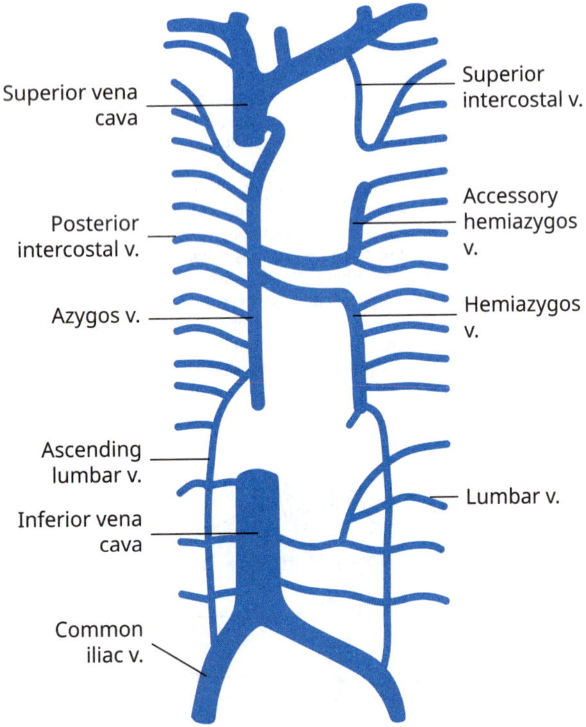

Figure 13.4 The azygos and hemiazygos system.

Technique

(See Figure 13.5.)

- Each fistula site has nuances in terms of its access. The article by Borg et al. (2022) is recommended for level-specific tips. We describe the general

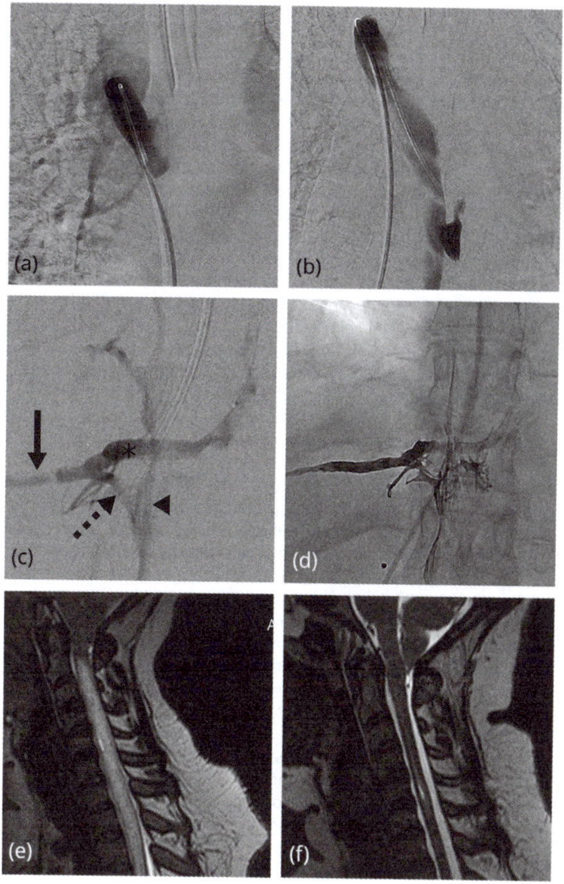

Figure 13.5 Transvenous embolisation of a cerebrospinal fluid–venous fistula. (a) Simmons catheter inserted into the azygos vein. (b) Catheter brought more inferiorly into the azygos using a Terumo wire. (c) Venogram via microcatheter (asterisk) positioned in the segmental vein. The solid arrow is the intercostal vein, the dashed arrow is the intervertertebral foraminal vein, and the arrowhead is the epidural plexus. (d) Onyx cast. (e) Pretreatment magnetic resonance imaging (MRI) demonstrating tonsillar descent and cord oedema. (f) Improvement of MRI appearances.

technique for thoracic and upper lumbar fistulas, which are the most common site.

- Embolisation can be performed under conscious sedation or GA, commonly as a day-case procedure.
- A 6 or 8 Fr vascular access sheath is inserted into the CFV, or alternatively the antecubital or IJV. Arterial access is not required.
- A guide catheter, e.g. a 6 Fr Benchmark, with an angled intermediate catheter such as Berenstein, Simmons, or Cobra tip is inserted into the sheath and navigated into the superior vena cava.
- To access the azygos vein, the catheter tip is angled posteriorly at the level of the right main bronchus. Gentle probing around the origin of the azygos is performed with an 0.035" Glidewire (Terumo). After accessing the azygos vein, it is advanced as inferiorly distally as possible, to about the level of T12. Subsequently, the diagnostic catheter or guide catheter is advanced over the wire. There is often a valve at this junction which may hinder catheterisation, but it can usually be crossed.
- If the fistula is on the right side, the catheter is kept in the azygos vein. If on the left, the hemiazygos or accessory hemiazygos systems need to be accessed across the midline and then superiorly and inferiorly, respectively. These connections can be visualised by venography.
- Once inside the relevant vein, venography is again performed, usually revealing stumps at the origins of each segmental tributary. These are used as the initial target for catheterisation. If a stump is not evident, then aim for the intervertebral foramen, seen on the unsubtracted fluoroscopy of the relevant level. The relevant level can also be accessed readily via entering the epidural venous system and navigating up/down or to the contralateral side.
- A DMSO-compatible microcatheter (e.g. Apollo or Marathon, Medtronic, or Sonic, Balt) is used to selectively catheterise the segmental vein over an 0.010" or 0.014" guidewire. The microcatheter is then tracked over a wire deeper into the segmental vein. The course is initially lateral and then anterior-to-posterior.
- When the microcatheter is close to the intervertebral foramen (having passed the anatomical landmark of the pedicle, i.e. in the proximal intercostal vein, approximately 1 cm from the site of the fistula), a venogram is again performed to reveal the intercostal vein and foraminal venous plexus. At this point, try to get as close as possible to the foramen, which may be achieved by directing the microwire inferiorly.
- As an important safety step, the image is completely demagnified, and time is taken to confirm the appropriate vertebral body side and level on the unsubtracted image, corresponding it with the myelogram report. *The fistula is not visible during the embolisation*, so this crucial step decreases the chance of treating the wrong level.
- LE (such as Onyx or Squid) is then injected. The embolisation cast should completely fill the foraminal plexus surrounding the nerve root and extend somewhat into the lateral epidural plexus, intercostal vein, and paraspinal vein. Entry into the epidural plexus is identified by flow medial to the pedicle.
- After satisfactory embolisation, haemostasis is achieved by manual compression.

Post-procedure

- CT may be performed immediately afterwards, confirming the position of the Onyx cast and to examine the pulmonary veins if embolism is suspected. However, this step is rarely necessary.
- If well, the patient may be discharged after a few hours (similar to catheter angiography). Routine analgesia is prescribed for pain.
- Patients are counselled on the risks of rebound intracranial hypertension (approximately 10% of cases).

Follow-up

- MRI spine and brain are performed at a delayed interval post-procedure, usually 3 months.
- Application of a headache score is recommended before and after the procedure for objective assessment of relief.

Complications

- Wrong site surgery: as the fistula cannot be directly visualised during the procedure, there is a risk of embolising the wrong level. It is crucial to confirm the site using anatomical landmarks. NB: be mindful that parallax during the procedure may lead to confusion regarding the catheterised level.
- Perforation of the spinal venous system: this is rare and is usually self-limiting. It can be treated by injecting LE and may be asymptomatic.
- Deaths or major complications: while theoretically possible, no reported cases in the literature have been described to date.
- Rebound intracranial hypertension: occurs in 10% of patients. Often manifests as headache, occasionally severe, and often in a different pattern to the preceding postural headaches. Other symptoms can include retro-orbital pressure and pulsatile tinnitus and can usually be treated successfully with a short course of acetazolamide.
- Pulmonary embolism: minute amounts of LE agent can embolise from the epidural venous system to the pulmonary arteries in 5–10%. As the absolute volume of LE is low, this does not generally have significant clinical consequences. In the series by Brinjikji et al. (2022), all patients in whom this occurred were asymptomatic, required no treatment, and were discharged the same day.
- Access site haematoma: usually resolves with manual pressure.
- Pain at the embolisation site: can typically be managed with simple analgesia.

Further reading

Borg N, Cutsforth-Gregory J, Oushy S, et al. Anatomy of spinal venous drainage for the neurointerventionalist: from puncture site to intervertebral foramen. AJNR Am J Neuroradiol. 2022;43(4):517–525.

Brinjikji W, Garza I, Whealy M, et al. Clinical and imaging outcomes of cerebrospinal fluid–venous fistula embolisation. J Neurointerv Surg. 2022;14(10):953–956.

Brinjikji W, Savastano LE, Atkinson JLD, Garza I, Farb R, Cutsforth-Gregory JK. A novel endovascular therapy for CSF hypotension secondary to CSF–venous fistulas. AJNR Am J Neuroradiol. 2021;42(5):882–887.

Venous thrombectomy

- CVST is a rare cause of cerebral haemorrhage or cerebral venous infarction, accounting for about 0.5–2% of strokes but with a higher prevalence in younger women. 78% are <50 years of age.
- CVST also occurred at an increased frequency during the COVID pandemic in hospitalised patients. Far more rarely, it occurred in association with COVID vaccination.
- Clinical presentation may include severe headache, symptoms or signs of intracranial hypertension, encephalopathy, focal neurological deficit, and seizures. Rarely (and typically in those with a delayed presentation), patients may arrive comatose.
- When diagnosed early and treated promptly, outcomes are generally favourable. However, some patients may deteriorate, with as many as 13% ultimately dying or remaining severely disabled despite adequate anticoagulation therapy. Many suffer cognitive problems and many do not return to work. Outcome is worse with deep venous involvement.
- There are a variety of causes, the most common being the later stages of pregnancy and the puerperium, contraceptive pill, coagulopathies, and intracranial infection. Often, it is multifactorial.
- Risk factors for deterioration include age >37 years, male sex, coma, mental status disorders, haemorrhage on the admission CT scan, thrombosis of the deep cerebral venous system, and thrombosis associated with underlying cancer.
- Retrospective series and case reports have demonstrated the safety and feasibility of EVT in selected patients. However, the only RCT (Thrombolysis or Anticoagulation for Cerebral Venous Thrombosis (TO-ACT)), which compared EVT to standard care in patients with anticipated poor outcomes, did not find improved functional outcome with EVT. There were several well-documented issues with this trial, including slow patient recruitment and variable endovascular techniques. Therefore, many large centres continue to offer EVT to certain patient subgroups with severe CVST on an individual basis.
- The SNIS Standards and Guidelines Committee states: 'For patients with cerebral venous sinus thrombosis, anticoagulation with heparin is front-line therapy; endovascular therapy may be considered particularly in cases of clinical deterioration despite medical therapy (Class IIa, Level B-R).'

Investigation

- Non-contrast cranial CT: may be normal in up to 25% but may reveal hyperdensity of the occluded sinuses or cortical veins or cerebral oedema. Parenchymal haemorrhage, intraventricular haemorrhage, and SAH are all possible.
- CT venography: demonstrates intraluminal filling defects indicative of a thrombus within the venous sinuses (which may be subtle in the deep venous system or cortical veins) and allows for the evaluation of venous vascular anatomy (Figure 13.6).
- MRI: has a higher sensitivity for detecting cerebral oedema and subtle haemorrhage, and thrombus within the sinuses or cortical veins. Small subcortical crescenteric areas of haemorrhage are characteristic. Signal change within the thrombus in the involved sinuses varies

with stage reflecting evolution from de-oxyhaemoglobin through to methaemoglobin.

- MR venography: this may be performed using multiplanar 3D time-of-flight or with multiplanar 3D gadolinium-enhanced T1-weighted imaging. The latter is more sensitive and is preferred.
- DSA is reserved when the diagnosis cannot be made on CT or MRI (extremely rare nowadays). It may reveal non-visualisation of the occluded dural sinus or cortical veins, intraluminal filling defects, and venous congestion (engorgement of cortical veins, prominence of medullary veins, or reversed flow within the cortical veins).

Treatment strategy

- Systemic anticoagulation is first line and is generally given even in the presence of ICH at baseline.
- Decompressive craniectomy is indicated for impending herniation and should be performed early, ideally within 12 h of admission.
- The precise indications for EVT remain undetermined. Below are some that have been published (Lee et al., 2018):
  - Clinical deterioration or progression of intracerebral haemorrhage/venous infarction despite anticoagulation.
  - Comatose presentation.
  - Deep cerebral venous thrombosis.
  - Posterior fossa involvement.
  - Major contraindications to anticoagulation, e.g. bleeding disorders, thrombocytopenia ($<100 \times 10^9$/L), and recent gastrointestinal haemorrhage.

Technique

(See Figure 13.6.)

- Technique varies widely between centres.
- GA is generally employed.
- Generally, systemic heparinisation will have already been initiated before the start of the procedure.
- Ultrasound is recommended for any vascular access in this patient cohort given that they are usually heparinised.
- A 4 or 5 Fr arterial catheter is inserted into the relevant ICA or vertebral artery for diagnostic cerebral angiography in the venous phase for diagnosis, navigation, and assessment of success.
- CFV access is generally successful. Direct jugular access is also possible but there is a small risk of consequent jugular thrombosis further impeding venous return.
- An 8 Fr guide catheter is navigated into the IJV or as far distally as the transverse sinus or torcular confluence.
- Newer guide catheters with soft tips and supportive shafts, e.g. Cerebase (Cerenovus), are recommended. Many of these can be safely tracked to the torcula if needed.
- Standard MT techniques such as stent retrievers, aspiration catheters, or combinations thereof can be used. The clot burden is often very high, and repeated passes may be necessary. Double stent-retriever techniques have been used successfully.

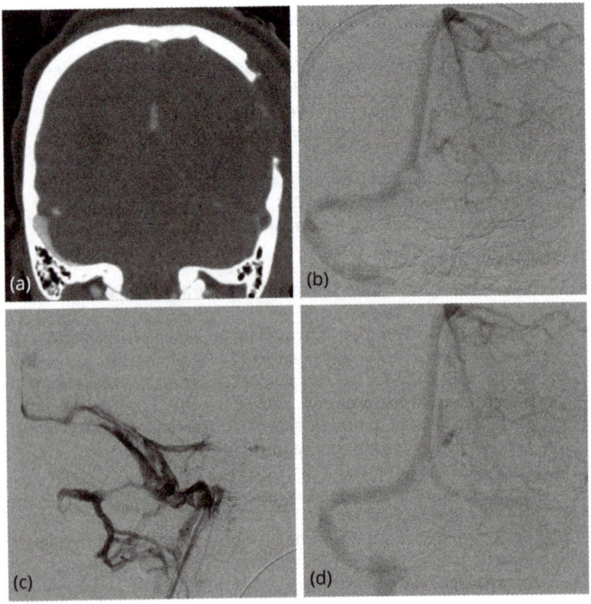

Figure 13.6 Venous thrombectomy. (a) Computed tomography venogram demonstrating thrombus within left transverse sinus. A decompressive craniectomy has already been undertaken. (b) Non-opacification of left transverse sinus confirmed on venous angiogram phase. (c) Venogram performed after thrombectomy. (d) Flow restored in the sinus (some clot still evident in confluence of sinuses).

- Even the deep venous system can be suitable for thrombectomy, although great care must be taken to avoid causing damage, as veins here can be small and fragile. Therefore, if undertaken at all, the use of aspiration thrombectomy, when feasible, or smaller, lower-profile stent retrievers is recommended.
- Adjuvant low-dose (10 mg recombinant tissue plasminogen activator) intrasinus thrombolysis may also be utilised (often a lot more may be required due to the excessive thrombus load), injected over 20 min or with an overnight infusion (as per local protocols).

Tips

- Unlike arterial thrombectomy, an angiographically perfect or near-perfect result is not the goal. The goal is to re-establish flow, and indeed often there can be a significant clinical improvement despite an irregular/ragged appearance to the sinus on follow-up venography.
- When using wires to navigate the venous system, it is recommended to form a J-tip to prevent catching in fragile cerebral veins.

Post-procedure

- These patients are typically already in HDU/ICU, and should be closely monitored after the procedure for any neurological change.
- They may require two or more EVT sessions during their hospital stay. This can be prompted by persistently increased ICPs/worsening venous infarct or haemorrhage/further clinical deterioration.
- These patients often have a surprisingly good clinical outcome (if managed aggressively), despite a poor appearance of the brain and venous system on imaging.

Follow-up

- Follow-up imaging should be performed as dictated by their clinical course. CT venography or MR venography is adequate. DSA to check vessel patency is rarely needed. They are at risk of chronic venous insufficiency, IIH, and DAVF development.
- Close coordination with stroke medicine, ICU, and often haematology is often required.

Further reading

Bousser MG, Ferro JM. Cerebral venous thrombosis: an update. Lancet Neurol. 2007;6(2):162–170.

Coutinho JM, Zuurbier SM, Bousser MG, et al. Effect of endovascular treatment with medical management vs standard care on severe cerebral venous thrombosis: the TO-ACT randomized clinical trial. JAMA Neurol. 2020;77(8):966–973.

Ferro JM, Canhão P, Stam J, Bousser MG, Barinagarrementeria F; ISCVT Investigators. Prognosis of cerebral vein and dural sinus thrombosis: results of the International Study on Cerebral Vein and Dural Sinus Thrombosis (ISCVT). Stroke. 2004;35(3):664–670.

Lee SK, Mokin M, Hetts SW, et al. Current endovascular strategies for cerebral venous thrombosis: report of the SNIS Standards and Guidelines Committee. J Neurointerv Surg. 2018;10(8):803–810.

Chapter 14

Spinal vascular lesions

Overview of spinal vascular lesions 494
Spinal dural arteriovenous fistula 497
Spinal epidural arteriovenous fistula 502
Spinal cord arteriovenous malformations 504
Vertebro-venous fistula 509
Spinal aneurysms 511

Overview of spinal vascular lesions

Various classification schemes exist for spinal vascular disorders; however, none are universally accepted. It is probably preferable to refer to each disorder by name. A schematic is provided in Figure 14.1.

Spinal dural arteriovenous fistulas

- The arteriovenous shunt is between a radiculomeningeal artery and a radicular vein. The shunt drains retrogradely into the perimedullary veins surrounding the spinal cord and resulting venous hypertension leads to chronic hypoxia.
- This is the most prevalent spinal vascular lesion, accounting for approximately 70% of cases.

Spinal epidural arteriovenous fistulas

- The fistula is between the epidural arterial arcade (or retrocorporeal arcade) and the epidural venous plexus.
- Despite the extradural drainage, there may be intradural reflux via perimedullary veins, and hence venous hypertension, myelopathy, and (rarely) SAH.

Intradural perimedullary arteriovenous fistulas

- These are intradural extramedullary lesions supplied by the anterior or posterolateral spinal arteries and drain into perimedullary veins without an intervening nidus, although there is often a varix at the shunt site.
- They are located on the anterior, posterior, or lateral cord pial surfaces, and typically in the upper cervical or thoracolumbar spine or the conus.

Intramedullary spinal arteriovenous malformations

- These comprise a nidus supplied by anterior and/or posterolateral spinal arteries and drain into perimedullary veins.
- The nidus frequently includes direct fistulas and aneurysms.

Metameric syndrome

- Also known as juvenile AVMs, these are high-flow lesions that consist of both intradural and extradural components (the entire metamere).
- They generally involve the spinal cord, vertebrae, and paraspinal muscles. Neural tissue is usually intermingled with the spinal component of the AVM nidus.

Spinal aneurysms

- Spinal aneurysms may be primary or, more commonly, associated with AVMs.

Spinal vascular tumours

Cavernous malformations (cavernomas)

- These are histologically identical to brain cavernous lesions. They consist of dilated endothelium-lined sinusoidal spaces.
- They account for about 10% of spinal vascular lesions. Associated cerebral cavernous lesions are present in about 40%.

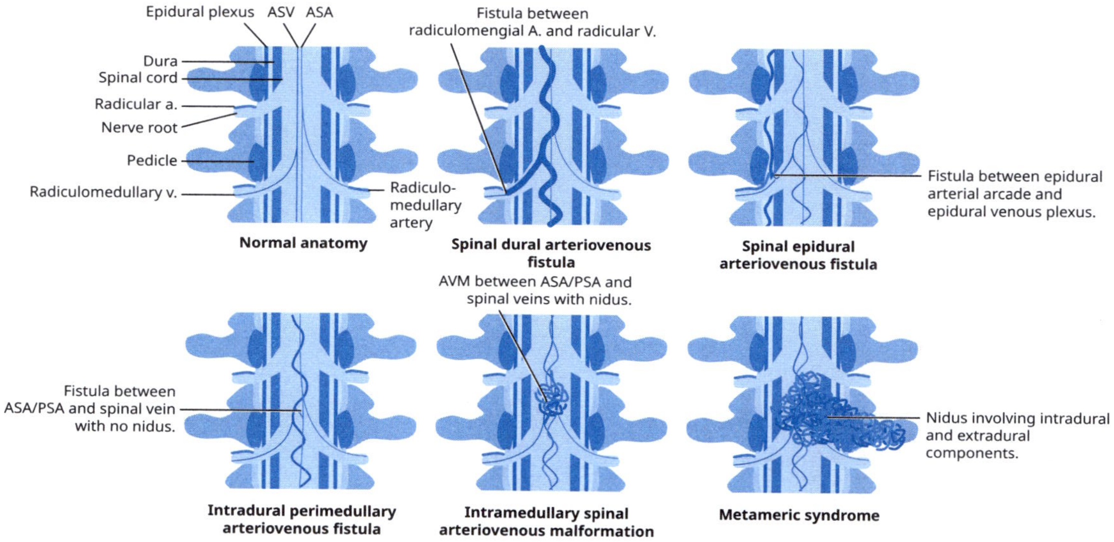

Figure 14.1 Types of spinal vascular malformations.

- Presentation is with acute haemorrhage or chronically progressive myelopathy. They are more common in women and typically in young adulthood.
- Diagnosis using MRI reveals a 'popcorn appearance' with heterogeneous signal intensities, a low T2 rim from haemosiderin, and hypointense blooming on gradient echo. There can be enhancement and cord expansion if recent haemorrhage.
- Surgical resection is generally possible for symptomatic lesions.

Other vascular tumours

- Primary tumours: aneurysmal bone cyst, angiofibroma, angiosarcoma, angiolipoma, haemangioblastoma, haemangioma, haemangiopericytoma, haemangioendothelioma, and osteoblastoma.
- Metastases: e.g. renal cell carcinoma, thyroid carcinoma, and hepatocellular carcinoma.

Further reading

Harrigan MR, Deveikis JP. Handbook of Cerebrovascular Disease and Neurointerventional Technique. 3rd ed. Humana Press; 2018.
Lasjaunias P, Berenstein A, ter Brugge KG, eds. Surgical Neuroangiography. Vol. 1. Springer; 2011.

Spinal dural arteriovenous fistula

The arteriovenous shunt occurs between a radiculomeningeal artery and a radicular vein (Figure 7.5). The shunt drains retrogradely through this vein to the perimedullary veins surrounding the spinal cord, causing venous hypertension that results in chronic hypoxia and progressive myelopathy. These are assumed to be acquired lesions but aetiology is unknown. Unlike cranial DAVF, venous thrombosis is not thought to be the main cause.

The location of the fistula is generally at the dura mater, close to the spinal nerve root, usually beneath the pedicle of the vertebral body.

Surgical disconnection of the leptomeningeal vein or embolisation of the fistula are both possible treatment options but surgery is more efficacious.

Clinical

- Typically, middle-aged to elderly men (mean age at diagnosis 66 years).
- Presentation consists of progressive myelopathy, paraesthesia, sensory loss, radicular pain, and autonomic symptoms such as urinary incontinence and erectile dysfunction. Upper or lower motor neurons may be affected.
- Symptoms usually progress insidiously, and delayed diagnosis is unfortunately common.
- Rapid onset of symptoms usually indicates venous infarction of the spinal cord. SAH does not occur.

Imaging

Magnetic resonance imaging

- MRI:
  - Dilated perimedullary vessels may be seen along the anterior, or more commonly, posterior surface, usually spanning three or more vertebral levels and best visualised on T2-weighted imaging.
  - Swelling and oedema of the spinal cord/conus on T2-weighted imaging and STIR may be seen due to venous congestion.
  - There may be contrast enhancement of the intramedullary signal change and the vessels. Note that a swollen cord *only* may be seen without obvious venous dilatation. Occasionally, the cord may appear normal.
  - The 'missing piece' sign is rare but sensitive for DAVF. It consists of a discrete non-enhancing segment of spinal cord (the 'missing piece') best seen on sagittal projections. It may be the only radiological evidence of the pathology.
- Time-resolved gadolinium-enhanced MRA (time-resolved imaging of contrast kinetics (TRICKS) or time-resolved angiography with interleaved stochastic trajectories (TWIST) sequences) can often identify the site of the fistula, thereby simplifying DSA. If this option is unavailable, a gadolinium-enhanced first-pass phase can often reveal early venous filling and even the shunt location.
- Contrast-enhanced CT of the spine is less sensitive than time-resolved MRI but may be beneficial when there is a contraindication to MRI, or when other diagnostic modalities have been exhausted and there is still clinical suspicion.

Digital subtraction angiography

- Techniques for spinal DSA are described in Chapter 7, 'Spinal angiography', p. 212.
- Stasis of contrast in the radiculomedullary arteries and anterior spinal artery suggests the presence of a fistula.
- When searching for the fistula, it is essential to perform selective injections at each segmental level. A level cannot be ruled out simply because it opacified due to aortic reflux or collateral circulation.
- It can be useful for surgical localisation to place coil(s) in the feeder at the time of angiography.

Indications for embolisation

- Most case series show a higher rate of cure after surgery versus endovascular. Nevertheless, spinal DSA is required for diagnosis and with the patient's prior consent might be attempted under the same anaesthetic if considered safe.
- Frail or elderly patients may benefit from decreased blood loss.
- If GA is contraindicated, the procedure can be performed under LA or sedation, although it can be harder due to patient movement. Embolic agents are also painful when injected.
- Patient preference.

Contraindications

- Branches supplying the spinal cord: radiculomedullary or radiculopial arteries supplying the spinal cord coincidentally originate from the same segmental artery in approximately 14% of cases. If present, this is a contraindication for embolisation due to the risk of spinal cord infarction. These arteries may be difficult to detect on standard angiography, but there is increased sensitivity with cone beam CT.
- A relative contraindication involves these branches arising from adjacent or contralateral arteries (to the DAVF).

Technique

(See Figure 14.2.)

- GA is recommended.
- IV heparinisation is achieved with ACT monitoring if available.
- A 6 Fr sheath is placed in the common femoral artery.
- If not already done, it is necessary to catheterise and perform angiography on the spinal levels above, below, and contralateral to the fistula to identify any branches supplying the spinal cord. Embolic material can migrate to these levels during embolisation.
- The segmental level is located and catheterised. A 4 or 5 Fr diagnostic catheter (depending on the size of the branch), such as a Cobra, Mikaelson, or Simmons 1 or 2, is typically sufficient for embolisation. If a more stable platform is needed, the catheter can be exchanged for a diagnostic catheter over an exchange-length wire. 5 or 6 Fr guide catheters can often be accommodated. These are very stable and can accommodate large or multiple devices. However, they may cause trauma to the vessel and can be difficult to insert into small branches.

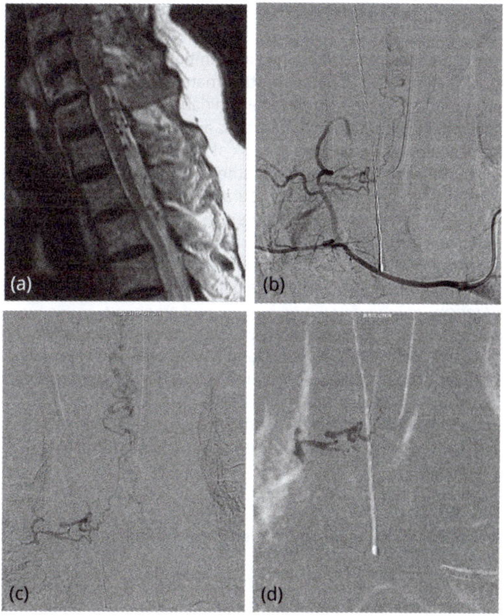

Figure 14.2 Embolisation of a spinal dural arteriovenous fistula (DAVF). (a) Sagittal T2-weighted magnetic resonance image demonstrates multiple engorged veins posterior to the cord. (b) Spinal angiography via the right supreme intercostal artery demonstrates a DAVF at the level of the neural foramen with drainage into spinal veins. (c) Selective angiography via the feeding spinal artery with a Magic 1.2 microcatheter. (d) Glue cast after embolisation with penetration into the proximal vein. Images courtesy of Dr Tufail Patankar.

- An RHV is attached to the catheter and connected to a heparinised saline flush.
- Once the site has been identified, magnified views with fast frame rates and respiratory arrest are performed. A 3D cone beam acquisition with 20% diluted contrast may be helpful to understand the anatomy. The catheter is likely wedged, so angiography must be performed gently.
- Carefully examine the anatomy of the injected area for medullary branches.
- The selection of microcatheter is based on the size and tortuosity of the dural branch supplying the fistula, and embolic agent:
  - DMSO-compatible microcatheters are essential for LEs, including the Marathon, Apollo, Echelon, Headway Duo, and Sonic. Use of the Scepter Mini balloon catheter or pressure cooker technique may reduce reflux and encourage forward flow.
  - n-BCA/lipiodol can be injected through most catheters. The Magic and Sonic 1.2 Fr are commonly selected due to their low profile.

- Using a roadmap, the microcatheter is navigated as close as possible to the nidus.
- A blank 'glue' roadmap is obtained and embolic material is injected.
  - As with all fistulas, the embolisation material *must* reach the proximal section of the vein. Proximal arterial ligation will result in recurrence.
  - Conversely, migration of the embolic agent too far downstream into the draining vein increases the risk of worsening venous ischaemia.
  - A wedged position of the microcatheter, to arrest antegrade flow, may help reduce reflux and encourage forward flow into the fistula. Alternatively balloon microcatheters, or proximal 'pressure cooker' coil-protected techniques may be employed.
- Once the injection has adequately penetrated the fistula, perform post-embolisation angiography from the delivery catheter to confirm fistula obliteration.
- Gently remove the microcatheter, ensuring no resistance is felt. If there is resistance, pull slowly, pausing for a few seconds between each tug. Ultimately, if the resistance is too high, it is better to cut off the catheter at the groin than to risk vessel avulsion.
- Aspirate the delivery catheter to remove any residual agent or thrombus.
- Utilise manual pressure or a vascular closure device for groin haemostasis.

Post-procedure

- Neurointensive care is recommended for 24 h with neurological monitoring.
- Post-procedure CT can be performed to confirm the intradural venous location of the embolic agent, prognostic of cure.
- Some centres advocate anticoagulation to reduce the risk of thrombosis. There is no evidence for or against.
- Follow-up MRI is performed at 3–6 months. If the MRI features are resolving, DSA may not be required. However, if MRI features persist, DSA is recommended.
- Similarly, if symptoms subside and then worsen, repeat angiography is indicated.

Tips

- Placing a coil in the lumbar or intercostal segmental artery distal to the radicular branch is optional but serves three purposes: (i) to prevent the embolic agent from entering muscular branches which can cause pain, (ii) to encourage the embolic agent to enter the fistula, and (iii) to act as a marker for surgical ligation in cases of embolisation failure.

Complications

- Injecting embolic material into a spinal cord branch poses a risk of cord infarction, which may result in paralysis, loss of sensation, dysaesthesia, pain, incontinence of the bladder and bowel, and loss of sexual function.
- Venous infarction may occur due to thrombosis of the draining perimedullary vein. Ensure that the agent does not penetrate too far downstream in the vein.

- Dissection or perforation of the segmental artery is rare. It can lead to a local haematoma, with a risk of retroperitoneal or retropleural complications. Embolisation of the branch should be performed.

Further reading

Adrianto Y, Yang KH, Koo HW, et al. Concomitant origin of the anterior or posterior spinal artery with the feeder of a spinal dural arteriovenous fistula (SDAVF). J Neurointerv Surg. 2017;9(4):405–410.

Spinal epidural arteriovenous fistula

The fistula is between the epidural arterial arcade (or retrocorporeal arcade) and the epidural venous plexus, with possible reflux into perimedullary veins.

These fistulas reside in the anterior (lower thoracic or lumbar) or lateral (upper thoracic and cervical) epidural spaces.

The aetiology is unknown. There is an association with prior surgery, and connective tissue disorders (e.g. neurofibromatosis type 1, Marfan's syndrome, fibromuscular dysplasia, and Ehlers–Danlos syndrome), although most are idiopathic.

Clinical features

- Despite the extradural drainage, there may be reflux into perimedullary veins, and hence venous hypertension, myelopathy, and even (rarely) SAH.
- Myelopathy may also occur in those without intradural reflux, due to compression of the thecal sac by a large, arterialised epidural venous pouch.
- Patients are typically younger than those with spinal DAVF, although a bimodal distribution has been reported; patients with intradural presentations are typically in their 50s, similar to DAVF in the thoracolumbar region. In contrast, those without intradural drainage usually present in their 20s, due to the mass effect of the fistula in the cervical and upper thoracic regions.

Imaging

- MRI features may be similar to DAVF, with cord oedema and perimedullary flow voids. Time-resolved MRI can identify the feeding arteries. CTA is also possible, reserved for those unable to tolerate MRI.
- DSA provides the diagnosis, differentiates between those with and without intradural drainage, and identifies radiculomedullary and radiculopial arteries coming off the same level.

Management

- EVT is considered first line.
- There are often multiple arterial feeders, large venous pouches, and there may be difficulty reaching the fistula. Multiple sessions may be required for complete occlusion of the fistula. In one series, 55% of fistulas were cured after the first session, rising to 92% after staged treatments, compared to 87% with surgery alone (Huang et al., 2013).
- A transarterial approach with n-BCA or LE agents may be attempted:
  - It is necessary to occlude the epidural pouch distal to the fistulous point, ideally up to communication with the paravertebral drainage. If the epidural sac remains arterialised, intradural drainage may recur.
  - If intradural reflux is present, it is important to introduce embolic material into the foot of the intradural vein. This may be a considerable distance from the epidural sac.
  - A considerable amount of agent may be required if the venous pouch is large. Adjuvant coils may be utilised to prevent collateral inflow from contralateral or adjacent segmental arteries.
- A transvenous approach is often possible:

  - This may be preferable if there are multiple arterial feeders and a high-flow fistula, and in high and mid- cervical fistulas, where there is risk of reflux into the vertebral or anterior spinal arteries.
  - Access can often be achieved via the azygos system (see Chapter 13, 'Cerebrospinal fluid–venous fistula embolisation', p. 483).
  - Occasionally, the epidural pouch is isolated and cannot be reached via the transvenous route.
  - Coiling and glue'LE may be attempted.
  - Direct percutaneous puncture of the epidural pouch may be possible, particularly if it is very large.
- Surgery can be challenging due to the anterior location of the fistulas. It is typically considered for cases that are difficult to treat with endovascular methods or when EVTs have failed.

Further reading

Brinjikji W, Yin R, Nasr DM, Lanzino G. Spinal epidural arteriovenous fistulas. J NeuroIntervent Surg. 2016;8(12):1305–1310.

Shetty GS, Singh V, Prasad SN, et al. Spinal epidural fistulas—a separate entity to dural fistulas with different angioarchitecture and treatment approach. World Neurosurg. 2021;149:e600–e611.

Takai K, Endo T, Yasuhara T, et al. Microsurgical versus endovascular treatment of spinal epidural arteriovenous fistulas with intradural venous drainage: a multicentre study of 81 patients. J Neurosurg Spine. 2020;33(3):381–391.

Spinal cord arteriovenous malformations

Intramedullary spinal arteriovenous malformation

These lesions comprise a nidus supplied by anterior and/or posterolateral arteries and drain into perimedullary veins. The nidus frequently includes direct fistulas and aneurysms.

These congenital lesions are similar to brain AVMs although are less common (1:6). Nonetheless, they are the second most common type of spinal vascular lesion.

Clinical

- Patients usually present in childhood or early adulthood.
- Acute presentation with SAH or cord haemorrhage may occur, resulting in severe pain in the back, neck, and legs. SAH can also migrate into the brain, resulting in headache, seizures, and loss of consciousness.
- The clinical presentation may alternatively consist of a gradual decline in function due to repeated minor haemorrhages.
- Arterial steal or pressure symptoms due to dilated vessels may occur, resulting in myelopathic symptoms of motor weakness, sensory disturbances, or radicular pain (from conus lesions).

Imaging

- MRI:
  - Dilated flow voids may be observed in and around the spinal cord.
  - Haemosiderin staining in the surrounding cord indicates prior haemorrhage.
  - Time-resolved MRA may define the feeding vessels, simplifying DSA.
- DSA: this is the gold standard for diagnosis and characterisation. It is necessary to identify all the supplying levels.

Pathophysiology

- Spinal AVMs are considered congenital.
- There are associations with other spinal vascular conditions, namely Klippel–Trenaunay–Weber syndrome and hereditary haemorrhagic telangiectasia.

Indications for embolisation

- Curative obliteration of the lesion due to the symptoms or the likelihood of progression.
- Partial treatment to alleviate symptoms or eliminate architectural weak points such as aneurysms may be performed when a complete cure is not possible.
- Preparation for adjunctive treatments such as surgery or radiotherapy.

Technique

(See Figure 14.3.)

- These are rare lesions and a full MDT discussion should take place to determine the aims and strategy of treatment. Seeking external expert review may be advisable, particularly if it is a non-emergency situation.
- GA is recommended.
- Intravenous heparinisation is achieved with ACT monitoring if available.
- A 6 Fr sheath is placed in the common femoral artery.

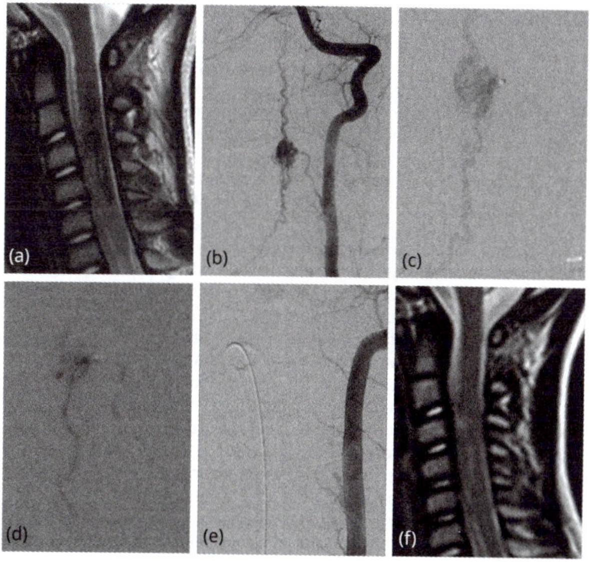

Figure 14.3 Embolisation of spinal arteriovenous malformation (AVM). A young patient presented with a severe neck ache and quadriparesis 2 months prior. (a) Sagittal T2 magnetic resonance imaging (MRI) shows upper cervical haematomyelia. (b) Left vertebral artery angiogram reveals a compact nidus fed by a spinal vessel. (c) Superselective microcatheter injection from the feeding pedicle. (d) Glue injection demonstrates minimal glue efflux into the anterior spinal axis. (e) Final angiography shows no residual AVM. (f) Follow-up T2 MRI after 2 weeks reveals resolution of the bleeding and disappearance of flow voids. Note that the T1 bright areas may represent thrombosis and/or glue deposited in the nidus. The patient remained neurologically intact.

- The relevant level is catheterised and the catheter connected to a heparinised saline flush. Magnified, superselective angiography at high frame rates is performed.
- Carefully examine the anatomy of the injected area on 2D angiography ± 3D cone beam CT.
  - It is crucial to understand the angioarchitecture of the lesion and the location of the anterior and posterior spinal arteries. If the plan is curative, the target is the AVM nidus and proximal part of the draining vein. Obliteration of the feeding arteries proximal to the nidus without occluding the vein is ineffective, as other arterial feeders will be recruited. Occlusion of the venous drainage without obliterating the nidus and feeding arteries creates a very high haemorrhage risk.
  - Posterior spinal arteries typically exhibit collateralisation, meaning that occlusion may not always be symptomatic. However, occlusion of an anterior spinal artery supplying the cord often leads to cord ischaemia.

  - Identification of branches of the anterior or posterior spinal arteries that solely supply the fistula (and thus *can* be occluded) is necessary through superselective microcatheter angiography. It is important to avoid reflux into the main anterior/posterior spinal artery branch.
- The selection of microcatheter is based on the size and tortuosity of the target branch supplying the AVM, along with the embolic agent.
- Agents used for AVM embolisation include:
  - n-BCA glue, advantageous in that it is highly thrombogenic and can be injected via low-profile catheters like the Magic. The objective is to achieve a complete cast of the fistulous connection and the proximal draining vein. It is usually the agent of choice.
  - LE agents can be injected more slowly and with greater control. However, the agent is more likely to penetrate into unwanted spinal branches during prolonged injections.
  - Coils: these have utility in the treatment of giant fistulas as a 'frame' for LE agents to slow down premature advancement into the vein. They may be used proximal to an injecting microcatheter in the 'pressure cooker' technique, to reduce flow in arterial feeders for symptomatic control, and as adjunctive treatment prior to embolisation or surgery.
  - Particles may be used to achieve symptomatic control or in presurgical embolisation. Recanalisation rates are high but morbidity is low.
- Using a roadmap, the microcatheter is navigated as close as possible to the fistulous point. It can be useful to 'wedge' the microcatheter, to avoid reflux of agent.
- A blank 'glue' roadmap is obtained and the embolic material is injected.
- Once embolisation is complete, gently remove the microcatheter, ensuring no resistance is felt. Aspirate the delivery catheter to remove any residual agent or thrombus.
- Post-embolisation angiography is then performed from the delivery catheter to confirm nidal obliteration.
- If necessary, additional feeders may be catheterised and embolised.
- Utilise manual pressure or a vascular closure device for groin haemostasis.

Post-procedure

- Neurointensive care is recommended for 24 h with neurological monitoring.
- Interval MRI is performed at 3–6 months. If the MRI features are resolving, DSA may not be required. If features persist, DSA is recommended.
- Similarly, if symptoms subside and then worsen, repeat angiography is indicated.

Complication avoidance and management

- If particles are used, caution must be exercised in those with high-flow shunts to avoid embolisation into the pulmonary circulation.
- Care must be exercised when removing microcatheters after n-BCA or LEs have been injected, as the microcatheter might adhere to the vessel. This may be avoided with detachable tip microcatheters and slow, steady traction. Ultimately, it may be preferable to leave the microcatheter in place rather than risk vascular avulsion; cut off the microcatheter at

the puncture site under slight tension to ensure it retracts below skin surface.

Intradural perimedullary arteriovenous fistulas

- These are intradural extramedullary lesions supplied by the anterior or posterolateral spinal arteries and draining into perimedullary veins without an intervening nidus, although there is often a varix at the shunt site.
- They are located on the anterior, posterior, or lateral cord pial surfaces, with the typical sites being the upper cervical or thoracolumbar spine or the conus.
- There are associations with other congenital spinal abnormalities such as diastematomyelia, hereditary haemorrhagic telangiectasia, Cobb syndrome, or Klippel–Trenaunay–Weber syndrome.
- Patients typically present in young adulthood with slow progressive myeloradiculopathy. SAH occurs in 20–40%, more commonly in high-flow lesions.

Categorisation

(See Spetzler et al., 2002.)

- Type A: supplied by the anterior spinal artery only with low flow and ascending venous drainage. This is the most common type.
- Type B: supplied by both the anterior and posterolateral spinal arteries, with ascending venous drainage. These are intermediate in size.
- Type C: supplied by dilated anterior and posterolateral spinal arteries, with ectatic segmental veins. These are large, high-flow lesions.

Imaging

- As with other spinal cord vascular lesions, diagnosis may be established with MRI/MRA, time-resolved MRA, CTA, and DSA.
- Type A lesions due to their small size and slow flow may be difficult to diagnose on all modalities.

Management

- Type A: surgical excision may be first line, as the arteries are often too small for superselective endovascular embolisation. This may also be the case for some smaller type B lesions.
- Types B and C: EVT, surgical treatment, or multimodal treatments are possible. EVT may be achieved with n-BCA glue, LE agents, sometimes with adjuvant coils.

Metameric syndromes

- Also known as juvenile AVMs, these are high-flow lesions that consist of both intradural and extradural components (the entire metamere). They can involve the spinal cord, vertebrae, and paraspinal muscles. Neural tissue is usually intermingled with the spinal component of the AVM nidus.
- Patients present in childhood or young adulthood. There is an association with Cobb syndrome (cutaneomeningospinal angiomatosis), a rare congenital disease consisting of spinal cord AVMs and vascular skin lesions (which may or may not be AVMs) within the dermatome corresponding to the spinal lesion.

- Often these are complex lesions with multiple feeders. They may therefore be difficult to fully characterise. All relevant feeding vessels require injection.
- Due to their complexity, treatment is high risk and typically, the goal is symptomatic relief rather than complete cure. This may involve multiple staged embolisation/surgical procedures.

Further reading

Brinjikji W, Lanzino G. Endovascular Treatment of Spinal Arteriovenous Malformations. Handb Clin Neurol. 2017;143:161–174.

Ji T, Guo Y, Shi L, Yu J. Study and therapeutic progress on spinal cord perimedullary arteriovenous fistulas. Biomed Rep. 2017;7(3):214–220.

Spetzler RF, Detwiler PW, Riina HA, Porter RW. Modified classification of spinal cord vascular lesions. J Neurosurg. 2002;96(2 Suppl):145–156.

Vertebro-venous fistula

- These shunts occur between the extracranial vertebral artery and adjacent vertebral veins.
- The most common aetiology is trauma. There are associations with connective tissue disorders, neurofibromatosis, and radiation therapy.
- Patients present due to the consequences of reduced arterial flow distal to the fistula with vertebrobasilar insufficiency and spinal cord ischaemia. With intradural reflux, venous hypertension may result in myelopathy or haemorrhage.
- Treatment may be endovascular or surgical. In the former, transarterial or transvenous approaches are possible:
  - A transvenous approach involves targeted occlusion of the fistula.
  - Transarterial involves occlusion of the vertebral artery. This can only be performed if the contralateral artery can provide sufficient flow. A test occlusion may be necessary.
  - A common approach is to occlude the vein and the artery (Figure 14.4).

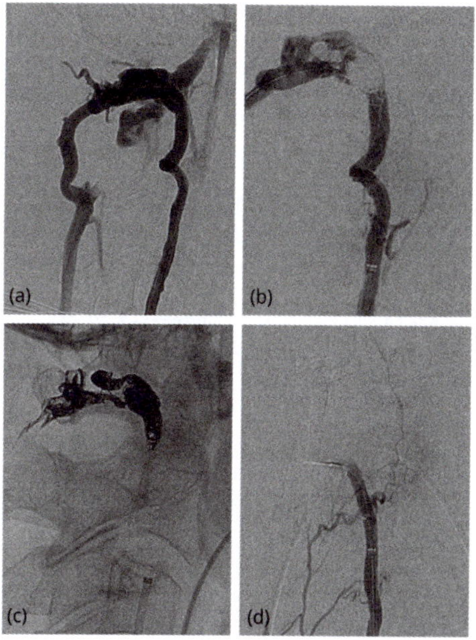

Figure 14.4 Embolisation of a vertebro-venous fistula. (a) Lateral vertebral angiogram demonstrates a fistula involving the suboccipital plexus. (b) A microcatheter has been passed transarterially through the fistula and coils have been detached across from the vein into the artery. (c) Onyx was then injected, detaching the fistula. (d) Final angiography demonstrates occlusion of the vertebral artery and fistula.

Further reading

Aljobeh A, Sorenson TJ, Bortolotti C, Cloft H, Lanzino G. Vertebral arteriovenous fistula: a review article. World Neurosurg. 2019;122:e1388–e1397. [Erratum in: World Neurosurg. 2020 May;137:505.]

Spinal aneurysms

Arteriovenous malformation-associated aneurysms

- For AVM-associated spinal aneurysms, direct intervention should be considered in cases of rupture, mass effect, or if AVM treatment is not feasible.
- Conversely, if complete AVM nidal resection is achieved, associated unruptured AVM aneurysms in difficult locations can often be managed conservatively, as regression is common.

Primary spinal cord aneurysm

(See Figure 14.5.)

- These are very rare, although likely underdiagnosed. They are probably the result of dissection and are associated with atherosclerotic, autoimmune, and connective tissue diseases.

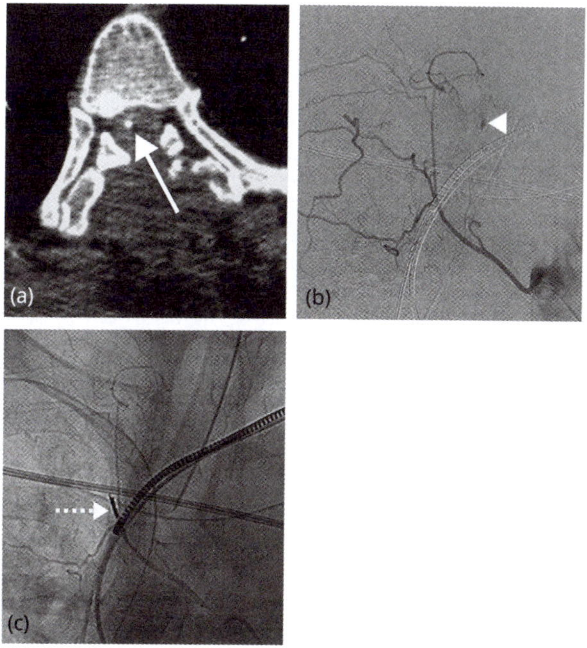

Figure 14.5 Embolisation of a spinal aneurysm. (a) Axial computed tomography angiography demonstrates enhancing focus anterior to the thoracic cord (arrow) in a patient presenting with back pain and paraplegia. (b) Spinal angiography via right T4 injection reveals an aneurysm of the anterior spinal artery (arrowhead). (c) Occlusion of the proximal feeding artery was sufficient to treat the aneurysm (dashed arrow).

- Typical presentation includes sudden onset of back pain, SAH or subdural haemorrhage, and weakness in the legs.
- Spinal CTA or MRA is typically diagnostic, with DSA confirmation.
- They are usually fusiform and located on the radiculomedullary or radiculopial arteries, usually the ascending limb.
- Treatment options include surgical trapping, endovascular embolisation, or conservative. EVT may utilise coil embolisation when the aneurysm has a neck, or it may involve sacrificing the affected branch (this may be achieved proximally). Conservative treatment is also possible, as spontaneous regression can occur. However, risk of rebleeding exists and treatment of symptomatic aneurysms is recommended when safe.

Further reading

Baldassarre B, Balestrino A, D'Andrea A, et al. Management of spinal aneurysms associated with arteriovenous malformations: systematic literature review and illustrative case. Eur Spine J. 2021;30(10):2767–2774.

Renieri L, Raz E, Lanzino G, et al. Spinal artery aneurysms: clinical presentation, radiological findings and outcome. J Neurointerv Surg. 2018;10(7):644–648.

Tumour embolisation

Paraganglioma embolisation *514*
Juvenile nasopharyngeal angiofibroma embolisation *521*
Meningioma embolisation *524*
Haemangioblastoma embolisation *528*
Spinal tumour embolisation *531*

Paraganglioma embolisation

- Paragangliomas in the neck and skull base are rare, typically slow-growing, highly vascular neuroendocrine tumours.
- The carotid body is the most common location, comprising 50–70% of head and neck paragangliomas. Jugular paragangliomas account for 15–25%. Tympanic and vagal paragangliomas are less common, making up 20% and 5%, respectively.
- Peak incidence occurs at the age of 30–50 years, but they are seen in younger ages in familial types.
- Only half demonstrate growth after diagnosis. Mean growth rate of jugulotympanic tumours is 0.4 mm per year; carotid body and vagal tumours grow at 1.6 mm per year. Predictors of growth are genetic status, age at presentation, and tumour origin (vagale > carotid body > jugular or tympanic).
- Although typically benign, 4–10% of paragangliomas have malignant potential. Vagal paragangliomas have the highest risk, with potential dissemination to lymph nodes, lung, liver, bone, and skin.
- 10–20% of sporadic and 80% of familial paragangliomas are multicentric.
- Genetic testing is necessary. Inheritance for linked genes is autosomal dominant with varying penetrance. Associated clinical syndromes include von Hippel–Lindau, multiple endocrine neoplasia types 2A and 2B, phaeochromocytomas, neurofibromatosis type 1, and Carney–Stratakis syndrome (paragangliomas + gastric stromal sarcoma).
- Carotid body tumours and jugular paragangliomas require complex surgical resections due to their high vascularity and the vicinity of CNs. These procedures carry the risk of CN damage, lengthy surgery, and significant blood loss.
- Stereotactic radiotherapy may be reserved for recurrent or unresectable tumours but is increasingly employed as primary therapy, particularly for jugular paragangliomas.
- Preoperative embolisation may be used to reduce intraoperative blood loss, surgical time, morbidity, and mortality. Embolisation of carotid body and jugular paragangliomas to reduce tumour vascularity is often performed for larger, more vascular tumours, although there is a lack of level I evidence for the technique and meta-analyses reveal mixed results.

Presentation

Carotid body paragangliomas

- Carotid body paragangliomas (or carotid body tumours or chemodectomas) arise from the paraganglion cells of the carotid body and present as painless, pulsatile, slowly enlarging neck masses, sometimes with CN palsies.
- Located at the carotid bifurcation on the anterior border of the sternocleidomastoid, they are movable from side to side but have limited vertical movement due to their attachment to the carotid artery. They characteristically splay the ECA anteriorly and ICA and jugular vein posteriorly.

Jugular paragangliomas

- Jugular paragangliomas (or glomus jugulare) are the commonest tumour of the jugular foramen. They arise from paraganglia along Jacobson's nerve (the tympanic branch of the glossopharyngeal nerve), or from Arnold's nerve (the mastoid branch of the vagus nerve).
- They present with pulsatile tinnitus, hearing loss, hoarseness, aural pain, and CN palsy. Otoscopy may reveal a reddish bulge behind an intact ear drum.

Vagal paragangliomas

- Vagal paragangliomas (or glomus vagale) present as a pulsatile neck mass, predominantly posterior to the angle of the mandible. They typically arise from the nodose ganglion (inferior vagal nerve), but can arise anywhere along the vagus nerve.
- Symptoms include hoarseness, dysphagia, and dysphonia. They displace the carotid artery anteriorly and jugular vein posteriorly but do not widen the carotid bifurcation.

Tympanic paragangliomas

- Tympanic paragangliomas (or glomus tympanicum) are located at the cochlear promontory and constitute the most common middle ear tumour.
- They present with pulsatile tinnitus and conductive hearing loss. A vascular tympanic membrane is seen on otoscopy. The tumour arises from the inferior tympanic nerve in the inferior tympanic canaliculus and is supplied by the inferior tympanic artery. Embolisation is not generally performed on these tumours.

Imaging

- Imaging is important to identify the site and tumour extent, potential invasion of the ICA, and involvement of venous sinuses.
- Workup includes MRI of the head and neck, CT of the skull base, and imaging of the thorax, abdomen, and pelvis (using MR or gallium positron emission tomography).
- MRI: paragangliomas are iso- to hypointense on T1-weighted imaging and hyperintense on T2-weighted imaging. They demonstrate a 'salt and pepper' appearance with punctate foci of haemorrhage or slow flow ('salt') and flow voids ('pepper'). There is avid contrast enhancement.
- CT: jugular paragangliomas are associated with 'moth-eaten' permeative bone destruction at the margins of the jugular foramen, differentiating them from schwannomas. Jugular paragangliomas may extend superiorly to the hypotympanum and mesotympanum, inferiorly to invade the jugular vein, laterally to the facial nerve canal, and medially to the cerebellopontine angle. Intracranial extension occurs in 15–20% (NB: vascular metastases e.g. renal cell, can appear identical).
- DSA (Figure 15.1): enlarged feeding arteries, an intense tumour blush, and early draining veins.

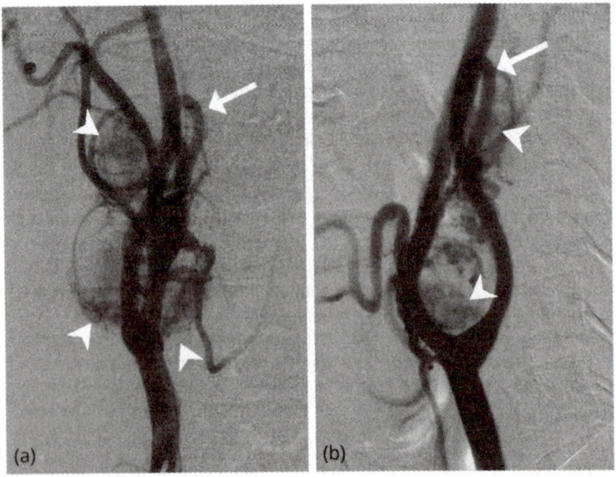

Figure 15.1 Carotid body tumour. (a) Digital subtraction angiography of the right common carotid artery with anteroposterior and (b) lateral views shows tumour blush (arrowheads) largely supplied by hypertrophied ascending pharyngeal artery (arrows). Images courtesy of Dr Neeraj Chaudhary.

Blood supply

- Carotid body tumours: arterial supply is from 1–2 mm of the carotid body (or glomic) artery, arising from the CCA in 75–85%, ECA in 8–10%, ICA in 4–7%, and ascending pharyngeal artery (APA) in 2–7%. The APA is almost always the major contributing artery. In addition, the facial, lingual, superior and inferior laryngeal, ascending cervical, and superior thyroid arteries are commonly involved.
- Jugular paragangliomas: arterial supply is predominantly from the APA via the inferior tympanic and jugular branches. These have dangerous anastomoses with the ICA and supply CNs VI, IX, X, and XI. There may be a contribution from the stylomastoid artery (which supplies the facial nerve). Additional supply may arise from the anterior tympanic branch of the IMA, superior tympanic artery from the petrous branch of the MMA, and the accessory meningeal artery (which can also supply the facial nerve and anastomoses with the ICA). In addition, there may be contributions from dural branches of the ICA (caroticotympanic) and from cerebellar arteries. These are considered too risky to embolise here.
- Vagal paragangliomas: arterial supply is from the musculospinal branch of the APA and muscular branches of the occipital artery. With extension to the skull base, there will be additional supply from the neuromeningeal trunk of the APA.

Preprocedural workup

- Pharmacological management of hypersecretion of catecholamines (in 4–10%) both prior to embolisation and before surgery is crucial to

prevent intraprocedural fluctuations of BP and acute hypertensive crisis. Beware also of the possibility of associated silent phaeochromocytomas.
- Embolisation is best performed 24–72 h prior to surgery as this achieves maximal thrombosis while minimising arterial re-canalisation from collateral feeding arteries.
- Endovascular or direct percutaneous approaches can be utilised for paraganglioma embolisation.

Pre-embolisation angiography assessment

- Angiography is performed on the ipsilateral ICA, ECA, vertebral, subclavian, costocervical, and thyrocervical arteries centred on the tumour location. Identify feeding arteries, assess tumour blush, and document baseline cerebral vascular anatomy. Assess for dangerous extracranial/intracranial anastomoses. These are always present but may be angiographically occult initially, only opening up as embolisation proceeds.
- Specific attention should be paid to the APA connections with the ipsilateral ICA via the tympanic arterial arcade and the inferolateral trunk branches and ipsilateral and contralateral connections of the APA with the vertebral artery via the odontoid arcade.
- If dangerous anastomoses are visible, these can be occluded first with microcoils.

Technique: transarterial

(See Figure 15.2.)

- Either LA or GA can be utilised, depending on the patient's ability to tolerate, and the complexity, of the procedure.
- Systemic heparinisation is achieved.
- Angiography is performed on all vessels thought to supply the tumour.
- A guide catheter is placed in the ECA and angiography performed.
- A microcatheter is advanced into the target artery under roadmap guidance. It is advisable to go as distal as possible, avoiding vessel injury or spasm in the branch vessel precluding distal access. Microcatheter angiography is performed to identify dangerous anastomoses.
- Particle embolisation is usually straightforward and relatively low risk. Embolisation of the arterial supply to CNs can be avoided by using particle sizes *at least* >100 μm (vasa nervorum are around 60–80 μm). A safe bet is size 250–350 μm. If significant venous shunting is present, then particle size can be increased to 300–500 μm. Inject the particulate mixture (particles dissolved in suspended in 50–70% iohexol solution) under subtracted fluoroscopy (blank roadmap) in gentle pulses, with free flow and without a wedged microcatheter position. The suspension is regularly agitated to avoid clumping and injected using 1 mL syringes which must be readily identified and not confused with syringes containing saline or contrast (use different colour syringes or apply stickers).
- Selective microcatheter angiography (following careful, gentle saline flushing of the microcatheter first to purge any particles) can be performed to assess not only the progression of the embolisation but to ensure that dangerous anastomoses are not opening up. Guide catheter angiography with an indwelling microcatheter may not show the true extent of embolisation.

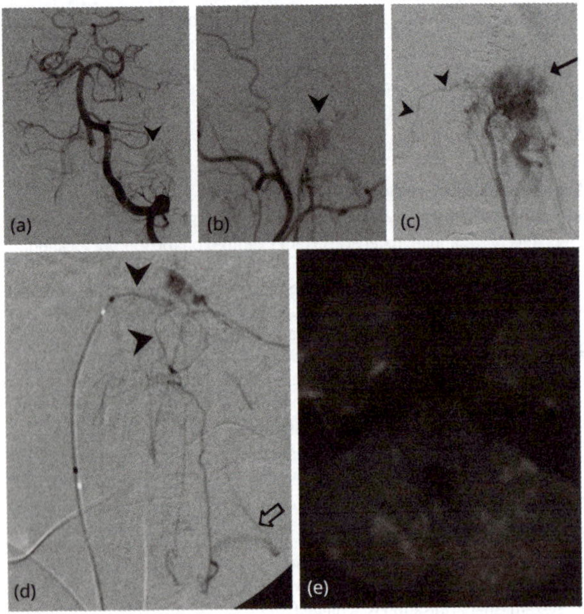

Figure 15.2 Presurgical embolisation of jugular paraganglioma tumour. (a) Tumour blush (arrowhead) is seen on anteroposterior (AP) view of left vertebral artery injection and (b) lateral view of the left external carotid artery injection. (c) Selective injection of the left ascending pharyngeal artery in AP view shows tumour blush (arrow) and collateralisation to the C1 arch (arrowheads). (d) Superselective microangiography of the left ascending pharyngeal artery neuromeningeal trunk branch lateral view shows collateralisation of the C1 arch (arrowheads) to the contralateral vertebral artery (open arrows). (e) If this connection is overlooked, it can lead to non-target embolisation as seen on post-embolisation diffusion-weighted magnetic resonance imaging sequence. Images courtesy of Dr Neeraj Chaudhary.

- Embolisation should cease when forward blood flow significantly decreases but before it stops altogether, to avoid reflux.
- The artery can then be occluded with detachable coils.

Technique: direct puncture

- GA is preferred to avoid pain during the injection of LEs.
- The patient's head is immobilised in an anatomically neutral position and the site of needle entry is draped in a sterile fashion.
- A guide catheter is placed in the ECA for intermittent angiographic visualisation of the tumour supply during embolisation.
- A balloon microcatheter may be positioned in the proximal ICA in carotid body tumours. This can be inflated during injection of LEs to avoid retrograde injection through small feeders into the ICA lumen. Maximum

balloon inflation time should be 3 min. The Hyperform or Hyperglide balloon microcatheter is preferred by the authors, positioned just distal to the carotid bulb, covering the tumour extent and a little more distal. IV heparinisation is necessary.

- An 18–20 G spinal needle is inserted into the centre of the tumour under biplanar fluoroscopic guidance utilising an arterial roadmap. Cone beam CT may also facilitate accurate positioning of the needle. If the needle is correctly sited removal of the stylet usually reveals continuous blood reflux. The hub of the spinal needle is then attached to a 20 cm DMSO-compatible Luer lock extension tube.
- Angiography may be performed via the needle to confirm tumour penetration.
- The dead space of the extension tubing and needle is flushed with DMSO. Ensure no air bubbles are injected.
- LE is injected under fluoroscopic guidance using the biplanar subtracted blank (glue) roadmap at a rate of 0.1–0.2 mL/min. Controlled injection may be aided by utilising the 'tap' technique—making small taps with the operator's thumb at the end of the syringe. If an unwanted vein or artery is entered, stop the injection and wait 20–30 s before reinjecting.
- Gradual penetration of the embolic agent is visualised with intermittent negative roadmaps. The duration of injection typically ranges from 10 to 90 min.
- Control angiography is obtained at the end of embolisation to assess the degree of embolisation and to decide whether further punctures are needed to complete the job.

Tips

- Tumour penetration and devascularisation is greater with LEs; however, CN injury is also more likely.
- Infiltration of LE beyond the tumour margins obscures the surgical boundaries and poses a risk of sparks generated by bipolar cautery during surgery and should be avoided.
- Higher-viscosity LEs reduce the risk of migration outside the tumour in those with rapid venous shunting. Choice of viscosity is based on the size of the feeder vessel being embolised and extent of penetration needed.
- Balloon microcatheters (e.g. the Scepter Mini) can be used for transarterial LE injection, but caution is required regarding non-target embolisation, as LEs, injected in an occluded flow situation, increase distal/anastomotic penetration.
- Direct percutaneous embolisation with LE may improve penetration of the tumour vascular bed compared to transarterial particulate embolisation.

Complication avoidance and management

- Beware of anastomosis and non-target embolisation (Figure 15.2).
- Postprocedural fever and pain is not uncommon but generally self-limiting.
- Stroke or CN palsy may rarely occur and require urgent management, often involving a MDT.
- Tumour swelling can occur due to necrosis post-embolisation. This is typically managed conservatively, with steroids in severe cases.

- Iatrogenic ICA injury during surgery leading to sacrifice of the vessel is a dreaded complication and should be anticipated. A BTO preoperatively in an awake patient can be undertaken if this considered a possibility.

Further reading

Gad A, Sayed A, Elwan H, et al. Carotid body tumours: a review of 25 years experience in diagnosis and management of 56 tumours. Ann Vasc Dis. 2014;7(3):292–299.

Texakalidis P, Charisis N, Giannopoulos S, et al. Role of preoperative embolisation in carotid body tumour surgery: a systematic review and meta-analysis. World Neurosurg. 2019;129:503–513.e2.

Juvenile nasopharyngeal angiofibroma embolisation

- Juvenile nasopharyngeal angiofibroma (JNA) is a rare, locally aggressive vascular tumour primarily affecting adolescent males but occasionally seen in older patients and pregnant women.
- It typically presents with unilateral nasal obstruction, epistaxis, and facial swelling.
- The tumour originates in the nasopharynx/posterior nasal cavity, adjacent to the sphenopalatine foramen and can expand to involve the paranasal sinuses, pterygopalatine fossa, infratemporal fossa, orbit, sella, and middle cranial fossa. It is a non-encapsulated, well-circumscribed polypoid mass composed of vascular and fibrous tissue. The tumour vessels are lined by a single layer of endothelial cells and lack a complete muscular layer and are therefore prone to haemorrhage.
- The rich vascular supply can cause massive, life-threatening haemorrhage during surgical removal. Preoperative embolisation is undertaken to reduce intraoperative blood loss and improve the surgical resection.

Investigation

- MRI allows assessment of the extent of orbital and intracranial tumour extension, demonstrating a mass centred on the sphenopalatine foramen returning intermediate T1-weighted imaging signal and heterogeneous T2-weighted imaging signal with vascular flow voids and avid gadolinium enhancement.
- CT reveals an enhancing mass centred on a widened sphenopalatine foramen which may bow/remodel bony adjacent structures, e.g. the posterior wall of the maxillary antrum.
- DSA defines the tumour blood supply and guides embolisation.

Blood supply

- Supply is usually from branches of the sphenopalatine artery and other distal IMA feeders, usually the middle meningeal, accessory meningeal, posterior deep temporal, and ascending pharyngeal arteries.
- With growth, it recruits from the facial artery, ascending palatine and ethmoidal branches of the ophthalmic artery, and dural branches of the ICA (mandibulovidian, pterygovaginal, inferolateral trunk, and meningohypophyseal trunk). Often supply is bilateral even if the tumour is well lateralised.

Technique

(See Figure 15.3.)

- Transarterial or direct puncture techniques are possible. Beware of dangerous anastomoses and CN supply.
- The transarterial technique is identical to that of paragangliomas (see 'Paraganglioma embolisation', p. 514). Particle sizes 250–350 μm are commonly used.
- Direct tumour puncture may be performed under GA via a transzygomatic, transnasal, transoral, or transbuccal approach. An 18–20 G DMSO-compatible needle is placed into the tumour under

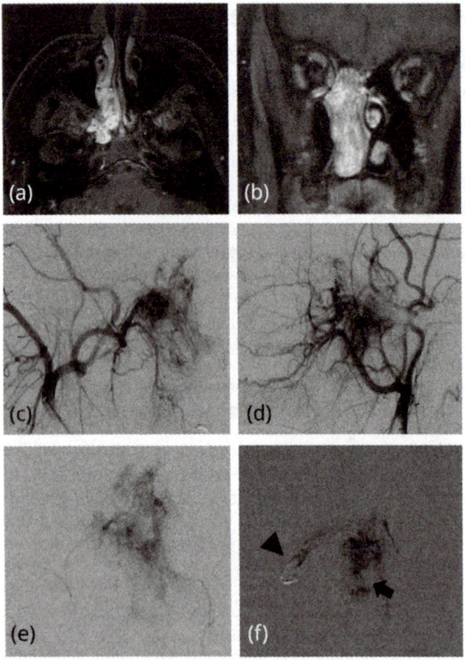

Figure 15.3 Juvenile nasopharyngeal embolisation. (a) A young man presented with 5-month history of nasal stuffiness and epistaxis. Post-contrast fat saturation axial and (b) coronal magnetic resonance images show a large hypervascular mass in the posterior right nasal cavity and nasopharynx extending into the sphenoid sinus. (c) Frontal and (d) lateral right external carotid artery (ECA) angiogram shows a hypervascular mass within the posterior right nasal cavity and nasopharynx extending into the sphenoid sinus with arterial supply from the sphenopalatine, accessory meningeal, and middle meningeal arteries. (e) Frontal right sphenopalatine artery angiogram shows filling of the hypervascular mass. (f) Spot frontal fluoroscopic image shows a balloon (arrowhead) in the sphenopalatine artery with ethylene vinyl alcohol (EVOH) in the tumour (thick black arrow). (g) Spot lateral fluoroscopic image shows a balloon in the accessory meningeal artery (arrowhead) after injection of EVOH into the tumour (thick arrow). (h) Frontal and (i) lateral right ECA angiogram after embolisation shows no filling of the hypervascular mass. Images courtesy of Dr Joseph Gemmete.

cone beam CT or fluoroscopic guidance. Contrast is injected through the needle to confirm its intratumoural placement. The hub of the spinal needle is then attached to a 20 cm DMSO-compatible Luer lock extension tube. Onyx or glue is then injected under negative roadmap guidance.

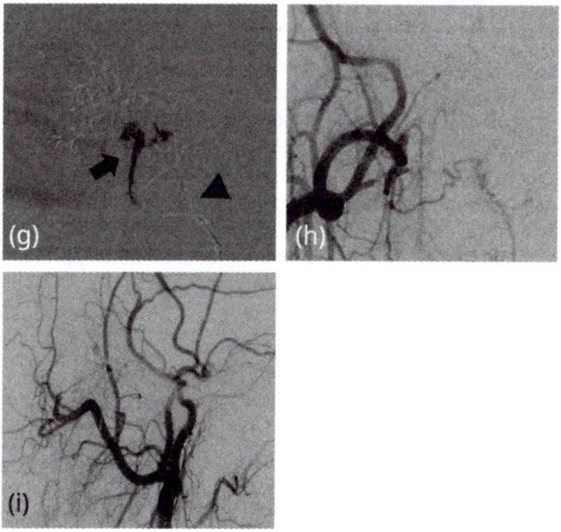

Figure 15.3 Continued

Tips

- To prevent non-target embolisation of the ICA or vertebral artery branches, coil or balloon occlusion can be utilised.

Postprocedural care

- The optimal time for surgical resection is 24–72 h following embolisation, allowing the maximum effect of tumour devascularisation while minimising the risk of collateral vessel formation.

Complication avoidance and management

- Postprocedural fever and pain can be managed with analgesics and antipyretics.
- Visual loss, stroke, or CN palsy, although rare, are serious complications and require urgent management, often involving a MDT.
- Tumour swelling can occur due to necrosis post-embolisation. This is typically managed conservatively, with steroids in severe cases.

Further reading

Kothari DS, Linker LA, Tham T, Maroda AJ, McElfresh JM, Fastenberg JH, Hachem RA, Elijovich L, Michael LM, Rangarajan SV. Preoperative embolization techniques in the treatment of juvenile nasopharyngeal angiofibroma: a systematic review. Otolaryngol Head Neck Surg. 2023;169(3):454–466.

Meningioma embolisation

- Meningiomas are vascular, typically slow-growing, tumours originating from arachnoidal meningothelial cap cells.
- Clinical presentation varies widely, often related to their size and location. Symptoms include headaches, seizures, or neurological deficits. They may be found incidentally in asymptomatic patients.
- Meningioma embolisation is performed to reduce tumour vascularity prior to surgical resection, making the surgery safer and easier. This is particularly important for large or highly vascular tumours, and those located in challenging anatomical locations.
- There is level III evidence only for efficacy.

Indications

- The decision to perform embolisation is based on risk:benefit analysis.

Contraindications

- Predominantly pial blood supply is a relative contraindication.
- Other general complications of angiography and embolisation, such as uncorrectable coagulopathy and renal dysfunction without the expectation of dialysis.

Imaging

- CT and MRI define tumour location, size, extent, and relation to nearby structures.
- These durally based, extra-axial, avidly and usually homogeneously enhancing masses are generally well circumscribed. They may contain cysts/areas of necrosis and can be lipomatous. 60% generate parenchymal oedema.
- CT: most are hyperdense on CT, less often isodense, and occasionally hypodense. Adjacent bone may be sclerotic and/or associated with cortical erosion. Intrinsic calcification is common.
- MRI: they are usually iso- or slightly hypointense on T1-weighted imaging and show variable T2 signal. 80% show vascular flow voids.
- DSA: arterial supply depends on location. A sunburst or radial blush appearing early with a prolonged vascular tumoural stain is characteristic. The venous phase is vital to assess possible sinus involvement and the consequences of venous redirected collateral flow, which can be important surgically.

Blood supply

- Most of the blood supply is derived from the dural vasculature, mainly the MMA. Occasionally, the blood supply may be pial, or choroidal (for intraventricular meningiomas).
- Convexity meningiomas: ipsilateral MMA ± contralateral MMA if close to midline. If there is erosion through the skull vault, there may be an additional supply from scalp arteries. Depending on location, additional supply may be from the superficial temporal, posterior auricular, and occipital arteries.

- Falcine meningiomas: artery of the falx cerebri from the anterior ethmoidal branch of the ophthalmic artery ± dural supply from pericallosal and/or callosomarginal arteries.
- Skull base meningiomas: olfactory groove and planum meningiomas receive a supply from ethmoidal branches of the ophthalmic artery.
- Cavernous sinus/parasellar meningiomas: cavernous ICA (inferolateral trunk, meningohypophyseal trunk), AMA, cavernous MMA, and recurrent meningeal branch of the ophthalmic artery.
- Middle cranial fossa/greater sphenoid wing meningiomas: sphenoidal branch of the MMA.
- Tentorial and posterior fossa meningiomas: marginal artery of the MHT, lateral clival branches of cavernous ICA, tentorial branches of the MMA, posterior meningeal and posterior falcine arteries. The latter may arise from the vertebral artery, PICA, or occipital arteries.
- Petroclival/cerebellopontine angle meningiomas: clival branches of the ICA, petrosal MMA, and the neuromeningeal trunk of the APA and AICA.
- Cerebellar convexity tumours: posterior meningeal artery, artery of the falx cerebelli and additionally, cerebellar arteries.

Technique

(See Figure 15.4.)

- The transarterial technique is similar to that of paragangliomas.
- Transfemoral or transradial access is gained and systemic heparinisation is achieved.
- Angiography of the relevant vessels (which might include ICA, ECA, and vertebral injections) is performed evaluating the feasibility of embolisation:
  - Embolisation may not be recommended if the tumour's blood supply is predominantly pial, given the potential for ischaemic complications.
  - Embolisation of deeply located skull base meningiomas with surgically poorly accessible feeders may be useful prior to surgical resection but carries significant risk because the feeders are often small dural vessels arising from the ICA or ophthalmic arteries, which have dangerous anastomoses and supply CNs. Subtotal embolisation of these might not usefully reduce blood loss and aggressive embolisation risks serious complications. Additionally, there is little point in embolising readily surgically accessible dural supply as is often the case with convexity meningiomas. Therefore, preoperative embolisation generally depends on a close dialogue with the referring team.
- A guide catheter is placed in the relevant artery. An intermediate catheter can also be utilised.
- Particles (polyvinyl alcohol (PVA) or spherical embolics such as tris-acryl gelatin microspheres), n-BCA glue, and EVOH (Onyx or Squid) can all be utilised. The selection of agent typically depends on the size, type, and location of the feeding vessel, as well as the vascularity of the tumour and operator preference. The choice of microcatheter depends on the agent used.
- At least 80% devascularisation by embolisation is necessary to make a difference.

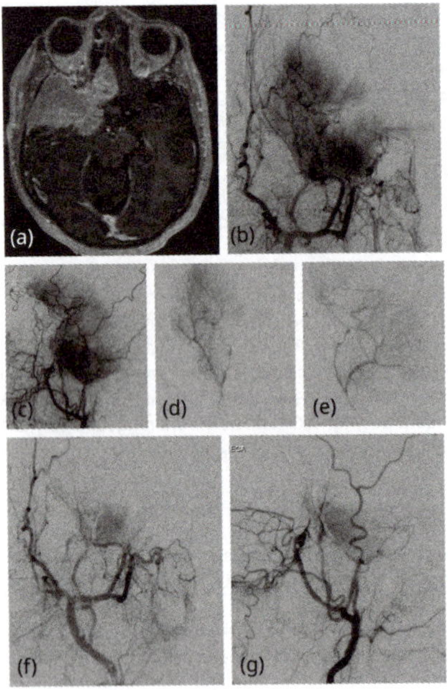

Figure 15.4 Embolisation of a sphenoid wing meningioma. (a) Axial contrast-enhanced magnetic resonance T1-weighted images axial show a large extra-axial mass arising from the dura of the sphenoid extending into the right temporal lobe, surrounding the right internal carotid artery, extending along the superior portion of the right orbit and cribriform plate. (b) Frontal and lateral (c) right external carotid artery (ECA) injection shows a hypervascular mass. (d) Frontal and (e) lateral right middle meningeal artery (MMA) angiogram shows filling of a portion of the hypervascular mass. (f) Frontal and lateral (g) right ECA angiogram after embolisation of the MMA and accessory meningeal artery with particles and coils shows reduced filling. Some vessels were not embolised due to their small calibre and risk of non-target embolisation to cranial nerves and the intracranial circulation. Images courtesy of Dr Joseph Gemmete.

Postprocedural care

- Consider steroids to reduce tumour-related swelling post embolisation.
- The optimal time for surgical resection after embolisation is generally within 48–96 h, allowing for maximal tumour devascularisation while minimising the risk of intraoperative bleeding and development of inflammation around the tumour or collateral arterial feeders.
- Gadolinium-enhanced MRI may provide good evaluation of the efficacy of the embolisation but is not routine.

Tips

- Use of a balloon catheter in the ICA or vertebral artery can help prevent reflux of the embolic material, thus reducing non-target embolisation and potential complications.

Complication avoidance and management

- Overall complication rates of preoperative embolisation range from 0% to 20% and include tumour haemorrhage, stroke, and CN palsy.
- Post-embolisation syndrome, characterised by fever and pain, can be managed with analgesics and anti-inflammatory medications.
- Neurological complications (stroke or CN palsy) are rare but if present require immediate evaluation and treatment. The risk is minimised with good angiographic technique and by preventing reflux into undesirable arterial territories. CN injury can be prevented by understanding their arterial supply and using larger particles to prevent devascularisation of the vasa nervorum.
- Haemorrhage and tumour swelling can occur and may necessitate additional surgical intervention or steroid administration.

Further reading

Friconnet G, Espíndola Ala VH, Lemnos L, et al. Pre-surgical embolisation of intracranial meningioma with Onyx: a safety and efficacy study. J Neuroradiol. 2020;47(5):353–357.

Jumah F, AbuRmilah A, Raju B, et al. Does preoperative embolisation improve outcomes of meningioma resection? A systematic review and meta-analysis. Neurosurg Rev. 2021;44(6):3151–3163.

Haemangioblastoma embolisation

- Haemangioblastomas are highly vascular WHO grade 1 tumours that occur typically in the cerebellum, brainstem, and spinal cord.
- They arise sporadically or in association with von Hippel–Lindau disease, the latter being more aggressive and prone to recurrence.
- The tumours are composed primarily of stromal and endothelial cells with reactive angiogenesis, leading to abundant and dilated blood vessels.
- Embolisation may be performed to reduce intraoperative blood loss and improve tumour resection. As the tumours are supplied by pial blood vessels, the risks are likely higher than those of dural blood supply. The risks need to be carefully weighed against the potential benefits.
- Defining the goals of embolisation requires discussion between the neurointerventional and neurosurgical teams.

Indications for embolisation

- Large cerebellar hemangioblastomas with significant solid tumour burden and deep arterial supply to minimise intraoperative blood loss, promote gross total resection, and soften the tumour for easier microdissection.

Contraindications

- Presence of significant en passage arterial supply or high risk of non-target embolisation.
- Risk of venous occlusion leading to haemorrhage, especially in tumours with early venous drainage similar to AVMs.

Investigation

- CT: reveals mass effect and potential hydrocephalus due to obstruction.
- CTA: recommended for mapping arterial supply.
- MRI: reveals a heterogeneously enhancing mass with solid and cystic components, and prominent flow voids indicating high vascularity.
- DSA: essential for defining the tumour's blood supply and planning embolisation. Typically shows a highly vascular lesion with rapid shunting and early venous drainage.

Blood supply

- Common feeders: SCA, PCA, and AICA. Occipital artery in rare cases. Feeding pedicles from the SCA are most commonly embolised.
- Pattern of supply: tumours often have a bilateral blood supply and multiple feeding arteries.

Technique

(See Figure 15.5.)

- A 5 or 6 Fr sheath is placed in the common femoral artery.
- Systemic heparinisation is achieved.
- Angiography is performed on all relevant vessels.
- A guide catheter is positioned in the relevant parent artery, typically the vertebral artery.

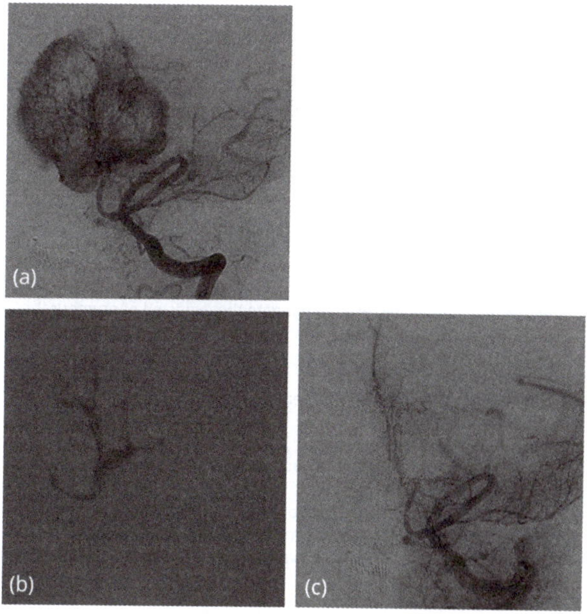

Figure 15.5 Haemangioblastoma embolisation. (a) Left vertebral artery injection demonstrates a large hypervascular posterior fossa tumour. (b) Injection of n-BCA glue via a posterior inferior cerebellar artery feeding vessel. (c) After embolisation the tumour is fully devascularised. Images courtesy of Dr Leve Joseph Sebastian.

- A microcatheter is then inserted and positioned as distal as possible inside the supplying artery. Choice of catheter depends on the embolic agent and the size of feeding artery.
- Microangiography is performed to confirm that only the tumour is supplied at this point.
- A blank 'glue' roadmap is instituted and the agent injected.
- Embolic agents include:
    - Co-polymer LE: preferred for its controlled forward flow and visibility during injection. It is often possible to embolise much of the tumour via one pedicle.
    - Glue: also commonly used. Multiple pedicles typically are injected.
    - PVA particles: used less frequently due to risk of shunting into venous drainage, potentially causing venous hypertension and haemorrhage.
    - Coils: used for parent artery sacrifice when suitable.
- During injection, watch carefully for reflux and stop injecting if it is too much.
- Angiography is repeated during embolisation to assess residual vascularisation.

- The goal is to reduce blood supply via parent artery sacrifice and tumour penetration. Significant reflux of embolic material must be avoided. It is also important to avoid occlusion of venous drainage to prevent tumour haemorrhage.
- To prevent non-target embolisation, the use of coils or balloon occlusion may be used.

Post-procedure

- The optimal timing for preoperative embolisation followed by surgery remains to be definitively established. 24–48 h is often chosen. Some studies suggest that when surgery is performed >72 h after embolisation, there is a tendency towards greater intraoperative blood loss.
- Steroids may be administered to mitigate the expected peritumoural oedema resulting from embolisation.

Complication avoidance and management

- Ischaemic stroke from non-target embolisation.
- Tumour haemorrhage from venous occlusion or excessive tumour penetration of embolic material.
- Postprocedural fever and pain: managed with analgesics and antipyretics.
- Neurological deficits due to CN involvement: often transient and managed conservatively. Steroids may be given.
- Tumour swelling due to necrosis: typically managed conservatively, with steroids if severe.

Outcomes

- A range of different outcomes exist in the literature with controversy as to whether routine preoperative embolisation is worth the risk.
- Complication rates vary from 0% to 20%. A systemic review in 2016 found a complication rate of 12%.
- A 2013 retrospective series of 46 embolised and 79 non-embolised cases found a lower rate of blood loss and transfusion in embolised patients, with no differences in complications.
- A systemic review in 2016, however, did not demonstrate reduced rates of operative complications or blood loss, or increased likelihood of total resection.

Further reading

Ampie L, Choy W, Lamano JB, et al. Safety and outcomes of preoperative embolisation of intracranial hemangioblastomas: a systematic review. Clin Neurol Neurosurg. 2016;150:143–151.

Spinal tumour embolisation

- Surgical intervention for spinal tumours typically involves decompressing the spinal cord, conducting radical tumour excision, and stabilising the spinal column using instrumentation.
- In cases involving highly vascular tumours, surgery can be challenging due to intraoperative bleeding. This not only restricts the extent of tumour resection but also elevates surgical risks, potentially leading to the discontinuation of surgery and suboptimal surgical outcomes.
- Preoperative embolisation is utilised for hypervascular spinal tumours to reduce surgical morbidity by minimising blood loss and reducing the need for blood transfusion. The goals are to shorten operative duration, control surgically inaccessible arterial feeders, enhance visualisation of the surgical field to reduce the risk of surgical complications, and improve the likelihood of complete surgical resection. Shorter hospital stay is also a potential benefit.
- Hypervascular spinal metastases most commonly include renal cell, neuroendocrine, and thyroid tumours.
- Primary hypervascular spinal tumours, such as haemangioblastomas, aneurysmal bone cyst, and osteoblastoma, may also be managed with preoperative embolisation.
- Embolisation can be performed transarterially or via direct puncture.

Indications

- Specific indications for preoperative endovascular embolisation of spinal tumours differ across medical centres and may encompass histological characteristics of the tumour and their hypervascularity.

Contraindications

- Radiculomedullary artery located close to the tumour-feeding artery.
- Other general complications of angiography and embolisation, such as uncorrectable coagulopathy and renal dysfunction without the expectation of dialysis.

Investigation

- MRI (Figure 15.6a): characterises bone lesions and demonstrates the lesion's extent, affected sites, and any medullary involvement.
- CT: precisely delineates anatomy and enables the detection of bone alterations, cortical reactions, and tumour calcification (these might be challenging to discern on MRI).
- Contrast-enhanced spinal CTA: aids in vascular mapping by providing information about tumour-feeding arteries.

Technique

(See Figure 15.6.)

- A 5 or 6 Fr sheath is placed in the common femoral artery.
- Systemic heparinisation is achieved.
- Spinal angiography is performed to delineate the extent of tumour vascularity, arterial supply routes, venous drainage patterns, and the identification of normal vasculature that should be preserved (radiculomedullary and radiculopial arteries—in particular, Adamkiewicz). Cone beam CT with 15% contrast can also help to identify such vessels.

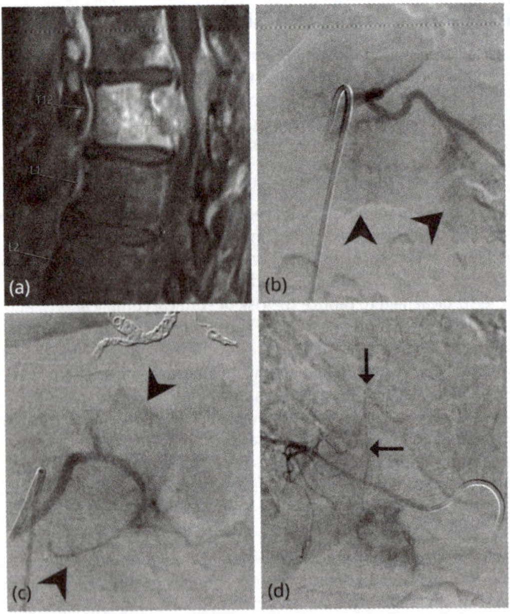

Figure 15.6 Spinal tumour embolisation. (a) Post-contrast sagittal magnetic resonance image of the thoracolumbar spine reveals invasion into the spinal column with epidural spread of locally aggressive renal carcinoma metastasis. (b) Tumour blush (arrowheads) is seen on selective angiography of the left T12 and left L1 (c) segmental arteries. These were sequentially embolised with particles and coils. (d) Selective angiography of the right T10 segmental artery reveals the classic hairpin-turn of the anterior spinal artery (arrows). This level therefore could not be embolised. Images courtesy of Dr Neeraj Chaudhary.

- Spinal angiography is performed at the levels likely to supply the tumour. Once the feeding artery is found, it is recommended to selectively catheterise at least two levels above and below to ensure a thorough evaluation of the tumour's vascular supply and identify branches that supply the spinal cord. Radiculomedullary arteries arising from spinal arteries supplying the tumour generally contraindicate spinal embolisation.
  - In cervical and upper thoracic tumours, inject the following arteries: vertebral, ECA, thyrocervical, and supreme intercostal arteries. Close attention should be paid to the presence of the artery of cervical enlargement (artery of Lazorthes). This typically arises from the cervical vertebral artery, but may arise from the deep cervical or supreme intercostal vessels.
  - In the lumbosacral region both iliac arteries, and the median sacral artery should be injected.

- The tumour-supplying segmental level is located and catheterised. A 4 or 5 Fr diagnostic catheter (depending on the size of the branch), such as a Cobra, Mikaelson, or Simmons 1 or 2, is typically sufficient for embolisation. If a more stable platform is needed, the catheter can be exchanged for a guide catheter over an exchange-length wire. 5 or 6 Fr guide catheters can sometimes be accommodated.
- Prior to embolisation, the segmental artery distal to the spinal branch may be occluded using detachable coils, helping to direct particles into the tumour mass, minimising unnecessary distal embolisation, and reducing postprocedural pain caused by muscle ischaemia.
- A microcatheter is then inserted and positioned as distal as possible in the branch supplying the tumour. The exact microcatheter depends on whether particles (larger) or glue/LEs (smaller) are used.
- Various embolic materials have been employed for spinal tumour embolisation, including gelatin sponge, PVA particles, coils, EVOH, and combinations thereof. The choice of embolic agent significantly relies on the neurointerventionalist's experience, preferences, and tumour vascular characteristics.
- A blank 'glue' roadmap is instituted and the agent injected.
- During injection, watch carefully for reflux and stop injecting if it is identified.
- Angiography is repeated during embolisation to assess how much tumour remains vascularised, and to look for radiculomedullary or radiculopial branches that initially were obscured due to preferential flow into the tumour.
- Once the tumour is adequately embolised, coils are deployed to occlude the segmental artery proximally to eliminate the anterograde pressure head in the feeding pedicle and reduce recanalisation prior to surgery (providing that no spinal supply is seen). They may also facilitate surgical level identification.

Tips

- In cases of moderately or hypervascularised tumours, particle embolisation is usually the choice of embolic agent.
- Typically, moderate-sized particles (150–300 μm) are preferred to mitigate the risk of transvenous material leakage and potential pulmonary embolism or over-embolisation.
- If embolisation poses an exceptionally high risk to the patient, the procedure should be abandoned.

Postprocedural care

- The optimal timing for preoperative embolisation followed by surgery remains to be definitively established. 24–48 h is often chosen due to concerns regarding the risks of rapid revascularisation and the potential for increased cord compression due to post-embolisation swelling or haemorrhage in patients with myelopathy. Some studies suggest that when surgery is performed >72 h after embolisation, there is a tendency towards greater intraoperative blood loss.
- Steroids may be administered to mitigate the expected peritumoural oedema resulting from embolisation.

Complication avoidance and management

- Preoperative embolisation of spinal tumours is generally regarded as a safe procedure. Major complications, including death, permanent neurological injury, arterial injury, and ischaemia of surrounding normal tissues, are exceedingly rare.
- Failure to identify radiculomedullary arteries along with subsequent embolic agent reflux, can result in spinal cord ischaemia with paralysis, anaesthesia, loss of bladder and bowel control, and sexual dysfunction.
- Careful attention should be given to longitudinal and retrocorporeal anastomoses.
- Even when embolisation is performed via a radicular artery that does not originate from a radiculomedullary artery, particle migration may occur through anastomoses, reaching an intercostal/lumbar artery at upper or lower levels, or contralaterally, which subsequently feeds an anterior or posterior radiculomedullary artery.
- It is not recommended to use particles <100 μm as they may inadvertently traverse non-visualised microanastomoses involving critical vessels. On the other hand, particles >300 μm can swiftly occlude proximal vessels or accumulate within the microcatheter.

Epistaxis and Middle meningeal artery embolisation

Epistaxis 536

Middle meningeal artery embolisation for chronic subdural haematoma 540

Epistaxis

- Around 6% of patients suffering epistaxis will require medical attention. The condition is most prevalent in those <20 and >40 years and is commonly associated with nasal trauma, recent surgery, or a predisposition to nosebleeds.
- 90% occur along the anterior nasal septal area (Kiesselbach's plexus within Little's area; see Chapter 2, 'Sphenopalatine artery', p. 28). This receives supply from the ECA (sphenopalatine, descending palatine, and superior labial branches) and ophthalmic artery (anterior and posterior ethmoidal branches).
- Posterior epistaxis is commonly arterial although it can also arise from Woodruff's venous plexus, located in the posterior aspect of the inferior meatus on the lateral wall of the nasal cavity. Posterior epistaxis has the added risks of aspiration and difficulties in attaining haemostasis, potentially requiring surgery or embolisation.

Primary epistaxis

- Constitutes 85% of cases and is typically idiopathic.

Secondary epistaxis

- Trauma: 17% of epistaxis visits, is the most prevalent cause.
- Coagulopathy.
- Vascular malformations: AVMs, such as those resulting from hereditary haemorrhagic telangiectasia.
- Iatrogenic: from anticoagulants, antiplatelet drugs, intranasal medications, and nasal procedures/operations.
- Neoplastic: sinonasal and nasopharyngeal tumours elevate vascularity and mucosal inflammation.
- Inflammatory: rhinosinusitis and chronic excoriation irritate the nasal mucosa.

Management

- Initial evaluation focuses on airway management, respiratory status, and haemodynamic stabilisation.
- Full blood count, metabolic and coagulation screening, and blood group and save are performed based on the severity of the haemorrhage and underlying conditions.
- Treatment approaches vary, with anterior epistaxis often managed with manual compression, haemostatic mesh insertion, and chemical or electric cauterisation. More severe cases may require anterior nasal packing. This is uncomfortable and may itself cause nasal trauma, aspiration, or airway obstruction.
- Posterior epistaxis is addressed with endoscopic cauterisation, anteroposterior tamponade, surgical arterial ligation, or endovascular embolisation.
- If intervention is required, many regard surgical arterial ligation to be the treatment of choice because of the rare but serious complications associated with embolisation.

Investigation

- CTA is the first-line non-invasive imaging modality:
  - Acquisition in both the arterial and tissue phases is recommended. The former defines the anatomy and can identify targets for treatment including extravasation, pseudo-aneurysms, and vascular malformations. The latter may more clearly reveal additional causes, e.g. tumours or post-traumatic/operative lesions.
  - However, certain factors can lead to poor visibility of small distal arterial branches on CTA including motion, bolus timing, presence of debris, surgical packing material, and dental amalgam/other metal artefacts.
  - A negative CTA should not automatically exclude DSA for high-risk patients.
- DSA: angiography of the ICA and ECA bilaterally is the gold standard for bleed localisation. It is sensitive for ongoing extravasation, may identify the cause, and also reveals dangerous ECA–ICA anastomoses as a precursor for embolisation.

Technique for embolisation

- GA is generally recommended, especially when the bleed threatens airway patency.
- Start with ICA angiography. It is important to exclude ICA bleeding sources and verify the choroidal blush (the landmark for the retinal artery). The nasal mucosa supply from ethmoidal arteries should also be assessed.
- Next, place a guide catheter into the ECA and perform angiography (Figure 16.1). Evaluate for vascular anomalies, ECA–ICA anastomoses, and epistaxis causes. Note that if the choroidal blush is present only on ECA angiography then the MMA cannot be occluded as it may be the only supply of the retinal artery via meningo-ophthalmic or meningolacrimal branches. There may also be retinal supply through more distal IMA anastomoses, namely the anterior deep temporal artery to the lacrimal artery or the sphenopalatine artery to the ethmoidal arteries. If dual ICA/ECA retinal supply is present, then the ECA anastomoses may be closed with large particles or coils initially to avoid non-target embolisation.
- Particle embolisation of the sphenopalatine and facial arteries is straightforward and relatively safe. Note: particle embolisation through branches of the ICA, ophthalmic arteries, and ascending pharyngeal branches is high risk and should be avoided. 250–350 μm particles provide a good balance between effectiveness and safety.
- Navigate a 0.017–0.027" microcatheter (the larger the better if it will fit in the vessel) within the IMA just distal to the origin of the infraorbital artery. Smaller microcatheters can be used but they tend to become quickly blocked. Embolisation should be at least distal to the AMA, MMA, and middle deep temporal artery. Embolising the latter risks causing postprocedural pain and trismus.
- Inject particles suspended in 50–75% contrast with saline utilising a blank roadmap until significant flow reduction has been achieved. Injection strength should be finely controlled to avoid reflux. A wedged catheter position should be avoided when injecting particles to prevent a build-up of pressure (which can open up dangerous anastomoses). The suspension is regularly agitated to avoid clumping.

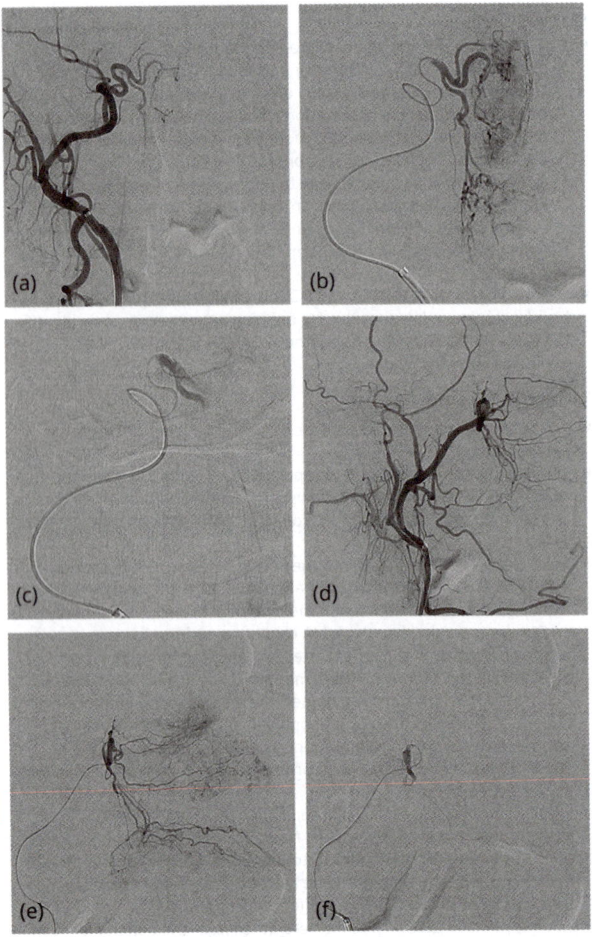

Figure 16.1 Epistaxis. (a) Anteroposterior external carotid artery angiogram of a patient with acute epistaxis. (b) Selective microcatheter angiography of the internal maxillary artery. Embolisation was performed with particles at this location. (c) Post embolisation microcatheter angiography. (d–f) Lateral views of the same case.

- Bilateral embolisation is employed if there is bilateral bleeding, in the setting of vascular pathologies such as hereditary haemorrhagic telangiectasia, and if the IMA receives collateral supply from the contralateral IMA across the midline.

Tips

- Particle size selection should be chosen based on the vessel being targeted, with a focus on minimising non-target embolisation.
- Particles <100 µm risk CN ischaemia and passage through dangerous anastomoses and are generally avoided.
- Particles 100–300 µm can be used when bleeding is thought to be in capillary beds and for super-selective embolisation of smaller vessels.
- The microcatheter should not be wedged when particles are used, as forward flow is required.

Complications

- Bleeding stops immediately in around 93–100%, dropping down to 77–95% when accounting for early rebleeds (3–33 days post-procedure). The long-term success rates are lowest in patients with hereditary haemorrhagic telangiectasia where repeated embolisations are often necessary due to the chronic nature of underlying vascular abnormalities.
- Minor transient complications of the procedure (20–60%) include headache, facial pain, jaw pain, trismus, facial oedema, numbness, cold hypersensitivity, paraesthesias, palatal ulceration, altered mental status, groin haematoma, groin pain, or fever.
- Local post-procedure pain, even in absence of ischaemic mucosal injury, is self-limiting and tends to be responsive to NSAIDs.
- Ischaemic complications:
  - The skin and mucosal surfaces of the facial and nasal/oral cavities should be evaluated during and/or after the procedure. The physician should look for discolouration or blanching, and changes in temperature. After awakening from anaesthesia, the patient should be re-examined to evaluate for pain and lack of sensation.
  - If there appears to be true ischaemia after embolisation, glyceryl trinitrate (50 mcg/mL), typically bilaterally, can be infused superselectively at the end of the procedure. As this works to dilate collateral arterial channels and increase perfusion, there is a small risk of rebleeding; however, this risk must be balanced with permanent ischaemic damage.
  - Post-procedure transient complications include skin slough, mucosal necrosis, and ischaemic sialadenitis.
  - Persistent complications encompass facial scarring, permanent monocular blindness, peripheral facial nerve paralysis, and cerebral infarction. Blindness and stroke are reported in <2%.
  - CN deficits, often due to soft tissue oedema, may be treated with a short course of methylprednisolone. Administration of methylprednisolone (250 mg IV every 6 h) may be helpful. Some patients can be discharged with a 6-day tapering dose of oral methylprednisolone.
- Rebleeds can occur due to the ethmoidal supply not being addressed during an initial procedure, requiring further ethmoidal ligation.

Further reading

Willems PWA, Farb RI, Agid R. Endovascular treatment of epistaxis. Am J Neuroradiol. 2009;30(9): 1637–1645.

Middle meningeal artery embolisation for chronic subdural haematoma

- Chronic subdural haematoma (cSDH) is characterised by an abnormal accumulation of blood products in the subdural space and typically exhibits a slow, indolent course of disease progression that nevertheless may be life-threatening. By 2030, the incidence of cSDH in the USA is projected to surpass that of primary brain tumours and metastases.
- Reported perioperative mortality after surgical treatment of cSDH, including burr-hole craniostomy, twist-drill drainage, and craniotomy, ranges from 1.2% to 11% across previously published cohorts, while in elderly patients overall 1-year mortality after diagnosis or treatment has been reported as high as 32%.
- The high incidence in the elderly is believed to be due to vascular endothelial fragility and increasing use of anticoagulant/antiplatelet medications.
- Multiple risk factors contribute to poor outcomes of cSDH, including a lower GCS score, age >65 years, frailty, male sex, chronic alcoholism, the presence of medical comorbidities, and coagulopathies.
- The initiating event may be clinical or subclinical trauma causing haemorrhage from the bridging veins in the potential space between the dura and arachnoid mater. This is followed by often-asymptomatic expansion in the subdural space. Repeated cycles of inflammation, fibrinolysis, and angiogenesis lead to vascular neomembrane formation. Elevated ICP due to the haematoma's constant growth ultimately leads to symptoms including gait disturbance and falls, mental deterioration, limb weakness, acute confusion, headache, drowsiness or coma, speech impairment, collapse, and seizure.
- The vascular neomembrane is located within and along the deep surface of the subdural collection. It is composed of border zone cells and proliferating, fragile, inner layer vessels that are prone to continued and recurrent bleeding. Vascular neomembranes are supplied by the MMA via a secondary anastomotic network of the periosteal layer and penetrating vessels through the meningeal layer of the dura.
- Embolisation is hypothesised to devascularise the membranes and inhibit recurrent bleeding from these fragile vessels, facilitating reabsorption of accumulated subdural fluid.
- RCT results (to date EMBOLISE, STEM, and MAGIC-MT) have demonstrated reductions in haematoma recurrence/progression, primarily for adjunctive (to surgical drainage) MMAE.

Clinical management

- Asymptomatic patients, or those with cSDH without brain compression or midline shift, are often managed conservatively.
  - This involves follow-up imaging, ICP control, and monitoring to detect clinical deterioration.
  - Conservative management primarily involves reversing anticoagulation. In urgent cases, antiplatelet agents are reversed with platelet transfusions.
  - Statins may reduce endothelial inflammation and reduce neomembrane formation.

    - Prophylactic antiepileptic drugs may lower seizure risk.
    - Steroids are usually ineffective.
- Surgical management involves twist-drill or burr holes under LA or GA, or craniotomies/mini-craniotomies normally performed under GA. The placement of drains is associated with significantly reduced re-operation rates without increasing complications.

Indications for embolisation

- As an adjunctive to surgical drainage to decrease recurrence (ideally under the same anaesthetic).
- Sole therapy in those with less severe symptoms or those who are not candidates for surgery.
- There is particular utility in those on antiplatelet or anticoagulant therapy.

Technique

- MMA embolisation can be performed on cooperative patients under LA or light sedation if particles or coils are used. Embolisation with LEs is painful, and GA is recommended (although injection of intra-arterial LA in the MMA can alternatively reduce this pain).
- Femoral or radial access is obtained and initially angiography of the ICA is performed to identify the ophthalmic artery origin, and important variants such as stapedial artery origin of the MMA. If the choroidal blush is not seen via the ICA injection, then most likely the retinal supply is from the MMA via a meningo-ophthalmic artery.
- The ECA is next catheterised and angiography performed (Figure 16.2). 'Cotton wool' staining and wispiness of distal MMA branches is commonly observed in branches supplying cSDH.
- The choice of microcatheter depends on the size of the MMA branches and the agent used. For particles, a 0.017–0.027" microcatheter is used. If the branches are very small, it may not be possible to use a catheter large enough for particle embolisation, and LE (0.013" microcatheter) or glue (0.09" microcatheter) must be used.
- Under roadmap guidance, the microcatheter, either alone or through an intermediate catheter, is navigated into the MMA and microangiography is undertaken.
- The choice of MMA branches is dependent on their likely contribution to the cSDH, the presence of collaterals, and the embolic agent utilised.
- MMA anatomy is extremely variable. Notably, anastomoses with the ophthalmic artery (meningo-ophthalmic and meningolacrimal branches) and ICA (inferolateral trunk) must be identified to avoid non-target embolisation. Refrain from embolisation of the petrosal MMA branch as this contributes to a vascular arcade supplying the facial nerve.
- Once the microcatheter is appropriately situated, embolisation is performed.
- PVA particles, typically 250–350 μm, suspended in 50–75% contrast with saline may be used. Embolisation is performed in a pulsatile fashion under negative roadmap guidance to confirm antegrade flow, slowing/stasis of flow, and prevention of reflux. As always, the smaller the microcatheter, the higher the risk of catheter blockage with particles. The suspension is regularly agitated to avoid clumping.
- LE agents, e.g. EVOH copolymer and n-BCA glue, may also be used. Advantages include the more permanent nature of these agents, the

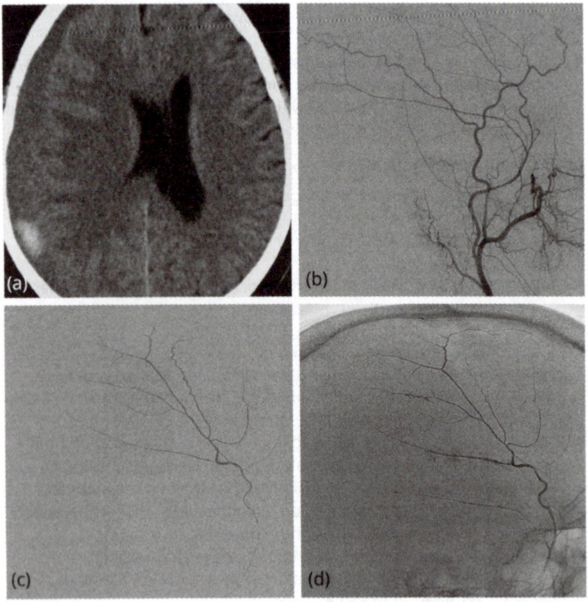

Figure 16.2 Middle meningeal embolisation for subdural haematoma. (a) Cranial computed tomography scan demonstrating right-sided subdural haematoma with mass effect. (b) Guide catheter positioned in the right external carotid artery. (c) Selective microcatheter angiogram of the middle meningeal artery (MMA). (d) Onyx cast after injection into the MMA achieving distal penetration. Note the 'cotton wool' appearances along some of the branches representing proliferating capillary vessels.

ability to embolise multiple divisions of the MMA via one branch, distal penetration, visibility, and potentially decreased procedural time. Disadvantages include increased cost (more with copolymers) and pain during injection (necessitating GA).

- Detachable coils may also be used for proximal ligation, usually after exhausting the above methods or for an uncooperative patient under LA/sedation.
- The above techniques may be used in combination for maximal efficacy.

Postprocedural care

- Outpatients may be discharged the following day. Day-case treatment has also been performed.
- When to restart anticoagulant/antiplatelet therapy depends on the severity of the SDH and the indication for the medication. It may be possible to restart these the day after embolisation.
- Unenhanced CT scans should be obtained to monitor changes in cSDH size, typically at 30 and 90 days.

Tips

- Squid-12 might be a good choice of LE agent as it is able to penetrate distally while possessing good radiopacity.
- Reflux of LE occurs rapidly once the branch is occluded and so embolisation must be performed slowly to avoid non-target embolisation.
- Simultaneous infusion of 5% glucose in water solution through the intermediate/guide catheter while injecting dilute 10–30% n-BCA ('sugar rush' technique) may improve distal penetration if glue is used.

Complications

- Overall complications have been reported at around 2%.
- Potential neurological complications include ischaemic stroke, visual loss, and CN palsies.
- Recurrence following MMA embolisation may result from supply from other dural branches from the ECA, ICA, or vertebral arteries.

Further reading

Chen H, McIntyre MK, Kan P, Gandhi D, Colasurdo M. Middle meningeal artery embolization for non-acute subdural hematoma: a meta-analysis of large randomized controlled trials. AJNR Am J Neuroradiol. 2025;46(10):2069–2074.

Link TW, Rapoport BI, Paine SM, Kamel H, Knopman J. Middle meningeal artery embolisation for chronic subdural hematoma: endovascular technique and radiographic findings. Interv Neuroradiol. 2018;24(4):455–462.

Majidi S, Matsoukas S, De Leacy RA, et al. Middle meningeal artery embolization for chronic subdural hematoma using N-butyl cyanoacrylate with D5W push technique. Neurosurgery. 2022;90(5):533–537.

Index

For the benefit of digital users, indexed terms that span two pages (e.g., 52–53) may, on occasion, appear on only one of those pages.

Tables and figures are indicated by an italic *t* and *f* following the page number.

3D/4D rotational angiography 216
3MAX, 4MAX and 5MAX (Penumbra) 121–22
11 SLS 298–99

A

abciximab 107, 146*t*
accessory meningeal artery 25–26
  anterior branch 25–26
Acclino/Credo stents 132
acetazolamide 479–82
acetic acid 137–39
activated clotting time (ACT) 109
activated partial thromboplastin time (APTT) 109
adrenocorticotropic hormone (ACTH) 476, 477
aggregation/coagulation process 101
air embolism 222–23
airway, breathing, circulation, disability and exposure (ABCDE) 320–21
Alberta Stroke Program Early CT Score (ASPECTS) 323, 323*f*
alfentanil 340–41
alteplase 330, 394–95
American Heart Association 112–13, 330–31, 341–42
American Stroke Association 341–42
Amplatz wire 117
anaesthesia for ischaemic stroke 339–42
  conscious sedation 339–40
  general anaesthesia 340–42
  local anaesthesia 339
  standards 339
analgesia 94–96
anastomoses 47
  intrinsic, axial and longitudinal 87–88
  short longitudinal 86–87
  see also cranial anastomoses, 'dangerous'
anastomotic vein of Labbé, posterior 69–70
anastomotic vein of Trolard, superior 69–70
aneurysmal rupture 223, 223*f*, 242
  intraprocedural 268–69, 269*f*
aneurysm-bridging stents 132
aneurysms 217
  ruptured (dissecting or blister type) 103
  unruptured 235–39, 330–31
  see also cerebral aneurysms
ANGEL-ASPECTS trial 335–36
ANGEL-REBOOT trial 365
angiographic technique 203–5
  cone beam computed tomography 205
  contrast injection 203–4
  digital subtraction angiography 204
  frame rate 204
  masks 204–5
  pulse rate 204
  roadmaps 204–5
angiography
  3D/4D rotational 216
  biplane 209–11
  catheter 313
  cerebral *see* cerebral angiography
  check 252
  diagnostic *see* diagnostic angiography
  digital subtraction *see* digital subtraction angiography (DSA)
  meningioma embolisation 525
  paediatric *see* paediatric angiography
  spinal *see* spinal angiography
  time-resolved angiography with interleaved stochastic trajectories (TWIST) 497
angioplasty
  balloon 314–15
  carotid artery stenting 403
  chemical 314
  intracranial atherosclerotic disease
    stenting 411–12
  rescue angioplasty 388–89
  stent first (antegrade approach) 356–57
  stent last (retrograde approach) 357–58, 358*f*, 359–62
  stent-retriever 315
  tandem carotid occlusion 361
Angio-Seal device 179
angular artery 14–15
antenatal imaging 469
anterior cerebral artery (ACA) 40–43, 40*f*
  A1 (pre-communicating) segment 40–41
  A2 (post-communicating) segment 42
  A3 (precallosal) segment 42
  A4 (supracallosal) segment 43
  A5 (postcallosal) segment 43
  angiogram of anterior circulation 41*f*
  anterior communicating artery 41–42
  callosomarginal artery 42
  dural branches 43
  frontopolar artery 42
  long callosal arteries 43
  medial lenticulostriate arteries 40–41
  orbitofrontal artery 42
  parietal branches 43
  pericallosal artery 42
  recurrent artery of Heubner 40–41
  short callosal perforating arteries 43
anterior cranial fossa dural arteriovenous fistula (DAVF) 439–40
  anatomy 439
  complication avoidance 440
  tips 440
  treatment 439–40, 439*f*

anterior inferior cerebellar artery (AICA) 52
lateral branch 52
medial branch 52
anticoagulation 108–13
coagulation pathway 108–9, 108*f*
coagulation tests 109
coil embolisation of intracranial aneurysms 247–48
direct oral anticoagulants for atrial fibrillation and aneurysm treatment 112–13
fluoroscopic-guided lumbar puncture 148
intravenous thrombolysis 330–31
low-molecular weight heparin 111
periprocedural anticoagulation 146–47, 146*t*
unfractionated heparin 109–11
warfarin 111–12
antiplatelet therapy 101
coil embolisation of intracranial aneurysms 249
flow diversion 287
fluoroscopic-guided lumbar puncture 148
intracranial atherosclerotic disease stenting 410–12
intravenous thrombolysis 330–31
periprocedural 146–47, 146*t*
stenting 280–81
tandem carotid occlusion 363–64
Woven Endobridge (WEB) intrasaccular device 298
antispasmodics 98–100
antithrombotics for secondary stroke prevention 395
aortic arch 8, 8*f*
variants 10–11, 11*f*
apixaban 146*t*
Apollo (Medtronic) 122–24, 455, 485–86, 498–500
arrhythmia 308
arterial anatomy *see* spinal arterial anatomy
arterial cord supply 77–81
cervical cord 77–81
iliolumbar artery 77–81
lumbar cord 77–81
median sacral artery 77–81
radicular arteries 77–81
radiculomedullary arteries 78–80
radiculopial arteries 80–81
segmental arteries 77–81
sulcal arteries 80
thoracic cord above T3 77–81
thoracic cord below T3 77–81
arterial dissection 242
arteriovenous fistula *see* intradural perimedullary arteriovenous fistula; spinal dural arteriovenous fistula (DAVF) ; spinal epidural arteriovenous fistula
arteriovenous malformations 218, 244
see also intramedullary spinal arteriovenous malformations; ruptured pial arteriovenous malformations (AVMs)
artery disease, peripheral 176
artery reocclusion 388–89
Artisse (Medtronic) 302
ARUBA trial 453
Asahi Chikai (Asahi) 118
ascending pharyngeal artery
inferior branch 19–20
middle branch 19–20
ASPECTS 334, 335–36
aspiration 346*f*
aspirin 102, 146*t*, 363–64, 407–8, 410–12
see also dual antiplatelet therapy (DAPT) (aspirin plus clopidogrel or ticagrelor)
Aspirin Reaction Units (ARU) 105–6
atherosclerotic disease 400–13
carotid artery stenting 400–5
intracranial atherosclerotic disease stenting 409–13
vertebral artery stenting 406–8
atherosclerotic stenosis 356–58
Atlas stent 132
atrial fibrillation 103, 112–13
atrial vein
lateral 71
medial 70
atropine 224*t*
ATTENTION trial 368–69, 370
auricular artery
deep 21
posterior 15
auricular branches, anterior 16
AURORA trial 334
autonomy, respect for 3
AXS Infinity LS (Stryker) 120–21
azygos system 484*f*

B

Ballast (Balt) 120–21
balloon angioplasty 314–15
balloon devices 125–28
angioplasty balloon catheters 127–28
balloon guide catheters 125
dual-lumen balloons 126–27
remodelling balloon catheters 125–27
single-lumen balloon catheters 125–26
balloon guide catheters 344–45
balloon inflation 389
balloon remodelling technique 253–55, 253*f*
balloon test occlusion 273–74, 274*f*
BAOCHE trial 368–69, 370
Barricade coil (Balt) 129–30
Barrow classification 421*t*, 422
basal (or lateral) tentorial artery 33–34
basal vein of Rosenthal (BVR) 71–72
BASICS trial 368–69
basilar artery 51–53
anterior inferior cerebellar artery (AICA) 52
asymmetric fusion 53
basilar tip 51
basilar trunk perforating arteries 51
caudal fusion (V shape) variant 53
complete occlusion 51
cranial fusion type variant (T-shape) 53
internal auditory (labyrinthine) artery 52
lateral branch 52
lateral (caudal marginal) division 52–53
long circumflex branches 51
medial branch 51, 52
medial (rostral) division 52–53
mid-basilar 51
paramedian branches 51

pontine paramedian perforators 51
posterior circulation angiogram 50*f*
proximal basilar 51
short circumflex branches 51
short pontine perforators 51
subarcuate branch 52
superior cerebellar artery (SCA) 52–53
superior vermian branch 52–53
variants 53
Wollschlaeger and Wollschlaeger, artery of 52–53
Basilar Artery on Computed Tomography Angiography (BATMAN) score 370
basilar occlusion 369
basilar strategy 371–74, 371*f*
basilar trunk perforating arteries
basilar tip 253*f*, 265
basilar trunk 265
median branches 51
mid-basilar 51
proximal basilar 51
Benchmark (Penumbra) 120–21
beneficence 3
bentracimab for ticagrelor reversal 104–5
Berenstein catheter 198, 385–86, 480–82
Bern score 153
BEST trial 368–69
beta-agonist inhaler 224*t*
biplane angiography 209–11
Birch vs University College London Hospital NHS Foundation Trust (2008) 4–5
Birmingham gauge (G) or gauge 116
blank 'glue' roadmap 498–500, 504–6, 528–30, 531–33
bleomycin 136
blood pressure management 97, 341, 394
blood sugar 395
Bobby (Microvention) 125, 344–45
Bolam vs Friern Hospital Management Committee (1957) 4–5
Borden classification 421*t*, 422
BossStent (Sonorous) 482
brachiocephalic artery 8, 104–5
brachiocephalic (or innominate) vein 63
bradycardia 405
brain arteriovenous malformations (bAVMs) 448–74
classification 451–52
copolymer liquid embolics 456–57
cross-sectional imaging 450
cyanoacrylate glue 456
detachable tip microcatheters 455
digital subtraction imaging 450
embolic materials 456–57
endovascular treatment complications 454
imaging 450
imaging follow-up 450
Lawton-Young supplementary classification 451, 451*t*
materials 455–57
microcatheters 455
natural history 448–49
non-detachable tip microcatheters 455
particles 457
Pollock-Flickinger radiosurgical classification 452
pre-radiosurgical embolisation of unruptured pial AVMs 467
presentation 448
ruptured AVMs 453
ruptured pial AVMs 458–64
Spetzler-Martin classification 451, 451*t*
stereotactic radiosurgery (STRS) 472–74
transvenous embolisation 465–66, 466*f*
treatment indications 453
unruptured AVMs 453
vein of Galen malformations (VOGMs) 468–71
brainstem veins 74
lateral mesencephalic veins 74
longitudinally orientated veins 74
midline group 74
peduncular veins 74
transversely orientated veins 74
breastfeeding and diagnostic angiography 196
bronchospasm 223–25
buccal artery 26

C

calcarine 56–57
calcified plaque 404
calcium channel blockers 103–4
callosal arteries, long 43
callosal perforating arteries, short 43
callosomarginal artery 42
cancer and paediatric thrombectomy 381–82
cangrelor 103–6, 363–64
capillary neovascularisation 89
capsular arteries of McConnell 33–34
cardiac complications and subarachnoid haemorrhage 308
cardiac disease and paediatric thrombectomy 381–82
Carney-Stratakis syndrome 514–20
carotid artery
aneurysm, giant internal 289*f*
left common , 10, 208
left internal and external 209
right common 9–10, 208
right external 208
right internal 208
see also carotid artery stenting; external carotid artery (ECA) I; external carotid artery (ECA) II; external carotid artery (ECA) III; internal carotid artery (ICA)
carotid artery stenting
angioplasty 403
calcified plaque 404
complications 405
evidence 401
follow-up imaging 404
indications 400
post-procedure 404
pros and cons 401
stenting 403
technique 401–3, 402*f*
tips 404
UK National Clinical Guidelines for Stroke 2023 400–1
vessel diameter mismatch 404
vessel tortuosity 404
carotid body paragangliomas 514–20, 516*f*
carotid cave 33

carotid occlusion
  with patent circle of Willis 337–38
  see also tandem carotid occlusion
carotid puncture, direct 386
carotid stents 131
carotid T-occlusion 352, 352*f*
carotid vascular access 187–88
  closure 187
  complications 187–88
  subtracted and unsubtracted angiograms 188*f*
  technique 187
Carotid Wallstent (Boston Scientific) 131
CASWEP trial 401–3
Catchview Mini (Balt) 134, 379–80
catheters 119–24
  angiography 119, 313
  common angiographic shapes 199*f*
  diagnostic angiography 198
  guide 119–21
  intermediate, distal access and reperfusion or aspiration 121–22
  kinking and knotting 220
  microcatheters 122–24
  select 119
  see also balloon devices
caudal fusion (V shape) variant 53
caudate head, medial 70
cavernous malformations (cavernomas) 494–96
cavernous segment 33–34
  anterior branch 33–34
cavernous sinuses 68
  branches 24–25
Cello (Medtronic) 344–45
cement injection 170
centimetres (unit measurements) 116
Cerebase (Cerenovus) 120–21, 480–82, 489–90
cerebellar artery
  anterior inferior 52
  superior 52–53
cerebellum veins 74–76
  deep group 76
  fissure veins 76
  inferior hemispheric veins 74–76
  paired inferior vermian veins 74–76
  petrosal surface drainage 74–76
  precentral 74–76
  suboccipital surface drainage 74–76
  superficial group 74–76
  superficial tonsillar veins 74–76
  superior hemispheric veins 74–76
  superior and inferior peduncle veins 76
  superior vermian veins 74–76
  tentorial surface drainage 74–76
cerebral amyloid angiopathy 245
cerebral aneurysms 228–315
  acutely ruptured aneurysms 234–35
  AVM-associated 'flow' aneurysms 261–62
  balloon test occlusion 273–74, 274*f*
  basilar tip 265
  basilar trunk 265
  blister aneurysms 233, 257, 258*f*
  clinical presentation 229–30
  coil dislodgment and/or migration 270, 271*f*
  coil embolisation of intracranial aneurysms 247–55
  coil stretching 271–72, 272*f*
  dissecting aneurysms 103, 233
  ELAPSS score 238*t*
  endovascular coil embolisation 228*f*
  epidemiology 229
  five-year risk of aneurysm rupture in ISUIA 235*t*
  flow diversion 228*f*, 286–97
  fusiform aneurysms 233, 256–57
  giant aneurysms 258–59, 259*f*
  giant serpentine aneurysms 259
  ICA cavernous segment location 262
  ICA PCOM segment 262–63
  infectious aneurysms 233, 260–61, 260*f*
  initial investigation 231
  intracranial aneurysms 233
  intraprocedural aneurysmal rupture 268–69, 269*f*
  intrasaccular devices 298–304
  intrasaccular embolisation 228*f*
  investigation and neuroscience centre 231
  investigations 231–32
  leucoencephalopathy, delayed 272
  locations 262–66
  neoplastic aneurysms 233
  paediatric aneurysms 277–79
  parent vessel occlusion 275–76, 276*f*
  pathophysiology 233
  patient information diagram 228, 228*f*
  periprocedural complications 267–72
  PHASE risk prediction score 237*t*
  posterior cerebral artery (PCA) 265–66
  pseudoaneurysms 233
  recurrent 301–2
  saccular aneurysms 233, 256
  screening 231–32
  small aneurysms 256, 256*f*
  spinal 244
  stent-assisted coil embolisation 228*f*
  stenting 280–85
  subarachnoid haemorrhage complications 305–9
  subarachnoid haemorrhage differential diagnosis 242–46
  subarachnoid haemorrhage grading 240–41
  symptoms and signs 229–30
  thromboembolic complications 267–68, 268*f*
  traumatic aneurysms 233, 261
  types 256–62
  unruptured intracranial aneurysms 235–39
  vasospasm and delayed cerebral ischaemia 310–15
cerebral angiography 206–11, 207*f*
  default position 209–11
  femoral artery to aortic arch 206
  great vessels selection 206–9

projections 209–11, 210*f*
projections, tips for 211
vessel selection tips 209
cerebral arteriopathy, focal 381–82
cerebral artery *see* anterior cerebral artery (ACA); middle cerebral artery (MCA); posterior cerebral artery (PCA)
cerebral ischaemia 305
delayed *see* vasospasm and delayed cerebral ischaemia
cerebral salt wasting 306–7
cerebral spinal fluid removal 313
cerebral vasospasm 98–99
cerebral veins
anterior 72
internal 72
cerebral venous sinus thrombosis (CVST) 488–91
cerebrospinal fluid-venous fistula 153
cerebrospinal fluid-venous fistula embolisation 483–87
access site haematoma 487
alternative treatment options 483
anatomy 483–84, 483*f*
azygos system 484*f*
complications 487
deaths or major complications 487
epidural (extradural) compartment 483–84
imaging follow-up 487
pain at embolisation site 487
paraspinal compartment 483–84
perforation of spinal venous system 487
post-procedure 487
pulmonary embolism 487
rebound intracranial hypertension 487
technique 485–86, 485*f*
wrong site surgery 487
cervical artery, ascending 60
cervical carotid stenting 103
cervical cord 77–81
cervical enlargement, artery of (artery of Lazorthes) 84
cervical myelopathy 416–17
cervical region, upper 60
cervical segment 30–32
cervical vein, deep 63
Charter of Fundamental Rights of the European Union (2000) 3
check angiography 252
chemical angioplasty 314
China Angioplasty & Stenting for Symptomatic Intracranial Severe Stenosis (CASSISS) trial 409
CHOICE 2 trial 394–95
CHOICE trial 343
choroidal artery
lateral posterior 56
medial posterior 56
choroidal segment, anterior 36–37
chronic kidney disease 196
chronic subdural haematoma (cSDH) *see* middle meningeal artery embolisation for chronic subdural haematoma (cSDH)
ciliary arteries, paraophthalmic segment 35
cilostazol 146*t*
Cincinnati segmental classification 30
cingulate gyri 70
Circle of Willis 38, 39*f*
circumflex artery
long 54–56
short 54–56
short pontine 51
circumflex branches
long 51
short 51
cisternography *see* static myelography and cisternography
clival artery, lateral 33–34
clopidogrel 103–6, 107, 146*t*, 407–8, 410–12
see also dual antiplatelet therapy (DAPT) (aspirin plus clopidogrel or ticagrelor)
clot composition 343
coagulation
pathway/coagulation cascade 108–9, 108*f*
tests 109
coaxial configuration 119–24
Cobb syndrome 82–83, 507–8
Cobra 213–14, 498–500, 531–33
Cochrane review (2023) 410
Cognard classification 421*t*, 422*f*
Cognard type 1 423
Cognard type 2a 423
Cognard type 2b 427, 430
Cognard types1-2a 426–27, 430
Cognard types 2b-5 423
Cognard types 3-5 427, 429*f*, 430
cognitive complications 308–9
coil dislodgment and/or migration 270, 271*f*
coil embolisation
adjunctive 281, 282*f*, 288–89
stent-assisted 103, 228*f*
see also coil embolisation of intracranial aneurysms
coil embolisation of intracranial aneurysms 247–55, 248*f*
accessing aneurysm 250
adjunctive embolisation techniques 252–55
aneurysm recurrence and re-haemorrhage 255
anticoagulation 247–48
antiplatelet usage 249
balloon remodelling technique 253–55, 253*f*
check angiography 252
coiling 250–52
double microcatheter technique 255
guide catheter placement 249–50
postoperative care 252
preoperative assessment 247
vascular access 247
coils 129–30, 504–6
features 129–30
filling 129–30
framing 129–30
haemangioblastoma embolisation 528–30
spinal tumour embolisation 531–33
stretching 271–72, 272*f*
temporary 389
collateral grading 324–25
collateral scoring 324, 325*f*
collicular arteries 54–56
common drugs 95–96
common pathway (CP) 108–9
communicating artery
anterior 41–42
posterior 54

communicating segment, posterior 36
communicating vein, posterior 72
computed tomography angiography (CTA) 324
contrast-enhanced spinal 531
epistaxis 537
haemangioblastoma embolisation 528
multiphase 324–25
vasospasm and delayed cerebral ischaemia 312–13
computed tomography (CT)
cone beam 205
contrast-enhanced 497
haemangioblastoma embolisation 528
ischaemic stroke 322–27, 322*f*
meningioma embolisation 524
paraganglioma embolisation 515
spinal tumour embolisation 531
computed tomography (CT)-guided lumbosacral nerve root injection 162–63
contraindications 162
equipment 162
indications 162
technique 162–63, 163*f*
tips 163
computed tomography (CT)-guided thoracolumbar spinal biopsy 166–67
complication avoidance and management 167
indications/ contraindications/ equipment 166
paraspinal approach 166–67
technique 166–67, 167*f*
tips 167
transpedicular approach 166–67, 167*f*
computed tomography perfusion (CTP) 325–27, 326*f*
CONDOR trial 423
condylar confluence, anterior 67
cone beam computed tomography 205
conscious sedation 339–40
consent 4–5
diagnostic angiography 194–95
free and informed 3, 4–5
paediatric angiography 216
contact aspiration, direct 345–47, 347*f*
continuous heparinised saline irrigation 201
Contour (Stryker) 302–3
contrast adverse reaction 195
contrast agents 216
contrast-induced acute kidney injury 225–26
contrast-induced encephalopathy 226, 395–96
contrast injection 203–4
contrast reaction, acute 223–25
convexity branches
anterior 24–25
posterior 24–25
Co-operative Aneurysm Study 313–14
Copernic (Balt) 126
copolymer liquid embolics 140–43, 456–57, 528–30
how to inject 141–43
Menox 140
Obtura 141
Onyx 140
PHIL 141
Squid 140
cord vascularisation, extrinsic 86–87
coronal segment 21–25
cortical drainage 70
costocervical trunk 9
COX-2 inhibitors 146*t*
cranial anastomoses, 'dangerous' 58–60
ascending cervical artery 60
ascending pharyngeal artery 60
ascending pharyngeal artery collaterals 58
internal maxillary artery (IMA) collaterals 58–59
musculospinal branch 60
occipital artery 60
orbital region 59–60
petronous-cavernous region 58–59
prevertebral branch 60
pterygovaginal artery 58–59
stylomastoid artery 60
upper cervical region 60
vidian artery 58–59
cranial dural arteriovenous fistula (DAVF) 416–45
aetiology 416
anterior cranial fossa DAVF 439–40
Barrow classification 421*t*, 422
Borden classification 421*t*, 422
classification 421–22
clinical presentation 416–17
Cognard classification 421*t*, 422*f*
Cognard type 1 423
Cognard type 2a 423
Cognard type 2b 427, 430
Cognard types 1-2a 426–27, 430
Cognard types 2b-5 423
Cognard types 3-5 427, 429*f*, 430
cross-sectional imaging 419
digital subtraction angiography 419
direct carotid-cavernous DAVF 444–45
endovascular treatment, principles of 426–29
epidemiology and demographics 416
follow-up imaging 419–20
imaging 419–20
indications for treatment 423–24
indirect cavernous sinus DAVF 441–43
intermittent manual compression 423
lateral foramen magnum DAVF 436–38
natural history 417–18
superior sagittal sinus DAVF 432, 432*f*
symptomatic or ruptured dural fistula 423–24
tentorial DAVF 433–35
transverse-sigmoid sinus DAVF 430–31, 431*f*
treatment complications 425
cranial fusion type (T shape) variant 53
cranial nerve palsies 306
oculomotor and abducens 416–17
cranial nerve supply 61, 61*t*

CREDO Stent (Acandis) 365–67, 372–74
CREST trial 401
cross-sectional imaging 450
Cushing's disease 476
cyanoacrylate glue 137–39, 456
complications 139
how to inject 138–39

D

dalteparin 111
Davidoff and Schechter, meningeal branch of 56–57
DAWN trial 334, 335*t*
decubitus myelogram, lateral 156*f*
deep/distal feeders 458–59
deep group of veins 76
deep vein thrombosis 112–13, 189
deep venous drainage 71*f*
DEFUSE trial 334, 335*t*
delivery wire perforation 294, 295*f*
dementia 416–17
dental artery
inferior 26
posterior superior 27
Derivo 2 (Acandis) 286–87
desmopressin for aspirin reversal 102
devices *see* equipment and devices
DEVT trial 332
diabetes insipidus 307
diagnostic angiography 194–226
acute contrast reaction 223–25
air embolism 222–23
aneurysm rupture 223, 223*f*
breastfeeding 196
catheter kinking and knotting 220
catheters 198
cerebral angiography 206–11
chronic kidney disease 196
consent 194–95
contrast adverse reaction 195
contrast-induced acute kidney injury 225–26
contrast-induced encephalopathy 226
emergency medication doses 224*t*
examination 194
exchange technique 201
flushing 200–1
history 194
hypertension, uncontrolled 195
iatrogenic vessel dissection 220–21
metformin 196
microcatheter angiography 202
microemboli 221
paediatric angiography 216
periprocedural details 194
post-procedure 197
pregnancy 196
preparation 195
pre-procedure 194
specific diseases 217–19
spinal angiography 212–15
syringes 200
technique 203–5
thrombocytopenia 196
thromboembolism 221–22
vasospasm 221
warfarin 195
wires 199–200
see also diagnostic angiography - complication management; diagnostic angiography - specific diseases
diagnostic angiography - complication management 220–26
acute contrast reaction 223–25
air embolism 222–23
aneurysm rupture 223
catheter kinking and knotting 220
contrast-induced acute kidney injury 225–26
contrast-induced encephalopathy 226
iatrogenic vessel dissection 220–21
microemboli 221
puncture site complications 220
thromoembolism 221–22
vasospasm 221
diagnostic angiography - specific diseases 217–19
aneurysms 217
angiography for stereotactic radiosurgery 219
arteriovenous malformations 218
dural arteriovenous fistula 218
intraparenchymal haemorrhage 218
moyamoya 218–19
perimesencephalic haemorrhage 217
reversible cerebral vasoconstriction syndrome 217–18
subarachnoid haemorrhage 217
vasculitis 218
diastematomyelia 507
diffusion-weighted imaging (DWI) 327–29
lesions 101
digital subtraction angiography (DSA) 204
brain arteriovenous malformations (bAVMs) 450
cerebral aneurysms 301–2
cranial dural arteriovenous fistula 419
epistaxis 537
haemangioblastoma embolisation 528
intramedullary spinal arteriovenous malformations 504
meningioma embolisation 524
paraganglioma embolisation 515
spinal dural arteriovenous fistula 498
dimethyl sulfoxide (DMSO)-compatible microcatheters 498–500
diphenhydramine 224*t*
diploic veins 69
dipryridamole 146*t*
direct carotid-cavernous dural arteriovenous fistula (DAVF) 444–45
anatomy 444
clinical 444
complication avoidance and management 445
tips 445
treatment 444–45, 445*f*
DIRECT- MT trial 332
direct oral coagulants (DOACs) 112–13
DIRECT SAFE trial 332
DISTAL trial 378
'don't move, don't breathe, don't swallow' instruction 203–4

double microcatheter technique 255
double stent retrieval 346*f*, 350–52, 351*f*
drugs and analgesia 94–113
  analgesia, sedation and general anaesthesia 94–96
  anticoagulation 108–13
  antispasmodics 98–100
  aspirin 102
  blood pressure control 97
  common drugs 95–96
  glycoprotein IIb/IIIa receptor inhibitors 107
  P2Y12 inhibitors 103–6
  platelet aggregation and coagulation 101
dual antiplatelet therapy (DAPT) (aspirin plus clopidogrel or ticagrelor) 103, 363–64, 401–3, 413, 480–82
Duo (Microvention) 455
dural arteriovenous fistula (DAVF) 218, 244, 497
  spinal 494, 495*f*, 497–501
  see also cranial dural arteriovenous fistula (DAVF)
dural branches 43
dural fistula, symptomatic or ruptured 423–24
dural tears, lateral 153
dural venous sinuses 64–68, 65*f*
  anterior condylar confluence 67
  cavernous 68
  confluence of sinuses (torcular Herophili) 64
  dural 64
  inferior petrosal 67
  inferior sagittal 64
  marginal 67
  occipital 17–18
  sigmoid 67
  sphenoparietal 67
  straight 64
  superior petrosal 67
  superior sagittal 64
  transverse (lateral) 67
  venous phase angiogram of internal carotid artery 66*f*
  see also dural venous sinus pressure monitoring and stenting
dural venous sinus pressure monitoring and stenting 479–82
  clinical presentation 479
  complication avoidance and management 482
  imaging 479
  modified Dandy criteria 479
  postprocedural care 482
  pressure measurement 480, 481*f*
  risks 480
  stenting, indications for 479
  symptoms and signs 479
  technique 480–82
  tips 482
  venous stenting 480–82, 481*f*
dynamic fluoroscopic myelography 153–57
  causes 153
  contraindications 154
  equipment 154
  imaging 153
  postprocedural care 156
  technique 154–56
  tips 156–57

E

ECASS4-EXTEND trial 331–32
Echelon (medtronic) 122–24, 498–500
Eclipse (Balt) 126, 127
ECST trial 401
ED-10 coil (Kaneka) 129–30
edoxaban 146*t*
ELAPSS score 238*t*
Embocure 463*f*
Emboguard (Cerenovus) 125,344–45
embolic materials 456–57
embolic stroke 405
embolisation
  cerebrospinal fluid-venous *see* cerebrospinal fluid-venous fistula embolisation
  endovascular coil 228*f*
  intramedullary spinal arteriovenous malformations 504
  intrasaccular 228*f*
  middle meningeal artery *see* middle meningeal embolisation for chronic subdural haematoma (cSDH)
  pre-radiosurgical of unruptured pial arteriovenous malformations (AVMs) 467
  presurgical targeted in ruptured pial arteriovenous malformations (AVMs) 458–59
  spinal dural arteriovenous fistula 498
  transvenous embolisation of arteriovenous malformations (AVMs) 465–66, 466*f*
  see also tumour embolisation
EMBOLISE trial 540–43
embolism to other vascular territories 389
Emboshield (Abbott) 131
Embotrap (Cerenovus) 348
Embovac/Large Bore Catheter (Cerenovus) 121–22
embryology of spinal vascular system 82–83
emergency medication doses 224*t*
emissary veins 69
encephalitis 319–20
encephalopathy, contrast-induced 226, 395–96
ENDOLOW trial 336
endovascular clipping 458–59
endovascular coil embolisation 228*f*
endovascular management principles 469–71, 470*f*
endovascular treatment 426–29
  characterisation 426
  Cognard type 2b 427
  Cognard types 1-2a 426–27
  Cognard types 3-5 427, 429*f*
  complications 454
  materials 426
  post-procedure 428–29
  transarterial technique 427–28
  transvenous technique 428
enoxaparin 111, 146*t*
Enterprise stent 132
Envoy (Cerenovus) 120–21
ephedrine 97
epidural arteriovenous fistula *see* spinal epidural arteriovenous fistula
epinephrine 224*t*
epistaxis 536–39
  complications 539
  embolisation technique 183*f*, 537–38
  investigation 537
  ischaemic complications 539

management 536
primary epistaxis 536
secondary epistaxis 536
tips 539
EPITHET trial 332
eptifibatide (Integrillin) 107, 363–64
equipment and devices 116–43
aneurysm-bridging stents 132
balloon devices 125–28
carotid stents 131
catheters 119–24
coils 129–30
copolymer liquid embolics 140–43
cyanoacrylate glue 137–39
flow diverters 133
guidewires 117–18
intrasaccular devices 134
neck-bridging devices 134
particles 135–36
sclerosants 136
sheaths 119–24
stent retrievers 134
erythema, diffuse 223–25
erythromycin 103–4
ESCAPE-MeVO trial 378
ethics 3
ethmoidal arteries, anterior and posterior 35
European Asymptomatic Carotid Surgery Trial (ACST) 401
European Convention on Human Rights (1950) 3
European Society of Minimally Invasive Neurological Therapy 332, 370–77
European Stroke Organisation 103, 111–13, 330–31, 332, 370–77
EXTEND trial 331–32
external carotid artery (ECA) I 12–16, 13*f*, 14*f*
facial artery 12–15
lateral ECA angiogram 14*f*
lingual artery 12
posterior auricular artery 15
proximal branches 13*f*
superficial temporal 15–16
superior thyroid artery 12
external carotid artery (ECA) II 17–20
ascending pharyngeal artery 18–20, 18*f*
occipital artery 17–18
external carotid artery (ECA) III 21–29
accessory meningeal artery 25–26
anterior deep temporal artery 26–27
anterior tympanic artery 21
buccal artery 26
deep auricular artery 21
descending palatine artery 28
first (mandibular) segment 21–29
foramen rotundum, artery of 27
inferior dental (or alveolar) artery 26
infraorbital artery 27
internal maxillary artery 23*f*
third (pterygopalatine) segment 21–29
internal medullary artery 22*f*
masseteric artery 26
middle deep temporal artery 26
middle meningeal artery 21–25
pharyngeal (pterygovaginal) artery 28
posterior superior dental artery 27
pterygoid artery 26
pterygoid canal (vidian artery), artery of 28
second (zygomatic or pterygoid) segment 21–29
sphenopalatine artery 28–29
superior orbital fissure, artery of 27
third (pterygopalatine) segment 21–29
external jugular vein (EJV) 62
external ventricular drain (EVD) 103–4
extracranial segment 21–25
extracranial veins 62–63
anterior jugular veins 62
deep cervical vein 63
external jugular vein 62
face, scalp and skull 62
internal jugular vein 62
pterygoid plexus 62
vertebral artery venous plexus 63
vertebral venous system 63
extramandibular branches 26
extraspinal venous system 91
extrinsic medullary veins 89–90
extrinsic pathway (EP) 108–9
extrinsic vascularisation of cord 86–87

F

facial artery 12–15
facial veins 62
Fargo Mini (Balt) 121–22, 138–39
femoral artery to aortic arch 206
femoral vascular access 176–81
cautions 176
complications 179–81
difficulty inserting introducer wire 177–78
difficulty inserting sheath 178
femoral puncture and sheath insertion 176–77
haemostasis closure devices 179
haemostasis, manual compression for 178–79
subtracted and unsubtracted angiography via femoral sheath 178*f*
fentanyl 96
fexofenadine 224*t*
fibrinolytic agents 146*t*
'first-pass effect' 353–54
Fisher grades 311
Fisher scale 241, 241*t*
fissure veins 76
FLAIR 327–29
flow diversion 133, 286–97
access 287–88
adjunctive coil embolisation 288–89
aneurysms and vessel assessment 288
antiplatelet therapy 287
complications 294–97
covering branch vessels 293–94
crossing aneurysm 292
delivery wire perforation 294
deployment 105, 289–91
device mal-deployment 291
devices 286–87
failure to occlude aneurysm 295–96

flow diversion (*cont.*)
imaging follow up 294
indications for flow-diverting stents 287
intracranial haemorrhage 297
ischaemia 294
late ischaemic complications 297
multiple devices 293
neointimal hyperplasia 296–97
paediatric aneurysms 278–79
patient aftercare and discharge 294
patient preparation 287
post-deployment manipulation 291–92
post-treatment rupture 296
stent 228*f*
stent migration 294–95
vessel apposition 291–92
FlowGate (Stryker) 344–45
flumazenil for midazolam reversal 95
fluoroscopic-guided lumbar puncture 148–50, 149*f*, 150*f*
antiplatelet and anticoagulant usage 148
contraindications 148
equipment 148
indications 148
technique 148–49, 156*f*
tips 149
fluoroscopic-guided lumbosacral nerve root injection and medial branch block 158–61
complication avoidance and management 161
contraindications 158
equipment 158
medial branch block technique 159–60, 160*f*
nerve root block technique 158–59
postprocedural care 161
tips 160
fluoroscopic-guided transpedicular thoracolumbar spinal biopsy 164–65
complication avoidance and management 165
contraindications 164
equipment 164
indications 164
postprocedural care 165
technique 164–65
tips 165
flushing
continuous heparinised saline irrigation 201
diagnostic angiography 200–1
'double flush' technique 200–1
hand 200–1
focal cerebral arteriopathy (FACA) 381–82
focal deficits 416–17
Foix-Alajouanine myelopathy 89–90
fondaparinux 146*t*
foramen lacerum, recurrent artery of 33–34
foramen rotundum, artery of 27
FRED (Microvention) 133, 286–87
French gauge (Fr) 116
frontal lobes, inferior 70
frontal and parietal terminal divisions, superficial temporal 16
frontal region, central 70
frontopolar artery 42
functional disorders 319–20
furosemide 224*t*
fusion, asymmetric 53

G

Galen, vein of *see* vein of Galen
gelatin sponge 531–33
general anaesthesia 94–96, 340–42
blood pressure management 341
giant internal carotid artery aneurysm 289*f*
Glidewire (Terumo) 117, 199–200, 485–86
Glubran (GEM) 137–39, 456
glyceryl trinitrate (GTN) 97, 99
glycoprotein IIb/IIIa receptor inhibitors 107, 146*t*, 363–64
gradient-recalled echo 327–29
great vessels selection 206–9
brachiocephalic artery 206
distal right subclavian branches 206–7
left common carotid artery 208
left distal subclavian branches 209
left internal and external carotid arteries 209
left subclavian artery 209
left vertebral artery 209
right common carotid artery 208
right external carotid artery 208
right internal carotid artery 208
right vertebral artery 207–8
groin haematoma 179–80
Guglielmi Detachable Coils 129–30
guide catheter placement 249–50
guidewires 117–18
microwires 117–18
standard diameter wires 117
'gun barrel' transpedicular approach 168*f*

H

haemangioblastoma embolisation 528–30
blood supply 528
complication avoidance and management 530
contraindications 528
indications for embolisation 528
investigation 528
outcomes 530
postprocedure 530
technique 528–30, 529*f*
tips 533
haematological disorders 381–82
haematoma
access site 185, 487
groin 179–80
venous vascular access 189
haemorrhagic conversion of infarct 392–93
haemorrhagic telangiectasia, hereditary 507
haemostasis 190
closure devices 179
manual compression 178–79
hand injections 203–4
Headway Duo (Micronvention) 122–24, 132, 379–80, 498–500
hemispheric veins
inferior 74–76
superior 74–76
heparin, unfractionated 146*t*

hereditary haemorrhagic telangiectasia 507
HERMES 334, 335–36, 378
Heubner, recurrent artery of 40–41
higher-dose intra-arterial protocol (milrinone) 99–100
Histoacryl (Braun) 137–39, 456
historical background 2
hives (urticaria) 223–25
hormonal/electrolyte complications, neurological 306–7
Hunt and Hess scale 240, 240*t*
Hybrid (Balt) 118
hydralazine 97
hydrocephalus 305
Hyperform (Medtronic) 126, 518–19
Hyperglide (Medtronic) 126, 518–19
hyperglycaemia 307
hyperperfusion syndrome 405
hypersomnolence 416–17
hypertension
  drug treatment 97
  hypertensive crisis 223–25
  idiopathic intracranial 479–82
  induced 394
  rebound intracranial 487
  uncontrolled in diagnostic angiography 195
hypoglossal artery, persistent 30–32
hypoglossal branch 19–20
hypoglycaemia 319–20
hyponatraemia 306
hypophyseal arteries
  posterior inferior 33–34
  superior 35
hypotension 223–25
  carotid artery stenting 405
  drug treatment 97

I

iatrogenic arterial dissection 391
iatrogenic vessel dissection 220–21
idiopathic intracranial hypertension (IIH) 479–82
iliolumbar artery 77–81
immune-mediated thrombocytopenia 110
inches (unit measurement) 116
indirect cavernous sinus dural arteriovenous fistula (DAVF) 441–43
  anatomy 441
  clinical 441
  complication avoidance and management 443
  tips 442–43
  treatment 441–42, 442*f*
infection 176, 381–82
inferior petrosal sinus sampling 476–78
  contraindications 476
  indications 476
  interpretation 477
  post-procedure 477
  risks 476
  technique 476–77, 477*f*
  tips 477–78
inferolateral trunk (ILT) 33–34
infraorbital artery 27
infratentorial veins 74–76, 75*f*
  brainstem veins 74
  cerebellum veins 74–76
  superior petrosal vein 76
inhalational anaesthetic agents 96
intermastoid oblique 211
intermittent manual compression 423
internal auditory (labyrinthine) artery 52
internal carotid artery (ICA) 30–37
  aberrant variant 30–32
  capsular arteries of McConnell 33–34
  caroticotympanic branch 32
  carotid cave 33
  cavernous segment 33–34, 262
  cervical segment 30–32
  choroidal segment, anterior 36–37
  ciliary arteries 35
  Cincinnati segmental classification 30
  clival artery, lateral 33–34
  ethmoidal arteries, anterior or posterior 35
  hypoglossal arteries, persistent 30–32
  hypophyseal artery
    posterior inferior 33–34
    superior 35
  inferolateral trunk (ILT) 33–34
  lacrimal artery 35
  mandibulovidian artery 32
  marginal artery of Bernasconi and Cassinari 33–34
  meningohypophyseal trunk (MHT) branch 33–34
  New York University segmental classification 30, 31*f*
  ophthalmic artery 34, 35
  otic artery 32–33
  paraophthalmic segment 35–36
  petrosal segment 32–33
  posterior communicating artery (PCOM) segment 36, 262–63
  proatlantal arteries 30–32
  recurrent artery of foramen lacerum 33–34
  retinal artery, central 35
  segmental classification 30
  stapedial artery, persistent 32–33
  tentorial artery, basal (or lateral) 33–34
  terminal segment 37
  trigeminal artery, persistent 34
  venous phase angiogram 66*f*
  web 362–63, 362*f*
internal maxillary artery (IMA) 21–29, 22*f*
  collaterals 58–59
International Covenant on Civil and Political Rights (1967) 3
intracranial aneurysms *see* coil embolisation of intracranial aneurysms
intracranial atherosclerotic disease (ICAD) 103
  acute, basilar stenting 373*f*
  see also intracranial atherosclerotic disease (ICAD) stenting; mechanical thrombectomy and intracranial atherosclerotic disease (ICAD)
intracranial atherosclerotic disease (ICAD) stenting 409–13
  postprocedural care 413
  technique 410–12, 411*f*
intracranial haemorrhage 297
  spontaneous 416–17

intradural perimedullary arteriovenous fistula 494, 495*f*, 507
  imaging 507
  management 507
  Type A 507
  Type B 507
  Type C 507
intramedullary spinal arteriovenous malformations 494, 495*f*, 504–7
  clinical 504
  complication avoidance and management 506–7
  embolisation, indications for 504
  imaging 504
  pathophysiology 504
  post-procedure 506
  technique 504–6, 505*f*
intranidal high-flow fistula, targeted occlusion of 460–61, 460*f*
intraparenchymal haemorrhage 218
intraprocedural aneurysmal rupture 268–69, 269*f*
intraprocedural subarachnoid haemorrhage 389–91, 390*f*
intrasaccular devices 134, 298–304, 299*f*
  Artisse (Medtronic) 302
  Contour (Stryker) 302–3
  Nautilus (EndoStream Medical) 303–4
  Neqstent (Stryker) 303
  see also Woven Endobridge (WEB) intrasaccular device
intrasaccular embolisation 228*f*
intravenous (IV) fluids 224*t*
intravenous thrombolysis 111–13, 330–33
  clinical pharmacology of thrombolytic agents 330
  complications 331
  contraindications 330–31
  evidence 330
  late-window thrombolysis 331–32
  mechanical thrombectomy 332
  paediatric 382
  post-thrombolysis care 332–33
  thrombolysis for stroke with witnessed onset 332
  thrombolysis for wake-up stroke/stroke of unknown time onset 331–32
intrinsic anastomoses, axial and longitudinal 87–88
intrinsic pathway (IP) 108–9
intrinsic spinal cord veins 89
intrinsic vascularisation of cord 87–88
ischaemia
  complications, late 297
  flow diversion 294
  leg 179
  stenting 284–85
  see also ischaemic stroke
ischaemic stroke 318–98
  Alberta Stroke Program Early CT Score (ASPECTS) 323, 323*f*
  anaesthesia 339–42
  antithrombotics for secondary stroke prevention 395
  blood pressure 394
  blood sugar 395
  clinical presentation 318–21
  clot composition 343
  collateral scoring 324, 325*f*
  computed tomography 322–27, 322*f*
  computed tomography angiography (CTA) 324
  computed tomography perfusion (CTP) 325–27, 326*f*
  contrast-induced encephalopathy 395–96
  essential information to gather 318–19
  examination 320–21
  functional and social history 318–19
  history 318–20
  hypertension, induced 394
  intravenous thrombolysis 330–33
  investigation 322–29
  magnetic resonance imaging 327–29, 328*f*
  mechanical thrombectomy complications 385–93
  mechanical thrombectomy and intracranial atherosclerotic disease (ICAD) 365–67
  mechanical thrombectomy principles 344–54
  medications and compliance 318–19
  medium and distal vessel thrombectomy 378–80
  modified Rankin Scale 319, 319*t*
  multiphase computed tomography angiography (CTA) and collateral grading 324–25
  neurological agents 394–95
  paediatric thrombectomy 381–84
  posterior circulation thrombectomy 368–77
  postprocedural care 394–96
  re-imaging after transfer 386–87
  re-occlusion 396
  reperfusion eligibility 318–19
  reperfusion injury 395
  risk factors and comorbidities 318–19
  stroke mimics 319–20
  symptom onset and course 318–19
  symptoms, nature of 318–19
  tandem carotid occlusion 355–64
  temperature control 395
  thrombectomy patient selection 334–38

J

'jailing' technique 132
JB 2 catheter 198
jugular branch 17–18
jugular paragangliomas 514–20
jugular vein
  anterior 62
  ascending pharyngeal artery 19–20
  external 62
  internal 62
juvenile nasopharyngeal angiofibroma embolisation 521–23
  blood supply 521
  complication avoidance and management 523

direct tumour puncture 521–22
investigation 521
postprocedural care 523
technique 521–22, 522*f*
tips 523
transarterial technique 521–22

K

ketamine 96
ketoconazole 103–4
kidney disease, chronic 196
kidney injury, contrast-induced, acute 225–26
Klippel-Trenaunay-Weber syndrome 507
kyphoplasty *see* vertebroplasty and kyphoplasty

L

labetalol 97, 224*t*
labial arteries, inferior and superior 14–15
lacrimal artery 35
laryngeal oedema 223–25
lateral foramen magnum dural arteriovenous fistula (DAVF) 436–38
anatomy 436
anterior condylar confluence/vein DAVF 436
clinical 436
complication avoidance 438
jugular foramen DAVF 436
locations 436
marginal sinus DAVF 436
posterior condylar canal DAVF 436
treatment 437–38, 437*f*
Lawton-Young supplementary classification 451, 451*t*
leg ischaemia 179
lenticulostriate arteries 44
medial 40–41
leucoencephalopathy, delayed 272
lidocaine 94, 94*t*, 176–77
lingual artery 12
Lipiodol (Guerbet) 137–39, 456
lipophilic statins 103–4
liquid embolic agents (LE) 504–7, 518–19
local anaesthesia (LA) 94, 339
lorazepam 224*t*
low-molecular-weight heparin (LMWH) 111
lumbar cord 77–81
lumbar enlargement, artery of (artery of Adamkiewicz) 84
lumbar puncture *see* fluoroscopic-guided lumbar puncture
lumbosacral nerve root injection *see* computed tomography (CT)-guided lumbosacral nerve root injection; fluoroscopic-guided lumbosacral nerve root injection and medial branch block
LVIS Evo stent 132

M

McConnell, capsular arteries of 33–34
Magic (Balt) 122–24, 137–39, 455, 498–500, 504–6
MAGIC-MT trial 540–43
magnetic resonance angiography (MRA) 327–29
time-resolved gadolinium-enhanced 497
magnetic resonance imaging (MRI) 327–29, 328*f*
haemangioblastoma embolisation 528
intramedullary spinal arteriovenous malformations 504
meningioma embolisation 524
paraganglioma embolisation 515
spinal dural arteriovenous fistula 497
spinal tumour embolisation 531
mandibulovidian artery 32
Manti catheter 198
Marathon (Medtronic) 122–24, 379–80, 455, 485–86, 498–500
marginal sinus 67
marginal territorial artery of Bernasconi and Cassinari 33–34
masseteric artery 26
masseteric muscular and buccal mucosal branches 14–15
mastoid branches 17–18
maxillary artery *see* internal maxillary artery (IMA)
mechanical tears in ventral dura 153
mechanical thrombectomy 112–13
intravenous thrombolysis 332
paediatric thrombectomy 382
see also mechanical thrombectomy complications; mechanical thrombectomy and intracranial atherosclerotic disease (ICAD); mechanical thrombectomy principles
mechanical thrombectomy complications 385–93
alternative access approaches 386
arch navigation, difficult 385–86
artery reocclusion 388–89
direct carotid puncture 386
embolism to other vascular territories 389
general advice 385
haemorrhagic conversion of infarct 392–93
hard stops 387
iatrogenic arterial dissection 391
intraprocedural subarachnoid haemorrhage 389–91, 390*f*
multiple passes and strategy change 386–87
optimising for success 386–87
postprocedural subarachnoid haemorrhage 392
relative stops 387
rescue angioplasty and stenting 388–89
stent detachment/retention 391–92
strategy modification 387
transradial access 386
mechanical thrombectomy and intracranial atherosclerotic disease (ICAD) 365–67
evidence 365
postprocedural management 367
recognition 365
technique 365–67, 366*f*

mechanical thrombectomy principles 344–54
access 344
aspiration 346*f*
balloon guide catheters 344–45
brachial access 344
carotid access 344
carotid T-occlusion 352, 352*f*
combined technique 346*f*, 349, 350*f*
direct contact aspiration 345–47, 347*f*
double stent retrieval 346*f*, 350–52, 351*f*
femoral access 344
mTICI and eTICI scores 353*t*
stent retrieval 346*f*
techniques 345, 346*f*
Thrombolysis in Cerebral Infarction scores 353–54
wrist access 344
medial branch block 158–61, 160*f*
medial (rostral) division 52–53
medial surfaces, peripheral 70
medium and distal vessel thrombectomy 378–80
evidence 330
imaging 379
indications 379
location (definition) 378
primary versus secondary (definition) 378–79
technical considerations 379–80
medium vessel occlusion 336
medullary veins 70–73
atrial vein
lateral 71
medial 70
basal vein of Rosenthal 71–72
caudate head, medial 70
cerebral veins
anterior 72
internal 72
extrinsic 89–90
posterior communicating vein 72
septal veins
anterior 70
posterior and middle 70
subependymal veins
lateral 71
medial 70
thalamostriate vein 71
vein of Galen 72–73
venous circle outflow 72
ventricular vein, inferior 71
meningeal artery
middle 21–25
posterior 47
meningeal blood supply, recurrent 36
meningeal branch of Davidoff and Schechter 56–57
meningeal veins 69
meningioma embolisation 524–27
blood supply 524–25
cavernous sinus/paraseller meningiomas 524–25
cerebellar convexity tumours 524–25
complication avoidance and management 527
contraindications 524
convexity meningiomas 524–25
falcine meningiomas 524–25
imaging 524
indications 524
middle cranial fossa/greater sphenoid wing meningiomas 524–25
petroclival/cerebellopontine angle meningiomas 524–25
postprocedural care 526
skull base meningiomas 524–25
technique 525, 526*f*
tentorial and posterior fossa meningiomas 524–25
tips 527
transarterial technique 525
meningitis 319–20
meningohypophyseal trunk (MHT) 33–34
meningolacrimal artery 36
meningo-ophthalmic orbital blood supply 35–36
Menox (Meril Life Sciences) 140
mental capacity 4–5
Merci (Stryker) 125, 344–45
mesencephalic veins, lateral 74
metabolic stroke 381–82
metacryloxysulfolane 137–39
metameric arteries 82–83
metameric syndrome 494, 495*f*, 507–8
spinal arteriovenous 82–83
metaraminol 97
metformin 196
methylprednisolone 539
microangiography 528–30
microcatheters 455, 528–30
angiography 202, 517–18
detachable tip 455
non-detachable tip 455
microemboli 221
microguidewires (microwires) 117–18, 202
midazolam 95
middle cerebral artery (MCA) 44–46, 45*f*
accessory 44
anterior temporal 44
duplicated 44
frontal branch 46
lenticulostriate arteries 44
M1 (horizontal) segment 44
M2 (insular) segment 44
M3 (opercular) segment 46
M4 (cortical) segment 46
parieto-occipital branch 46
parieto-occipital branch 46, 56–57
temporal branch 46
watershed zone 46
middle cerebral (Sylvian) vein, superficial 69–70
middle meningeal artery embolisation for chronic subdural haematoma (cSDH) 540–43, 542*f*
clinical management 540–41
complications 543
indications for 541
postprocedural care 542
technique 541–42
tips 543
midline group of veins 74
migraine with aura 319–20
Mikaelson 498–500, 531–33
millimetres (unit measurement) 116
milrinone 99–100
MiniTrek (Abbott) 127–28
Mirage (Medtronic) 118
'missing piece' sign 497
MIVI Q (MIVI Neuroscience) 121–22
modified Dandy criteria 479
Modified Glasgow Outcome score 305–9
modified Rankin Scale (mRS) 319, 319*t*, 336–37
Montgomery vs Lanarkshire Health Board (2015) 4–5
morphine 95

MOSTE trial 336
Moyamoya ('puff of smoke') 218–19, 381–82
MRCLEAN-LATE trial 334, 335*t*
mTICI and eTICI scores 353*t*
multiple endocrine neoplasia types 2A and 2B 514–20
muscular branches
ascending pharyngeal artery 19–20
descending 17–18
occipital artery 17–18
musculospinal branch 19–20, 60
myelography *see* static myelography and cisternography
myelopathy 212
Myers loop or infracalcarine 54–57

N

naloxone for morphine reversal 95
Nantes intravenous protocol (milrinone) 99–100
nasal artery
lateral 14–15
posterior lateral 29
nasopharyngeal angiofibroma embolisation *see* juvenile nasopharyngeal angiofibroma embolisation
National Institute for Health and Care Excellence (NICE) 103–4, 234–35, 410
National Institutes of Health Stroke Scale (NIHSS) score 320–21, 336, 368–69
Nautilus (EndoStream Medical) 303–4
Navian (Medtronic) 121–22
n-BCA/lipiodol 498–500, 502–3, 504–7, 525, 541–42
N-butyl-cyanoacrylate 456
neck-bridging devices 134
neointimal hyperplasia 296–97
neonatal imaging 469
Neqstent (Stryker) 303
nerve root sleeve leaks, distal 153
neurofibromatosis type 1 514–20
neurogenic pulmonary oedema 307
neurological agents 394–95
neurological complications 305–6
neuromeningeal trunk 19–20
Neuron Max (Penumbra) 120–21
neuropathic pain, left leg 163*f*
NeuroSpeed (Acandis) 127–28, 365–67, 372–74
neurovascular anatomy 8–91
anterior cerebral artery 40–43
basilar artery 51–53
circle of Willis 38, 39*f*
cranial nerve supply 61, 61*t*
'dangerous' cranial anastomoses 58–60
diploic veins 69
dural venous veins 64–68
emissary veins 69
external carotid artery (ECA) I 12–16
external carotid artery (ECA) II 17–20
external carotid artery (ECA) III 21–29
extracranial veins 62–63
infratentorial veins 74–76
internal carotid artery 30–37
medullary veins 70–73
meningeal veins 69
middle cerebral artery 44–46
posterior cerebral artery 54–57
spinal arterial anatomy 84–88
spinal vascular anatomy 77–81
spinal vascular system embryology 82–83
spinal venous anatomy 89–91
supratentorial veins 69–70
thoracic aorta 8–34
vertebral artery 47–50
Neva (Vesalio) 348
New York University segmental classification 30, 31*f*
n-hexyl cyanoacrylate 137–39
Nimbus (Cerenovus) 134, 348, 371–72
nimodipine 98
Nitinol stents 131
nitroglycerine 224*t*, 539
non-maleficence 3
non-steroidal anti-inflammatory drugs (NSAIDs) 146*t*
non-vascular procedures 146–74
anticoagulation/antiplatelets 146–47, 146*t*
CT-guided lumbosacral nerve root injection 162–63
CT-guided thoracolumbar spinal biopsy 166–67
dynamic fluoroscopic myelography 153–57
equipment 146
fluoroscopic-guided lumbar puncture 148–50
fluoroscopic-guided lumbosacral nerve root injection and medial branch block 158–61
fluoroscopic-guided transpedicular thoracolumbar spinal biopsy 164–65
percutaneous venolymphatic malformations 172–74
periprocedural management 146–47
standard management 146
static myelography and cisternography 151–52
vertebroplasty and kyphoplasty 168–71
noradrenaline 97
North American Symptomatic Carotid Endarterectomy Trial (NASCET) 400–1
novel oral anticoagulants (NOACs) 146*t*
Nuremberg Code (1949) 3

O

Obtura 141
occipital artery 17–18, 60
cutaneous branch 17–18
occipital cortex, medial 70
occipital lobes 54–57
inferior 70
occipital sinus 17–18
occlusion
balloon test 273–74, 274*f*
basilar 369
carotid 337–38
carotid T 352, 352*f*
complete 51
deep surgically inaccessible feeders 458, 459*f*
intranidal high-flow fistula 460–61, 460*f*
parent vessel 275–76, 276*f*

occlusion (*cont.*)
  perinidal/nidal aneurysms or pseudoaneurysms 461–62, 461*f*
  V4 isolated 369
  see also tandem carotid occlusion
Offset (Stryker) 345–47
omeprazole 103–4
Onyx Liquid Embolic System (Medtronic) 140, 141–43, 456–57, 465–66, 485–86, 525
ophthalmic artery 34, 35
ophthalmic orbital blood supply, dorsal 35–36
ophthalmic symptoms 416–17
optic radiation or supracalcarine 54–57
OPTIMAS trial 395
orbital blood supply variants 36
orbital fissure, superior 27
orbital region 59–60
orbitofrontal artery 42
otic artery 32–33
Oviedo Convention 4–5

P

P2Y12 inhibitors 103–6, 146*t*
P64/P48 (Phenox) 133, 286–87
paediatric aneurysms 277–79
  differences from adults 277
  dissecting aneurysms 277
  flow diversion 278–79
  fusiform aneurysms 278
  giant aneurysms 277
  management of incidental brain aneurysms 277
  pathophysiology of formation 277
  saccular aneurysms 278
  treatment considerations 278
paediatric angiography 216
  3D/4D rotational angiography 216
  complication avoidance 216
  consent 216
  contrast agents 216
  radiation dose 216
  vascular access 216
paediatric patients 330–31
paediatric thrombectomy 381–84
  aetiology 381–82
  clinical presentation 381
  complications 383
  contraindications 383
  device selection 383
  dissection 381–82
  imaging 382
  intravenous thrombolysis 382
  mechanical thrombectomy indications 382
  outcomes 383–84
  postprocedural care 383
  procedural considerations 383
paediatric vascular access 190–91
  haemostasis 190
  radial 191
  transfemoral 190
  umbilical 191
paired inferior vermian veins 74–76
palatine artery
  ascending 14–15
  descending 28
paraganglioma embolisation 514–20
  blood supply 516
  carotid body paragangliomas 514, 516*f*, 516
  complication avoidance and management 519–20
  direct puncture technique 518–19
  imaging 515
  jugular paragangliomas 515, 516
  pre-embolisation angiography assessment 517
  preprocedural workup 516–17
  presentation 514–15
  tips 519
  transarterial technique 517–18, 518*f*
  tympanic paragangliomas 515
  vagal paragangliomas 515, 516
paragangliomas
  carotid body 514–20, 516*f*
  familial 514–20
  jugular 514–20
  sporadic 514–20
  vagal 514–20
  see also paraganglioma embolisation
paramedian arteries 24–25
paramedian branches 51
paraophthalmic segment 35–36
paraterminal gyri 70
parent vessel occlusion 275–76, 276*f*
parietal branches 43
parietal region 70
Parkinsonism 416–17
particles 135–36, 457, 504–6
  embolisation 517–18
paternalism 3
PC400 coil (Penumbra) 129–30
PC-ASPECTS 323, 369, 370
peduncle veins, superior and inferior 76
peduncular perforating branches 56
peduncular veins 74
pentoxifylline 146*t*
Percherone, artery of 54–56
Perclose (Abbott) device 179
percutaneous venolymphatic malformations 172–74
  complications 174
  contraindications 172
  equipment 172
  postprocedural care 173
  technique 172–73, 173*f*
  tips 173–74
pericallosal artery 42
pericallosal (or splenial) branches, posterior 56–57
perimesencephalic haemorrhage 217, 243–44
perinatal stroke 381–82
perinidal/nidal aneurysms or pseudoaneurysms, targeted occlusion of 461–62, 461*f*
peripheral artery disease 176
peripheral medial surfaces 70
periprocedural management 146–47, 194
  anticoagulation/antiplatelets 146–47, 146*t*
  equipment 146
  standard management 146
persistent hypoglossal artery 30–32
persistent stapedial artery 32–33
persistent trigeminal artery 34

petronous-cavernous region 58–59
petrosal branches 24–25
petrosal segment 32–33
 caroticotypmanic 32
petrosal sinuses
 inferior 67
 sampling *see* inferior petrosal sinus sampling
 superior 67
petrosal surface drainage 74–76
petrosal vein, superior 76
petrosquamosal branch 24–25
phaeochromocytomas 514–20
 silent 516–17
pharyngeal artery 28
 ascending 18–20, 18*f*, 58, 60
PHASE risk prediction score 237*t*
Phenom series of microcatheters 122–24
phenylephrine 97
PHIL (Precipitating Hydrophobic Injectable Liquid) (Microvention) 141, 456–57
phosphodiesterase inhibitors 146*t*
physical integrity 3
pial network 86–87
Pipeline Embolisation device (Medtronic) 286–87
pITA (Phenox) 127–28
plasmin 330
platelet aggregation and coagulation 101
platelet function testing 105–6
pneumonia, aspiration and ventilator-associated 308
Pollock-Flickinger radiosurgical classification 452
polyvinyl alcohol (PVA) 525, 528–30, 531–33
pontine circumflex arteries, short 51
pontine perforators 51
 paramedian 51
posterior branch 25–26, 33–34
posterior cerebral artery (PCA) 54–57, 55*f*, 265–66
 anterior, middle and posterior temporal branches 56–57
 calcarine branch 56–57
 collicular arteries 54–56
 hippocampal branch 56–57
 lateral posterior choroidal artery 56
 long and short circumflex arteries 54–56
 medial posterior choroidal artery 56
 meningeal branch of Davidoff and Schecter 56–57
 Myers loop or infracalcarine 54–57
 occipital lobe 54–57
 optic radiation or supracalcarine 54–57
 P1 segment 54–56
 P2 segment 56
 P3 segment 56–57
 P4 segment 56–57
 parieto-occipital branch 56–57
 peduncular perforating branches 56
 Percheron, artery of 54–56
 posterior communicating artery 54
 posterior pericallosal (or splenial) branches 56–57
 posterior thalamoperforators 54–56
 strategy 374–75
 thalamogeniculate perforators 56
 thrombectomy 369
 variants 57
posterior circulation thrombectomy 368–77
 acute intracranial atherosclerotic disease basilar stenting 373*f*
 basilar occlusion 369
 evidence 368–69
 imaging 370
 indications 369
 posterior cerebral artery (PCA) strategy 374–75
 posterior cerebral artery (PCA) thrombectomy 369
 proximal basilar strategy 372–74
 tandem occlusion 375–77, 376*f*
 technique 370–77
 top of basilar strategy 371–72, 371*f*
 V4 occlusion, isolated 369
 V4 strategy 374
posterior inferior cerebellar artery (PICA) 48–50
posterior inferior hypophyseal artery 33–34
Posterior (POST)-NIHSS 320–21
posterior superior dental artery 27
postprocedural subarachnoid haemorrhage 392
prasugrel 103–6, 107, 146*t*
precentral cerebellar vein 74–76
Precise (Cordis) 482
pregnancy
 diagnostic angiography 196
 intravenous thrombolysis 330–31
pre-radiosurgical embolisation of unruptured pial arteriovenous malformations (AVMs) 467
'pressure cooker' technique 142–43, 427–28, 462–64, 498–500, 504–6
presurgical targeted embolisation of ruptured pial arteriovenous malformations (AVMs) 458–59
prevertebral branch 60
prilocaine 94, 94*t*
prior surgery or procedures and femoral vascular access 176
privacy 3
proatlantal arteries 30–32
PROFATE trial 344–45
PROPHET-II 186
propofol 96, 340–41
protamine
 low-molecular-weight heparin (LMWH) reversal 111
 unfractionated heparin (UFH) reversal 109–11
PROTECT-MT trial 344–45
Protegé Everflex (Covidien) 482
prothrombin 108–9
prothrombin time (PT) 109
pseudoaneurysm 180
psychological complications 309

pterional segment 21–25
pterygoid artery 26
pterygoid canal, artery of (vidian artery) 28
pterygoid plexus 62
pterygovaginal artery 58–59
pulmonary
complications 307–8
pulmonary embolism 487
pulmonary oedema 223–25
pulsatile tinnitus 416–17
pulse rate 204
pump injections 203–4
pure radicular arteries 84

R

radial artery spasm 98–99
radial perforating arteries 87–88
radial vascular access 182–86
access site haematoma 185
closure 184
complications 185–86
digital subtraction angiography via radial sheath 183*f*
high take-off radial artery 184–85
paediatric 191
radial artery loops 184–85
radial artery occlusion 184–85, 186
radial artery perforation 185–86
radial artery size 182
radial 'cocktail' 182–84
spasm and catheter entrapment 185
technique 182–84
tips 184–85
radiation dose in paediatric angiography 216
radiation exposure 212
radicular arteries 77–81, 84
radicular veins 90–91
radiculomedullary arteries 78–80, 84, 86–87
radiculopial arteries 80–81, 84, 86–87
REACT (Medtronic) 121–22
rebleeding 305–6
rebound intracranial hypertension 487
recurrent artery of foramen lacerum 33–34
recurrent artery of Heubner 40–41
recurrent meningeal blood supply 36
RED (Penumbra) 121–22
remifentanil/fentanyl 340–41
renal complications 308
reperfusion injury 395
rescue angioplasty 388–89
RESCUE-Japan LIMIT trial 335–36
respiratory distress syndrome, acute 307
restenosis, late 405
retinal artery, central 35
retroperitoneal haemorrhage 180–81
reverse transorbital oblique 209–11
reversible cerebral vasoconstriction syndrome 217–18, 242
RIST (Medtronic) 120–21
rivaroxaban 146*t*
ruptured aneurysms (dissecting or blister type) 103
ruptured pial arteriovenous malformations (AVMs) 458–64
deep/distal feeders 458–59
embocure 463*f*
occlusion of deep surgically inaccessible feeders 458, 459*f*
palliative treatment 464
presurgical targeted embolisation 458–59
targeted occlusion of intranidal high-flow fistula 460–61, 460*f*
targeted occlusion of perinidal/nidal aneurysms or pseudo-aneurysms 461–62, 461*f*

S

sacral artery, median 77–81
'safe triangle' 159*f*
sagittal sinus
inferior 64
see also superior sagittal sinus
salbutamol 224*t*
SaveChildS trial 383–84
scalp veins 62
scapular artery, dorsal 9
Scepter Mini (Microvention) 127, 498–500
sclerosants 136
Scottish Intracranial Vascular Malformation Study (SIVMS) 416
sedation 94–96
segmental arteries 77–81
seizures/convulsions/epilepsy 223–25, 306, 319–20
SELECT-2 trial 335–36
selective serotonin reuptake inhibitors (SSRIs) 146*t*
SENDit (Penumbra) 345–47
septal (or medial sphenopalatine) artery, posterior 29
septal veins
anterior 70
posterior and middle 70
severe bleeding disorders 176
sheaths 119–24
long 119–21
vascular 119
sickle cell disease 245
sigmoid sinuses 67
silent phaeochromocytomas 516–17
SILK (Balt) 133
SILK Vista (Balt) 286–87
Simmons catheter 1 or 2 182–84, 198, 199*f*, 220, 385–86, 498–500, 531–33
sinuses *see* dural venous sinuses
SKIP trial 332
skull veins 62
SL 10 coil (Stryker) 122–24, 129–30
SMART (Cordis) 482
Society of NeuroInterventional Surgery (SNIS) Standards and Guidelines Committee 112–13, 488–91
sodium tetradecyl sulphate (STS) 136
Sofia (Microvention) 121–22
Solitaire (Medtronic) 132, 348
Sonic (Balt) 122–24, 137–39, 455, 485–86, 498–500
space-occupying lesions 319–20
spasm and catheter entrapment 185
Spetzler-Martin classification 451, 451*t*
sphenopalatine artery 28–29
sphenoparietal sinus 67
SpiderFX (Medtronic) 131
Spif Flow coil (Balt) 129–30
spinal aneurysms 244, 494
spinal angiography 212–15, 214*f*, 531–33

complications 215
indications 212
pre-procedure 212
risks 212
technique 213–14
tips 214–15
wrongly labelled or missing levels 215
spinal arterial anatomy 84–88, 85*f*
anterior spinal artery (ASA) (longitudinal ventral system) 86
extrinsic vascularisation of cord 86–87
pial network (posterolateral longitudinal system) 86–87
pure radicular arteries 84
radial perforating arteries 87–88
radiculomedullary arteries 84–87
radiculopial arteries 84, 86–87
sulcal arteries 87
supply of spinal arteries 84
spinal arteriovenous metameric syndrome 82–83
spinal artery 47
anterior (longitudinal ventral system) 48–50, 86
C6-C1 segmental 47
lateral 48–50
see also spinal arterial anatomy
spinal cerebrospinal fluid (CSF) leaks 154*f*, 155*f*
spinal cord arteriovenous malformations 244, 504–8
intradural perimedullary arteriovenous fistula 507
intramedullary spinal arteriovenous malformations 504–7
metameric syndromes 507–8
spinal cord infarction 215
spinal cord vascularisation, intrinsic 87–88
spinal cord veins, intrinsic 89
spinal dural arteriovenous fistula (DAVF) 494, 495*f*, 497–501
clinical 497
complications 500–1
contraindications 498
digital subtraction angiography 498
embolisation, indications for 498
imaging 497–98
MRI 497
post-procedure 500
technique 498–500, 499*f*
tips 500
spinal epidural arteriovenous fistula 494, 495*f*, 502–3
clinical features 502
imaging 502
management 502–3
transarterial approach 502–3
spinal haemorrhage 212
spinal tumour embolisation 531–34
complication avoidance and management 534
contraindications 531
hypervascular spinal metastases 531–34
indications 531
investigation 531
postprocedural care 533
primary hypervascular spinal tumours 531–34
technique 531–33, 532*f*
tips 533
spinal vascular anatomy summary 77–81
arterial cord supply 77–81
arterial and venous systems 78*f*, 79*f*
venous drainage of spinal cord 81
spinal vascular lesions 494–512, 495*f*
aneurysms 494
arteriovenous malformations 504–8
cavernous malformations (cavernomas) 494–96
dural arteriovenous fistula 494, 495*f*, 497–501
epidural arteriovenous fistula 494, 495*f*, 502–3
intradural perimedullary arteriovenous fistula 494, 495*f*
intramedullary arteriovenous malformations 494, 495*f*
metameric syndrome 494, 495*f*
metastases 496
normal anatomy 495*f*
primary tumours 496
vasular tumours 494–96
vertebro-venous fistula 509–10, 509*f*
spinal vascular system 82–83
spinal venous anatomy 89–91
extrinsic medullary veins 89–90
intrinsic spinal cord veins 89
radicular veins 90–91
spinal and extraspinal venous system 91
Squid (Balt) 140, 141–43, 456–57, 465–66, 485–86, 525
stapedial artery, persistent 32–33
static myelography and cisternography 151–52
complication avoidance and management 151–52
contraindications 151
equipment 151
technique 151
tips 151
STEM trial 540–43
Stenting and Aggressive Medical Management for Preventing Recurrent Stroke in Symptomatic Stenosis (SAMMPRIS) trials 406, 409
stents/stenting 280–85
access 280
adjunctive coil embolisation 281, 282*f*
aneurysm-bridging 132
aneurysm and vessel assessment 280–81
antiplatelet therapy 280–81
braided 132, 280–81
carotid 131
complications 284–85
deployment 282–83
detachment/retention 391–92
failure to occlude aneurysm 285
flow-diverting 287
imaging follow-up 284
indications 280
ischaemia 284–85
laser-cut 102, 132
late ischaemic complications 285
late migration 285
mechanical thrombectomy complications 388–89

stents/stenting (*cont.*)
  migration 294–95
  neurointervention 132
  occlusion rates 280–81
  patient aftercare and discharge 284
  personal experience with device 280–81
  resheathability 132, 280–81
  retrieval 134, 346*f*, 347–52
  size of vessels and landing zones 280–81
  stent-assisted coil embolisation 103, 228*f*
  stent design 280
  stent-retriever angioplasty 315
  tandem carotid occlusion 361–62
  thrombosis, acute 405
  visibility 280–81
  Y-stenting 283–84, 283*f*
  see also vertebral artery stenting
stereotactic radiosurgery (STRS) 472–74
  angiography for 219
  clinical and radiological follow-up 473–74
  indications 472
  mechanism 472
  outcomes and complications 473, 474*f*
  treatment planning 473
'stiff chest' syndrome 96
straight sinus 64
stroke mimics 381–82
Stroke Thrombolysis Trialists' Collaboration (IST-3) Collaborative Group 330
stylomastoid artery 17–18, 60
stylomastoid branch 15
subarachnoid haemorrhage 217
  intraprocedural 389–91, 390*f*
  intravenous thrombolysis 330–31
  postprocedural 392
  see also subarachnoid haemorrhage complications; subarachnoid haemorrhage differential diagnosis; subarachnoid haemorrhage grading
subarachnoid haemorrhage complications 305–9
  cardiac complications 308
  cognitive complications 308–9
  hormonal/electrolyte complications 306–7
  neurological complications 305–6
  psychological complications 309
  pulmonary complications 307–8
  renal complications 308
subarachnoid haemorrhage differential diagnosis 242–46
  aneurysmal rupture 242
  arterial dissection 242
  arteriovenous malformation 244
  cerebral amyloid angiopathy 245
  drugs 245
  dural arteriovenous fistula 244
  idiopathic 246
  perimesencephalic haemorrhage 243–44
  reversible cerebral vasoconstriction syndrome 242
  sickle cell disease 245
  spinal aneurysms 244
  spinal arteriovenous malformation 244
  traumatic brain injury 242
  tumours and cavernomas 245
  vasculitis 242
  venous infarction 245
subarachnoid haemorrhage grading 240–41
  Fisher scale 241, 241*t*
  Hunt and Hess scale 240, 240*t*
  World Federation of Neurological Surgeons (WFNS) grading scale 240, 240*t*
subarcuate branch 52
subclavian artery
  left 10, 209
  right 9
subclavian branches
  distal left 209
  distal right 206–7
subclavian vein 63
subependymal veins
  lateral 71
  medial 70
submandibular gland branches 14–15
submental artery 14–15
submentovertex 211
suboccipital surface drainage 74–76
sulcal arteries 80, 87
superficial group of veins 74–76
superficial middle cerebral (Sylvian) vein (SMV) 69–70
superficial tonsillar veins 74–76
superior anastomotic vein of Trolard 69–70
superior branch
  ascending pharyngeal artery 19–20
  cavernous segment 33–34
  inferolateral trunk (ILT) 25–26
superior cerebellar artery (SCA) 52–53
superior sagittal sinus 64
superior sagittal sinus dural arteriovenous fistula (DAVF) 432, 432*f*
  anatomy 432
  complication avoidance 432
  tips 432
  treatment 432
supratentorial veins 69–70
  anterior septal vein 70
  cortical drainage 70
  lateral subependymal veins 71
  medial atrial vein 70
  medial caudate head 70
  posterior anastomotic vein of Labbé 69–70
  posterior and middle septal veins 70
  superficial middle cerebral (Sylvian) vein 69–70
  superior anastomotic vein of Trolard 69–70
supratrochlear artery 35
Surpass Evolve (Stryker) 133, 286–87
susceptibility weighted imaging (SWI) 327–29
suxamethonium/rocuronium 340–41
SWIFT-DIRECT trial 332
Swiss Registry 336
symptomatic or ruptured dural fistula 423–24
Synchro (Stryker) 118
syncope 319–20
syndrome of inappropriate antidiuretic hormone secretion (SIADH) 306
syringes 200

T

T2 weighted imaging 327–29
Takotsubo cardiomyopathy 308
tandem carotid occlusion 375–77, 376*f*
  angioplasty 361
  angioplasty and stent first (antegrade approach) 356–57
  angioplasty and stent last (retrograde approach) 357–58, 358*f*, 359–62
  antiplatelet regimen after stenting 363–64
  with atherosclerotic stenosis 356
  conservative management 360–61
  with dissection 359–62, 359*f*
  initial technique 355–56
  with internal carotid artery web 362–63, 362*f*
  stenting 361–62
  types 355
tantalum 137–39
targeted occlusion of intranidal high-flow fistula 460–61, 460*f*
targeted occlusion of perinidal/nidal aneurysms or pseudoaneurysms 461–62, 461*f*
Target Nano coil (Stryker) 129–30
TECNO trial 394–95
temperature control 395
temporal artery
  anterior 44
  anterior deep 26–27
  middle deep 26
  posterior deep 16
temporal lobes, inferior 70
temporal segment 21–25
tenecteplase (metalyse) 330, 394–95
tentorial dural arteriovenous fistula (DAVF) 433–35
  anatomy 433
  classification (Lawton) 433
  complication avoidance 435
  tips 435
  treatment 433–34, 434*f*
tentorial surface drainage 74–76
terminal branches 26
terminal segment 37
Terumo wire 480–82
Tetra coil (Stryker) 129–30
thalamogeniculate perforators 56
thalamoperforators, posterior 54–56
thalamostriate vein 71
THAWS trial 331–32
thoracic aorta 8–34
  aortic arch 8, 8*f*
  aortic arch variants 10–11, 11*f*
  brachiocephalic artery 8
  left common carotid artery 10
  left subclavian artery 10
  right common carotid artery 9–10
  right subclavian artery 9
thoracic cord above T3 77–81
thoracic cord below T3 77–81
thoracic (or mammary) artery, internal 9
thoracolumbar enlargement vein 89–90
thoracolumbar spinal biopsy *see* computed tomography (CT)-guided thoracolumbar spinal biopsy
thrombectomy
  mechanical *see* mechanical thrombectomy
  medium and distal vessel 378–80
  paediatric 381–84
  posterior cerebral artery (PCA) 369
  posterior circulation 368–77
  venous 488–91
  see also thrombectomy patient selection
thrombectomy patient selection 334–38
  6-24 hours 334
  carotid occlusion with patent circle of Willis 337–38
  large core 335–36
  less than 6 hours: RCTs and HERMES 334
  medium vessel occlusion 336
  mRS score, high pre-morbid 336–37
  NIHSS score, low 336
thrombin 108–9
thrombin time (TT) 109
thrombocytopenia 196
  immune-mediated 110
thromboembolic complications 267–68, 268*f*, 301
thromboembolism 221–22
  venous 307–8
thrombolysis *see* intravenous thrombolysis
Thrombolysis in Cerebral Infarction scores 353–54
Thrombolysis or Anticoagulation for Cerebral Venous Thrombosis (TOACT) trial 488–91
thrombosis
  acute stent 405
  cerebral venous sinus 488–91
  venous 425
thrombus 330
thyrocervical trunk 9
thyroid artery, superior 12
ticagrelor 103–6, 107, 146*t*
  see also dual antiplatelet therapy (DAPT) (aspirin plus clopidogrel or ticagrelor)
ticlopidine 146*t*
Tigertriever 13 134, 348, 379–80
time-resolved angiography with interleaved stochastic trajectories (TWIST) 497
time-resolved gadolinium-enhanced magnetic resonance angiography (MRA) 497
tirofiban 107, 363–64
TITAN registry 363–64
tonsillar branch 14–15
tonsillar veins, superficial 74–76
topiramate 479–82
Townes view 209–11
Trak-21 122–24
transarterial technique 427–28
transcranial Doppler 312
Transend (Stryker Neurovascular) 118
Transform (Stryker) 126
transorbital oblique 209–11
transosseous branch 17–18
transpedicular thoracolumbar spinal biopsy *see* fluoroscopic-guided transpedicular thoracolumbar spinal biopsy
transvenous embolisation of arteriovenous malformations (AVMs) 465–66, 466*f*

transvenous technique 428
transverse facial artery, superficial temporal 16
transverse (lateral) sinuses 67
transversely orientated veins 74
transverse-sigmoid sinus dural arteriovenous fistula (DAVF) 430–31, 431*f*
anatomy 430
Cognard type 2b 430
Cognard types 1-2a 430
Cognard types 3-5 430
tips 430–31
traumatic brain injury 242
Traxcess (Microvention) 118
Trek (Abbott) 127–28
Trevo (Stryker) 122–24, 348
triaxial configuration 119–24
trigeminal artery, persistent 34
trigeminocardiac reflex 142–43, 425
tris-acryl gelatin microspheres 525
Trolard, superior anastomotic vein of 69–70
Trufill (Cerenovus) 137–39
tumour embolisation 514–34
haemangioblastoma 528–30
juvenile nasopharyngeal angiofibroma 521–23
meningioma 524–27
paraganglioma 514–20
spinal 531–34
tumours and cavernomas 245
Turbridge (Microport) 286–87
tympanic artery
anterior 16, 21
inferior 19–20

U

UK National Clinical Guidelines for Stroke 2023 400–1, 406, 410
unfractionated heparin (UFH) 109–11
reversal 109–11
United Nations Universal Declaration of Human Rights (1948) 3
units of measurement 116
Universal Declaration on Bioethics and Human Rights (UNESCO) 3

V

V 4 occlusion, isolated 369
V 4 strategy 374
VacLok (Merit Medical) 345–47
vagal paragangliomas 514–20
vascular access 176–91
carotid 187–88
femoral 176–81
paediatric 190–91
paediatric angiography 216
radial 182–86
venous 189
vasculitis 218, 242
VASOGRADE criteria 311
vasospasm 221
vasospasm, cerebral 98–99
vasospasm and delayed cerebral ischaemia 310–15
balloon angioplasty 314–15
catheter angiography 313
cerebral spinal fluid removal 313
chemical angioplasty 314
clinical presentation 311
CT angiography and perfusion 312–13
delayed cerebral ischaemia (definition) 310
diagnosis 311–13
incidence and patho-physiology 310–11
management 313–15
pharmacological management 313–14
physiological management 313
stent-retriever angioplasty 315
transcranial Doppler 312
vasospasm/angiospasm (definition) 310
Vectra (Stryker) 121–22
vein of Galen 72–73
vein of Galen malformations (VOGMs) 468–71
aetiology 468
anatomy 468
antenatal imaging 469
choroidal type 468
clinical presentation 468
endovascular management principles 469–71, 470*f*
imaging 469
mural type 468
neonatal imaging 469
veins
lateral group of 74
longitudinally orientated 74
venous circle 72
outflow 72
venous drainage of the spinal cord 81
venous infarction 245, 416–17, 500–1
venous procedures 476–91
cerebrospinal fluid-venous fistula embolisation 483–87
dural venous sinus pressure monitoring and stenting 479–82
inferior petrosal sinus sampling 476–78
venous thrombectomy 488–91
venous sinus stenosis 479–82
venous thrombectomy 488–91
computed tomography (CT) venography 488–89
digital subtraction angiography (DSA) 488–89
imaging follow-up 491
investigation 488–89
magnetic resonance imaging (MRI) 488–89
magnetic resonance (MR) venography 488–89
non-contrast cranial CT 488–89
post-procedure 491
technique 489–90, 490*f*
tips 476
treatment strategy 489
venous thromboembolism 307–8
venous thrombosis 425
venous vascular access 187–89
closure 189
complications 189
deep vein thrombosis 189
haematoma 189
technique 189
ventral dura, mechanical tears in 153
ventral ophthalmic orbital blood supply 35–36
ventricular drain, external 103–4
ventricular vein, inferior 71
verapamil 98–99
VerifyNow-P2Y12 Assay reference ranges 105–6
VerifyNow PRU Test 105–6

vermian branch, superior 52–53
vermian veins
  paired inferior 74–76
  superior 74–76
vertebral artery 47–50, 48*f*
  anterior meningeal branch of 47
  anterior spinal artery 48–50
  C6-C1 segmental spinal arteries 47
  lateral spinal artery 48–50
  left 209
  PICA 48–50
  posterior meningeal artery 47
  right 207–8
  right subclavian artery 9
  V1 (preforaminal) segment 47
  V2 (foraminal) segment 47
  V3 (extracranial) segment 47
  V4 (intracranial) segment 47–50
  venous plexus 63
  see also vertebral artery stenting
Vertebral Artery Ischaemia Stenting Trial (VIST) 406
vertebral artery stenting 406–8
  evidence 406
  imaging follow-up 408
  postprocedural care 408
  technique 407–8, 407*f*
  tips 408
  UK National Clinical Guidelines for Stroke 2023 406
Vertebral Artery Stenting Trial (VAST) 406
vertebral metastases 169*f*
vertebral venous system 63
vertebral ('vert') catheter 198
vertebroplasty and kyphoplasty 168–71
  complication avoidance and management 171
  contraindications 168
  equipment 168
  postprocedural care 171
  technique 168–70, 168*f*, 169*f*
  tips 171
vessel diameter mismatch 404
vessel dissection 179
vessel tortuosity 404
VIA microcatheter 122–24, 298–99
vidian artery 58–59
Visual Analogue Scale pain score 158–59
Vitesse Intracranial Stent Study for Ischaemic Stroke Therapy (VISSIT) trial 409
von Hippel-Lindau syndrome 514–20, 528–30

W

WAKE-UP trial 331–32
Wallstent (Boston Scientific) 482
Walrus (Q'Apel) 125, 344–45
warfarin 111–12, 146*t*, 195
watershed zone 46
WEAVE trial 103
Wedge (Microvention/Terumo) 345–47
Wingspan Stent System Post Market Surveillance (WEAVE) trial 409
wires 199–200
  standard diameter 117
Wollschlaeger and Wollschlaeger, artery of 52–53
World Federation of Neurological Surgeons (WFNS) grading scale 240, 240*t*
World Health Organization (WHO) Surgical Safety Checklist 195, 197
Woven Endobridge (WEB) intrasaccular device 298–302, 300*f*
  access 298
  aneurysm occlusion, satisfactory 301–2
  antiplatelets 298
  catheterisation and deployment 301
  compaction 301–2
  complications 301
  deployment 299–301
  device migration 301–2
  device selection 298–99
  follow-up 301–2
  indications 298
  morbidity, device-related 301
  non-symmetrical branches at base of aneurysm 301
  parent artery impingement 301
  recurrent aneurysms 301–2
  retreatment rate 301
  rupture during deployment 301
  thromboembolic complications 301
Woven Endobridge (WEB) Occlusion Scale 301–2

X

XT series (Stryker) 122–24

Z

Zilver (Cook Medical) 131, 482
Zoom 71 (Imperative Care) 121–22
zygomatico-orbital artery 16